Fourth Edition

Medical Terminology

A Living Language

Bonnie F. Fremgen, PhD
Adjunct Professor
University of Notre Dame
Notre Dame, IN

Suzanne S. Frucht, PhD
Associate Professor
Northwest Missouri State University
Maryville, MO

PEARSON

Prentice
Hall

Upper Saddle River, New Jersey 07458

Library of Congress Cataloging-in-Publication Data

Fremgen, Bonnie F.
  Medical terminology : a living language / Bonnie F. Fremgen,
Suzanne S. Frucht.—4th ed.
      p. ; cm.
  Includes bibliographical references and index.
  ISBN-13: 978-0-13-158998-8
  ISBN-10: 0-13-158998-9
  1. Medicine—Terminology.
  [DNLM: 1. Medicine—Terminology—English.   W 15 F869m 2009]
I. Frucht, Suzanne S.   II. Title.
  R123.F697 2009
  610.1'4—dc22

                                                    2007052267

Publisher: Julie Levin Alexander
Assistant to Publisher: Regina Bruno
Executive Editor: Mark Cohen
Associate Editor: Melissa Kerian
Editorial Assistant: Nicole Ragonese
Media Editor: John J. Jordan
Development Editor: Danielle Doller
Managing Production Editor: Patrick Walsh
Production Liaison: Christina Zingone
Production Editor: Bruce Hobart, Pine Tree Composition
Manufacturing Manager: Ilene Sanford
Manufacturing Buyer: Pat Brown
Design Coordinator: Mary Siener
Cover Designer: Ilze Lemesis
Interior Designer: Wanda España
Director of Marketing: Karen Allman
Executive Marketing Manager: Katrin Beacom
New Media Project Manager: Stephen Hartner
New Media Production: Horus Development
Director, Image Resource Center: Melinda Patelli
Manager, Rights and Permissions: Zina Arabia
Manager, Visual Research: Beth Brenzel
Manager, Cover Visual Research & Permissions: Karen Sanatar
Image Permission Coordinator: Craig A. Jones
Composition: Pine Tree Composition, Inc.
Printer/Binder: Quebecor World
Cover Printer: Phoenix Color Corp.
Cover Photo: Getty Images, Inc.-Stockbyte

Dedication

To my husband for his love and encouragement.
Bonnie Fremgen

To my husband, Rick, and my daughter,
Kristin, for their love, support, and friendship.
Suzanne Frucht

Pearson Education LTD.
Pearson Education Australia PTY, Limited
Pearson Education Singapore, Pte. Ltd
Pearson Education North Asia Ltd
Pearson Education, Upper Saddle River, NJ

Pearson Educación de Mexico, S.A. de C.V.
Pearson Education—Japan
Pearson Education Malaysia, Pte. Ltd
Pearson Education Canada, Ltd.

10 9 8 7 6 5
ISBN-13: 978-0-13-158998-8
ISBN-10: 0-13-158998-9

Welcome!

Welcome to the fascinating study of medical language—a vital part of your preparation for a career as a health professional. We are glad that you have joined us. Throughout your career, in a variety of settings, you will use medical terminology to communicate with co-workers and patients. Employing a carefully constructed learning system, **Medical Terminology: A Living Language** has helped thousands of readers gain a successful grasp of medical language within a real-world context.

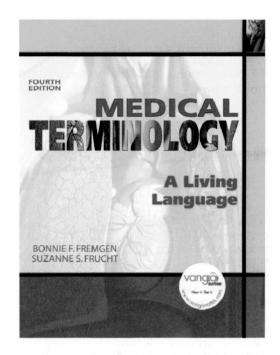

In developing this book we had six goals in mind:

1. To provide a clear introduction to the basic rules of using word parts to form medical terms.
2. To use phonetic pronunciations that will help you easily pronounce terms by spelling out the word part according to the way it sounds.
3. To help you understand medical terminology within the context of the human body systems. Realizing that this book is designed for a terminology course and not an anatomy & physiology course, we have aimed to stick to only the basics.
4. To help you visualize medical language with an abundance of real-life photographs and accurate illustrations.
5. To provide you with a wealth of practice applications at the end of each chapter to help you review and master the content as you go along.
6. To create rich multimedia practice opportunities for you by way of the bonus DVD-ROM, online study guide (**www.prenhall.com/fremgen**), and online course options which provide quizzes, games, videos, and audio pronunciations.

Please turn the page to get a visual glimpse of what makes this book an ideal guide to your exploration of medical terminology.

A Guide to What Makes This Book Special

Streamlined Content

14 chapters and only the most essential anatomy & physiology coverage makes this book a perfect mid-sized fit for a one-term course.

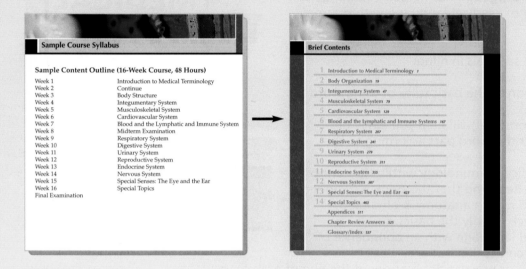

Sample Course Syllabus

Sample Content Outline (16-Week Course, 48 Hours)

Brief Contents

Chapter-Opening Page Spreads

"At a Glance" and "Illustrated" pages begin each chapter, providing a quick, visual snapshot of what's covered.

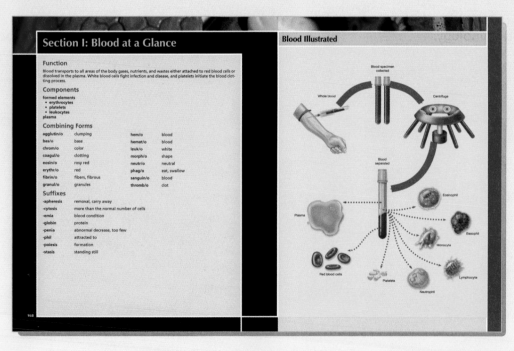

Section I: Blood at a Glance

Function

Blood transports to all areas of the body gases, nutrients, and wastes either attached to red blood cells or dissolved in the plasma. White blood cells fight infection and disease, and platelets initiate the blood clotting process.

Components

formed elements
- erythrocytes
- platelets
- leukocytes
plasma

Combining Forms

agglutin/o	clumping	hem/o	blood
bas/o	base	hemat/o	blood
chrom/o	color	leuk/o	white
coagul/o	clotting	morph/o	shape
eosin/o	rosy red	neutr/o	neutral
erythr/o	red	phag/o	eat, swallow
fibrin/o	fibers, fibrous	sanguin/o	blood
granul/o	granules	thromb/o	clot

Suffixes

-apheresis	removal, carry away
-cytosis	more than the normal number of cells
-emia	blood condition
-globin	protein
-penia	abnormal decrease, too few
-phil	attracted to
-poiesis	formation
-stasis	standing still

Blood Illustrated

Key Terms and Pronunciations

Every subsection starts with a list of key terms and pronunciations for those words that will be covered in that section. This sets the stage for comprehension and mastery.

Med Term Tips

This popular feature offers tidbits of noteworthy information about medical terms that engage learners.

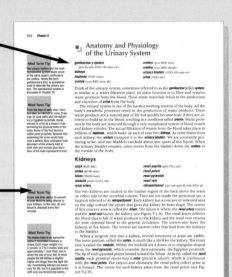

Medically-Accurate Illustrations

Concepts come to life with vibrant, clear, consistent, and scientifically precise images.

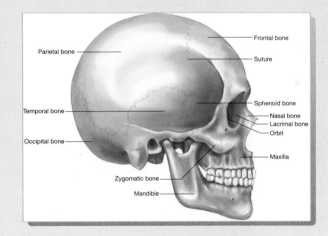

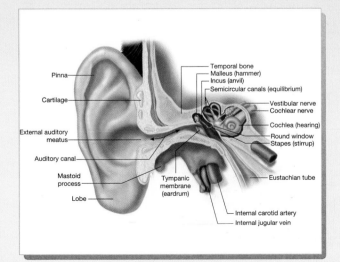

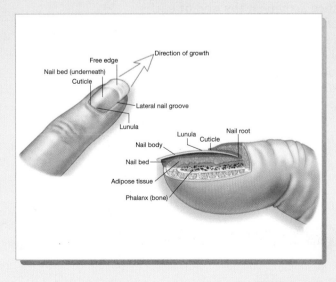

Word Tables

Study lists are categorized and presented in a clear, logical, color-coded format that eases the learning process.

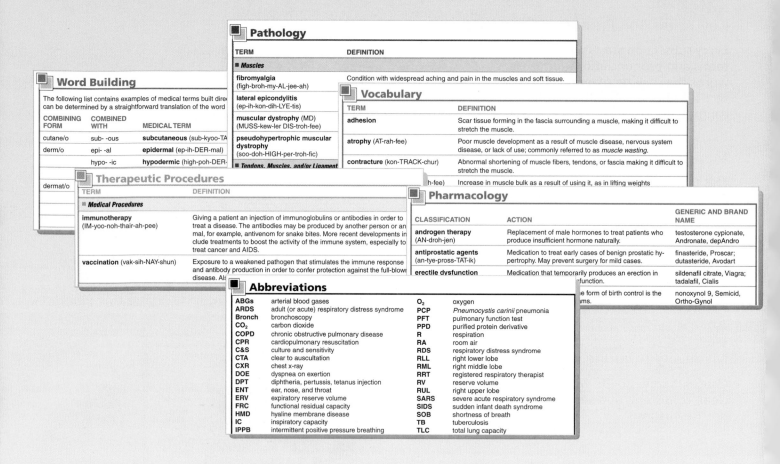

Word Building

The following list contains examples of medical terms built dire...
can be determined by a straightforward translation of the word...

COMBINING FORM	COMBINED WITH	MEDICAL TERM
cutane/o	sub- -ous	**subcutaneous** (sub-kyoo-TA...
derm/o	epi- -al	**epidermal** (ep-ih-DER-mal)
	hypo- -ic	**hypodermic** (high-poh-DER-...
dermat/o		

Pathology

TERM	DEFINITION
■ *Muscles*	
fibromyalgia (figh-broh-my-AL-jee-ah)	Condition with widespread aching and pain in the muscles and soft tissue.
lateral epicondylitis (ep-ih-kon-dih-LYE-tis)	
muscular dystrophy (MD) (MUSS-kew-ler DIS-troh-fee)	
pseudohypertrophic muscular dystrophy (soo-doh-HIGH-per-troh-fic)	
■ *Tendons, Muscles, and/or Ligament*	

Vocabulary

TERM	DEFINITION
adhesion	Scar tissue forming in the fascia surrounding a muscle, making it difficult to stretch the muscle.
atrophy (AT-rah-fee)	Poor muscle development as a result of muscle disease, nervous system disease, or lack of use; commonly referred to as *muscle wasting*.
contracture (kon-TRACK-chur)	Abnormal shortening of muscle fibers, tendons, or fascia making it difficult to stretch the muscle.
...h-fee)	Increase in muscle bulk as a result of using it, as in lifting weights

Therapeutic Procedures

TERM	DEFINITION
■ *Medical Procedures*	
immunotherapy (IM-yoo-noh-thair-ah-pee)	Giving a patient an injection of immunoglobulins or antibodies in order to treat a disease. The antibodies may be produced by another person or an... mal, for example, antivenom for snake bites. More recent developments in... clude treatments to boost the activity of the immune system, especially to treat cancer and AIDS.
vaccination (vak-sih-NAY-shun)	Exposure to a weakened pathogen that stimulates the immune response and antibody production in order to confer protection against the full-blow... disease. Als...

Pharmacology

CLASSIFICATION	ACTION	GENERIC AND BRAND NAME
androgen therapy (AN-droh-jen)	Replacement of male hormones to treat patients who produce insufficient hormone naturally.	testosterone cypionate, Andronate, depAndro
antiprostatic agents (an-tye-pross-TAT-ik)	Medication to treat early cases of benign prostatic hypertrophy. May prevent surgery for mild cases.	finasteride, Proscar; dutasteride, Avodart
erectile dysfunction	Medication that temporarily produces an erection in... ...function.	sildenafil citrate, Viagra; tadalafil, Cialis
	...e form of birth control is the ...ms.	nonoxynol 9, Semicid, Ortho-Gynol

Abbreviations

ABGs	arterial blood gases	**O₂**	oxygen
ARDS	adult (or acute) respiratory distress syndrome	**PCP**	*Pneumocystis carinii* pneumonia
Bronch	bronchoscopy	**PFT**	pulmonary function test
CO₂	carbon dioxide	**PPD**	purified protein derivative
COPD	chronic obstructive pulmonary disease	**R**	respiration
CPR	cardiopulmonary resuscitation	**RA**	room air
C&S	culture and sensitivity	**RDS**	respiratory distress syndrome
CTA	clear to auscultation	**RLL**	right lower lobe
CXR	chest x-ray	**RML**	right middle lobe
DOE	dyspnea on exertion	**RRT**	registered respiratory therapist
DPT	diphtheria, pertussis, tetanus injection	**RV**	reserve volume
ENT	ear, nose, and throat	**RUL**	right upper lobe
ERV	expiratory reserve volume	**SARS**	severe acute respiratory syndrome
FRC	functional residual capacity	**SIDS**	sudden infant death syndrome
HMD	hyaline membrane disease	**SOB**	shortness of breath
IC	inspiratory capacity	**TB**	tuberculosis
IPPB	intermittent positive pressure breathing	**TLC**	total lung capacity

Terminology Checklist

A practice activity at the end of each chapter prompts students to master each key term. This feature is enhanced with an audioglossary available on the accompanying DVD-ROM and website at www.prenhall.com/fremgen.

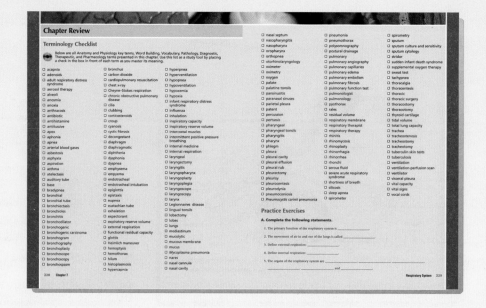

Workbook Section

Case studies and study review questions at the end of each chapter are presented in many different formats including fill-in-the-blank, matching, and labeling to promote comprehension and retention. Answers are found at the end of the book. Here are some examples:

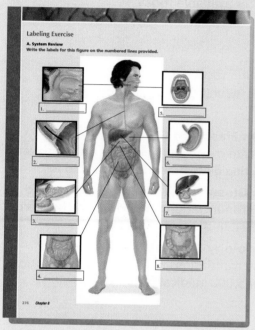

Labeling Exercises – A visual challenge to reinforce readers' grasp of anatomy & physiology concepts.

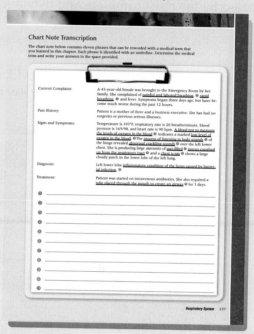

Chart Note Transcription – A slice-of-real-life exercise that asks readers to replace lay terms in a medical chart with the proper medical term.

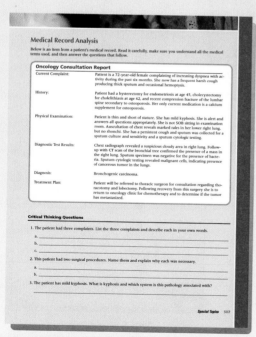

Medical Record Analysis – Scenarios that use critical thinking questions to help readers develop a firmer understanding of the terminology in context.

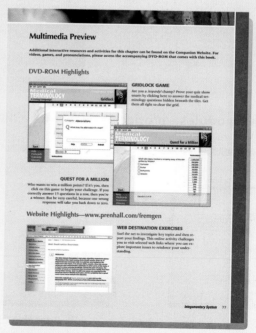

Multimedia Preview – Pages that conclude each chapter and direct readers to the wealth of features on the student DVD-ROM and website. This is a gateway to deeper understanding.

The Total Teaching and Learning Package

We are committed to providing students and instructors with exactly the tools they need to be successful in the classroom and beyond. To this end, *Medical Terminology: A Living Language* is supported by the most complete and dynamic set of resources available today.

Student DVD-ROM

A bonus DVD-ROM is included with every text, and provides 12 different interactive game modules, animations, videos, an audio glossary, and more. Here are some highlights:

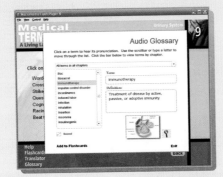

- **Custom Flashcard Generator** – allows students to create and print their own flashcards by selecting glossary terms on which to focus.
- **Audio Glossary** – provides definitions and audio pronunciations of each of the key terms presented in the text.
- **Terminology Translator** – Contains the Spanish translations and audio pronunciations of over 5,000 medical terms.

Pathology Spotlights – a video library that provides a mini-documentary profile of selected diseases and procedures presented within each chapter.

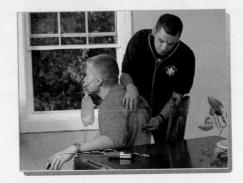

12 different game modules – provide students with a diverse and fun array of study tools.

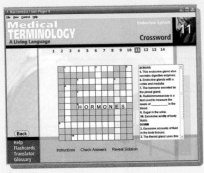

Crossword

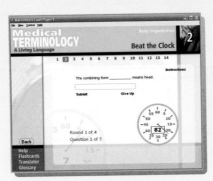

Beat the Clock

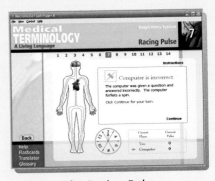

The Racing Pulse

Online Learning

No medical terminology textbook has as full a selection of web-based resources as *Medical Terminology: A Living Language*. Whether you are looking for a basic Internet study experience, a robust, self-paced online course delivery system, or anything in between we offer the solution that suits your needs.

MyMedTermLab

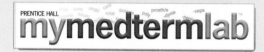

The most complete, dynamic online medical terminology course available today! Compatable within any learning management system, this revolutionary, self-paced program engages students with activities, assessments, and rich media that is unmatched in the market. Features include:

- Integrated e-book – Provides a one-to-one match with the text and allows readers to access videos and animations straight from the "page."
- Interactive modules – Designed for readers to step through a self-paced tutorial program screen by screen.

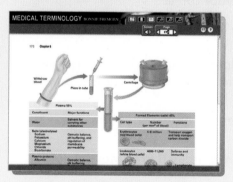

e-book

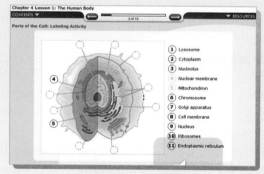

Interactive Modules

Companion Website

Our most basic online option, this is a free-access online study guide located at **www.prenhall.com/fremgen**. It contains:

- Quizzes in multiple-choice, true/false, labelling, fill-in, and essay formats. Instant feedback and explanations are provided and results can be emailed to instructors.
- An audio glossary in which key terms are pronounced.

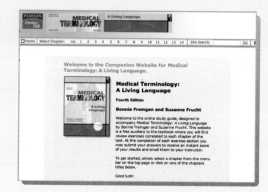

Tools for the Instructor

Medical Terminology: A Living Language offers a rich array of ancillary materials to benefit instructors and help infuse a spark in the classroom. The full complement of supplemental teaching materials is available to all qualified instructors from your Pearson Health sales representative. (**www.prenhall.com/replocator**)

Instructor's Resource Manual

This manual contains a wealth of material to help faculty plan and manage the medical terminology course. It includes:

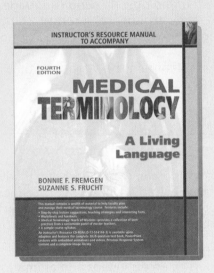

- *Medical Terminology Pearls of Wisdom*, a collection of best teaching practices shared by a national panel of master medical terminology educators.
- Step-by-step lectures, outlines, and daily lesson plans organized by learning objective.
- A syllabus conversion guide to help instructors transition from the 3rd edition of this text.
- A sample syllabus.
- A complete test bank of nearly 3,000 questions.

Instructor's Media Library

A multi-disc set containing all the electronic resources necessary to manage your course.

- The complete test bank of nearly 3,000 questions that allows instructors to generate customized exams and quizzes.
- A comprehensive, turn-key lecture package in PowerPoint format containing discussion points, along with embedded color images from the textbook as well as bonus animations and videos to help infuse an extra spark into the classroom experience.
- PowerPoint content to support instructors who wish to use Classroom Response System. For more information visit **www.prenhall.com/prs**.
- A complete image library that includes every photograph and illustration contained in the textbook; provided three ways: with labels, with leader lines only, and unlabeled.

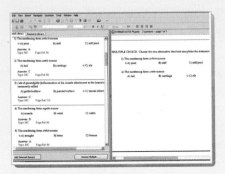

Test Bank

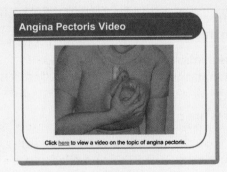

Videos

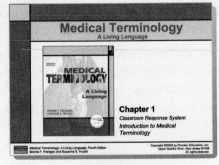

PowerPoint Lectures

Preface

Since the first edition of **Medical Terminology: A Living Language** was published it has been noted for its "clean" and logical format that promotes learning. In this revised edition, we have built upon this strength by enhancing many features to make this text an ideal choice for semester-or quarter-length courses.

Features of the New Edition

This edition contains new features that facilitate student mastery, while maintaining the best aspects of previous editions. Each chapter is arranged in a similar format and the content has been reorganized with an emphasis on maintaining consistency and accuracy. All terms have been reevaluated to ensure they remain in current use and reflect the newest technologies and procedures.

- An all-new art program carefully crafted by a team of medically trained illustrators with attention to precision brings medical terminology to life and makes learning more fun and effective.
- System At A Glance chapter-opening feature provides a quick reference for each topic being discussed in terms of its function, organs, combining forms, suffixes, and prefixes.
- System Illustrated chapter-opening feature provides full-color drawings of each system with detailed art of organs to be discussed in the chapter.
- Chapter 2 includes a new section on Body Regions to help readers better understand this important information.
- The pharmacology tables have been expanded to include commonly used generic and brand names.
- Practice Exercises increased by 20% over the 3rd edition.
- New labeling activities at the end of chapters help readers practice their ability to identify the organs in each body system.

Chapter Format

Every chapter begins with learning objectives followed by new System At A Glance and System Illustrated features that give readers a brief glimpse into the anatomy, physiology, and terminology associated with that system. The chapter text, supported by a wealth of tables and diagrams follows. Beginning in Chapter 2, color-coded tables then provide a series of easy-to-use study lists. Throughout each chapter readers will also find Med Term Tips, which are intended to stimulate interest by describing quick facts about medical terms. Each chapter concludes with a comprehensive workbook section featuring case studies, quizzes, and worksheets.

The end-of-chapter activities have been significantly expanded in this edition and answers at the end of the text provide immediate feedback. Activities include:

- **Terminology Checklist**—This feature includes an alphabetical listing of each term from the chapter. Students are encouraged to listen to the audio pronunciation of each term on the accompanying DVD-ROM and check off each term as they master how to say it correctly.

- **Medical Record Analysis**–Students apply practical use of medical terminology for each body system by reading a realistic case scenario and responding to critical thinking questions about it.
- **Chart Note Transcription**–Students read a patient scenario and then replace lay phrases used to describe maladies, procedures, tests, and conditions with the accurate medical terms.
- **Practice Exercises**–These include a variety of questions that allow students to test their knowledge of chapter material.
- **Labeling Exercises**–These new activities require students to correctly label system and anatomy art from the chapter to practice identifying parts of organs and systems discussed.

Organization of the Book

Introductory Chapter. Chapter 1 contains information necessary for an understanding of how medical terms are formed. This includes learning about word roots, combining forms, prefixes, and suffixes, and general rules for building medical terms. Readers will also learn about terminology for medical records and the different health care settings. Chapter 2 presents terminology relating to the body organization, including organs and body systems. Here readers will first encounter word building tables, a feature found in each remaining chapter that lists medical terms and their respective word parts.

Anatomy and Physiology Chapters. Chapters 3 through 13 are organized by body system. Each chapter begins with a System At A Glance which lists combining forms, prefixes, and/or suffixes with their meanings and is followed by System Illustrated overview of the organs in the system. The anatomy and physiology section is divided into the various components of the system, and each subsection begins with a list of key medical terms accompanied by a pronunciation guide. Key terms are boldfaced the first time they appear in the narrative. A word building table and medical terms with pronunciations follow each anatomy and physiology section. For ease of learning, the medical terms are divided into four separate sections: vocabulary, pathology, diagnostic procedures, and therapeutic procedures. Pharmacology and abbreviations sections then follow to complete the chapter.

Special Topics Chapter. Chapter 14 contains timely information and appropriate medical terms relevant to the following medical specialties: pharmacology, mental health, diagnostic imaging, rehabilitation services, surgery, and oncology. Knowledge of these topics is necessary for the well-rounded health care worker.

Appendices. The appendices contain helpful reference lists of word parts and definitions. This information is intended for quick access. There are four appendices: Abbreviations; Combining Forms; Prefixes; and Suffixes. The Combining Forms, Prefixes, and Suffixes appendices present English-to-medical and then medical-to-English conversions. Finally, all of the key terms appear again in the glossary/index at the end of the text.

Teaching and Learning Package

To enhance the teaching and learning process, an attractive media-focused resource package for both students and faculty accompanies *Medical Terminology: A Living Language.* The full complement of supplemental teaching materials is available to all qualified instructors from your Pearson Health sales representative.

Student DVD-ROM

The bonus student DVD-ROM is packaged with every copy of the textbook. It includes:

- Custom flashcard generator that allows students to easily create custom study aids for additional practice.
- Audio Glossary that challenges readers to practice and listen to correct pronunciations of terms presented in the text.
- Terminology Translator containing the Spanish translations and audio pronunciations of over 5,000 medical terms.
- Interactive exercises, games, and activities that quiz students on spelling, word building concepts, anatomy, and more.
- Pathology Spotlight videos providing a mini-documentary profile of selected diseases presented within each chapter.

Companion Website

Students and faculty will both benefit from the bonus Companion Website at www.prenhall.com/fremgen. This website serves as a text-specific, interactive online workbook to accompany *Medical Terminology: A Living Language*. Featuring an automatic scoring and feedback function, the Companion Website is organized in correspondence with the chapters of the text. Highlights include:

- A variety of multiple-choice, true/false, labeling, and fill-in-the-blank quizzes
- Internet links that relate to chapter content
- An audio glossary with pronunciations of key terms
- Case studies that allow students to apply their knowledge of the chapter content

The website instantly tabulates student results and allows those results to be sent to instructors via e-mail. Alternatively, the results can be saved and printed.

MyMedTermLab

MyMedTermLab is the most complete, dynamic online medical terminology course available today. Compatable within any learning management system, this revolutionary, self-paced program engages students in activities, assessments, and rich media that is unmatched in the market. Features include:

- Integrated e-book provides a one-to-one match with the text and allows readers to access videos and animations straight from the "page."
- Interactive modules designed for readers to step through a self-paced tutorial program screen by screen.
- A customizable test bank containing nearly 3,000 questions.
- PowerPoint lectures with embedded video clips and animations
- A full array of course management tools.

For more information, a demonstration, or a discussion about customizable options for our online course systems, please contact your Pearson Health sales representative.

Instructor's Resource Manual

This guide contains a wealth of material to help faculty plan and manage the medical terminology course. It includes:

- Step-by-step lectures, outlines, and daily lesson plans organized by learning objectives
- Worksheets, lecture suggestions and content correlations to the instructional media materials
- *Medical Terminology Pearls of Wisdom*, a collection of best teaching practices shared by a national panel of master medical terminology educators
- A syllabus conversion guide to help instructors transition from the 3rd edition of this text
- A sample syllabus
- A nearly 3,000-question test bank

Instructor's Media Library

A multi-disc set containing all the electronic resources necessary to manage your course. It includes:

- The nearly 3,000-question test bank that allows instructors to generate customized exams and quizzes
- A comprehensive, turn-key lecture package in PowerPoint format containing discussion points, along with embedded color images from the textbook as well as bonus animations and videos to help infuse an extra spark into the classroom experience.
- PowerPoint content to support instructors who wish to use Personal Response Systems. For more information visit www.prenhall.com/prs.
- A complete image library that includes every photograph and illustration containing in the textbook.

About the Authors

Bonnie F. Fremgen

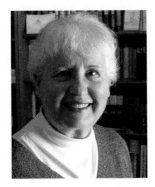

Bonnie F. Fremgen is a former associate dean of the Allied Health Program at Robert Morris College. She has taught medical law and ethics courses as well as clinical and administrative topics. In addition, she has served as an advisor for students' career planning. She has broad interests and experiences in the health care field, including hospitals, nursing homes, and physicians' offices.

Dr. Fremgen holds a nursing degree as well as a master's in health care administration. She received her PhD from the College of Education at the University of Illinois. She has performed postdoctoral studies in Medical Law at Loyola University Law School in Chicago. She has authored five textbooks with Prentice Hall.

Suzanne S. Frucht

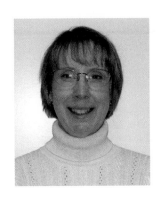

Suzanne S. Frucht is an Associate Professor of Physiology at Northwest Missouri State University (NWMSU). She holds baccalaureate degrees in biological sciences and physical therapy from Indiana University, an MS in biological sciences at NWMSU, and a PhD in molecular biology and biochemistry from the University of Missouri-Kansas City.

For 14 years she worked full-time as a physical therapist in various health care settings, including acute care hospitals, extended care facilities, and home health. Based on her educational and clinical experience she was invited to teach medical terminology part-time in 1988 and became a full-time faculty member three years later as she discovered her love for the challenge of teaching. She teaches a variety of courses including medical terminology, human anatomy, human physiology, and animal anatomy and physiology. She received the Governor's Award for Excellence in Teaching in 2003.

About the Illustrators

Marcelo Oliver is president and founder of Body Scientific International Llc. He holds an MFA degree in Medical and Biological Illustration from University of Michigan. For the past 15 years, his passion has been to condense complex anatomical information into visual education tools for students, patients, and medical professionals. For seven years he worked as a medical illustrator and creative director developing anatomical charts used for student and patient education. In the years that followed, he created educational and marketing tools for medical device companies prior to founding Body Scientific International, Llc.

Body Scientific's lead artists in this publication were medical illustrators Liana Bauman and Katie Burgess. Both hold an Master of Science degrees in Biomedical Visualization degree from the University of Illinois at Chicago. Their contribution in the publication was key in the creation and editing of artwork throughout.

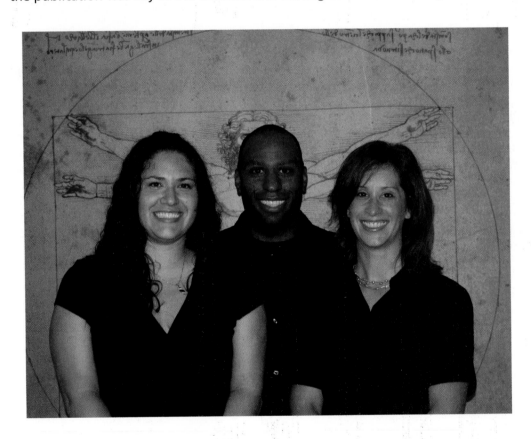

Our Development Team

We would like to express deep gratitude to our 95 colleagues from schools across the country that have provided us with hundreds of hours of their time over the years to help us tailor this book to suit the dynamic needs of instructors and students. These individuals have reviewed manuscript chapters and illustrations for content, accuracy, level, and utility. We sincerely thank you and feel that *Medical Terminology: A Living Language* has benefited immeasurably from your efforts, insights, encouragement, and selfless willingness to share your expertise as educators.

Reviewers of the 4th Edition

Yvonne Alles, MBA, RMT
Department Coordinator
Davenport University
Grand Rapids, Michigan

Steve Arinder, BS, MPH
Chair, Health Education
    Division
Meridian Community College
Meridian, Mississippi

K. William Avery, BSMT, JD, PhD
Chair and Professor, Allied
    Health
City College
Gainesville, Florida

Michael Battaglia, MS
Instructor
Greenville Technical College
Taylors, South Carolina

Barbara J Behrens, PTA, MS
PTA Program Coordinator
Mercer County Community
    College
Trenton, New Jersey

Norma J Bird, M.Ed., BS, CMA
Program Coordinator, Medical
    Assisting
Idaho State University College
    of Technology
Pocatello, Idaho

Trina Blaschko, RHIT
Instructor
Chippewa Valley Technical
    College
Eau Claire, Wisconsin

Bradley S. Bowden, PhD
Professor
Alfred University
Alfred, New York

Lyndal M. Curry, M.A., R.P.
EMS Degree Program
    Coordinator
University of South Alabama
Mobile, Alabama

Nancy Dancs, P.T.
Instructor
Waukesha County Technical
    College
Pewaukee, Wisconsin

Antoinette Deshaies, RN, BSPA
Adjunct Faculty
Glendale Community College
Glendale, Arizona

Carol Eckert, RN, MSN
Director, Nursing Education
Southwestern Illinois College
Belleville, Illinois

**Mildred K. Fuller, Ph.D.,
    MT(ASCP), CLS(NCA)**
Chair, Allied Health
Norfolk State University
Norfolk, Virginia

Deborah Galanski-Maciak
Davenport University
Grand Rapids, Michigan

**Steven B. Goldschmidt, DC,
    CCFC**
Instructor
North Hennepin Community
    College
Brooklyn Park, Minnesota

Mary Hartman, MS, OTR/L
Director, OTA Program
Genesee Community College
Batavia, New York

Joyce B. Harvey, Ph.D, RHIA
Associate Professor
Norfolk State University
Norfolk, Virginia

**Beulah A. Hofmann, RN, BSN,
    MSN, CMA**
Associate Professor
Chair, Nursing Department
Ivy Tech Community College
    of Indiana
Greencastle, Indiana

Susan Jackson, EdS
Instructor
Valdosta Technical College
Valdosta, Georgia

Mark Jaffe, DPM, MHSA
Assistant Professor
Nova Southeastern University
Ft. Lauderdale, Florida

Carol Lee Jarrell, MLT,AHI
Department Chair, Medical
Brown Mackie College
Merrillville, Indiana

Robin Jones, RHIA
Coordinator, Health
    Information Technology
Meridian Community College
Meridian, Mississippi

Julie A. Leu, CPC
Billing Compliance Coordinator
Creighton University
Omaha, Nebraska

Jeanne W. Lovelock, RN, MSN
Assistant Professor
Piedmont Virginia Community
    College
Charlottesville, Virginia

Jan Martin, R.T.(R)
Clinical Coordinator,
    Radiologic Technology
Ogeechee Tech College
Statesboro, Georgia

Leslie M. Mazzola, MA
Instructor
Cuyahoga Community College
Parma, Ohio

Michelle C. McCranie, CPhT
Instructor
Ogeechee Technical College
Statesboro, Georgia

Patricia Moody, RN
Instructor
Athens Technical College
Athens, Georgia

Catherine Moran, Ph.D.
Professor
Breyer State University
Birmingham, Alabama

Judy Ortiz MHS, MS, PA-C
Academic Coordinator/
    Associate Professor
Pacific University
Hillsboro, Oregon

Dave Peruski, RN, MSA, MSN
Program Coordinator, Nursing
Delta College
University Center, Michigan

Carolyn Ragsdale CST, BS
Instructor, Surgical Technology
Parkland College
Champaign, Illinois

Ellen Rosen, RN, MN
Adjunct Professor
Glendale Community College
Glendale, California

**Georgette Rosenfeld, Ph.D.,
RN, RRT**
Program Director, Respiratory
Care & Pharmacy Technician
Indian River Community
College
Fort Pierce, Florida

Brian L. Rutledge, MHSA
Instructor
Hinds Community College
Jackson, Mississippi

**Sue Shibley, M.Ed., CMT,
CCS-P, CPC**
North Idaho College
Instructor
Coeur d'Alene, Idaho

Misty Shuler, RHIA
Chair of Administrative
Medical Systems
Technologies
Asheville Buncombe Technical
Community College
Asheville, North Carolina

Donna Stern
Manager, Clinical Trials
Programs
University of California
San Diego Extension
La Jolla, California

**Annmary Thomas, MEd,
NREMT-P**
Assistant Professor
Community College
of Philadelphia
Philadelphia, Pennsylvania

Joan Ann Verderame, RN, MA
Program Director, Surgical
Technology
Bergen Community College
Paramus, New Jersey

Twila Wallace, MEd
Instructor
Central Community College
Columbus, Nebraska

Linda Walter, RN, MSN
Instructor
Northwestern Michigan
College
Traverse City, Michigan

Jean Watson, PhD
Faculty, Health Occupations
Clark College
Vancouver, Washington

Twila Weiszbrod, MPA
Adjunct Faculty
College of the Sequoias
Visalia, California

Lynn C. Wimett, RN, ANP, EdD
Chair, Post Licensure Programs
In Nursing
Regis University
Denver, Colorado

Kathy Zaiken, Pharm.D.
Assistant Professor
Massachusetts College
of Pharmacy and Health
Sciences
Boston, Massachusetts

Reviewers of Earlier Editions

**Rachael C. Alstatter, Program
Director**
Southern Ohio College
Fairfield, Ohio

Beverly A. Baker, DA, CST
Western Iowa Technical
Community College
Sioux City, Iowa

**Nancy Ridinger Bean, Health
Assistant Instructor**
Wythe County Vocational
School
Wytheville, Virginia

Deborah J. Bedford, CMA, AAS
Program Coordinator
Medical Assisting Program
North Seattle Community
College
Seattle, Washington

Pam Besser, Ph.D.
Professor of Rhetoric
Jefferson Community College
Louisville, Kentucky

Richard T. Boan, PhD
Coordinator
Allied Health Sciences
Midlands Technical College
Columbia, SC

**Susan W. Boggs, RN, BSN,
CNOR**
Program Coordinator
Surgical Technology
Piedmont Technical College
Greenwood, SC

Joan Walker Brittingham
Program Coordinator
Adult Education and Training
Sussex Tech Adult Division
Georgetown, Delaware

**Phyills J. Broughton, Curriculum
Coordinator**
Pitt Community College
Greenville, North Carolina

Barbara Bussard, Instructor
Southwestern Michigan
College
Dowagiac, Michigan

Toni Cade, MBA, RHIA, CCS
Assistant Professor
University of Louisiana
at Lafayette
Lafayette, Louisiana

Gloria H. Coats, RN, MSN
Nursing Instructor
Modesto Junior College
Modesto, CA

**Theresa H. deBeche, RN, MN,
CNS**
Head, Division of Nursing
and Allied Health
Louisiana State University
at Eunice
Eunice, LA

**Bonnie Deister, MS, BSN,
CMA-C**
Chairperson, Medical Assisting
& EMT-Paramedic
Department
Broome Community College
Binghamton, New York

Jamie Erskine, Ph.D., R.D.
Associate Professor
Department of Community
Health and Nutrition
University of Northern
Colorado
Greeley, Colorado

**Debra Getting, Practical
Nursing Instructor**
Norwest Iowa Community
College
Sheldon, Iowa

Ann Queen Giles, MHS, CMA
Program Director
Medical Assisting Program
Western Piedmont Community
College
Morganton, North Carolina

Brenda L. Gleason, MSN
Assistant Professor
Nursing
Iowa Central Community
College
Fort Dodge, IA

Linda S. Gott, RN, MS
Coordinator, Academy
for Health Professions
Pensacola High School
Pensacola, Florida

Martha Grove, Staff Educator
Human & Organization
Development
Mercy Regional Health System
Cincinnati, Ohio

Kathryn Gruber
Applied Sciences
Globe College
Oakdale, Minnesota

Karen R. Hardney, M.S., Ed.
Recruitment Director
College of Health Sciences
Chicago State University
Chicago, Illinois

Kimberley Hontz , RN
Antonelli Medical and
Professional Institute
Pottstown, Pennsylvania

Pamela S. Huber, M.S., MT(ASCP)
Assistant Professor
Medical Laboratory
    Technology Department
Erie Community College
Williamsville, New York

Eva I. Irwin
Instructor and Clinical
    Coordinator
Ivy Tech State College
Indianapolis, Indiana

Virginia J. Johnson, CMA
Program Director
Lakeland Academy
Minneapolis, Minnesota

Marcie C. Jones, BS, CMA
Program Director, Medical
    Assisting
Gwinnett Technical Institute
Lawrenceville, GA

Gertrude A. Kenny, BSN, RN, CMA
Associate Dean of Allied
    Health
Baker College of Muskegon
Muskegon, Michigan

Dianne K. Kuiti, RN
Medical Instructor-Medical
    Office Administrator
Duluth Business University
Duluth, Minnesota

Andrew La Marca, EMT-P
EMT and Paramedic
    Instructor/Coordinator
Mobile Life Support Services
Middletown, New York

Norma Longoria, BS, COI
Instructor
Health & Medical
    Administrative Service
Nursing/Allied Health Division
South Texas Community
    College
McAllen, TX

Lola McGourty, MSN, RN
Bossier Parish Community
    College
Bossier City, Louisiana

Connie Morgan
Program Chair, Medical
    Assisting Program
Ivy Tech State College
Kokomo., Indiana

Katrina B. Myricks
Instructor
Business and Office Technology
Holmes Community College
Ridgeland, MS

Pam Ncu, CMA
Program Department Head
International Business College
Fort Wayne, Indiana

Tina M. Peer, BSN, RN
Nursing and Allied Health
    Instructor
College of Southern Idaho
Twin Falls, ID
Sylvania, Ohio

Sister Marguerite Polcyn, OSF, PhD
Professor of Health Education
Lourdes College
Sylvania, OH

Vicki Prater, CMA, RMA, RAHA
Medical Program Director
Concorde Career Institute
San Bernardino, California

LuAnn Reicks, RNC, BS, MSN
Professor/Practical Nursing
    Coordinator
Iowa Central Community
    College
Fort Dodge, IA

Linda Reigel
Assistant Professor
Department of Business
Glenville State College
Glenville, West Virginia

Connie Smith, RPh
Coordinator, Advanced
    Practice Experience
Instructor
University of Louisiana at
    Monroe School of Pharmacy
Monroe, LA

Karen Snipe, CPhT, ASBA, MAEd
Pharmacy Technician Program
    Coordinator
Trident Technical College
Charleston, SC

Janet Stehling, RHIA
Instructor
Health Information Technology
McLennan College
Lorena, Texas

Marilyn Turner, RN, CMA
Program Director, Medical
    Assisting
Allied Health Department
    Chair
Ogeechee Technical College
Statesboro, GA

Kathy Wallington
Director, Medical Assisting
    Department
Phillips Junior College
Campbell, California

Sara J. Wellman, RHIT
Clinical Coordinator
Health Information Technology
    Program
Indiana University Northwest
Gary, Indiana

Leesa Whicker, BA, CMA
Instructor
Central Piedmont Community
    College
Charlotte, NC

A Commitment to Accuracy

As a student embarking on a career in health care you probably already know how critically important it is to be precise in your work. Patients and co-workers will be counting on you to avoid errors on a daily basis. Likewise, we owe it to you – the reader – to ensure accuracy in this book. We have gone to great lengths to verify that the information provided in *Medical Terminology: A Living Language* is complete and correct. To this end, here are the steps we have taken:

1. **Editorial Review**–We have assembled a large team of developmental consultants (listed on the preceding pages) to critique every word and every image in this book. No fewer than 12 content experts have read each chapter for accuracy. In addition, some members of our developmental team were specifically assigned to focus on the precision of each illustration that appears in the book.

2. **Medical Illustrations**–A team of medically-trained illustrators was hired to prepare each piece of art that graces the pages of this book. These illustrators have a higher level of scientific education than the artists for most textbooks, and they worked directly with the authors and members of our development team to make sure that their work was clear, correct, and consistent with what is described in the text

3. **Accurate Ancillaries**–Realizing that the teaching and learning ancillaries are often as vital to instruction as the book itself, we took extra steps to ensure accuracy and consistency within these components. Textbook co-author Suzanne Frucht served the dual role of editor/author of each of the ancillary components. She wrote or edited every test question, every PowerPoint slide, and every element of the student DVD-ROM and online courses. Her goal was to guarantee a tight mesh between the content in the book and the content in these additional resources. Finally, we assigned some members of our development team to specifically focus on critiquing every bit of content that comprises the instructional ancillary resources to confirm accuracy.

While our intent and actions have been directed at creating an error-free text, we have established a process for correcting any mistakes that may have slipped past our editors. Pearson takes this issue seriously and therefore welcomes any and all feedback that you can provide along the lines of helping us enhance the accuracy of this text. If you identify any errors that need to be corrected in a subsequent printing, please sending them to:

Pearson Health Editorial
Medical Terminology Corrections
One Lake Street
Upper Saddle River, NJ 07458

Thank you for helping Pearson to reach its goal of providing the most accurate medical terminology textbooks available.

Contents

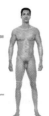
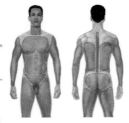
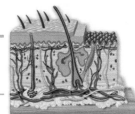

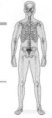
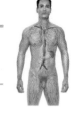

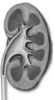

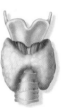

12 Nervous System 387

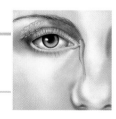

13 Special Senses: The Eye and Ear 423

14 Special Topics 463

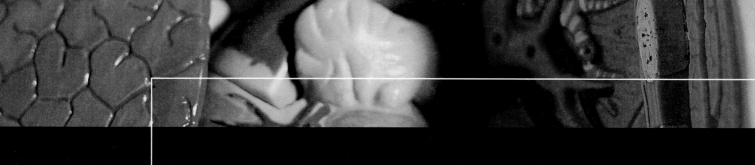

1

Introduction to Medical Terminology

Learning Objectives

Upon completion of this chapter, you will be able to:

- Discuss the four parts of medical terms.
- Recognize word roots and combining forms.
- Identify the most common prefixes and suffixes.
- Define word building and describe a strategy for translating medical terms.
- State the importance of correct spelling of medical terms.
- State the rules for determining singular and plural endings.
- Discuss the importance of using caution with abbreviations.
- Recognize the documents found in a medical record.
- Recognize the different healthcare settings.
- Understand the importance of confidentiality.

Medical Terminology at a Glance

Learning medical terminology can initially seem like studying a strange new language. However, once you understand some of the basic rules as to how medical terms are formed using word building, it will become much like piecing together a puzzle. The general guidelines for forming words; an understanding of word roots, combining forms, prefixes, and suffixes; pronunciation; and spelling are discussed in this chapter. Chapter 2 introduces you to terms used to describe the body as a whole. Chapters 3 through 13 each focus on a specific body system and present new combining forms, prefixes, and suffixes, as well as exercises to help you gain experience building new medical terms. Finally, Chapter 14 includes the terminology for several important areas of patient care. In addition, "Med Term Tips" are sprinkled throughout all of the chapters to assist in clarifying some of the material. New medical terms discussed in each section are listed separately at the beginning of the section, and each chapter contains numerous pathological, diagnostic, treatment, and surgical terms. You can use these lists as an additional study tool for previewing and reviewing terms.

Understanding medical terms requires you to be able to put words together or build words from their parts. It is impossible to memorize thousands of medical terms; however, once you understand the basics, you can distinguish the meaning of medical terms by analyzing their prefixes, suffixes, and word roots. Remember that there will always be some exceptions to every rule, and medical terminology is no different. We will attempt to point out these exceptions where they exist. Most medical terms, however, do follow the general rule that there is a **word root** or fundamental meaning for the word, a **prefix** and a **suffix** that modify the meaning of the word root, and sometimes a **combining vowel** to connect other word parts. You will be amazed at the seemingly difficult words you will be able to build and understand when you follow the simple steps in word building (see Figure 1.1 ■).

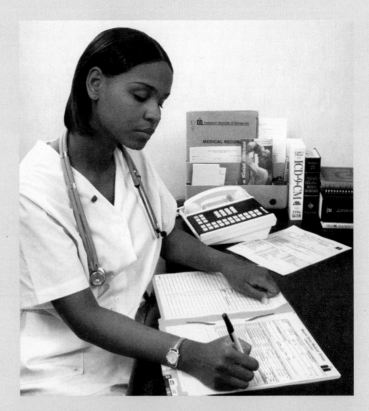

■ **Figure 1.1** Nurse completing a patient report. Healthcare workers use medical terminology in order to accurately and efficiently communicate patient information to each other.

Building Medical Terms from Word Parts

Four different word parts or elements can be used to construct medical terms:

1. The **word root** is the foundation of the word.
2. A **prefix** is at the beginning of the word.
3. A **suffix** is at the end of the word.
4. The **combining vowel** is a vowel (usually o) that links the word root to another word root or a suffix.

cardiogram = record of the heart

pericardium = around the heart

card**itis** = inflammation of the heart
cardi**o**my**o**pathy = disease of the heart muscle

The following sections on word roots, combining vowels and forms, prefixes, and suffixes will consider each of these word parts in more detail and present examples of some of those most commonly used.

Word Roots

The word root is the foundation of a medical term and provides us with the general meaning of the word. The word root often indicates the body system or part of the body that is being discussed, such as *cardi* for heart. At other times the word root may be an action. For example, the word root *cis* means to cut (as in incision).

A term may have more than one word root. For example, **osteoarthritis** (oss tee oh ar THRY tis) combines the word root *oste* meaning bone and *arthr* meaning the joints. When the suffix *-itis*, meaning inflammation, is added, we have the entire word, meaning an inflammation involving bone at the joints.

Combining Vowel/Form

To make it possible to pronounce long medical terms with ease and to combine several word parts, a combining vowel is used. This is most often the vowel *o*. Combining vowels are utilized in two places: between a word root and a suffix or between two word roots.

To decide whether to use a combining vowel between a word root and suffix, first look at the suffix. If it begins with a vowel, do not use the combining vowel. If, however, the suffix begins with a consonant, then use a combining vowel. For example: To combine *arthr* with *-scope* will require a combining vowel: **arthroscope** (AR throh scope). But to combine *arthr* with *-itis* does not require a combining vowel: **arthritis** (ar THRY tis).

The combining vowel is typically kept between two word roots, even if the second word root begins with a vowel. For example, in forming the term **gastroenteritis** (gas troh en ter EYE tis) the combining vowel is kept between the two word roots *gastr* and *enter* (gastrenteritis is incorrect). As you can tell from pronouncing these two terms, the combining vowel makes the pronunciation easier.

When writing a word root by itself, its **combining form** is typically used. This consists of the word root and its combining vowel written in a word root/vowel form, for example, *cardi/o*. Since it is often simpler to pronounce word roots when they appear in their combining form, this format is used throughout this book.

Common Combining Forms

Some commonly used word roots in their combining form, their meaning, and examples of their use follow. Review the examples to observe when a combining vowel was kept and when it was dropped according to the rules presented on the preceding page.

Combining Form	Meaning	Example (Definition)
aden/o	gland	adenopathy (gland disease)
carcin/o	cancer	carcinoma (cancerous tumor)
cardi/o	heart	cardiac (pertaining to the heart)
chem/o	chemical	chemotherapy (treatment with chemicals)
cis/o	to cut	incision (process of cutting into)
dermat/o	skin	dermatology (study of the skin)
enter/o	small intestine	enteric (pertaining to the small intestine)
gastr/o	stomach	gastric (pertaining to the stomach)
gynec/o	female	gynecology (study of females)
hemat/o	blood	hematic (pertaining to the blood)
hydr/o	water	hydrocele (protrusion of water [in the scrotum])
immun/o	immune	immunology (study of immunity)
laryng/o	voice box	laryngeal (pertaining to the voice box)
morph/o	shape	morphology (study of shape)
nephr/o	kidney	nephromegaly (enlarged kidney)
neur/o	nerve	neural (pertaining to a nerve)
ophthalm/o	eye	ophthalmic (pertaining to the eye)
ot/o	ear	otic (pertaining to the ear)
path/o	disease	pathology (study of disease)
pulmon/o	lung	pulmonary (pertaining to the lungs)
rhin/o	nose	rhinoplasty (surgical repair of the nose)
ur/o	urine, urinary tract	urology (study of the urinary tract)

Prefixes

A new medical term is formed when a prefix is added to the front of the term. Prefixes frequently give information about the location of an organ, the number of parts, or the time (frequency). For example, the prefix *bi-* stands for two of something, such as **bilateral** (bye LAH ter al), which means having two sides. However, not every term will have a prefix.

Common Prefixes

Some of the more common prefixes, their meanings, and examples of their use follow. When written by themselves, prefixes are followed by a hyphen.

Prefix	Meaning	Example (Definition)
a-	without, away from	aphasia (without speech)
an-	without	anoxia (without oxygen)
ante-	before, in front of	antepartum (before birth)

anti-	against	antibiotic (against life)
auto-	self	autograft (a graft from one's own body)
brady-	slow	bradycardia (slow heartbeat)
✱dys-	painful, difficult	dyspnea (difficulty breathing)
endo-	within, inner	endoscope (instrument to view within)
epi-	upon, over	epigastric (upon or over the stomach)
eu-	normal, good	eupnea (normal breathing)
hetero-	different	heterograft (a graft from another person's body)
homo-	same	homozygous (having two identical genes)
hyper-	over, above	hypertrophy (overdevelopment)
hypo-	under, below	hypoglossal (under the tongue)
infra-	under, beneath, below	infraorbital (below, under the eye socket)
inter-	among, between	intervertebral (between the vertebrae)
intra-	within, inside	intravenous (inside, within a vein)
macro-	large	macrocephalic (having a large head)
micro-	small	microcephalic (having a small head)
neo-	new	neonate (newborn)
pan-	all	pancarditis (inflammation of all the heart)
para-	beside, beyond, near	paranasal (near or alongside the nose)
per-	through	percutaneous (through the skin)
peri-	around	pericardial (around the heart)
post-	after	postpartum (after birth)
pre-	before, in front of	prefrontal (in front of the frontal bone)
pseudo-	false	pseudocyesis (false pregnancy)
retro-	backward, behind	retrograde (movement in a backward direction)
sub-	below, under	subcutaneous (under, below the skin)
super-	above, excess	supernumerary (above the normal number)
supra-	above	suprapubic (above the pubic bone)
tachy-	rapid, fast	tachycardia (fast heartbeat)
trans-	through, across	transurethral (across the urethra)
ultra-	beyond, excess	ultrasound (high-frequency sound waves)

Med Term Tip

Be very careful with prefixes; many have similar spellings but very different meanings. For example:

anti- means "against"; *ante-* means "before"
inter- means "between"; *intra-* means "inside"
per- means "through"; *peri-* means "around"

Number Prefixes

Some common prefixes pertaining to the number of items or measurement, their meanings, and examples of their use follow.

Prefix	Meaning	Example (Definition)
bi-	two	bilateral (two sides)
hemi-	half	hemiplegia (paralysis of one side/half of the body)
mono-	one	monoplegia (paralysis of one extremity)
multi-	many	multigravida (woman pregnant more than once)
nulli-	none	nulligravida (woman with no pregnancies)
poly-	many	polyuria (large amounts of urine)

quad-	four	quadriplegia (paralysis of all four extremities)
semi-	partial, half	semiconscious (partially conscious)
tri-	three	triceps (muscle with three heads)
uni-	one	unilateral (one side)

Suffixes

A suffix is attached to the end of a word to add meaning, such as a condition, disease, or procedure. For example, the suffix *-itis*, which means inflammation, when added to *cardi-* forms the new word **carditis** (car DYE tis), which means inflammation of the heart. Every medical term *must* have a suffix. The majority of the time, the suffix is added to a word root, as in carditis above. However, terms can also be built from a suffix added directly to a prefix, without a word root. For example, the term **dystrophy** (DIS troh fee), which means abnormal development, is built from the prefix *dys-* (meaning abnormal) and the suffix *-trophy* (meaning development).

Med Term Tip

Remember, if a suffix begins with a vowel, the combining vowel is dropped: for example, *mastitis* rather than *mastoitis*.

Common Suffixes

Some common suffixes, their meanings, and examples of their use follow. When written by themselves, suffixes are preceded by a hyphen.

Suffix	Meaning	Example (Definition)
-algia	pain	gastralgia (stomach pain)
-cele	hernia, protrusion	cystocele (protrusion of the bladder)
-cise	cut	excise (to cut out)
-cyte	cell	erythrocyte (red cell)
-dynia	pain	cardiodynia (heart pain)
-ectasis	dilation	bronchiectasis (dilated bronchi)
-gen	that which produces	mutagen (that which produces mutations)
-genesis	produces, generates	osteogenesis (produces bone)
-genic	producing, produced by	carcinogenic (producing cancer)
-ia	state, condition	hemiplegia (condition of being half paralyzed)
-iasis	abnormal condition	lithiasis (abnormal condition of stones)
-ism	state of	hypothyroidism (state of low thyroid)
-itis	inflammation	cellulitis (inflammation of cells)
-logist	one who studies	cardiologist (one who studies the heart)
-logy	study of	cardiology (study of the heart)
-lysis	destruction	osteolysis (bone destruction)
-malacia	abnormal softening	chondromalacia (abnormal cartilage softening)
-megaly	enlargement, large	cardiomegaly (enlarged heart)
-oma	tumor, mass	carcinoma (cancerous tumor)
-osis	abnormal condition	cyanosis (abnormal condition of being blue)
-pathy	disease	myopathy (muscle disease)
-plasia	development, growth	dysplasia (abnormal development)
-plasm	formation, development	neoplasm (new formation)
-ptosis	drooping	proctoptosis (drooping rectum)

-rrhage	excessive, abnormal flow	hemorrhage (excessive bleeding)
-rrhea	discharge, flow	rhinorrhea (discharge from the nose)
-rrhexis	rupture	hysterorrhexis (ruptured uterus)
-sclerosis	hardening	arteriosclerosis (hardening of an artery)
-stenosis	narrowing	angiostenosis (narrowing of a vessel)
-therapy	treatment	chemotherapy (treatment with chemicals)
-trophy	nourishment, development	hypertrophy (excessive development)

Adjective Suffixes

The following suffixes are used to convert a word root into an adjective. These suffixes usually are translated as *pertaining to*.

Suffix	Meaning	Example (Definition)
-ac	pertaining to	cardiac (pertaining to the heart)
-al	pertaining to	duodenal (pertaining to the duodenum)
-an	pertaining to	ovarian (pertaining to the ovary)
-ar	pertaining to	ventricular (pertaining to a ventricle)
-ary	pertaining to	pulmonary (pertaining to the lungs)
-eal	pertaining to	esophageal (pertaining to the esophagus)
-iac	pertaining to	chondriac (pertaining to cartilage)
-ic	pertaining to	gastric (pertaining to the stomach)
-ical	pertaining to	neurological (pertaining to the study of the nerves)
-ile	pertaining to	penile (pertaining to the penis)
-ior	pertaining to	superior (pertaining to above)
-ory	pertaining to	auditory (pertaining to hearing)
-ose	pertaining to	adipose (pertaining to fat)
-ous	pertaining to	intravenous (pertaining to within a vein)
-tic	pertaining to	acoustic (pertaining to hearing)

Surgical Suffixes

The following suffixes indicate surgical procedures.

Suffix	Meaning	Example (Definition)
-centesis	puncture to withdraw fluid	arthrocentesis (puncture to withdraw fluid from a joint)
-ectomy	surgical removal	gastrectomy (surgically remove the stomach)
-ostomy	surgically create an opening	colostomy (surgically create an opening for the colon through the abdominal wall)
-otomy	cutting into	thoracotomy (cutting into the chest)
-pexy	surgical fixation	nephropexy (surgical fixation of a kidney)
-plasty	surgical repair	dermatoplasty (surgical repair of the skin)
-rrhaphy	suture	myorrhaphy (suture together muscle)

Med Term Tip

Surgical suffixes have very specific meanings:

-otomy means "to cut into"
-ostomy means "to create a new opening"
-ectomy means "to cut out" or "remove"

Procedural Suffixes

The following suffixes indicate procedural processes or instruments.

Suffix	Meaning	Example (Definition)
-gram	record or picture	electrocardiogram (record of heart's electricity)
-graph	instrument for recording	electrocardiograph (instrument for recording the heart's electrical activity)
-graphy	process of recording	electrocardiography (process of recording the heart's electrical activity)
-meter	instrument for measuring	audiometer (instrument to measure hearing)
-metry	process of measuring	audiometry (process of measuring hearing)
-scope	instrument for viewing	gastroscope (instrument to view stomach)
-scopy	process of visually examining	gastroscopy (process of visually examining the stomach)

Word Building

Word building consists of putting together several word elements to form a variety of terms. The combining form of a word may be added to another combining form along with a suffix to create a new descriptive term. For example, adding *hyster/o* (meaning uterus) to *salping/o* (meaning fallopian tubes) along with the suffix *-ectomy* (meaning surgical removal of) forms **hysterosalpingectomy** (hiss-ter-oh-sal-pin-JEK-toh-mee), the removal of both the uterus and the fallopian tubes. You will note that the combining vowel *o* is dropped when adding the suffix *-ectomy* since two vowels are not necessary.

Interpreting Medical Terms

The following strategy is a reliable method for puzzling out the meaning of an unfamiliar medical term.

Med Term Tip

To gain a quick understanding of a term, it may be helpful to you to read from the end of the word (or the suffix) back to the beginning (the prefix), and then pick up the word root. For example, *pericarditis* reads inflammation (*-itis*) surrounding (*peri-*) the heart (*cardi/o*).

Step	Example
1. Divide the term into its word parts.	gastr/o/enter/o/logy
2. Define each word part.	gastr = stomach
	o = combining vowel, no meaning
	enter = small intestine
	o = combining vowel, no meaning
	-logy = study of
3. Combine the meaning of the word parts.	stomach, small intestine, study of

Pronunciation

You will hear different pronunciations for the same terms depending on where people were born or educated. As long as it is clear which term people are discussing, differing pronunciations are acceptable. Some people are difficult to understand over the telephone or on a transcription tape. If you have any doubt about a term being discussed, ask for the term to be spelled. For example, it is often difficult to hear the difference between the terms **abduction** and **adduction**. However, since the terms refer to opposite directions of movement, it is very important to double check if there is any question about which term was used.

Each new term in this book is introduced in boldface type, with the phonetic or "sounds like" pronunciation in parentheses immediately following. The part of the word that should receive the greatest emphasis during pronunciation appears in capital letters: for example, **pericarditis** (per ih car DYE tis). Toward the end of Chapters 2 through 14 is a Terminology Checklist. This is a list of all the key terms from the chapter. Each term is also pronounced on the CD-ROM packaged with this book. Listen to each word, then pronounce it silently to yourself or out loud. Check each term off the list as you master it. This list also serves as a review list for all the terms introduced in each chapter.

Spelling

Although you will hear differing pronunciations of the same term, there will be only one correct spelling. If you have any doubt about the spelling of a term or of its meaning, always look it up in a medical dictionary. If only one letter of the word is changed, it could make a critical difference for the patient. For example, imagine the problem that could arise if you note for insurance purposes that a portion of a patient's **ileum**, or small intestine, was removed when in reality he had surgery for removal of a piece of his **ilium**, or hip bone.

Some words have the same beginning sounds but are spelled differently. Examples include the following:

Med Term Tip

If you have any doubt about the meaning or spelling of a word, look it up in your medical dictionary. Even experienced medical personnel still need to look up a few words.

Sounds like *si*

psy	**psychiatry** (sigh-KIGH-ah-tree)
cy	**cytology** (sigh-TALL-oh-gee)

Sounds like *dis*

dys	**dyspepsia** (dis-PEP-see-ah)
dis	**dislocation** (dis-low-KAY-shun)

 # Singular and Plural Endings

Many medical terms originate from Greek and Latin words. The rules for forming the singular and plural forms of some words follow the rules of these languages rather than English. For example, the heart has a left atrium and a right atrium for a total of two *atria*, not two *atriums*. Other words, such as *virus* and *viruses*, are changed from singular to plural by following English rules. Each medical term needs to be considered individually when changing from the singular to the plural form. The following examples illustrate how to form plurals.

Words ending in	Singular	Plural
-a	vertebra	vertebrae
-ax	thorax	thoraces
-ex or -ix	appendix	appendices
-is	metastasis	metastases
-ma	sarcoma	sarcomata
-nx	phalanx	phalanges
-on	ganglion	ganglia
-us	nucleus	nuclei
-um	ovum	ova
-y	biopsy	biopsies

Abbreviations

Abbreviations are commonly used in the medical profession as a way of saving time. However, some abbreviations can be confusing, such as *SM* for simple mastectomy and *sm* for small. Use of the incorrect abbreviation can result in problems for a patient, as well as with insurance records and processing. If you have any concern that you will confuse someone by using an abbreviation, spell out the word instead. It is never acceptable to use one's own abbreviations. All types of healthcare facilities will have a list of approved abbreviations, and it is extremely important that you become familiar with this list and follow it closely. Throughout the book abbreviations are included, when possible, immediately following terms. In addition, a list of common abbreviations for each body system is given in each chapter. Finally, Appendix I provides a complete alphabetical listing of all the abbreviations used in this text.

 # The Medical Record

The **medical record** or chart documents the details of a patient's hospital stay. Each healthcare professional who has contact with the patient in any capacity completes the appropriate report of that contact and adds it to the medical chart. This results in a permanent physical record of the patient's day-to-day condition, when and what services he or she received, and the response to treatment. Each institution adopts a specific format for each document and its location within the chart. This is necessary because each healthcare professional must be able to locate quickly and efficiently the information he or she needs in order to provide proper care for the patient. The medical record is also a legal document. Therefore, it is essential that all chart components be completely filled out and signed. Each page must contain the proper patient identification information: the patient's name, age, gender, physician, admission date, and identification number.

While the patient is still in the hospital, a unit clerk is usually responsible for placing documents in the proper place. After discharge, the medical records department ensures that all documents are present, complete, signed, and in the correct order. If a person is readmitted, especially for the same diagnosis, parts of this previous chart can be pulled and added to the current chart for reference (see Figure 1.2 ■). Physicians' offices and other outpatient care providers such as clinics and therapists also maintain a medical record detailing each patient's visit to their facility.

A list of the most common elements of a hospital chart with a brief description of each follows.

History and Physical—Written or dictated by the admitting physician; details the patient's history, results of the physician's examination, initial diagnoses, and physician's plan of treatment

Physician's Orders—Complete list of the care, medications, tests, and treatments the physician orders for the patient

Nurse's Notes—Record of the patient's care throughout the day; includes vital signs, treatment specifics, patient's response to treatment, and patient's condition

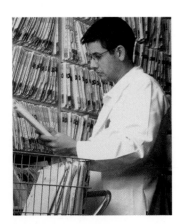

■ **Figure 1.2** Health information professionals maintain accurate, orderly, and permanent patient records. Medical records are securely stored and available for future reference.

Physician's Progress Notes—Physician's daily record of the patient's condition, results of the physician's examinations, summary of test results, updated assessment and diagnoses, and further plans for the patient's care

Consultation Reports—Reports given by specialists whom the physician has asked to evaluate the patient

Ancillary Reports—Reports from various treatments and therapies the patient has received, such as rehabilitation, social services, or respiratory therapy

Diagnostic Reports—Results of diagnostic tests performed on the patient, principally from the clinical lab (for example, blood tests) and medical imaging (for example, X-rays and ultrasound)

Informed Consent—Document voluntarily signed by the patient or a responsible party that clearly describes the purpose, methods, procedures, benefits, and risks of a diagnostic or treatment procedure

Operative Report—Report from the surgeon detailing an operation; includes a pre- and postoperative diagnosis, specific details of the surgical procedure itself, and how the patient tolerated the procedure

Anesthesiologist's Report—Relates the details regarding the substances (such as medications and fluids) given to a patient, the patient's response to anesthesia, and vital signs during surgery

Pathologist's Report—Report given by a pathologist who studies tissue removed from the patient (for example, bone marrow, blood, or tissue biopsy)

Discharge Summary—Comprehensive outline of the patient's entire hospital stay; includes condition at time of admission, admitting diagnosis, test results, treatments and patient's response, final diagnosis, and follow-up plans

Healthcare Settings

The use of medical terminology is widespread. It provides healthcare professionals with a precise and efficient method of communicating very specific patient information to one another, regardless of whether they are in the same type of facility (see Figure 1.3 ■). Descriptions follow of the different types of settings where medical terminology is used.

Acute Care or General Hospitals—Provide services to diagnose (laboratory, diagnostic imaging) and treat (surgery, medications, therapy) diseases for a short period of time; in addition, they usually provide emergency and obstetrical care

Specialty Care Hospitals—Provide care for very specific types of diseases; for example, a psychiatric hospital

Nursing Homes or Long-Term Care Facilities—Provide long-term care for patients who need extra time to recover from an illness or injury before returning home, or for persons who can no longer care for themselves

Ambulatory Care, Surgical Centers, or Outpatient Clinics—Provide services that do not require overnight hospitalization; the services range from simple surgeries to diagnostic testing or therapy

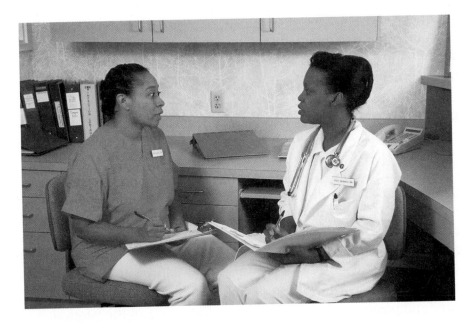

Figure 1.3 A nurse and medical assistant review a patient's chart and plan his or her daily care.

Physicians' Offices—Provide diagnostic and treatment services in a private office setting

Health Maintenance Organization (HMO)—Provides a wide range of services by a group of primary-care physicians, specialists, and other healthcare professionals in a prepaid system

Home Health Care—Provides nursing, therapy, personal care, or housekeeping services in the patient's own home

Rehabilitation Centers—Provide intensive physical and occupational therapy; they include inpatient and outpatient treatment

Hospice—Provides supportive treatment to terminally ill patients and their families

 # Confidentiality

Anyone who works with medical terminology and is involved in the medical profession must have a firm understanding of confidentiality. Any information or record relating to a patient must be considered privileged. This means that you have a moral and legal responsibility to keep all information about the patient confidential. If you are asked to supply documentation relating to a patient, the proper authorization form must be signed by the patient. Give only the specific information that the patient has authorized. The Health Insurance Portability and Accountability Act of 1996 (HIPAA) set federal standards that provide patients with more protection of their medical records and health information, better access to their own records, and greater control over how their health information is used and to whom it is disclosed.

Chapter Review

Terminology Checklist

Below are all key terms presented in this chapter. Use this list as a study tool by placing a check in the box in front of each term as you master its meaning.

- ☐ acute care hospitals
- ☐ ambulatory care centers
- ☐ ancillary reports
- ☐ anesthesiologist's report
- ☐ combining form
- ☐ combining vowel
- ☐ consultation report
- ☐ diagnostic reports
- ☐ discharge summary
- ☐ general hospitals
- ☐ health maintenance organization (HMO)

- ☐ history and physical
- ☐ home health care
- ☐ hospices
- ☐ informed consent
- ☐ long-term care facilities
- ☐ medical record
- ☐ nurse's notes
- ☐ nursing homes
- ☐ operative report
- ☐ outpatient clinics
- ☐ pathologist's report

- ☐ physicians' offices
- ☐ physician's orders
- ☐ physician's progress notes
- ☐ prefix
- ☐ rehabilitation centers
- ☐ specialty care hospitals
- ☐ suffix
- ☐ surgical centers
- ☐ word root

Practice Exercises

A. Complete the following statements.

1. The combination of a word root and the combining vowel is called a(n) _____.

2. The vowel that connects two word roots or a suffix with a word root is usually a(n) _____.

3. A word part used at the end of a word root to change the meaning of the word is called a(n) _____.

4. A(n) _____ is used at the beginning of a word to indicate number, location, or time.

5. Although the pronunciation of medical terms may differ slightly from one person to another, the _____ must never change.

6. The four components of a medical term are _____, _____, _____, and _____.

B. Define the following combining forms.

1. aden/o _____

2. carcin/o _____

3. cardi/o _____

4. chem/o _____

5. cis/o _____

6. dermat/o _____

7. enter/o _____

8. gastr/o _____

9. gynec/o _____

10. hemat/o _____

11. hydr/o _____

12. immun/o _____

13. laryng/o _____

14. morph/o _____

15. nephr/o _____

16. neur/o _____

17. ophthalm/o _____

18. ot/o _____

19. pulmon/o _____

20. rhin/o _____

21. ur/o _____

C. Define the following suffixes.

1. -plasty _____

2. -stenosis _____

3. -itis _____

4. -al _____

5. -algia _____

6. -otomy _____

7. -megaly _____

8. -ectomy _____

9. -rrhage _____

10. -centesis _____

11. -gram _____

12. -ac _____

13. -malacia _____

14. -ism _____

15. -rrhaphy _____

16. -ostomy _____

17. -pexy _____

18. -rrhea _____

19. -scopy _____

20. -oma _____

D. Join a combining form and a suffix to form words with the following meanings.

1. study of lungs _____

2. pain relating to a nerve _____

3. nose discharge or flow _____

4. abnormal softening of a kidney _____

5. enlarged heart _____

6. cutting into the stomach _____

7. inflammation of the skin _____

8. surgical removal of the voice box _____

9. surgical repair of a joint _____

10. gland disease _____

E. Write a prefix for each of the following expressions.

1. within, inside _____

2. large _____

3. before, in front of _____

4. around _____

5. new _____

6. without _____

7. half _____

8. painful, difficult _____

9. above _____

10. over, above _____

11. many _____

12. slow _____

13. self _____

14. across _____

15. two _____

F. Circle the prefixes in the following terms and define in the space provided.

1. tachycardia _____

2. pseudocyesis _____

3. hypoglycemia _____

4. intercostal _____

5. eupnea _____

6. postoperative _____

7. monoplegia _____

8. subcutaneous _____

G. Change the following singular terms to plural terms.

1. metastasis _____

2. ovum _____

3. diverticulum _____

4. atrium _____

5. diagnosis _____

6. vertebra _____

H. Use the suffix -ology, meaning *the study of*, to write a term for each medical specialty.

1. heart _____

2. stomach _____

3. skin _____

4. eye _____

5. urinary tract _____

6. kidney _____

7. blood _____

8. female _____

9. nerve _____

10. disease _____

I. Build a medical term by combining the word parts requested in each question.

For example, use the combining form for *spleen* with the suffix meaning *enlargement* to form a word meaning *enlargement of the spleen* (answer: *splenomegaly*).

1. combining form for *heart* _____
   suffix meaning *abnormal softening* _____
   term meaning *softening of the heart*

2. word root form for *stomach* _____
   suffix meaning *to surgically create an opening* _____
   term meaning *creating an opening into the stomach*

3. combining form for *nose* _____
   suffix meaning *surgical repair* _____
   term meaning *surgical repair of the nose*

4. prefix meaning *over, above* _____
   suffix meaning *nourishment, development* _____
   term meaning *overdevelopment*

5. combining form meaning *disease* _____
   suffix meaning *the study of* _____
   term meaning *the study of disease*

6. word root meaning *gland* _____
   suffix for *tumor/mass* _____
   term meaning *gland tumor or mass*

7. combining form meaning *stomach* _____
   combining form meaning *small intestine* _____
   suffix meaning *study of* _____
   term meaning *study of stomach and small intestine*

8. word root meaning *ear* _____
   suffix meaning *inflammation* _____
   term meaning *ear inflammation*

9. prefix meaning *water* _____
   suffix meaning *treatment* _____
   term meaning *water treatment*

10. combining form meaning *cancer* _____
    suffix meaning *that which produces* _____
    term meaning *that which produces cancer*

J. Match each definition to its term.

1. _____ Provides services for a short period of time

2. _____ Complete outline of a patient's entire hospital stay

3. _____ Describes purpose, methods, benefits, and risks of procedure

4. _____ Contains updated assessment, diagnoses, and further plans for care

5. _____ Provides supportive care to terminally ill patients and families

6. _____ Written by the admitting physician

7. _____ Reports results from study of tissue removed from the patient

8. _____ Written by the surgeon

9. _____ Provides services not requiring overnight hospital stay

10. _____ Report given by a specialist

11. _____ Record of a patient's care through the day

12. _____ Clinical lab and medical imaging reports

13. _____ Provides intensive physical and occupational therapy

14. _____ Report of treatment/therapy the patient received

15. _____ Provides care for patients who need more time to recover

a. rehabilitation center

b. nurse's notes

c. ancillary report

d. hospice

e. discharge summary

f. physician's progress notes

g. ambulatory care center

h. diagnostic report

i. long-term care facility

j. informed consent

k. history and physical

l. acute care hospital

m. pathologist's report

n. consultation report

o. operative report

Multimedia Preview

Additional interactive resources and activities for this chapter can be found on the Companion Website. For videos, games, and pronunciations, please access the accompanying DVD-ROM that comes with this book.

DVD-ROM Highlights

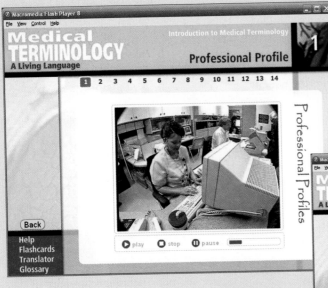

PROFESSIONAL PROFILE: MEDICAL TRANSCRIPTIONIST

Get a glimpse of what medical transcriptionists do on the job each day by watching a video profile of this exciting career field. Each chapter presents a brief segment featuring a different health profession that you may chose to explore.

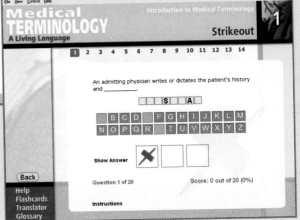

STRIKEOUT!

Click on the alphabet tiles to fill in the empty squares in the word or phrase to complete the sentence. This game quizzes your vocabulary and spelling. But choose your letters carefully because three strikes and you're out!

Website Highlights—www.prenhall.com/fremgen

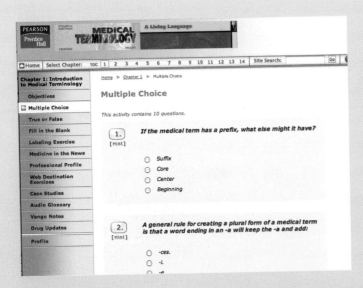

MULTIPLE CHOICE QUIZ

Take advantage of the free-access on-line study guide that accompanies your textbook. You'll find a multiple-choice quiz that provides instant feedback that allows you to check your score and see what you got right or wrong. By clicking on this URL you'll also access links to download mp3 audio reviews, current news articles, and an audio glossary.

2

Body Organization

Learning Objectives

Upon completion of this chapter, you will be able to:

- Recognize the combining forms introduced in this chapter.
- Correctly spell and pronounce medical terms and anatomical structures relating to body structure.
- Discuss the organization of the body in terms of cells, tissues, organs, and systems.
- Describe the common features of cells.
- Define the four types of tissues.
- List the major organs found in the twelve organ systems.
- Describe the anatomical position.
- Define the body planes.
- Identify regions of the body.
- Define directional and positional terms.
- List the body cavities and their contents.
- Locate and describe the nine anatomical and four clinical divisions of the abdomen.
- Build body organization medical terms from word parts.
- Interpret abbreviations associated with body organization.

Body Organization at a Glance

Arrangement

The body is organized into levels. Each level is built from the one below it. In other words, the body as a whole is composed of systems, a system is composed of organs, an organ is composed of tissues, and tissues are composed of cells.

Levels

cells   tissues   organs   systems   body

Combining Forms

abdomin/o	abdomen	muscul/o	muscle
adip/o	fat	neur/o	nerve
anter/o	front	organ/o	organ
brachi/o	arm	oste/o	bone
caud/o	tail	pelv/o	pelvis
cephal/o	head	peritone/o	peritoneum
cervic/o	neck	pleur/o	pleura
chondr/o	cartilage	poster/o	back
crani/o	skull	proxim/o	near to
crur/o	leg	pub/o	genital region
cyt/o	cell	somat/o	body
dist/o	away from	spin/o	spine
dors/o	back of body	super/o	above
epitheli/o	epithelium	system/o	system
glute/o	buttock	thorac/o	chest
hist/o	tissue	ventr/o	belly
infer/o	below	vertebr/o	vertebra
later/o	side	viscer/o	internal organ
medi/o	middle		

Med Term Tip

The prefixes and suffixes introduced in Chapter 1 will be used over and over again in your medical terminology course, making it easier to recognize new terms more quickly. Beginning with this chapter new combining forms, prefixes, and suffixes will appear at the beginning of each chapter.

Body Organization Illustrated

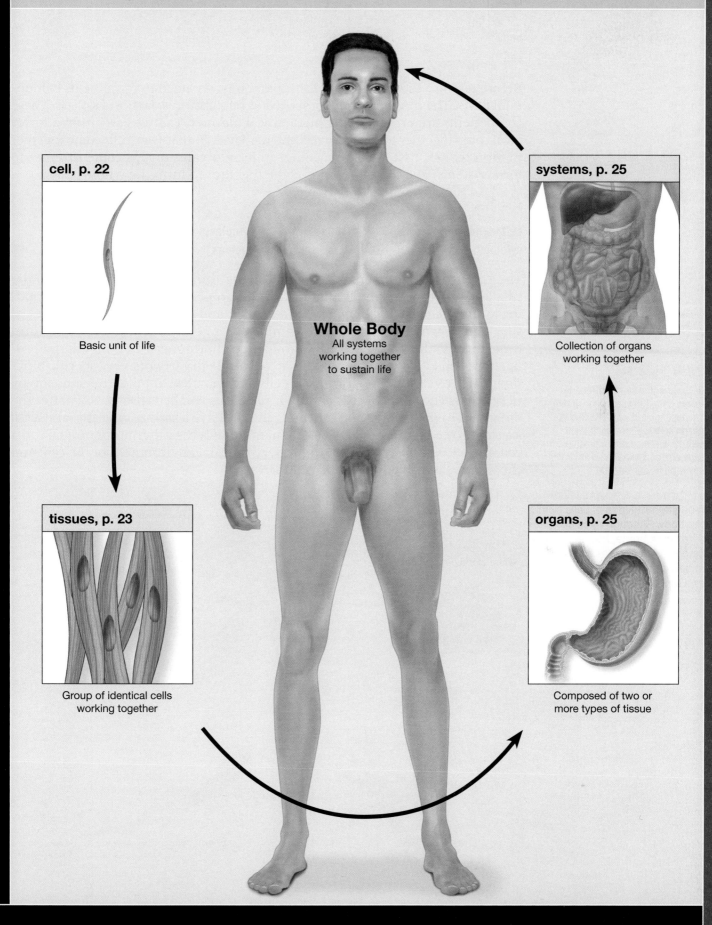

cell, p. 22

Basic unit of life

tissues, p. 23

Group of identical cells working together

Whole Body
All systems working together to sustain life

systems, p. 25

Collection of organs working together

organs, p. 25

Composed of two or more types of tissue

Levels of Body Organization

body	organs	tissues
cell	systems	

Before taking a look at the whole human body, we need to examine its component parts. The human **body** is composed of **cells**, **tissues**, **organs**, and **systems**. These components are arranged in a hierarchical manner. That is, parts from a lower level come together to form the next higher level. In that way, cells come together to form tissues, tissues come together to form organs, organs come together to form systems, and all the systems come together to form the whole body.

Cells

cell membrane	cytoplasm (SIGH-toh-plazm)
cytology (sigh-TALL-oh-jee)	nucleus

The cell is the fundamental unit of all living things. In other words, it is the smallest structure of a body that has all the properties of being alive: responding to stimuli, engaging in metabolic activities, and reproducing itself. All the tissues and organs in the body are composed of cells. Individual cells perform functions for the body such as reproduction, hormone secretion, energy production, and excretion. Special cells are also able to carry out very specific functions, such as contraction by muscle cells and electrical impulse transmission by nerve cells. The study of cells and their functions is called **cytology**. No matter the difference in their shape and function, all cells have a **nucleus**, **cytoplasm**, and a **cell membrane** (see Figure 2.1 ■). The cell membrane is the outermost boundary of a cell. It encloses the cytoplasm, the watery internal environment of the cell, and the nucleus which contains the cell's DNA.

Med Term Tip

Cells were first seen by Robert Hooke over 300 years ago. To him, the rectangular shapes looked like prison cells, so he named them cells. It was a common practice for early anatomists to name an organ solely on its appearance.

■ **Figure 2.1** Examples of four different types of cells from the body. Although each cell has a cell membrane, nucleus, and cytoplasm, each has a unique shape depending on its location and function.

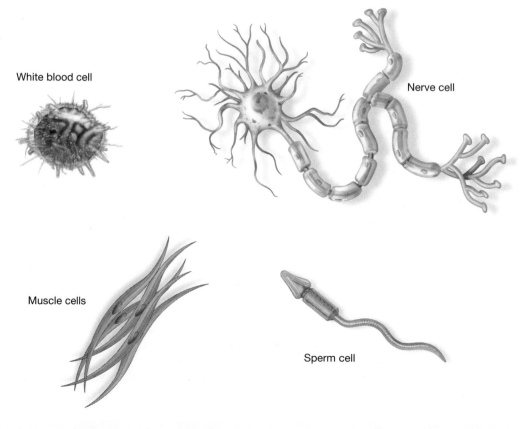

White blood cell

Nerve cell

Muscle cells

Sperm cell

Tissues

connective tissue
epithelial tissue (ep-ih-THEE-lee-al)
histology (hiss-TALL-oh-jee)

muscle tissue
nervous tissue

Histology is the study of tissue. A tissue is formed when like cells are grouped together and function together to perform a specific activity. The body has four types of tissue: **muscle tissue**, **epithelial tissue**, **connective tissue**, and **nervous tissue**.

Muscle Tissue

cardiac muscle
muscle fibers

skeletal muscle
smooth muscle

Muscle tissue produces movement in the body through contraction, or shortening in length, and is composed of individual muscle cells called **muscle fibers** (see Figure 2.2 ■). Muscle tissue forms one of three basic types of muscles: **skeletal muscle**, **smooth muscle**, or **cardiac muscle**. Skeletal muscle is attached to bone. Smooth muscle is found in internal organs such as the intestine, uterus, and blood vessels. Cardiac muscle is found only in the heart.

Epithelial Tissue

epithelium (ep-ih-THEE-lee-um)

Epithelial tissue, or **epithelium**, is found throughout the body and is composed of close-packed cells that form the covering for and lining of body structures. For example, both the top layer of skin and the lining of the stomach are epithelial tissue (see Figure 2.2). In addition to forming a protective barrier, epithelial tissue may be specialized to absorb substances (such as nutrients from the intestine), secrete substances (such as sweat glands), or excrete wastes (such as the kidney tubules).

Connective Tissue

adipose (ADD-ih-pohs)
bone

cartilage (CAR-tih-lij)
tendons

Connective tissue is the supporting and protecting tissue in body structures. Because connective tissue performs many different functions depending on its location, it appears in many different forms so that each is able to perform the task required at that location. For example, **bone** provides structural support for the whole body. **Cartilage** is the shock absorber in joints. **Tendons** tightly connect skeletal muscles to bones. **Adipose** provides protective padding around body structures (see Figure 2.2).

Nervous Tissue

brain
nerves

neurons
spinal cord

Nervous tissue is composed of cells called **neurons** (see Figure 2.2). This tissue forms the **brain**, **spinal cord**, and a network of **nerves** throughout the entire body. This allows for the conduction of electrical impulses to send information between the brain and the rest of the body.

Med Term Tip

The term *epithelium* comes from the prefix *epi-* meaning "on top of" and the combining form *theli/o* meaning "nipple" (referring to any projection from the surface).

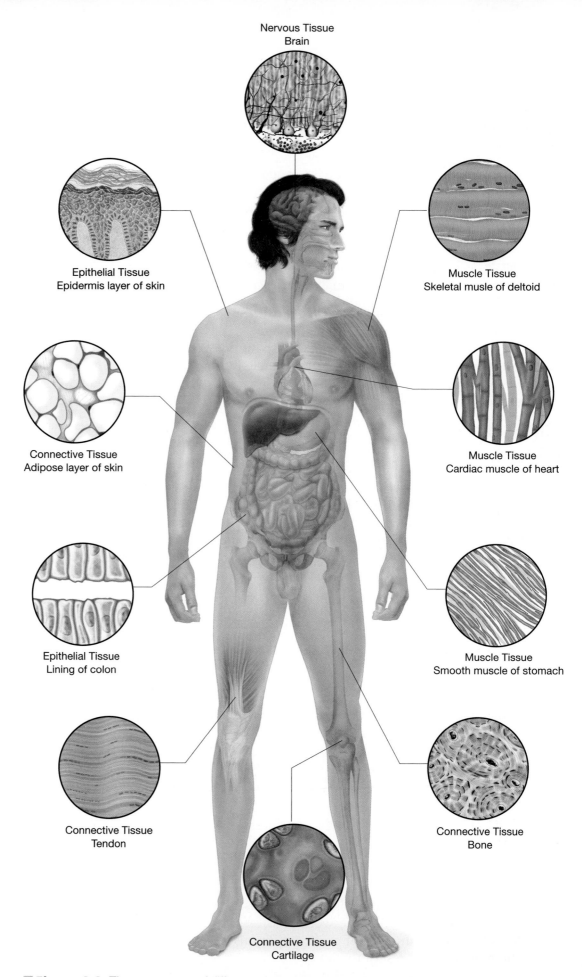

Nervous Tissue
Brain

Epithelial Tissue
Epidermis layer of skin

Muscle Tissue
Skeletal musle of deltoid

Connective Tissue
Adipose layer of skin

Muscle Tissue
Cardiac muscle of heart

Epithelial Tissue
Lining of colon

Muscle Tissue
Smooth muscle of stomach

Connective Tissue
Tendon

Connective Tissue
Bone

Connective Tissue
Cartilage

Figure 2.2 The appearance of different types of tissues—muscle, epithelial, nervous, connective—and their location within the body.

Organs and Systems

Organs are composed of several different types of tissue that work as a unit to perform special functions. For example, the stomach contains smooth muscle tissue, nervous tissue, and epithelial tissue that allow it to contract to mix food with digestive juices.

A system is composed of several organs working in a coordinated manner to perform a complex function or functions. To continue our example, the stomach plus the other digestive system organs—the oral cavity, esophagus, liver, pancreas, small intestine, and colon—work together to ingest, digest, and absorb our food.

Table 2.1 ■ presents the organ systems that will be studied in this textbook along with the major organs found in each system, the system functions, and the medical specialties that treat conditions of that system.

Table 2.1	**Organ Systems of the Human Body**	
SYSTEM/MEDICAL SPECIALTY	**STRUCTURES**	**FUNCTIONS**
Integumentary (in-teg-you-MEN-tah-ree) **dermatology** (der-mah-TALL-oh-jee)	• skin • hair • nails • sweat glands • sebaceous glands	Forms protective two-way barrier and aids in temperature regulation.
Musculoskeletal (MS) (mus-qu-low-SKEL-et-all) **orthopedics** (or-thoh-PEE-diks) **orthopedic surgery** (or-the-PEE-dik)	• bones • joints • muscles	Skeleton supports and protects the body, forms blood cells, and stores minerals. Muscles produce movement.

Table 2.1   Organ Systems of the Human Body (continued)

SYSTEM/MEDICAL SPECIALTY	STRUCTURES	FUNCTIONS
Cardiovascular (CV) (car-dee-oh-VAS-kew-lar) **cardiology** (car-dee-ALL-oh-jee)	• heart • arteries • veins	Pumps blood throughout the entire body to transport nutrients, oxygen, and wastes.
Blood (**Hematic** System) (he-MAT-tik) **hematology** (hee-mah-TALL-oh-jee)	• plasma • erythrocytes • leukocytes • platelets	Transports oxygen, protects against pathogens, and controls bleeding.
Lymphatic (lim-FAT-ik) **immunology** (im-yoo-NALL-oh-jee)	• lymph nodes • lymphatic vessels • spleen • thymus gland • tonsils	Protects the body from disease and invasion from pathogens.

Table 2.1	Organ Systems of the Human Body (continued)	
SYSTEM/MEDICAL SPECIALTY	**STRUCTURES**	**FUNCTIONS**
Respiratory **otorhinolaryngology** (ENT) (oh-toh-rye-noh-lair-ing-GALL-oh-jee) **pulmonology** (pull-mon-ALL-oh-jee) **thoracic surgery** (tho-RASS-ik)	• nasal cavity • pharynx • larynx • trachea • bronchial tubes • lungs	Obtains oxygen and removes carbon dioxide from the body.
Digestive or **Gastrointestinal** (GI) **gastroenterology** (gas-troh-en-ter-ALL-oh-jee) **proctology** (prok-TOL-oh-jee)	• oral cavity • pharynx • esophagus • stomach • small intestine • colon • liver • gallbladder • pancreas • salivary glands	Ingests, digests, and absorbs nutrients for the body.
Urinary (YOO-rih-nair-ee) **nephrology** (neh-FROL-oh-jee) **urology** (yoo-RALL-oh-jee)	• kidneys • ureters • urinary bladder • urethra	Filters waste products out of the blood and removes them from the body.

Table 2.1   Organ Systems of the Human Body (continued)

SYSTEM/MEDICAL SPECIALTY	STRUCTURES	FUNCTIONS
Female reproductive **gynecology** (GYN) (gigh-neh-KOL-oh-jee) **obstetrics** (OB) (ob-STET-riks)	• ovary • fallopian tubes • uterus • vagina • vulva • breasts	Produces eggs for reproduction and provides place for growing baby.
Male reproductive **urology** (yoo-RALL-oh-jee)	• testes • epididymis • vas deferens • penis • seminal vesicles • prostate gland • bulbourethral gland	Produces sperm for reproduction.
Endocrine (EN-doh-krin) **endocrinology** (en-doh-krin-ALL-oh-jee)	• pituitary gland • pineal gland • thyroid gland • parathyroid glands • thymus gland • adrenal glands • pancreas • ovaries • testes	Regulates metabolic activities of the body.

Table 2.1	Organ Systems of the Human Body	
SYSTEM/MEDICAL SPECIALTY	**STRUCTURES**	**FUNCTIONS**
Nervous **neurology** (noo-RAL-oh-jee) **neurosurgery** (noo-roh-SIR-jer-ee)	• brain • spinal cord • nerves	Receives sensory information and coordinates the body's response.
Special senses **ophthalmology** (off-thal-MALL-oh-jee)	• eye	Vision
otorhinolaryngology (ENT) (oh-toh-rye-noh-lair-ing-GALL-oh-jee)	• ear	Hearing and balance

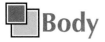

Body

anatomical position

As seen from the previous sections, the body is the sum of all the systems, organs, tissues, and cells found in it. It is important to learn the anatomical terminology that applies to the body as a whole in order to correctly identify specific locations and directions when dealing with patients. The **anatomical position** is used when describing the positions and relationships of structures in the human body. A body in the anatomical position is standing erect with the arms at the side of the body, the palms of the hands facing forward, and the eyes looking straight ahead. In addition, the legs are parallel with the feet, and the toes are pointing forward (see Figure 2.3 ■). For descriptive purposes the assumption is always that the person is in the anatomical position even if the body or parts of the body are in any other position.

Body Planes

coronal plane (kor-RONE-al)	**longitudinal section**
coronal section	**median plane**
cross-section	**sagittal plane** (SAJ-ih-tal)
frontal plane	**sagittal section**
frontal section	**transverse plane**
horizontal plane	**transverse section**

The terminology for body planes is used to assist medical personnel in describing the body and its parts. To understand body planes, imagine cuts slicing through the body at various angles. This imaginary slicing allows us to use more specific language when describing parts of the body. These body planes, illustrated in Figure 2.4 ■, include the following:

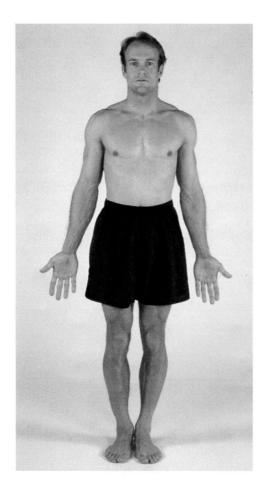

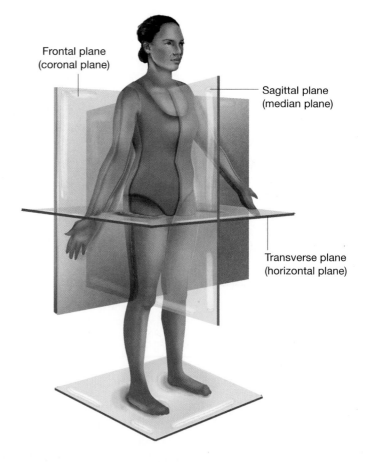

■ **Figure 2.3** The anatomical position: standing erect, gazing straight ahead, arms down at sides, palms facing forward, fingers extended, legs together, and toes pointing forward.

■ **Figure 2.4** The planes of the body. The sagittal plane is vertical from front to back, the frontal plane is vertical from left to right, and the transverse plane is horizontal.

1. **Sagittal plane:** This vertical plane, also called the **median plane**, runs lengthwise from front to back and divides the body or any of its parts into right and left portions. The right and left sides do not have to be equal. A cut along the sagittal plane yields a **sagittal section** view of the inside of the body.
2. **Frontal plane:** The frontal, or **coronal plane**, divides the body into front and back portions. In other words, this is a vertical lengthwise plane running from side to side. A cut along the frontal plane yields a **frontal** or **coronal section** view of the inside of the body.
3. **Transverse plane:** The transverse, or **horizontal plane**, is a crosswise plane that runs parallel to the ground. This imaginary cut would divide the body or its parts into upper and lower portions. A cut along the transverse plane yields a **transverse section** view of the inside of the body.

The terms **cross-section** and **longitudinal section** are frequently used to describe internal views of structures. A longitudinal section is produced by a lengthwise slice along the long axis of a structure. A cross-section view is produced by a slice perpendicular to the long axis of the structure.

Body Regions

abdominal region (ab-DOM-ih-nal)	**lower extremities**
brachial region (BRAY-kee-all)	**pelvic region** (PELL-vik)
cephalic region (she-FAL-ik)	**pubic region** (PEW-bik)
cervical region (SER-vih-kal)	**thoracic region** (tho-RASS-ik)
crural region (KREW-ral)	**trunk**
dorsum (DOOR-sum)	**upper extremities**
gluteal region (GLOO-tee-all)	**vertebral region** (VER-tee-bral)

The body is divided into large regions that can easily be identified externally. The **cephalic region** is the entire head. The neck is the **cervical region** and connects the head to the **trunk** (the torso). The trunk is further subdivided into different anterior and posterior regions. The anterior side consists of the **thoracic** (the chest), **abdominal**, **pelvic**, and **pubic** (genital) **regions**. The posterior side consists of the **dorsum** (the back), **vertebral region**, and **gluteal** (buttock) **region**. The **upper extremities** (UE) and **lower extremities** (LE) are attached to the trunk. The upper extremities or **brachial regions** are the arms. The lower extremities or **crural regions** are the legs. See Figure 2.5 ■ to locate each region on the body.

> **Med Term Tip**
>
> As you learn medical terminology, it is important that you remember not to use common phrases and terms any longer. Many people commonly use the term *stomach* (an organ) when they actually mean *abdomen* (a body region).

Body Cavities

abdominal cavity	**pericardial cavity** (pair-ih-CAR-dee-al)
abdominopelvic cavity	**peritoneum** (pair-ih-toh-NEE-um)
(ab-dom-ih-noh-PELL-vik)	**pleura** (PLOO-rah)
cranial cavity (KRAY-nee-al)	**pleural cavity** (PLOO-ral)
diaphragm (DYE-ah-fram)	**spinal cavity**
mediastinum (mee-dee-ass-TYE-num)	**thoracic cavity**
parietal layer (pah-RYE-eh-tal)	**viscera** (VISS-er-ah)
parietal peritoneum	**visceral layer** (VISS-er-al)
parietal pleura	**visceral peritoneum**
pelvic cavity	**visceral pleura**

The body is not a solid structure; it has many open spaces or cavities. The cavities are part of the normal body structure and are illustrated in Figure 2.6 ■. We

Figure 2.5 Anterior and posterior views of the body illustrating the location of various body regions.

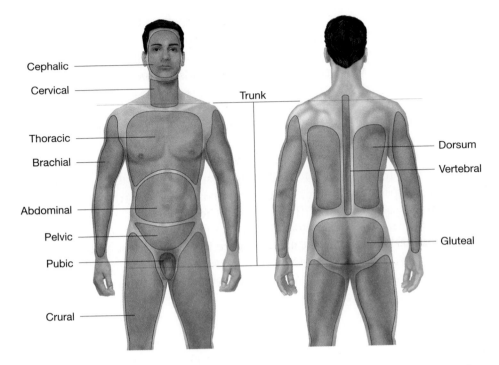

can divide the body into four major cavities—two dorsal cavities and two ventral cavities.

The dorsal cavities include the **cranial cavity**, containing the brain, and the **spinal cavity**, containing the spinal cord.

The ventral cavities include the **thoracic cavity** and the **abdominopelvic cavity**. The thoracic cavity contains the two lungs and a central region between them called the **mediastinum**. The heart, aorta, esophagus, trachea, and thymus gland are located in the mediastinum. There is an actual physical wall between the thoracic cavity and the abdominopelvic cavity called the **diaphragm**. The diaphragm is a muscle used for breathing. The abdominopelvic cavity is generally subdivided into a superior **abdominal cavity** and an inferior **pelvic cavity**. The organs of the digestive, excretory, and reproductive systems are located in these cavities. The organs

Figure 2.6 The dorsal (red) and ventral (blue) body cavities.

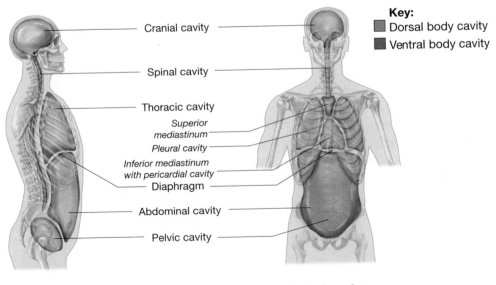

within the ventral cavities are referred to as a group as the internal organs or **viscera**. Table 2.2 ■ describes the body cavities and their major organs.

All of the cavities are lined by, and the viscera are encased in, a two-layer membrane called the **pleura** in the thoracic cavity and the **peritoneum** in the abdominopelvic cavity. The outer layer that lines the cavities is called the **parietal layer** (i.e., **parietal pleura** and **parietal peritoneum**), and the inner layer that encases the viscera is called the **visceral layer** (i.e., **visceral pleura** and **visceral peritoneum**).

Within the thoracic cavity, the pleura is subdivided, forming the **pleural cavity**, containing the lungs, and the **pericardial cavity**, containing the heart. The larger abdominopelvic cavity is usually subdivided into regions so different areas can be precisely referred to. Two different methods of subdividing this cavity are used: the anatomical divisions and the clinical divisions. Choose a method partly on personal preference and partly on which system best describes the patient's condition. See Table 2.3 ■ for a description of these methods for dividing the abdominopelvic cavity.

Directional and Positional Terms

Directional terms assist medical personnel in discussing the position or location of a patient's complaint. Directional or positional terms also help to describe one process, organ, or system as it relates to another. Table 2.4 ■ presents commonly used terms for describing the position of the body or its parts. They are listed in pairs that have opposite meanings: for example, superior versus inferior, anterior versus posterior, medial versus lateral, proximal versus distal, superficial versus deep, and supine versus prone. Directional terms are illustrated in Figure 2.7 ■.

Med Term Tip

The kidneys are the only major abdominopelvic organ located outside the sac formed by the peritoneum. Because they are found behind this sac, their position is referred to as *retroperitoneal*.

Med Term Tip

Remember when using location or direction terms, it is assumed that the patient is in the anatomical position unless otherwise noted.

Table 2.2	Body Cavities and Their Major Organs
CAVITY	**MAJOR ORGANS**

Dorsal cavities
  Cranial cavity
  Spinal cavity
	Brain
	Spinal cord

Ventral cavities Thoracic cavity	Pleural cavity: lungs Pericardial cavity: heart Mediastinum: heart, esophagus, trachea, thymus gland, aorta
Abdominopelvic cavity Abdominal cavity	Stomach, spleen, liver, gallbladder, pancreas, and portions of the small intestines and colon
Pelvic cavity	Urinary bladder, ureters, urethra, and portions of the small intestines and colon *Female:* uterus, ovaries, fallopian tubes, vagina *Male:* prostate gland, seminal vesicles, portion of the vas deferens

Table 2.3   Methods of Subdividing the Abdominopelvic Cavity

Anatomical Divisions of the Abdomen

- **Right hypochondriac** (high-poh-KON-dree-ak): Right lateral region of upper row beneath the lower ribs.

- **Epigastric** (ep-ih-GAS-trik): Middle area of upper row above the stomach.

- **Left hypochondriac:** Left lateral region of the upper row beneath the lower ribs.

- **Right lumbar:** Right lateral region of the middle row at the waist.

- **Umbilical** (um-BILL-ih-kal): Central area over the navel.

- **Left lumbar:** Left lateral region of the middle row at the waist.

- **Right iliac** (ILL-ee-ak): Right lateral region of the lower row at the groin.

- **Hypogastric** (high-poh-GAS-trik): Middle region of the lower row beneath the navel.

- **Left iliac:** Left lateral region of the lower row at the groin.

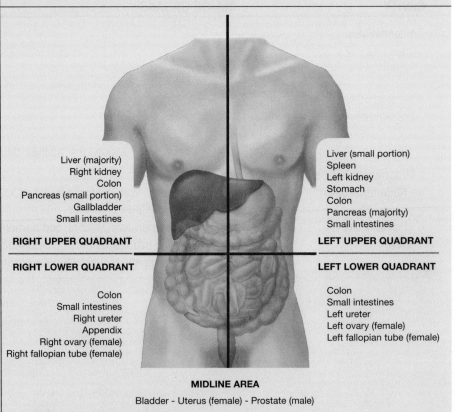

Right hypochondriac region	Epigastric region	Left hypochondriac region
Right lumbar region	Umbilical region	Left lumbar region
Right iliac region	Hypogastric region	Left iliac region

Med Term Tip

To visualize the nine anatomical divisions, imagine a tic-tac-toe diagram over this region.

Med Term Tip

The term *hypochondriac*, literally meaning "under the cartilage" (of the ribs), has come to refer to a person who believes he or she is sick when there is no obvious cause for illness. These patients commonly complain of aches and pains in the hypochondriac region.

Clinical Divisions of the Abdomen

- **Right upper quadrant (RUQ):** Contains majority of liver, gallbladder, small portion of pancreas, right kidney, small intestines, and colon.

- **Right lower quadrant (RLQ):** Contains small intestines and colon, right ovary and fallopian tube, appendix, and right ureter.

- **Left upper quadrant (LUQ):** Contains small portion of liver, spleen, stomach, majority of pancreas, left kidney, small intestines, and colon.

- **Left lower quadrant (LLQ):** Contains small intestines and colon, left ovary and fallopian tube, and left ureter.

- Midline organs: uterus, bladder, prostate gland.

Liver (majority)
Right kidney
Colon
Pancreas (small portion)
Gallbladder
Small intestines

RIGHT UPPER QUADRANT

RIGHT LOWER QUADRANT

Colon
Small intestines
Right ureter
Appendix
Right ovary (female)
Right fallopian tube (female)

Liver (small portion)
Spleen
Left kidney
Stomach
Colon
Pancreas (majority)
Small intestines

LEFT UPPER QUADRANT

LEFT LOWER QUADRANT

Colon
Small intestines
Left ureter
Left ovary (female)
Left fallopian tube (female)

MIDLINE AREA

Bladder - Uterus (female) - Prostate (male)

Figure 2.7 Anterior and lateral views of the body illustrating directional terms.

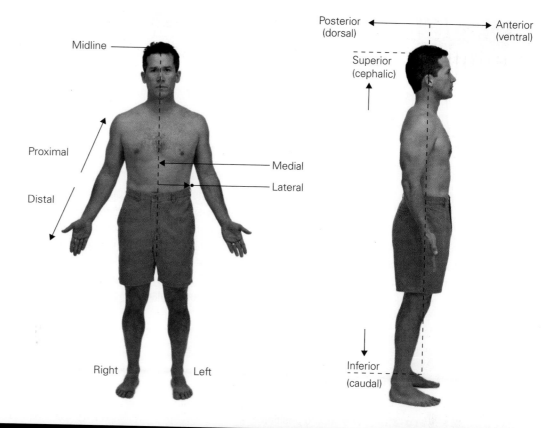

Table 2.4	Terms for Describing Body Position
superior (soo-PEE-ree-or) or **cephalic** (seh-FAL-ik)	More toward the head, or above another structure. (see Figure 2.7 ■). *Example:* The adrenal glands are superior to the kidneys.
inferior (in-FEE-ree-or) or **caudal** (KAWD-al)	More toward the feet or tail, or below another structure. (see Figure 2.7). *Example:* The intestine is inferior to the heart.
anterior (an-TEE-ree-or) or **ventral** (VEN-tral)	More toward the front or belly-side of the body. (see Figure 2.7). *Example:* The navel is located on the anterior surface of the body.
posterior (poss-TEE-ree-or) or **dorsal** (DOR-sal)	More toward the back or spinal cord side of the body. (see Figure 2.7). *Example:* The posterior wall of the right kidney was excised.
medial (MEE-dee-al)	Refers to the middle or near the middle of the body or the structure. (see Figure 2.7). *Example:* The heart is medially located in the chest cavity.
lateral (lat) (LAT-er-al)	Refers to the side. (see Figure 2.7). *Example:* The ovaries are located lateral to the uterus.
proximal (PROK-sim-al)	Located nearer to the point of attachment to the body. (see Figure 2.7). *Example:* In the anatomical position, the elbow is proximal to the hand.
distal (DISS-tal)	Located farther away from the point of attachment to the body. (see Figure 2.7). *Example:* The hand is distal to the elbow.
apex (AY-peks)	Tip or summit of an organ. *Example:* We hear the heart beat by listening over the apex of the heart.

Table 2.4	Terms for Describing Body Position
base	Bottom or lower part of an organ. *Example:* On the X-ray, a fracture was noted at the base of the skull.
superficial	More toward the surface of the body. *Example:* The cut was superficial.
deep	Further away from the surface of the body. *Example:* An incision into an abdominal organ is a deep incision.
supine (soo-PINE)	The body lying horizontally and facing upward (see Figure 2.8A ▆). *Example:* The patient is in the supine position for abdominal surgery.
prone (PROHN)	The body lying horizontally and facing downward (see Figure 2.8B ▆). *Example:* The patient is placed in the prone position for spinal surgery.

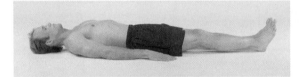

■ **Figure 2.8A** The supine position.

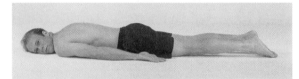

■ **Figure 2.8B** The prone position.

Word Building

When using medical terms to indicate different areas of the body or organs, it is usually necessary to turn the combining form into an adjective. For example, *gastr/o* becomes *gastric* or *ventr/o* becomes *ventral*. This is done by adding an adjective suffix to the combining form that translates as *pertaining to*. The following list contains examples of frequently used medical terms relating to body structure that are built directly from word parts. It is important to study this list because there are no rules about which of the several *pertaining to* suffixes to use.

COMBINING FORM	SUFFIX	MEDICAL TERM	DEFINITION
abdomin/o	-al	**abdominal** (ab-DOM-ih-nal)	pertaining to the abdomen
anter/o	-ior	**anterior** (an-TEE-ree-or)	pertaining to the front
brachi/o	-al	**brachial** (BRAY-kee-all)	pertaining to the arm
caud/o	-al	**caudal** (KAWD-al)	pertaining to the tail
cephal/o	-ic	**cephalic** (she-FAL-ik)	pertaining to the head
cervic/o	-al	**cervical** (SER-vih-kal)	pertaining to the neck
crani/o	-al	**cranial** (KRAY-nee-al)	pertaining to the skull
crur/o	-al	**crural** (KREW-ral)	pertaining to the leg
dist/o	-al	**distal** (DISS-tal)	pertaining to away
dors/o	-al	**dorsal** (DOR-sal)	pertaining to the back of body
epitheli/o	-al	**epithelial** (ep-ih-THEE-lee-al)	pertaining to the epithelium
glute/o	-al	**gluteal** (GLOO-tee-all)	pertaining to the buttocks
infer/o	-ior	**inferior** (in-FEE-ree-or)	pertaining to below

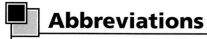

Word Building *(continued)*

COMBINING FORM	SUFFIX	MEDICAL TERM	DEFINITION
later/o	-al	**lateral** (LAT-er-al)	pertaining to the side
medi/o	-al	**medial** (MEE-dee-al)	pertaining to the middle
muscul/o	-ar	**muscular** (MUSS-kew-lar)	pertaining to muscles
neur/o	-al	**neural** (NOO-ral)	pertaining to nerves
organ/o	-ic	**organic** (or-GAN-ik)	pertaining to organs
pelv/o	-ic	**pelvic** (PELL-vik)	pertaining to the pelvis
peritone/o	-al	**peritoneal** (pair-ih-toe-NEE-all)	pertaining to the peritoneum
pleur/o	-al	**pleural** (PLOO-ral)	pertaining to the pleura
poster/o	-ior	**posterior** (poss-TEE-ree-or)	pertaining to the back
proxim/o	-al	**proximal** (PROK-sim-al)	pertaining to near
pub/o	-ic	**pubic** (PEW-bik)	pertaining to the genital region
somat/o	-ic	**somatic** (so-MAT-ik)	pertaining to the body
spin/o	-al	**spinal**	pertaining to the spine
super/o	-ior	**superior** (soo-PEE-ree-or)	pertaining to above
system/o	-ic	**systemic** (sis-TEM-ik)	pertaining to systems
thorac/o	-ic	**thoracic** (tho-RASS-ik)	pertaining to the chest
ventr/o	-al	**ventral** (VEN-tral)	pertaining to the belly side
vertebr/o	-al	**vertebral** (VER-the-bral)	pertaining to the vertebrae
viscer/o	-al	**visceral** (VISS-er-al)	pertaining to internal organs

Abbreviations

AP	anteroposterior	**lat**	lateral	**OB**	obstetrics
CV	cardiovascular	**LE**	lower extremity	**PA**	posteroanterior
ENT	ear, nose, and throat	**LLQ**	left lower quadrant	**RLQ**	right lower quadrant
GI	gastrointestinal	**LUQ**	left upper quadrant	**RUQ**	right upper quadrant
GYN	gynecology	**MS**	musculoskeletal	**UE**	upper extremity

Chapter Review

Terminology Checklist

Below are all Body Organization key terms presented in this chapter. Use this list as a study tool by placing a check in the box in front of each term as you master its meaning.

- [ ] abdominal
- [ ] abdominal cavity
- [ ] abdominal region
- [ ] abdominopelvic cavity
- [ ] adipose
- [ ] anatomical position
- [ ] anterior
- [ ] apex
- [ ] base
- [ ] blood
- [ ] body
- [ ] bone
- [ ] brachial
- [ ] brachial region
- [ ] brain
- [ ] cardiac muscle
- [ ] cardiology
- [ ] cardiovascular system
- [ ] cartilage
- [ ] caudal
- [ ] cell
- [ ] cell membrane
- [ ] cephalic
- [ ] cephalic region
- [ ] cervical
- [ ] cervical region
- [ ] connective tissue
- [ ] coronal plane
- [ ] coronal section
- [ ] cranial
- [ ] cranial cavity
- [ ] cross-section
- [ ] crural
- [ ] crural region
- [ ] cytology
- [ ] cytoplasm
- [ ] deep
- [ ] dermatology
- [ ] diaphragm

- [ ] digestive system
- [ ] distal
- [ ] dorsal
- [ ] dorsum
- [ ] endocrine system
- [ ] endocrinology
- [ ] epigastric
- [ ] epithelial
- [ ] epithelial tissue
- [ ] epithelium
- [ ] female reproductive system
- [ ] frontal plane
- [ ] frontal section
- [ ] gastroenterology
- [ ] gastrointestinal system
- [ ] gluteal
- [ ] gluteal region
- [ ] gynecology
- [ ] hematic system
- [ ] hematology
- [ ] histology
- [ ] horizontal plane
- [ ] hypogastric
- [ ] immunology
- [ ] inferior
- [ ] integumentary system
- [ ] lateral
- [ ] left hypochondriac
- [ ] left iliac
- [ ] left lower quadrant
- [ ] left lumbar
- [ ] left upper quadrant
- [ ] longitudinal section
- [ ] lower extremities
- [ ] lymphatic system
- [ ] male reproductive system
- [ ] medial
- [ ] median plane
- [ ] mediastinum

- [ ] muscle fibers
- [ ] muscle tissue
- [ ] muscular
- [ ] musculoskeletal system
- [ ] nephrology
- [ ] nerves
- [ ] nervous system
- [ ] nervous tissue
- [ ] neural
- [ ] neurology
- [ ] neurons
- [ ] neurosurgery
- [ ] nucleus
- [ ] obstetrics
- [ ] ophthalmology
- [ ] organic
- [ ] organs
- [ ] orthopedic surgery
- [ ] orthopedics
- [ ] otorhinolaryngology
- [ ] parietal layer
- [ ] parietal peritoneum
- [ ] parietal pleura
- [ ] pelvic
- [ ] pelvic cavity
- [ ] pelvic region
- [ ] pericardial cavity
- [ ] peritoneal
- [ ] peritoneum
- [ ] pleura
- [ ] pleural
- [ ] pleural cavity
- [ ] posterior
- [ ] proctology
- [ ] prone
- [ ] proximal
- [ ] pubic
- [ ] pubic region
- [ ] pulmonology

- ☐ respiratory system
- ☐ right hypochondriac
- ☐ right iliac
- ☐ right lower quadrant
- ☐ right lumbar
- ☐ right upper quadrant
- ☐ sagittal plane
- ☐ sagittal section
- ☐ skeletal muscle
- ☐ smooth muscle
- ☐ somatic
- ☐ special senses
- ☐ spinal
- ☐ spinal cavity

- ☐ spinal cord
- ☐ superficial
- ☐ superior
- ☐ supine
- ☐ systemic
- ☐ systems
- ☐ tendons
- ☐ thoracic
- ☐ thoracic cavity
- ☐ thoracic region
- ☐ thoracic surgery
- ☐ tissues
- ☐ transverse plane
- ☐ transverse section

- ☐ trunk
- ☐ umbilical
- ☐ upper extremities
- ☐ urinary system
- ☐ urology
- ☐ ventral
- ☐ vertebral
- ☐ vertebral region
- ☐ viscera
- ☐ visceral
- ☐ visceral layer
- ☐ visceral peritoneum
- ☐ visceral pleura

Practice Exercises

A. Complete the following statements.

1. The levels of organization of the body in order from smallest to largest are: _____, _____, _____, _____, _____.

2. No matter its shape, all cells have a _____, _____, and _____.

3. _____ is the study of tissue.

4. _____ tissue lines internal organs and serves as a covering for the skin.

5. In the _____ position the body is standing erect with arms at sides and palms facing forward.

6. The _____ quadrant of the abdomen contains the appendix.

7. The dorsal cavities are the _____ cavity and the _____ cavity.

8. There are _____ anatomical divisions in the abdominal cavity.

9. The _____ region of the abdominal cavity is located in the right lower lateral region near the groin.

10. Within the thoracic cavity the lungs are found in the _____ cavity and the heart is found in the _____ cavity.

B. Match each body plane to its definition.

1. _____ frontal plane

    a. divides the body into right and left

2. _____ sagittal plane

    b. divides the body into upper and lower

3. _____ transverse plane

    c. divides the body into anterior and posterior

C. Match each term to its definition.

1. _____ distal

2. _____ prone

3. _____ lateral

4. _____ inferior

5. _____ deep

6. _____ apex

7. _____ base

8. _____ posterior

9. _____ superficial

10. _____ supine

11. _____ anterior

12. _____ medial

13. _____ proximal

14. _____ superior

a. away from the surface

b. toward the surface

c. located closer to point of attachment to the body

d. caudal

e. tip or summit of an organ

f. lying face down

g. cephalic

h. ventral

i. dorsal

j. lying face up

k. to the side

l. middle

m. bottom or lower part of an organ

n. located further away from point of attachment to the body

D. Circle the prefixes in the following terms and define in the space provided.

1. epigastric _____

2. intervertebral _____

3. intramuscular _____

4. pericardium _____

5. hypochondriac _____

6. retroperitoneal _____

7. substernal _____

8. transurethral _____

E. Build terms for each expression using the correct prefixes, suffixes, and combining forms.

1. pertaining to spinal cord side _____

2. pertaining to the chest _____

3. pertaining to above _____

4. pertaining to the tail _____

5. pertaining to internal organs _____

6. pertaining to the side _____

7. pertaining to away from _____

8. pertaining to nerves _____

9. pertaining to systems _____

10. pertaining to the muscles _____

11. pertaining to the belly side _____

12. pertaining to the front _____

13. pertaining to the head _____

14. pertaining to middle _____

F. Write the abbreviations for the following terms.

1. musculoskeletal _____

2. lateral _____

3. right upper quadrant _____

4. cardiovascular _____

5. gastrointestinal _____

6. anteroposterior _____

7. obstetrics _____

8. left lower quadrant _____

G. Define the following combining forms.

1. viscer/o _____

2. poster/o _____

3. abdomin/o _____

4. thorac/o _____

5. medi/o _____

6. ventr/o _____

7. anter/o _____

8. hist/o _____

9. epitheli/o _____

10. crani/o _____

11. somat/o _____

12. proxim/o _____

13. cephal/o _____

H. For each organ listed below, identify the name of the system it belongs to and then match it to its function.

Organ	System	Function
1. _____ skin	_____	a. supports the body
2. _____ heart	_____	b. provides place for growing baby
3. _____ stomach	_____	c. filters waste products from blood
4. _____ uterus	_____	d. provides two-way barrier
5. _____ bones	_____	e. produces movement
6. _____ lungs	_____	f. produces sperm
7. _____ kidney	_____	g. ingest, digest, absorb nutrients
8. _____ testes	_____	h. coordinates body's response
9. _____ brain	_____	i. pumps blood through blood vessels
10. _____ muscles	_____	j. obtains oxygen

I. Match each organ to its body cavity.

1. _____ gallbladder   a. right upper quadrant

2. _____ appendix   b. left upper quadrant

3. _____ urinary bladder   c. right lower quadrant

4. _____ small intestines   d. left lower quadrant

5. _____ right kidney   e. all quadrants

6. _____ left ovary   f. midline structure

7. _____ stomach

8. _____ colon

9. _____ right ureter

10. _____ pancreas (majority)

J. For each term below, write the corresponding body region.

1. head _____   5. neck _____

2. genitals _____   6. arm _____

3. leg _____   7. back _____

4. buttocks _____   8. chest _____

K. Use the following terms in the sentences that follow.

cardiology   otorhinolaryngology   urology   gynecology

ophthalmology   gastroenterology   dermatology   orthopedics

1. John is a musician who plays an electric bass guitar and is experiencing difficulty in hearing soft voices. He would consult a physician in _____.

2. Ruth is a stock trader with the Chicago Board of Trade. She has had a pounding and racing heartbeat. She would consult a physician specializing in _____.

3. Mary Ann is experiencing excessive bleeding from the uterus. She would consult a _____ doctor.

4. Jose has fractured his wrist in a fall. He would be seen for an examination by a physician in _____.

5. A physician who performs eye exams specializes in the field of _____.

6. When her daughter had repeated bladder infections, Mrs. Cortez sought the opinion of a specialist in _____.

7. Martha could not get rid of a persistent skin rash with over-the-counter creams. She decided to make an appointment with a specialist in _____.

8. After reviewing his X-ray, the specialist in _____ informed Mr. Sparks that he had a stomach ulcer.

Labeling Exercise

A. Body Organization Review
Write the labels for this figure on the numbered lines provided.

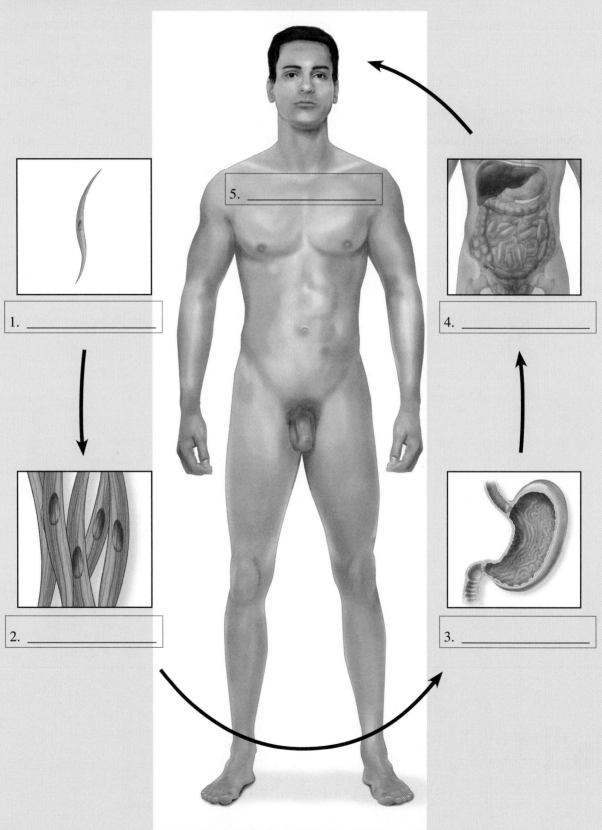

5. _____

1. _____

2. _____

3. _____

4. _____

B. Anatomy Challenge

1. Write the labels for this figure on the numbered lines provided.

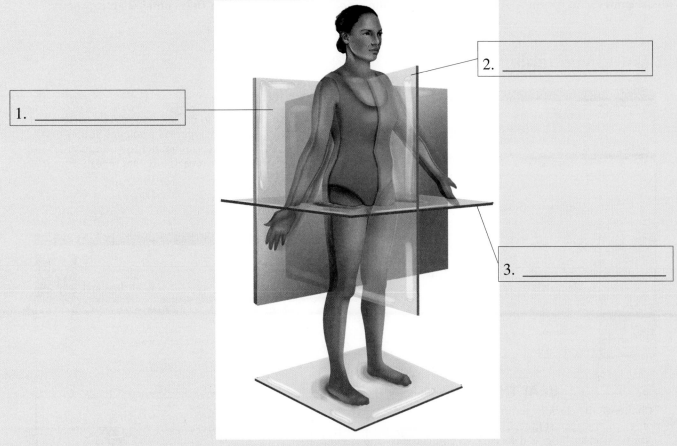

1. _____

2. _____

3. _____

2. Write the labels for this figure on the numbered lines provided.

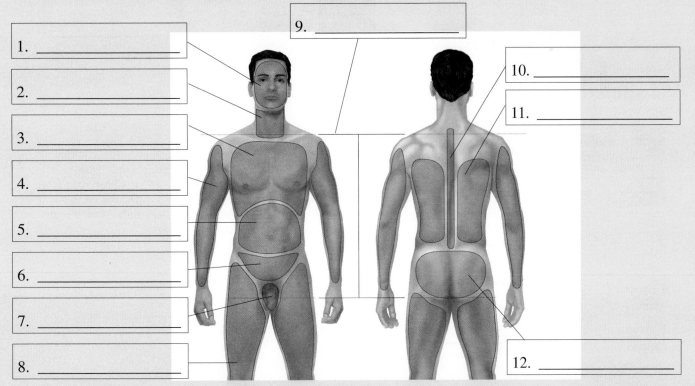

1. _____

2. _____

3. _____

4. _____

5. _____

6. _____

7. _____

8. _____

9. _____

10. _____

11. _____

12. _____

Multimedia Preview

Additional interactive resources and activities for this chapter can be found on the Companion Website. For videos, games, and pronunciations, please access the accompanying DVD-ROM that comes with this book.

DVD-ROM Highlights

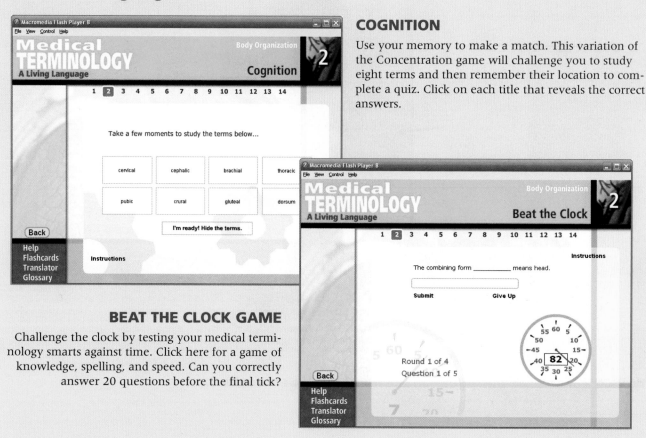

COGNITION

Use your memory to make a match. This variation of the Concentration game will challenge you to study eight terms and then remember their location to complete a quiz. Click on each title that reveals the correct answers.

BEAT THE CLOCK GAME

Challenge the clock by testing your medical terminology smarts against time. Click here for a game of knowledge, spelling, and speed. Can you correctly answer 20 questions before the final tick?

Website Highlights—www.prenhall.com/fremgen

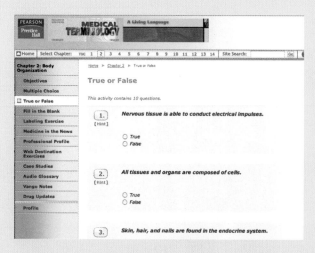

TRUE/FALSE QUIZ

Take advantage of the free-access on-line study guide that accompanies your textbook. You'll find a true/false quiz that provides instant feedback that allows you to check your score and see what you got right or wrong. By clicking on this URL you'll also access links to download mp3 audio reviews, current news articles, and an audio glossary.

3

Integumentary System

Learning Objectives

Upon completion of this chapter, you will be able to:

- Identify and define the combining forms, prefixes, and suffixes introduced in this chapter.
- Correctly spell and pronounce medical terms and major anatomical structures relating to the integumentary system.
- List and describe the three layers of skin and their functions.
- List and describe the four purposes of the skin.
- List and describe the accessory organs of the skin.
- Build and define integumentary system medical terms from word parts.
- Identify and define integumentary system vocabulary terms.
- Identify and define selected integumentary system pathology terms.
- Identify and define selected integumentary system diagnostic procedures.
- Identify and define selected integumentary system therapeutic procedures.
- Identify and define selected medications relating to the integumentary system.
- Define selected abbreviations associated with the integumentary system.

Integumentary System at a Glance

Function

The skin provides a protective two-way barrier between our internal environment and the outside world. It also plays an important role in temperature regulation, houses sensory receptors to detect the environment around us and secretes important fluids.

Organs

skin   hair   nails   sebaceous glands   sweat glands

Combining Forms

albin/o	white	**melan/o**	black
bi/o	life	**myc/o**	fungus
cry/o	cold	**necr/o**	death
cutane/o	skin	**onych/o**	nail
cyan/o	blue	**pil/o**	hair
derm/o	skin	**phot/o**	light
dermat/o	skin	**py/o**	pus
diaphor/o	profuse sweating	**rhytid/o**	wrinkle
electr/o	electricity	**scler/o**	hard
erythr/o	red	**seb/o**	oil
hidr/o	sweat	**trich/o**	hair
ichthy/o	scaly, dry	**ungu/o**	nail
kerat/o	hard, horny	**vesic/o**	bladder
leuk/o	white	**xer/o**	dry
lip/o	fat		

Suffixes

-derma	skin
-opsy	view of
-tome	instrument used to cut

Prefixes

allo-	other, different from usual
xeno-	strange, foreign

Integumentary System Illustrated

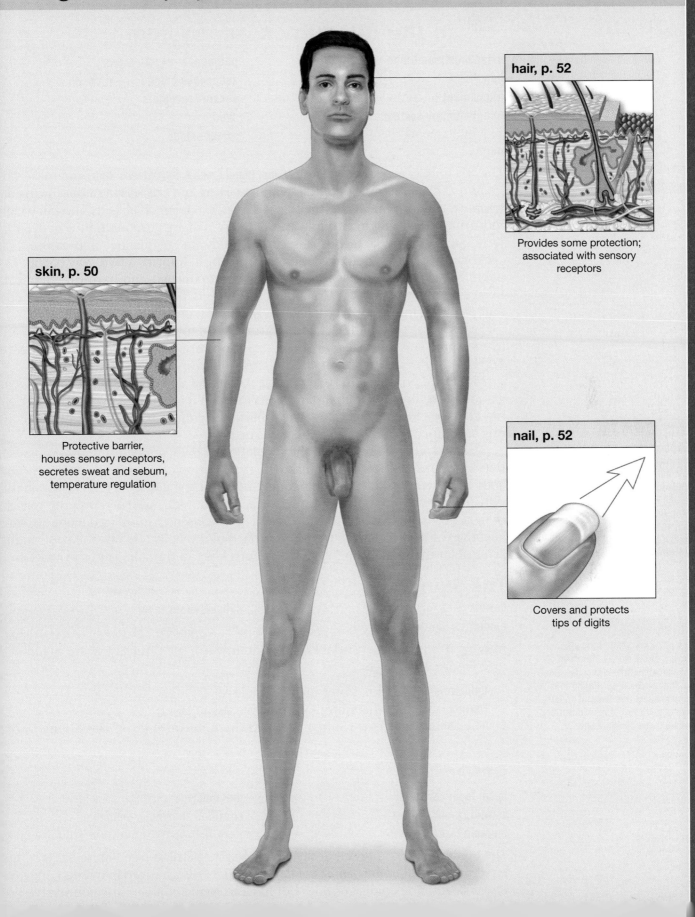

hair, p. 52

Provides some protection; associated with sensory receptors

skin, p. 50

Protective barrier, houses sensory receptors, secretes sweat and sebum, temperature regulation

nail, p. 52

Covers and protects tips of digits

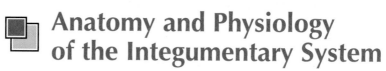

Anatomy and Physiology of the Integumentary System

cutaneous membrane (kew-TAY-nee-us)
hair
integument (in-TEG-you-mint)
integumentary system
   (in-teg-you-MEN-tah-ree)
nails

pathogens (PATH-oh-jenz)
sebaceous glands (see-BAY-shus)
sensory receptors
skin
sweat glands

The **skin** and its accessory organs—**sweat glands**, **sebaceous glands**, **hair**, and **nails**—are known as the **integumentary system**, with **integument** and **cutaneous membrane** being alternate terms for skin. In fact, the skin is the largest organ of the body and can weigh more than 20 pounds in an adult. The skin serves many purposes for the body: protecting, housing nerve receptors, secreting fluids, and regulating temperature.

The primary function of the skin is protection. It forms a two-way barrier capable of keeping **pathogens** (disease-causing organisms) and harmful chemicals from entering the body. It also stops critical body fluids from escaping the body and prevents injury to the internal organs lying underneath the skin.

Sensory receptors that detect temperature, pain, touch, and pressure are located in the skin. The messages for these sensations are conveyed to the spinal cord and brain from the nerve endings in the middle layer of the skin.

Fluids are produced in two types of skin glands: sweat and sebaceous. Sweat glands assist the body in maintaining its internal temperature by creating a cooling effect as sweat evaporates. The sebaceous glands, or oil glands, produce an oily substance that lubricates the skin surface.

The structure of skin aids in the regulation of body temperature through a variety of means. As noted previously, the evaporation of sweat cools the body. The body also lowers its internal temperature by dilating superficial blood vessels in the skin. This brings more blood to the surface of the skin, which allows the release of heat. If the body needs to conserve heat, it constricts superficial blood vessels, keeping warm blood away from the surface of the body. Finally, the continuous layer of fat that makes up the subcutaneous layer of the skin acts as insulation.

The Skin

dermis (DER-mis)
epidermis (ep-ih-DER-mis)

subcutaneous layer (sub-kyoo-TAY-nee-us)

Moving from the outer surface of the skin inward, the three layers are as follows (see Figure 3.1 ■):

1. **Epidermis** is the thin, outer membrane layer.
2. **Dermis** is the middle, fibrous connective tissue layer.
3. The **subcutaneous layer** (Subcu, Subq) is the innermost layer, containing fatty tissue.

Epidermis

basal layer (BAY-sal)
keratin (KAIR-ah-tin)
melanin (MEL-ah-nin)

melanocytes (mel-AN-oh-sights)
stratified squamous epithelium (STRAT-
   ih-fyde SKWAY-mus ep-ih-THEE-lee-um)

The epidermis is composed of **stratified squamous epithelium** (see Figure 3.2 ■). This type of epithelial tissue consists of flat scale-like cells arranged in overlapping layers or strata. The epidermis does not have a blood supply or any connective tissue, so it is dependent for nourishment on the deeper layers of skin.

Med Term Tip

Flushing of the skin, a normal response to an increase in environmental temperature or to a fever, is caused by an increased blood flow to the skin of the face and neck. However, in some people, it is also a response to embarrassment called blushing and is not easily controlled.

Med Term Tip

An understanding of the different layers of the skin is important for healthcare workers because much of the terminology relating to types of injections and medical conditions, such as burns, is described using these designations.

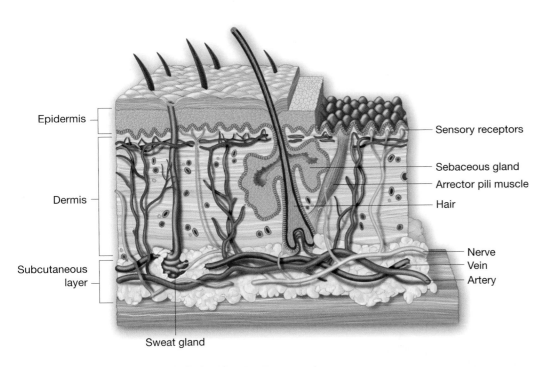

Epidermis

Dermis

Subcutaneous layer

Sweat gland

Sensory receptors

Sebaceous gland

Arrector pili muscle

Hair

Nerve

Vein

Artery

■ **Figure 3.1** Skin structure, including the three layers of the skin and the accessory organs: sweat gland, sebaceous gland, and hair.

The deepest layer within the epidermis is called the **basal layer**. Cells in this layer continually grow and multiply. New cells that are forming push the old cells toward the outer layer of the epidermis. During this process the cells shrink, die, and become filled with a hard protein called **keratin**. These dead, overlapping, keratinized cells allow the skin to act as an effective barrier to infection and also make it waterproof.

The basal layer also contains special cells called **melanocytes**, which produce the black pigment **melanin**. Not only is this pigment responsible for the color of the skin, but it also protects against damage from the ultraviolet rays of the sun. This damage may be in the form of leatherlike skin and wrinkles, which are not hazardous, or it may be one of several forms of skin cancer. Dark-skinned people have more melanin and are generally less likely to get wrinkles or skin cancer.

Med Term Tip

We lose 30,000 to 50,000 old dead skin cells per minute and replace them with new younger cells. In fact, because of this process, our skin is replaced entirely about every seven years.

Med Term Tip

A suntan can be thought of as a protective response to the rays of the sun. However, when the melanin in the skin is not able to absorb all the rays of the sun, the skin burns and DNA may be permanently and dangerously damaged.

■ **Figure 3.2** Photomicrograph of the epidermis layer of the skin.

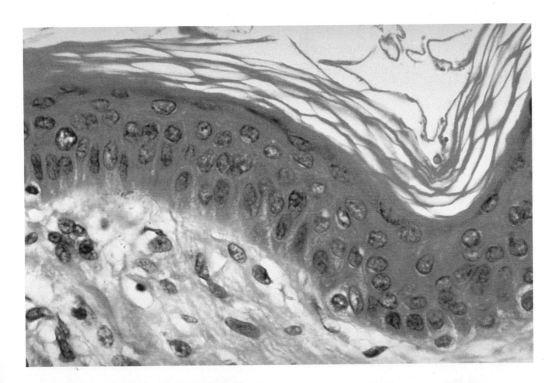

Dermis

collagen fibers (KOL-ah-jen)   **corium** (KOH-ree-um)

Med Term Tip

Ridges formed in the dermis of our fingertips are what give each of us unique fingerprints. These do not change during a person's lifetime and so are a reliable means of identification. In fact, fingerprints are still visible on Egyptian mummies.

The dermis, also referred to as the **corium**, is the middle layer of skin, located between the epidermis and the subcutaneous layer. Its name means "true skin." Unlike the thinner epidermis, the dermis is living tissue with a very good blood supply. The dermis itself is composed of connective tissue and **collagen fibers**. Collagen fibers are made from a strong, fibrous protein present in connective tissue, forming a flexible "glue" that gives connective tissue its strength. The dermis houses hair follicles, sweat glands, sebaceous glands, blood vessels, lymph vessels, sensory receptors, nerve fibers, and muscle fibers.

Subcutaneous Layer

hypodermis (high-poh-DER-mis)   **lipocytes** (LIP-oh-sights)

The third and deepest layer of the skin is the subcutaneous layer, also called the **hypodermis**. This layer of tissue, composed of fat cells called **lipocytes**, protects the deeper tissues of the body and acts as insulation for heat and cold.

Accessory Organs

The accessory organs of the skin are the anatomical structures located within the dermis, including the hair, nails, sebaceous glands, and sweat glands.

Hair

arrector pili (ah-REK-tor pee-lie)   **hair root**
hair follicle (FALL-ikl)   **hair shaft**

Med Term Tip

Our hair turns gray as part of the normal aging process when we no longer produce melanin.

The fibers that make up hair are composed of the protein keratin, the same hard protein material that fills the cells of the epidermis. The process of hair formation is much like the process of growth in the epidermal layer of the skin. The deeper cells in the **hair root** force older keratinized cells to move upward, forming the **hair shaft**. The hair shaft grows toward the skin surface within the **hair follicle**. Melanin gives hair its color. Sebaceous glands release oil directly into the hair follicle. Each hair has a small slip of smooth muscle attached to it called the **arrector pili** muscle (see Figure 3.3 ▪). When this muscle contracts the hair shaft stands up and results in "goose bumps."

Nails

cuticle (KEW-tikl)   **nail bed**
free edge   **nail body**
lunula (LOO-nyoo-lah)   **nail root**

Med Term Tip

Because of its rich blood supply and light color, the nail bed is an excellent place to check patients for low oxygen levels in their blood. Deoxygenated blood is a very dark purple-red and gives skin a bluish tinge called *cyanosis*.

Nails are a flat plate of keratin called the **nail body** that covers the ends of fingers and toes. The nail body is connected to the tissue underneath by the **nail bed**. Nails grow longer from the **nail root**, which is found at the base of the nail and is covered and protected by the soft tissue **cuticle**. The **free edge** is the exposed edge that is trimmed when nails become too long. The light-colored half-moon area at the base of the nail is the **lunula** (see Figure 3.4 ▪).

Sebaceous Glands

sebum

Sebaceous glands, found in the dermis, secrete the oil **sebum**, which lubricates the hair and skin, thereby helping to prevent drying and cracking. These glands secrete

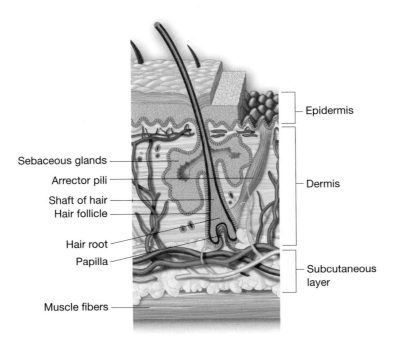

sebum directly into hair follicles, rather than a duct (see Figure 3.1). Secretion from the sebaceous glands increases during adolescence, playing a role in the development of acne. Sebum secretion begins to diminish as age increases. A loss of sebum in old age, along with sun exposure, can account for wrinkles and dry skin.

Sweat Glands

apocrine glands (APP-oh-krin)
perspiration
sudoriferous glands (sue-doh-RIF-er-us)

sweat duct
sweat pore

About two million sweat glands, also called **sudoriferous glands**, are found throughout the body. These highly coiled glands are located in the dermis. Sweat travels to the surface of the skin in a **sweat duct**. The surface opening of a sweat duct is called a **sweat pore** (see Figure 3.1).

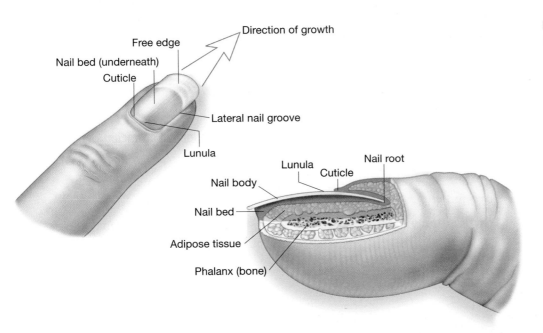

■ **Figure 3.4** External and internal structures of nails.

Med Term Tip

Word Watch — be careful when using *hydro-* meaning "water" and *hidr/o* meaning "sweat."

Sweat glands function to cool the body as sweat evaporates. Sweat or **perspiration** contains a small amount of waste product but is normally colorless and odorless. However, there are sweat glands called **apocrine glands** in the pubic and underarm areas that secrete a thicker sweat, which can produce an odor when it comes into contact with bacteria on the skin. This is what we recognize as body odor.

Word Building

The following list contains examples of medical terms built directly from word parts. The definition for these terms can be determined by a straightforward translation of the word parts.

COMBINING FORM	COMBINED WITH	MEDICAL TERM	DEFINITION
cutane/o	sub- -ous	**subcutaneous** (sub-kyoo-TAY-neeus)	pertaining to under the skin
derm/o	epi- -al	**epidermal** (ep-ih-DER-mal)	pertaining to upon the skin
	hypo- -ic	**hypodermic** (high-poh-DER-mik)	pertaining to under the skin
	intra- -al	**intradermal** (in-trah-DER-mal)	pertaining to within the skin
dermat/o	-itis	**dermatitis** (der-mah-TYE-tis)	inflammation of the skin
	-logist	**dermatologist** (der-mah-TALL-oh-jist)	specialist in skin
	-osis	**dermatosis** (der-mah-TOH-sis)	abnormal condition of skin
	-pathy	**dermatopathy** (der-mah-TOP-ah-thee)	skin disease
	-plasty	**dermatoplasty** (DER-mah-toh-plas-tee)	surgical repair of the skin
hidr/o	an- -osis	**anhidrosis** (an-hi-DROH-sis)	abnormal condition of no sweat
	hyper- -osis	**hyperhidrosis** (high-per-hi-DROH-sis)	abnormal condition of excessive sweat
lip/o	-ectomy	**lipectomy** (lih-PECK-toh-mee)	removal of fat
	-oma	**lipoma** (lip-OH-mah)	fatty mass
melan/o	-oma	**melanoma** (mel-ah-NOH-mah)	black tumor
	-cyte	**melanocyte** (meh-LAN-oh-sight)	black cell
necr/o	-osis	**necrosis** (neh-KROH-sis)	abnormal condition of death
onych/o	-ectomy	**onychectomy** (on-ee-KECK-toh-mee)	removal of a nail
	-malacia	**onychomalacia** (on-ih-koh-mah-LAY-she-ah)	softening of nails
	myc/o -osis	**onychomycosis** (on-ih-koh-my-KOH-sis)	abnormal condition of nail fungus
	-phagia	**onychophagia** (on-ih-koh-FAY-jee-ah)	nail eating (nail biting)
py/o	-genic	**pyogenic** (pye-oh-JEN-ik)	pus forming
rhytid/o	-ectomy	**rhytidectomy** (rit-ih-DECK-toh-mee)	removal of wrinkles
	-plasty	**rhytidoplasty** (RIT-ih-doh-plas-tee)	surgical repair of wrinkles
seb/o	-rrhea	**seborrhea** (seb-or-EE-ah)	oily discharge

Word Building *(continued)*

COMBINING FORM	COMBINED WITH	MEDICAL TERM	DEFINITION
trich/o	myc/o -osis	**trichomycosis** (trik-oh-my-KOH-sis)	abnormal condition of hair fungus
ungu/o	-al	**ungual** (UNG-gwal)	pertaining to the nails

SUFFIX	COMBINED WITH	MEDICAL TERM	MEANING
-derma	erythr/o	**erythroderma** (eh-rith-roh-DER-mah)	red skin
	ichthy/o	**ichthyoderma** (ick-thee-oh-DER-mah)	scaly and dry skin
	leuk/o	**leukoderma** (loo-koh-DER-mah)	white skin
	py/o	**pyoderma** (pye-oh-DER-mah)	pus skin
	scler/o	**scleroderma** (sklair-ah-DER-mah)	hard skin
	xer/o	**xeroderma** (zee-roh-DER-mah)	dry skin

Vocabulary

TERM	DEFINITION
abrasion (ah-BRAY-zhun)	A scraping away of the skin surface by friction.
cicatrix (SICK-ah-trix)	A scar.
comedo (KOM-ee-do)	Collection of hardened sebum in hair follicle. Also called a *blackhead*.
contusion	Injury caused by a blow to the body; causes swelling, pain, and bruising. The skin is not broken.
cyanosis (sigh-ah-NOH-sis)	Bluish tint to the skin caused by deoxygenated blood.

■ **Figure 3.5** A cyanotic infant. Note the bluish tinge to the skin around the lips, chin, and nose. *(St. Bartholomew's Hospital, London/Photo Researchers, Inc.)*

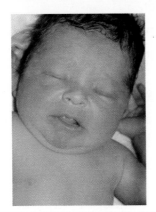

depigmentation (dee-pig-men-TAY-shun)	Loss of normal skin color or pigment.
dermatology (Derm, derm) (der-mah-TALL-oh-jee)	Branch of medicine involving diagnosis and treatment of conditions and diseases of the integumentary system. Physician is a *dermatologist*.
diaphoresis (dye-ah-for-REE-sis)	Profuse sweating.

Vocabulary *(continued)*

TERM	DEFINITION
ecchymosis (ek-ih-MOH-sis)	Skin discoloration caused by blood collecting under the skin following blunt trauma to the skin. A bruise (see Figure 3.6A ■).
erythema (er-ih-THEE-mah)	Redness or flushing of the skin.
eschar (ESH-shar)	A thick layer of dead tissue and tissue fluid that develops over a deep burn area.
hirsutism (HER-soot-izm)	Excessive hair growth over the body.
hyperemia (high-per-EE-mee-ah)	Redness of the skin due to increased blood flow.
hyperpigmentation (high-per-pig-men-TAY-shun)	Abnormal amount of pigmentation in the skin.
keloid (KEE-loyd)	Formation of a raised and thickened hypertrophic scar after an injury or surgery.

■ **Figure 3.7** Keloids, hypertrophic scarring on the back. *(Martin Rotker/ Phototake NYC)*

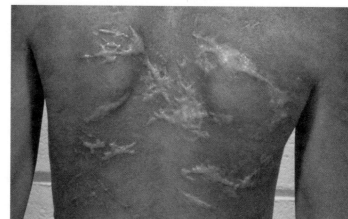

TERM	DEFINITION
keratosis (kair-ah-TOH-sis)	Term for any skin condition involving an overgrowth and thickening of the epidermis layer.
lesion (LEE-shun)	A general term for a wound, injury, or abnormality.
nevus (NEV-us)	Pigmented skin blemish, birthmark, or mole. Usually benign but may become cancerous.
pallor (PAL-or)	Abnormal paleness of the skin.
petechiae (peh-TEE-kee-eye)	Pinpoint purple or red spots from minute hemorrhages under the skin (see Figure 3.6B ■).

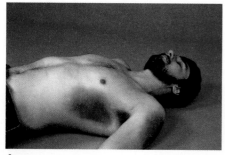

A.

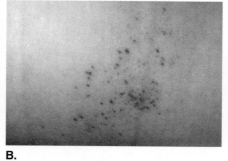

B.

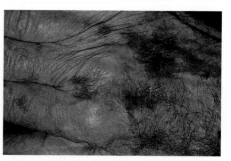

C.

■ **Figure 3.6** A) Male lying supine with large ecchymosis on lateral rib cage and shoulder. B) Petechiae, pinpoint skin hemorrhages. *(Custom Medical Stock Photo, Inc.)* C) Purpura, hemorrhaging into the skin due to fragile blood vessels. *(Caroll H. Weiss/Camera M.D. Studios)*

Vocabulary *(continued)*

TERM	DEFINITION
photosensitivity (foh-toh-sen-sih-TIH-vih-tee)	Condition in which the skin reacts abnormally when exposed to light, such as the ultraviolet (UV) rays of the sun.
plastic surgery	Surgical specialty involved in repair, reconstruction, or improvement of body structures such as the skin that are damaged, missing, or misshapen. Physician is a *plastic surgeon*.
pruritus (proo-RIGH-tus)	Severe itching.
purpura (PER-pew-rah)	Hemorrhages into the skin due to fragile blood vessels. Commonly seen in elderly people (see Figure 3.6C ■). **Med Term Tip** *Purpura* comes from the Latin word for "purple," which refers to the color of these pinpoint hemorrhages.
purulent (PYUR-yoo-lent)	Containing pus or an infection that is producing pus. Pus consists of dead bacteria, white blood cells, and tissue debris.
strawberry hemangioma (hee-man-jee-OH-ma) ■ **Figure 3.8** Strawberry hemangioma, a birthmark caused by a collection of blood vessels in the skin. *(H.C. Robinson/Science Photo Library/Photo Researchers, Inc.)*	Congenital collection of dilated blood vessels causing a red birthmark that fades a few months after birth.
suppurative (SUP-pure-a-tiv)	Containing or producing pus.
urticaria (er-tih-KAY-ree-ah)	Also called *hives;* a skin eruption of pale reddish wheals with severe itching. Usually associated with food allergy, stress, or drug reactions.
verruca (ver-ROO-kah)	Commonly called *warts;* a benign growth caused by a virus. Has a rough surface that is removed by chemicals and/or laser therapy.

Pathology

■ Surface Lesions

cyst (SIST)

Fluid-filled sac under the skin (see Figures 3.9A & 3.9B ■).

A
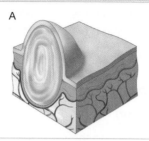

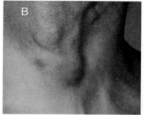

(Bart's Medical Library/Phototake NYC)

---

fissure (FISH-er)

Crack-like lesion or groove on the skin (see Figures 3.9C & 3.9D ■).

C
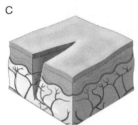

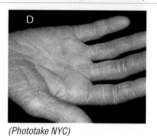

(Phototake NYC)

---

laceration   A torn or jagged wound; incorrectly used to describe a cut.

---

macule (MACK-yool)

Flat, discolored area that is flush with the skin surface. An example would be a freckle or a birthmark (see Figures 3.9E & 3.9F ■).

E
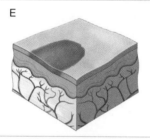

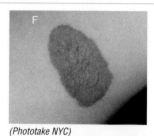

(Phototake NYC)

---

nodule (NOD-yool)

Firm, solid mass of cells in the skin larger than 0.5 cm in diameter (see Figures 3.9G & 3.9H ■).

G
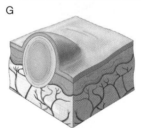

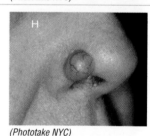

(Phototake NYC)

---

papule (PAP-yool)

Small, solid, circular raised spot on the surface of the skin less than 0.5 cm in diameter (see Figures 3.9I & 3.9J ■).

I
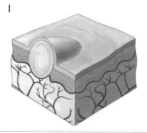

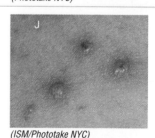

(ISM/Phototake NYC)

---

pustule (PUS-tyool)

Raised spot on the skin containing pus (see Figures 3.9E and 3.9K & 3.9L ■).

K
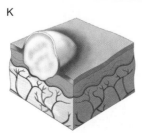

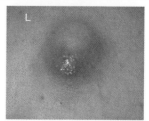

(P. Marazzi/Science Photo Library/Photo Researchers, Inc.)

Pathology *(continued)*

ulcer (ULL-ser) Open sore or lesion in skin or mucous membrane (see Figures 3.9M & 3.9N ■).	M 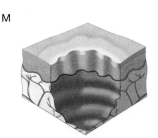	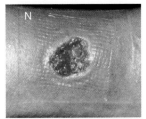 *(Dr. P. Marazzi/Photo Researchers, Inc.)*
vesicle (VESS-ikl) A blister; small, fluid-filled raised spot on the skin (see Figures 3.9O & 3.9P ■).	O 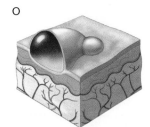	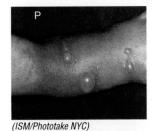 *(ISM/Phototake NYC)*
wheal (WEEL) Small, round, swollen area on the skin; typically seen in allergic skin reactions such as *hives* and usually accompanied by urticaria (see Figures 3.9Q & 3.9R ■).	Q 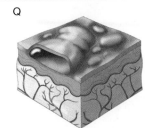	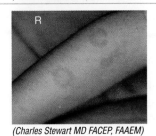 *(Charles Stewart MD FACEP, FAAEM)*

TERM	DEFINITION
■ *Skin*	
abscess (AB-sess)	A collection of pus in the skin.
acne (ACK-nee)	Inflammatory disease of the sebaceous glands and hair follicles resulting in papules and pustules.
acne rosacea (ACK-nee roh-ZAY-she-ah)	Chronic form of acne seen in adults involving redness, tiny pimples, and broken blood vessels, primarily on the nose and cheeks.
acne vulgaris (ACK-nee vul-GAY-ris)	Common form of acne seen in teenagers. Characterized by comedo, papules, and pustules.
albinism (al-BIH-nizm)	A genetic condition in which the body is unable to make melanin. Characterized by white hair and skin and red pupils due to the lack of pigment. The person with albinism is called an *albino*.
basal cell carcinoma (BCC) (BAY-sal sell kar-sin-NOH-ma)	Cancerous tumor of the basal cell layer of the epidermis. A frequent type of skin cancer that rarely metastasizes or spreads. These cancers can arise on sun exposed skin.

■ **Figure 3.10** Basal cell carcinoma. A frequent type of skin cancer that rarely metastasizes.
(ISM/Phototake NYC)

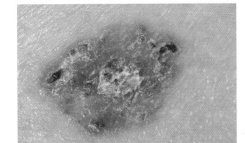

Pathology *(continued)*

TERM	DEFINITION
burn	Damage to the skin that can result from exposure to open fire, electricity, ultraviolet light from the sun, or caustic chemicals. Seriousness depends on the amount of body surface involved and the depth of the burn. Depth of the burns is determined by the amount of damage to each layer skin and burns are categorized as 1st degree, 2nd degree, or 3rd degree. See Figure 3.11 ▓ for a description of the damage associated with each degree of burn. Extent of a burn is estimated using the Rule of Nines (see Figure 3.12 ▓).

Superficial
First Degree

Skin reddened

(Moynahan Medical Center)

Partial thickness
Second Degree

Blisters

(Charles Stewart MD FACEP, FAAEM)

Full thickness
Third Degree

Charring

▓ **Figure 3.11** Comparison of the level of skin damage as a result of the three different degrees of burns.

■ **Figure 3.12** Rule of Nines. A method for determining percentage of body burned. Each differently colored section represents a percentage of the body surface. All sections added together will equal 100%.

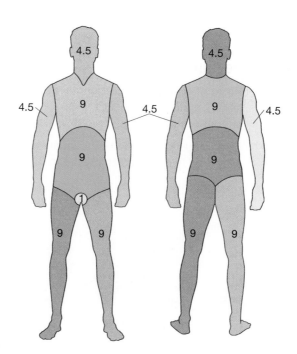

■ **Pathology** *(continued)*

TERM	DEFINITION
cellulitis (sell-you-LYE-tis)	A diffuse, acute infection and inflammation of the connective tissue found in the skin.
decubitus ulcer (decub) (dee-KYOO-bih-tus)	Open sore caused by pressure over bony prominences cutting off the blood flow to the overlying skin. These can appear in bedridden patients who lie in one position too long and can be difficult to heal. Also called *bedsore* or *pressure sore*. **Med Term Tip** *Decubitus* comes from the Latin word *decumbo*, meaning "lying down," which leads to the use of the term for a bedsore or pressure sore.
dry gangrene (GANG-green)	Late stages of gangrene characterized by the affected area becoming dried, blackened, and shriveled; referred to as *mummified*.
eczema (EK-zeh-mah)	Superficial dermatitis of unknown cause accompanied by redness, vesicles, itching, and crusting.
gangrene (GANG-green)	Tissue necrosis usually due to deficient blood supply.
ichthyosis (ick-thee-OH-sis)	Condition in which the skin becomes dry, scaly, and keratinized.
impetigo (im-peh-TYE-goh)	A highly infectious bacterial infection of the skin with pustules that rupture and become crusted over.

■ **Figure 3.13** Impetigo, a highly contagious bacterial infection. Note the extensive crusting around the eye.
(Bart's Medical Library/Phototake NYC)

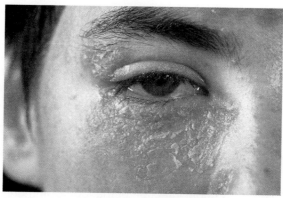

Pathology *(continued)*

TERM	DEFINITION
Kaposi's sarcoma (KAP-oh-seez sar-KOH-mah)	Form of skin cancer frequently seen in acquired immunodeficiency syndrome (AIDS) patients. Consists of brownish-purple papules that spread from the skin and metastasize to internal organs.
malignant melanoma (MM) (mah-LIG-nant mel-a-NOH-ma)	Dangerous form of skin cancer caused by an uncontrolled growth of melanocytes. May quickly metastasize or spread to internal organs.

■ **Figure 3.14** Malignant melanoma. This tumor demonstrates the highly characteristic color of this tumor. *(ISM/Phototake NYC)*

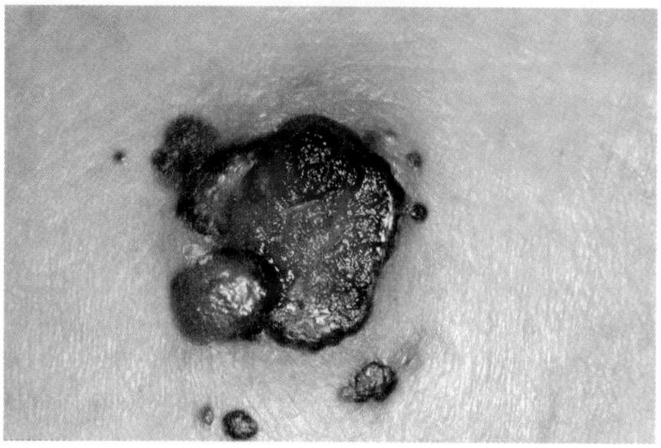

TERM	DEFINITION
pediculosis (peh-dik-you-LOH-sis)	Infestation with lice. The eggs laid by the lice are called nits and cling tightly to hair.
psoriasis (soh-RYE-ah-sis)	Chronic inflammatory condition consisting of papules forming "silvery scale" patches with circular borders.

■ **Figure 3.15** Psoriasis. This photograph demonstrates the characteristic white skin patches of this condition.

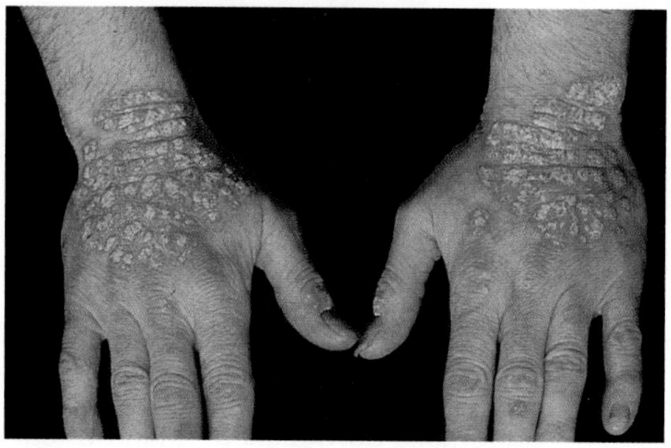

TERM	DEFINITION
rubella (roo-BELL-ah)	Contagious viral skin infection. Commonly called *German measles.*
scabies (SKAY-bees)	Contagious skin disease caused by an egg-laying mite that burrows through the skin and causes redness and intense itching; often seen in children.
sebaceous cyst (see-BAY-shus SIST)	Sac under the skin filled with sebum or oil from a sebaceous gland. This can grow to a large size and may need to be excised.
squamous cell carcinoma (SCC) (SKWAY-mus sell kar-sih-NOH-mah)	Cancer of the epidermis layer of skin that may invade deeper tissue and metastasize. Often begins as a sore that does not heal.
systemic lupus erythematosus (SLE) (sis-TEM-ik LOO-pus air-ih-them-ah-TOH-sis)	Chronic disease of the connective tissue that injures the skin, joints, kidneys, nervous system, and mucous membranes. May produce a characteristic red, scaly butterfly rash across the cheeks and nose.
tinea (TIN-ee-ah)	Fungal skin disease resulting in itching, scaling lesions.
tinea capitis (TIN-ee-ah CAP-it-is)	Fungal infection of the scalp. Commonly called *ringworm.*
tinea pedis (TIN-ee-ah PED-is)	Fungal infection of the foot. Commonly called *athlete's foot.*

Pathology *(continued)*

TERM	DEFINITION
varicella (VAIR-ih-chell-a)	Contagious viral skin infection. Commonly called *chickenpox*.

Figure 3.16 Varicella or chicken pox, a viral skin infection. In this photograph, the rash is beginning to form scabs.

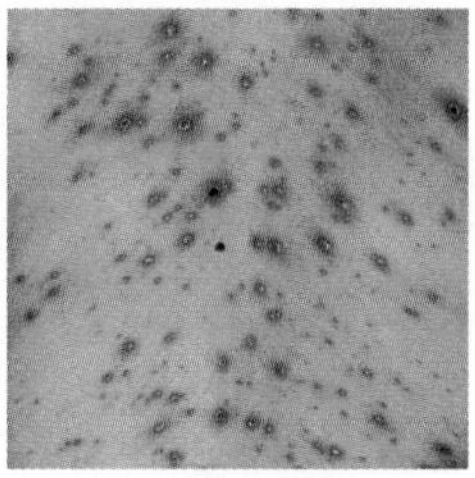

TERM	DEFINITION
vitiligo (vit-ill-EYE-go)	Disappearance of pigment from the skin in patches, causing a milk-white appearance. Also called *leukoderma*.
wet gangrene (GANG-green)	An area of gangrene that becomes secondarily infected by pus-producing bacteria.
■ Hair	
alopecia (al-oh-PEE-she-ah)	Absence or loss of hair, especially of the head. Commonly called *baldness*.
carbuncle (CAR-bung-kl)	Furuncle involving several hair follicles.
furuncle (FOO-rung-kl)	Bacterial infection of a hair follicle. Characterized by redness, pain, and swelling. Also called a *boil*.
■ Nails	
onychia (oh-NICK-ee-ah)	Infected nail bed.
paronychia (pair-oh-NICK-ee-ah)	Infection of the skin fold around a nail.

Diagnostic Procedures

TERM	DEFINITION
■ Clinical Laboratory Tests	
culture and sensitivity (C&S)	A laboratory test that grows a colony of bacteria removed from an infected area in order to identify the specific infecting bacteria and then determine its sensitivity to a variety of antibiotics.
■ Biopsy Procedures	
biopsy (BX, bx) (BYE-op-see)	A piece of tissue is removed by syringe and needle, knife, punch, or brush to examine under a microscope. Used to aid in diagnosis.

Med Term Tip

Word Watch — be careful when using *bi-* meaning "two" and *bi/o* meaning "life."

TERM	DEFINITION
exfoliative cytology (ex-FOH-lee-ah-tiv sigh-TALL-oh-jee)	Scraping cells from tissue and then examining them under a microscope.
frozen section (FS)	A thin piece of tissue is cut from a frozen specimen for rapid examination under a microscope.
fungal scrapings	Scrapings, taken with a curette or scraper, of tissue from lesions are placed on a growth medium and examined under a microscope to identify fungal growth.

Therapeutic Procedures

TERM	DEFINITION

Skin Grafting

TERM	DEFINITION
allograft (AL-oh-graft)	Skin graft from one person to another; donor is usually a cadaver.
autograft (AW-toh-graft) ■ **Figure 3.17** A freshly applied autograft. Note that the donor skin has been perforated so that it can be stretched to cover a larger burned area. *(Courtesy of Dr. William Dominic, Community Regional Medical Center)*	Skin graft from a person's own body.
dermatome (DER-mah-tohm)	Instrument for cutting the skin or thin transplants of skin.
dermatoplasty (DER-mah-toh-plas-tee)	Skin grafting; transplantation of skin.
heterograft (HET-ur-oh-graft)	Skin graft from an animal of another species (usually a pig) to a human. Also called *xenograft.*
skin graft (SG)	The transfer of skin from a normal area to cover another site. Used to treat burn victims and after some surgical procedures. Also called *dermatoplasty.*
xenograft (ZEN-oh-graft)	Skin graft from an animal of another species (usually a pig) to a human. Also called *heterograft.*

Surgical Procedures

TERM	DEFINITION
cauterization (kaw-ter-ih-ZAY-shun)	Destruction of tissue by using caustic chemicals, electric currents, heat, or by freezing.
cryosurgery (cry-oh-SER-jer-ee)	The use of extreme cold to freeze and destroy tissue.
curettage (koo-REH-tahz)	Removal of superficial skin lesions with a curette (surgical instrument shaped like a spoon) or scraper.
debridement (de-BREED-mint)	Removal of foreign material and dead or damaged tissue from a wound.
electrocautery (ee-leck-troh-KAW-teh-ree)	To destroy tissue with an electric current.
incision and drainage (I&D)	Making an incision to create an opening for the drainage of material such as pus.

Plastic Surgery Procedures

TERM	DEFINITION
chemabrasion (kee-moh-BRAY-zhun)	Abrasion using chemicals. Also called a *chemical peel.*
dermabrasion (DERM-ah-bray-shun)	Abrasion or rubbing using wire brushes or sandpaper. Performed to remove acne scars, tattoos, and scar tissue.
laser therapy	Removal of skin lesions and birthmarks using a laser beam that emits intense heat and power at a close range. The laser converts frequencies of light into one small, powerful beam.
liposuction (LIP-oh-suck-shun)	Removal of fat beneath the skin by means of suction.
rhytidectomy (rit-ih-DECK-toh-mee)	Surgical removal of excess skin to eliminate wrinkles. Commonly referred to as a *face lift.*

Pharmacology

CLASSIFICATION	ACTION	GENERIC AND BRAND NAMES
anesthetics (an-es-THET-tics)	Applied to the skin to deaden pain.	lidocaine, Xylocaine; procaine, Novocain
antibiotics (an-tye-bye-AW-tics)	Kill bacteria causing skin infections.	bacitracin/neomycin/polymixinB, Neosporin ointment
antifungals (an-tye-FUNG-alls)	Kill fungi infecting the skin.	miconazole, Monistat; clotrimazole, Lotrimin
antiparasitics (an-tye-pair-ah-SIT-tics)	Kill mites or lice.	lindane, Kwell; permethrin, Nix
antipruritics (an-tye-proo-RIGH-tiks)	Reduce severe itching.	diphenhydramine, Benadryl; camphor/pramoxine/zinc, Caladryl
antiseptics (an-tye-SEP-tics)	Used to kill bacteria in skin cuts and wounds or at a surgical site.	isopropyl alcohol; hydrogen peroxide
anti-virals	Treats herpes simplex infection.	valacyclovir, Valtrex; famcyclovir, Famvir; acyclovir, Zovirax
corticosteroid cream	Specific type of powerful anti-inflammatory cream.	hydrocortisone, Cortaid; triamcinolone, Kenalog

Abbreviations

BCC	basal cell carcinoma	**MM**	malignant melanoma
BX, bx	biopsy	**SCC**	squamous cell carcinoma
C&S	culture and sensitivity	**SG**	skin graft
decub	decubitus ulcer	**SLE**	systemic lupus erythematosus
Derm, derm	dermatology	**STSG**	split-thickness skin graft
FS	frozen section	**subcu, SC, sc,**	subcutaneous
HSV	herpes simplex virus	**subq**	
I&D	incision and drainage	**UV**	ultraviolet
ID	intradermal		

Med Term Tip

Word Watch—be careful when using the abbreviation *ID* meaning "intradermal" and *I&D* meaning "incision and drainage."

Chapter Review

Terminology Checklist

 Below are all anatomy and physiology key terms, word building, vocabulary, pathology, diagnostic, therapeutic, and pharmacology terms presented in this chapter. Use this list as a study tool by placing a check in the box in front of each term as you master its meaning.

- ☐ abrasion
- ☐ abscess
- ☐ acne
- ☐ acne rosacea
- ☐ acne vulgaris
- ☐ albinism
- ☐ allograft
- ☐ alopecia
- ☐ anesthetics
- ☐ anhidrosis
- ☐ antibiotics
- ☐ antifungals
- ☐ antiparasitics
- ☐ antipruritics
- ☐ antiseptics
- ☐ anti-virals
- ☐ apocrine glands
- ☐ arrector pili
- ☐ autograft
- ☐ basal cell carcinoma
- ☐ basal layer
- ☐ biopsy
- ☐ burn
- ☐ carbuncle
- ☐ cauterization
- ☐ cellulitis
- ☐ chemabrasion
- ☐ cicatrix
- ☐ collagen fibers
- ☐ comedo
- ☐ contusion
- ☐ corium
- ☐ corticosteroid cream
- ☐ cryosurgery
- ☐ culture and sensitivity
- ☐ curettage
- ☐ cutaneous membrane
- ☐ cuticle

- ☐ cyanosis
- ☐ cyst
- ☐ debridement
- ☐ decubitus ulcer
- ☐ depigmentation
- ☐ dermabrasion
- ☐ dermatitis
- ☐ dermatologist
- ☐ dermatology
- ☐ dermatome
- ☐ dermatopathy
- ☐ dermatoplasty
- ☐ dermatosis
- ☐ dermis
- ☐ diaphoresis
- ☐ dry gangrene
- ☐ ecchymosis
- ☐ eczema
- ☐ electrocautery
- ☐ epidermal
- ☐ epidermis
- ☐ erythema
- ☐ erythroderma
- ☐ eschar
- ☐ exfoliative cytology
- ☐ fissure
- ☐ free edge
- ☐ frozen section
- ☐ fungal scrapings
- ☐ furuncle
- ☐ gangrene
- ☐ hair
- ☐ hair follicle
- ☐ hair root
- ☐ hair shaft
- ☐ heterograft
- ☐ hirsutism
- ☐ hyperemia

- ☐ hyperhidrosis
- ☐ hyperpigmentation
- ☐ hypodermic
- ☐ hypodermis
- ☐ ichthyoderma
- ☐ ichthyosis
- ☐ impetigo
- ☐ incision and drainage
- ☐ integument
- ☐ integumentary system
- ☐ intradermal
- ☐ Kaposi's sarcoma
- ☐ keloid
- ☐ keratin
- ☐ keratosis
- ☐ laceration
- ☐ laser therapy
- ☐ lesion
- ☐ leukoderma
- ☐ lipectomy
- ☐ lipocytes
- ☐ lipoma
- ☐ liposuction
- ☐ lunula
- ☐ macule
- ☐ malignant melanoma
- ☐ melanin
- ☐ melanocytes
- ☐ melanoma
- ☐ nail bed
- ☐ nail body
- ☐ nail root
- ☐ nails
- ☐ necrosis
- ☐ nevus
- ☐ nodule
- ☐ onychectomy
- ☐ onychia

☐ onychomalacia	☐ rhytidectomy	☐ sweat duct
☐ onychomycosis	☐ rhytidoplasty	☐ sweat glands
☐ onychophagia	☐ rubella	☐ sweat pore
☐ pallor	☐ scabies	☐ systemic lupus erythematosus
☐ papule	☐ scleroderma	☐ tinea
☐ paronychia	☐ sebaceous cyst	☐ tinea capitis
☐ pathogens	☐ sebaceous gland	☐ tinea pedis
☐ pediculosis	☐ seborrhea	☐ trichomycosis
☐ perspiration	☐ sebum	☐ ulcer
☐ petechiae	☐ sensory receptors	☐ ungual
☐ photosensitivity	☐ skin	☐ urticaria
☐ plastic surgery	☐ skin graft	☐ varicella
☐ pruritus	☐ squamous cell carcinoma	☐ verruca
☐ psoriasis	☐ stratified squamous epithelium	☐ vesicle
☐ purpura	☐ strawberry hemangioma	☐ vitiligo
☐ purulent	☐ subcutaneous	☐ wet gangrene
☐ pustule	☐ subcutaneous layer	☐ wheal
☐ pyoderma	☐ sudoriferous glands	☐ xenograft
☐ pyogenic	☐ suppurative	☐ xeroderma

Practice Exercises

A. Complete the following statements.

1. The three layers of skin in order starting with the most superficial layer are _____, _____,

   and _____.

2. The _____ layer is the only living layer of the epidermis.

3. The subcutaneous layer of skin is composed primarily of _____.

4. Sensory receptors are located in the _____ layer of skin.

5. Nails and hair are composed of a hard protein called _____.

6. _____ is the pigment that gives skin its color.

7. Another name for the dermis is _____.

8. The nail body is connected to underlying tissue by the _____.

9. _____ glands release their product directly into hair follicles while _____ glands release

   their product into a duct.

10. _____ glands are sweat glands found in the underarm and pubic areas.

B. State the terms described using the combining forms provided.

The combining form *dermat/o* refers to the skin. Use it to write a term that means:

1. inflammation of the skin _____

2. any abnormal skin condition _____

3. an instrument for cutting the skin _____

4. specialist in skin _____

5. surgical repair of the skin _____

6. study of the skin _____

The combining form *melan/o* means black. Use it to write a term that means a:

7. black tumor _____

8. black cell _____

The suffix *-derma* means skin. Use it to write a term that means:

9. scaly skin _____

10. white skin _____

11. red skin _____

The combining form *onych/o* refers to the nail. Use it to write a term that means:

12. softening of the nails _____

13. infection around the nail _____

14. nail eating (biting) _____

15. removal of the nail _____

C. Define the following combining forms and use them to form integumentary terms.

		Definition	Integumentary term
1.	cry/o	_____	_____
2.	cutane/o	_____	_____
3.	diaphor/o	_____	_____
4.	py/o	_____	_____
5.	cyan/o	_____	_____
6.	ungu/o	_____	_____
7.	lip/o	_____	_____
8.	hidr/o	_____	_____
9.	rhytid/o	_____	_____
10.	seb/o	_____	_____
11.	trich/o	_____	_____
12.	necr/o	_____	_____

D. Define the following terms.

1. macule _____

2. papule _____

3. cyst _____

4. fissure _____

5. pustule _____

6. wheal _____

7. vesicle _____

8. ulcer _____

9. nodule _____

10. laceration _____

E. Describe the following types of burns.

1. first degree _____

2. second degree _____

3. third degree _____

F. Match each term to its definition.

1. ____ eczema		a.	decubitus ulcer
2. ____ nevus		b.	lack of skin pigment
3. ____ lipoma		c.	acne commonly seen in adults
4. ____ urticaria		d.	hardened skin
5. ____ bedsore		e.	redness, vesicles, itching, crusts
6. ____ acne rosacea		f.	birthmark
7. ____ acne vulgaris		g.	excessive hair growth
8. ____ hirsutism		h.	caused by deficient blood supply
9. ____ alopecia		i.	fatty tumor
10. ____ gangrene		j.	hives
11. ____ scleroderma		k.	baldness
12. ____ albinism		l.	acne of adolescence

G. Match each term to its definition.

1. ____ debridement
2. ____ cauterization
3. ____ chemabrasion
4. ____ dermatoplasty
5. ____ liposuction
6. ____ rhytidectomy
7. ____ curettage
8. ____ dermabrasion
9. ____ dermatome
10. ____ cryosurgery

a. surgical removal of wrinkled skin
b. instrument to cut thin slices of skin
c. removal of fat with suction
d. use extreme cold to destroy tissue
e. skin grafting
f. removal of lesions with scraper
g. removal of skin with brushes
h. removal of damaged skin
i. destruction of tissue with electric current
j. chemical peel

H. Write the abbreviations for the following terms.

1. frozen section _____
2. incision and drainage _____
3. intradermal _____
4. subcutaneous _____
5. ultraviolet _____
6. biopsy _____

I. Identify the following abbreviations.

1. C & S _____

2. BCC _____

3. derm _____

4. SG _____

5. decub _____

6. MM _____

J. Use the following terms in the sentences that follow.

impetigo	tinea	keloid	exfoliative cytology	xeroderma
petechiae	frozen section	paronychia	scabies	Kaposi's sarcoma

1. The winter climates can cause dry skin. The medical term for this is _____.

2. Kim has experienced small pinpoint purplish spots caused by bleeding under the skin. This is called _____.

3. Janet has a fungal skin disease. This is called _____.

4. A contagious skin disease caused by a mite is _____.

5. An infection around the entire nail is called _____.

6. A form of skin cancer affecting AIDS patients is called _____.

7. Latrivia has a bacterial skin infection that results in pustules crusting and rupturing. It is called _____.

8. James's burn scar became a hypertrophic _____.

9. For a(n) _____ test, cells scraped off the skin are examined under a microscope.

10. During surgery a _____ was ordered for a rapid exam of tissue cut from a tumor.

K. Use the following prefixes to write a word that means

epi-   sub-   intra-   hypo-

1. under the skin _____ or _____

2. within the skin _____

3. on the skin _____

L. Distinguish between the following types of skin graft.

1. allograft _____

2. heterograft _____

3. autograft _____

4. xenograft _____

M. Fill in the classification for each drug description, then match the brand name.

Drug Description	Classification	Brand Name
1. _____ kills fungi	_____	a. Kwell
2. _____ reduces severe itching	_____	b. Cortaid
3. _____ kills mites and lice	_____	c. Valtrex
4. _____ treats herpes simplex infection	_____	d. Benadryl
5. _____ powerful anti-inflammatory	_____	e. Neosporin
6. _____ deadens pain	_____	f. Monistat
7. _____ kills bacteria	_____	g. Xylocaine

Medical Record Analysis

Below is an item from a patient's medical record. Read it carefully, make sure you understand all the medical terms used, and then answer the questions that follow.

Dermatology Consultation Report

Reason for Consultation:	Evaluate patient for excision of recurrent basal cell carcinoma, left cheek.
History of Present Illness:	Patient is a 74-year-old male first seen by his regular physician five years ago for persistent facial lesions. Biopsies revealed basal cell carcinoma in two lesions, one on the nasal tip and the other on the left cheek. These were excised and healed with a normal cicatrix. The patient noted that the left cheek lesion returned approximately one year ago. Patient admits to not following his physician's advice to use sunscreen and a hat. Patient reports pruritus and states the lesion is growing larger. Patient has been referred for dermatology evaluation regarding deep excision of the lesion and dermatoplasty.
Past Medical History:	Patient's activity level is severely restricted due to congestive heart failure (CHF) with dyspnea, lower extremity edema, and cyanosis. He takes several cardiac medications daily and occasionally requires oxygen by nasal cannula. History is negative for other types of cancer.
Results of Physical Exam:	Examination revealed a 10 × 14 mm lesion on left cheek 20 mm anterior to the ear. The lesion displays marked erythema and poorly defined borders. The area immediately around the lesion shows depigmentation with vesicles. There is a well-healed cicatrix on the nasal tip with no evidence of the neoplasm returning.
Assessment:	Even without a biopsy, this is most likely a recurrence of this patient's basal cell carcinoma.
Recommendations:	Due to the lesion's size, shape, and reoccurrence, recommend deep excision of the neoplasm through the epidermis and dermis layers. The patient will then require dermatoplasty. The most likely donor site will be the proximal-medial thigh. This patient is at high risk for basal cell carcinoma and should never go outside without sunscreen and a hat. I have discussed the surgical procedure with the patient, and he fully understands the procedure, risks, and alternate treatment choices. In light of his cardiac status, if he decides to proceed with the surgery, he will need a thorough workup by his cardiologist.

Critical Thinking Questions

1. Which of the following symptoms was reported by the patient?
   a. easy bruising
   b. excessive scarring
   c. intense itching
   d. yellow skin

2. In your own words, describe the lesion on the patient's face. _____

_____

_____

3. What advice did this patient fail to follow? _____

_____

What happened, in part, because he did not follow instructions? _____

_____

4. This patient has a serious health condition other than his facial lesion. Name that condition and describe it in

your own words. _____

_____

What is the abbreviation for this condition? _____

This patient has three symptoms of this condition. List the three symptoms and describe each in your own
words. This condition and its symptoms use terminology that has not been introduced yet. You will need to
use your text as a reference to answer this question.

_____

_____

_____

5. What procedure was performed on the original lesion that confirmed the diagnosis? Explain, in your own

words, what this procedure involves. _____

_____

6. Briefly describe, in your own words, the two stages of the surgical procedure the physician recommends.

_____

_____

_____

Chart Note Transcription

The chart note below contains ten phrases that can be reworded with a medical term that you learned in this chapter. Each phrase is identified with an underline. Determine the medical term and write your answers in the spaces provided.

Current Complaint:	A 64-year-old female with an <u>open sore</u> ❶ on her right leg is seen by the <u>specialist in treating diseases of the skin</u>. ❷
Past History:	Patient states she first noticed an area of pain, <u>severe itching</u>, ❸ and <u>redness of the skin</u> ❹ just below her right knee about six weeks ago. One week later <u>raised spots containing pus</u> ❺ appeared. Patient states the raised spots containing pus ruptured and the open sore appeared.
Signs and Symptoms:	Patient has a deep open sore 5 × 3 cm: It is 4 cm distal to the knee on the lateral aspect of the right leg. It appears to extend into the <u>middle skin layer</u>, ❻ and the edges show signs of <u>tissue death</u>. ❼ The open sore has a small amount of drainage but there is no odor. A <u>sample of the drainage that was grown in the lab to identify the microorganism and determine the best antibiotic</u> ❽ of the drainage revealed *Staphylococcus* bacteria in the open sore.
Diagnosis:	<u>Inflammation of connective tissue in the skin.</u> ❾
Treatment:	<u>Removal of damaged tissue</u> ❿ of the open sore followed by application of an antibiotic cream. Patient was instructed to return to the specialist in treating diseases of the skin's office in two weeks, or sooner if the open sore does not heal, or if it begins draining pus.

❶ _____

❷ _____

❸ _____

❹ _____

❺ _____

❻ _____

❼ _____

❽ _____

❾ _____

❿ _____

Labeling Exercise

A. System Review

Write the labels for this figure on the numbered lines provided.

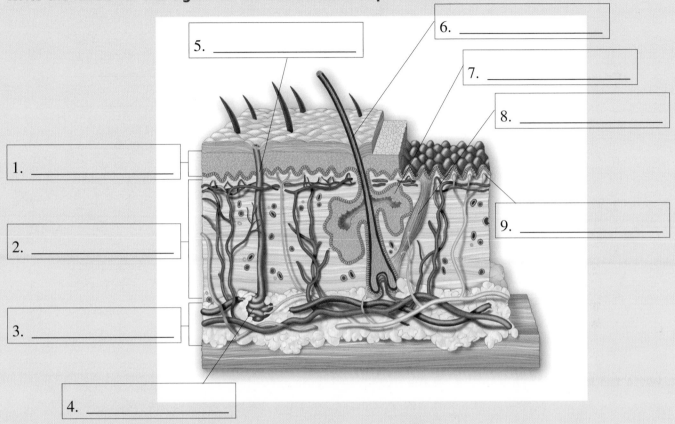

5. _____

6. _____

7. _____

8. _____

1. _____

9. _____

2. _____

3. _____

4. _____

B. Anatomy Challenge

1. Write the labels for this figure on the numbered lines provided.

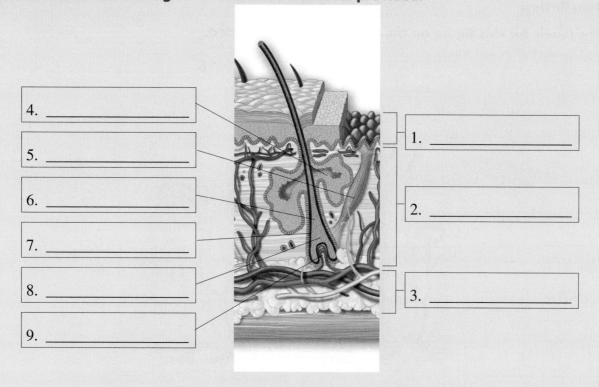

4. _____

5. _____

6. _____

7. _____

8. _____

9. _____

1. _____

2. _____

3. _____

2. Write the labels for this figure on the numbered lines provided.

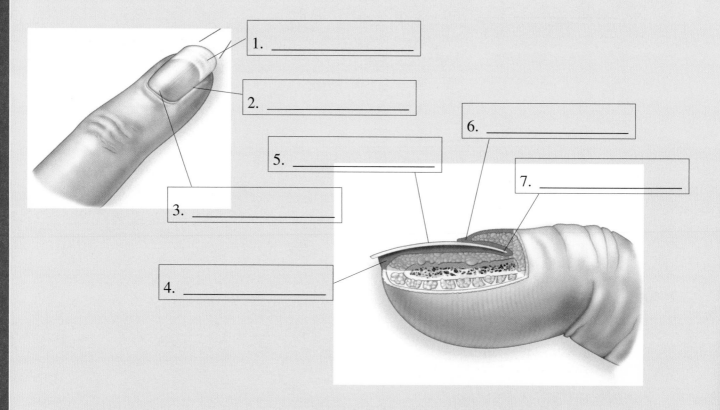

1. _____

2. _____

3. _____

4. _____

5. _____

6. _____

7. _____

Multimedia Preview

Additional interactive resources and activities for this chapter can be found on the Companion Website. For videos, games, and pronunciations, please access the accompanying DVD-ROM that comes with this book.

DVD-ROM Highlights

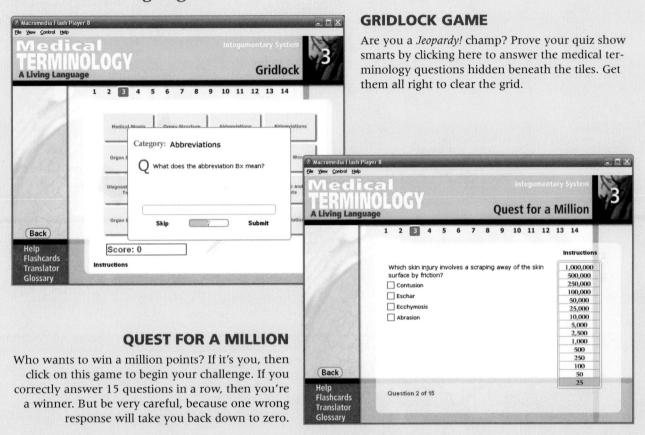

GRIDLOCK GAME

Are you a *Jeopardy!* champ? Prove your quiz show smarts by clicking here to answer the medical terminology questions hidden beneath the tiles. Get them all right to clear the grid.

QUEST FOR A MILLION

Who wants to win a million points? If it's you, then click on this game to begin your challenge. If you correctly answer 15 questions in a row, then you're a winner. But be very careful, because one wrong response will take you back down to zero.

Website Highlights—www.prenhall.com/fremgen

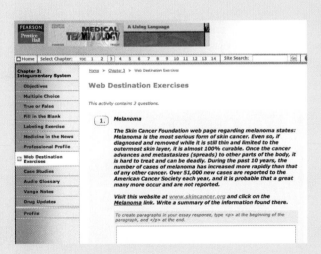

WEB DESTINATION EXERCISES

Surf the net to investigate key topics and then report your findings. This online activity challenges you to visit selected web links where you can explore important issues to reinforce your understanding.

4 Musculoskeletal System

Learning Objectives

Upon completion of this chapter, you will be able to:

- Identify and define the combining forms, prefixes, and suffixes introduced in this chapter.

- Correctly spell and pronounce medical terms and major anatomical structures relating to the musculoskeletal system.

- Locate and describe the major organs of the musculoskeletal system and their functions.

- Correctly place bones in either the axial or the appendicular skeleton.

- List and describe the components of a long bone.

- Identify bony projections and depressions.

- Identify the parts of a synovial joint.

- Describe the characteristics of the three types of muscle tissue.

- Use movement terminology correctly.

- Build and define musculoskeletal system medical terms from word parts.

- Identify and define musculoskeletal system vocabulary terms.

- Identify and define selected musculoskeletal system pathology terms.

- Identify and define selected musculoskeletal system diagnostic procedures.

- Identify and define selected musculoskeletal system therapeutic procedures.

- Identify and define selected medications relating to the musculoskeletal system.

- Define selected abbreviations associated with the musculoskeletal system.

Section I: Skeletal System at a Glance

Function

The skeletal system consists of 206 bones that make up the internal framework of the body, called the skeleton. The skeleton supports the body, protects internal organs, serves as a point of attachment for skeletal muscles for body movement, produces blood cells, and stores minerals.

Organs

bones   joints

Combining Forms

ankyl/o	stiff joint	metacarp/o	metacarpals
arthr/o	joint	metatars/o	metatarsals
articul/o	joint	myel/o	bone marrow, spinal cord
burs/o	sac	orth/o	straight
carp/o	wrist	oste/o	bone
cervic/o	neck	patell/o	patella
chondr/o	cartilage	ped/o	child, foot
clavicul/o	clavicle	pelv/o	pelvis
coccyg/o	coccyx	phalang/o	phalanges
cortic/o	outer portion	pod/o	foot
cost/o	rib	pub/o	pubis
crani/o	skull	radi/o	radius
femor/o	femur	sacr/o	sacrum
fibul/o	fibula	scapul/o	scapula
humer/o	humerus	scoli/o	crooked, bent
ili/o	ilium	spondyl/o	vertebrae
ischi/o	ischium	stern/o	sternum
kyph/o	hump	synovi/o	synovial membrane
lamin/o	lamina, part of vertebra	synov/o	synovial membrane
lord/o	bent backwards	tars/o	ankle
lumb/o	loin	thorac/o	chest
mandibul/o	mandible	tibi/o	tibia
maxill/o	maxilla	uln/o	ulna
medull/o	inner portion	vertebr/o	vertebra

Suffixes

-blast	immature, embryonic
-clasia	to surgically break
-desis	stabilize, fuse
-listhesis	slipping
-porosis	porous

Skeletal System Illustrated

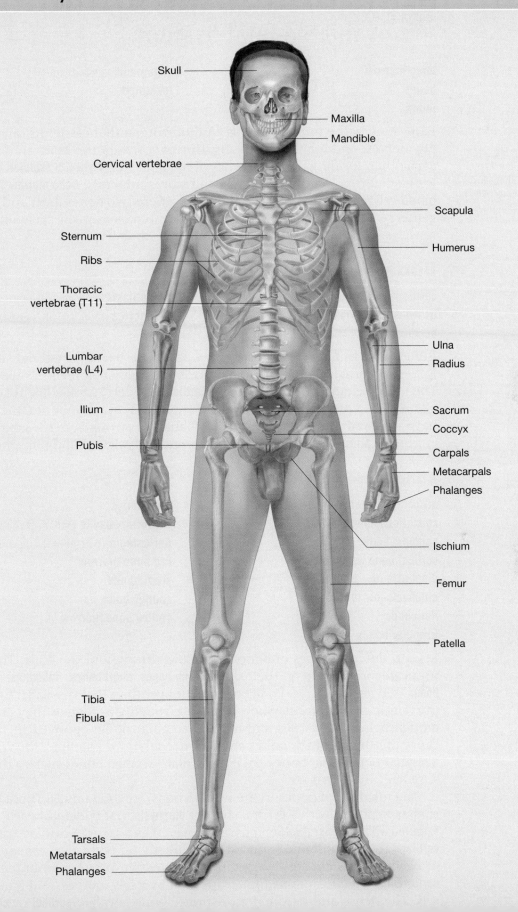

Skull

Maxilla

Mandible

Cervical vertebrae

Scapula

Sternum

Humerus

Ribs

Thoracic vertebrae (T11)

Ulna

Radius

Lumbar vertebrae (L4)

Ilium

Sacrum

Coccyx

Pubis

Carpals

Metacarpals

Phalanges

Ischium

Femur

Patella

Tibia

Fibula

Tarsals

Metatarsals

Phalanges

Anatomy and Physiology of the Skeletal System

bone marrow	ligaments (LIG-ah-ments)
bones	skeleton
joints	

Each bone in the human body is a unique organ that carries its own blood supply, nerves, and lymphatic vessels. However, when the **bones** are connected to each other, forming the framework of the body, it is called a **skeleton**. In addition, the skeleton protects vital organs and stores minerals. **Bone marrow** is the site of blood cell production. A **joint** is the place where two bones meet and are held together by **ligaments**. This gives flexibility to the skeleton. The skeleton, joints, and muscles work together to produce movement.

Bones

cartilage (CAR-tih-lij)	osteoblasts (OSS-tee-oh-blasts)
osseous tissue (OSS-ee-us)	osteocytes (OSS-tee-oh-sights)
ossification (oss-sih-fih-KAY-shun)	

Bones, also called **osseous tissue**, are one of the hardest materials in the body. Bones are formed from a gradual process beginning before birth called **ossification**. The fetal skeleton is formed from a **cartilage** model. This flexible tissue is gradually replaced by **osteoblasts**, immature bone cells. In adult bones, the osteoblasts have matured into **osteocytes**. The formation of strong bones is greatly dependent on an adequate supply of minerals such as calcium and phosphorus.

Bone Structure

articular cartilage (ar-TIK-yoo-lar)	long bones
cancellous bone (CAN-sell-us)	medullary cavity (MED-you-lair-ee)
compact bone	periosteum (pair-ee-AH-stee-um)
cortical bone (KOR-ti-kal)	red bone marrow
diaphysis (dye-AFF-ih-sis)	short bones
epiphysis (eh-PIFF-ih-sis)	spongy bone
flat bones	yellow bone marrow
irregular bones	

Several different types of bones are found throughout the body. They fall into four categories based on their shape: **long bones**, **short bones**, **flat bones**, and **irregular bones** (see Figure 4.1 ■). Long bones are longer than they are wide. Examples are the femur and humerus. Short bones are roughly as long as they are wide; examples being the carpals and tarsals. Irregular bones received their name because the shapes of the bones are very irregular; for example, the vertebrae are irregular bones. Flat bones are usually plate-shaped bones such as the sternum, scapulae, and pelvis.

The majority of bones in the human body are long bones. These bones have similar structure with a central shaft or **diaphysis** that widens at each end, which is called an **epiphysis**. Each epiphysis is covered by a layer of cartilage called **articular cartilage** to prevent bone from rubbing directly on bone. The remaining surface of each bone is covered with a thin connective tissue membrane called the **periosteum**, which contains numerous blood vessels, nerves, and lymphatic vessels. The dense and hard exterior surface bone is called **cortical** or **compact bone**.

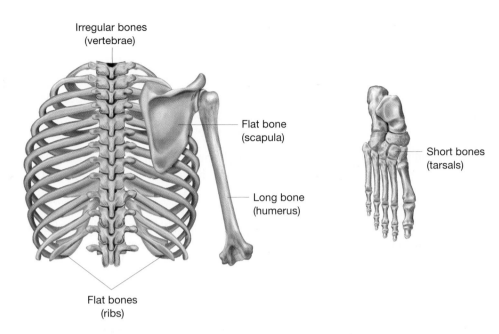

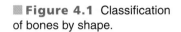**Figure 4.1** Classification of bones by shape.

Cancellous or **spongy bone** is found inside the bone. As its name indicates, spongy bone has spaces in it, giving it a spongelike appearance. These spaces contain **red bone marrow**. Red bone marrow manufactures most of the blood cells and is found in some parts of all bones.

The center of the diaphysis contains an open canal called the **medullary cavity**. This cavity contains **yellow bone marrow**, which is mainly fat cells. Figure 4.2 ▨ contains an illustration of the structure of long bones.

Bone Projections and Depressions

condyle (KON-dile)	**neck**
epicondyle (ep-ih-KON-dile)	**process**
fissure (FISH-er)	**sinus** (SIGH-nus)
foramen (for-AY-men)	**trochanter** (tro-KAN-ter)
fossa (FOSS-ah)	**tubercle** (TOO-ber-kl)
head	**tuberosity** (too-ber-OSS-ih-tee)

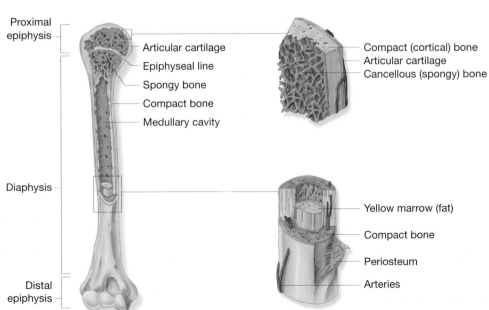

Figure 4.2 Components of a long bone. The entire long bone is on the left side accompanied by a blow-up of the proximal epiphysis and a section of the diaphysis.

Bones have many projections and depressions. Some are rounded and smooth in order to articulate with another bone in a joint. Others are rough to provide muscles with attachment points. The general term for any bony projection is a **process**. Then there are specific terms to describe the different shapes and locations of various processes. These terms are commonly used on operative reports and in physicians' records for clear identification of areas on the individual bones. Some of the common bony processes include the following:

1. The **head** is a large smooth ball-shaped end on a long bone. It may be separated from the body or shaft of the bone by a narrow area called the **neck**.
2. A **condyle** refers to a smooth rounded portion at the end of a bone.
3. The **epicondyle** is a projection located above or on a condyle.
4. The **trochanter** refers to a large rough process for the attachment of a muscle.
5. A **tubercle** is a small, rough process that provides the attachment for tendons and muscles.
6. The **tuberosity** is a large, rough process that provides the attachment of tendons and muscles.

See Figure 4.3 ■ for an illustration of the processes found on the femur.

In addition, bones have hollow regions or depressions. The most common depressions are as follows:

1. A **sinus**, which is a hollow cavity within a bone.
2. A **foramen**, which is a smooth round opening for nerves and blood vessels.
3. A **fossa**, which consists of a shallow cavity or depression on the surface of a bone.
4. A **fissure**, which is a slit-type opening.

■ **Figure 4.3** Bony processes found on the femur.

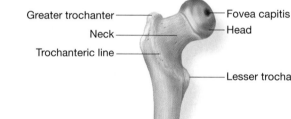

Greater trochanter

Neck

Trochanteric line

Fovea capitis

Head

Lesser trochanter

Patellar surface

Lateral epicondyle

Lateral condyle

Medial epicondyle

Medial condyle

Skeleton

appendicular skeleton (app-en-DIK-yoo-lar)   **axial skeleton** (AK-see-al)

The human skeleton has two divisions: the **axial skeleton** and the **appendicular skeleton**. Figures 4.4 and 4.8 illustrate the axial and appendicular skeletons.

Med Term Tip

Newborn infants have about 300 bones at birth that will fuse into 206 bones as an adult.

Axial Skeleton

cervical vertebrae
coccyx (COCK-six)
cranium (KRAY-nee-um)
ethmoid bone (ETH-moyd)
facial bones
frontal bone
hyoid bone (HIGH-oyd)
intervertebral disc (in-ter-VER-teh-bral)
lacrimal bone (LACK-rim-al)
lumbar vertebrae
mandible (MAN-dih-bl)
maxilla (mack-SIH-lah)
nasal bone

occipital bone (ock-SIP-eh-tal)
palatine bone (PAL-ah-tine)
parietal bone (pah-RYE-eh-tal)
rib cage
sacrum (SAY-crum)
sphenoid bone (SFEE-noyd)
sternum (STER-num)
temporal bone (TEM-por-al)
thoracic vertebrae
vertebral column (VER-teh-bral)
vomer bone (VOH-mer)
zygomatic bone (zeye-go-MAT-ik)

The axial skeleton includes the bones in the head, neck, spine, chest, and trunk of the body (see Figure 4.4 ■). These bones form the central axis for the whole body and protect many of the internal organs such as the brain, lungs, and heart.

The head or skull is divided into two parts consisting of the **cranium** and **facial bones**. These bones surround and protect the brain, eyes, ears, nasal cavity, and oral cavity from injury. The muscles for chewing and moving the head are attached to the cranial bones. The cranium encases the brain and consists of the **frontal**, **parietal**, **temporal**, **ethmoid**, **sphenoid**, and **occipital bones**. The facial bones surround the mouth, nose, and eyes and include the **mandible**, **maxilla**, **zygomatic**, **vomer**, **palatine**, **nasal**, and **lacrimal bones**. The cranial and facial bones are illustrated in Figure 4.5 ■ and described in Table 4.1 ■.

The **hyoid bone** is a single U-shaped bone suspended in the neck between the mandible and larynx. It is a point of attachment for swallowing and speech muscles.

The trunk of the body consists of the **vertebral column**, **sternum**, and **rib cage**. The vertebral or spinal column is divided into five sections: **cervical vertebrae**, **thoracic vertebrae**, **lumbar vertebrae**, **sacrum**, and **coccyx** (see Figure 4.6 ■ and Table 4.2 ■). Located between each pair of vertebrae, from the cervical through the lumbar regions, is an **intervertebral disc**. Each disc is composed of fibrocartilage to provide a cushion between the vertebrae. The rib cage has twelve pairs of ribs attached at the back to the vertebral column. Ten of the pairs are also attached to the sternum in the front (see Figure 4.7 ■). The lowest two pairs are called *floating ribs* and are attached only to the vertebral column. The rib cage serves to provide support for organs, such as the heart and lungs.

Med Term Tip

The term *coccyx* comes from the Greek word for the cuckoo because the shape of these small bones extending off the sacrum resembles this bird's bill.

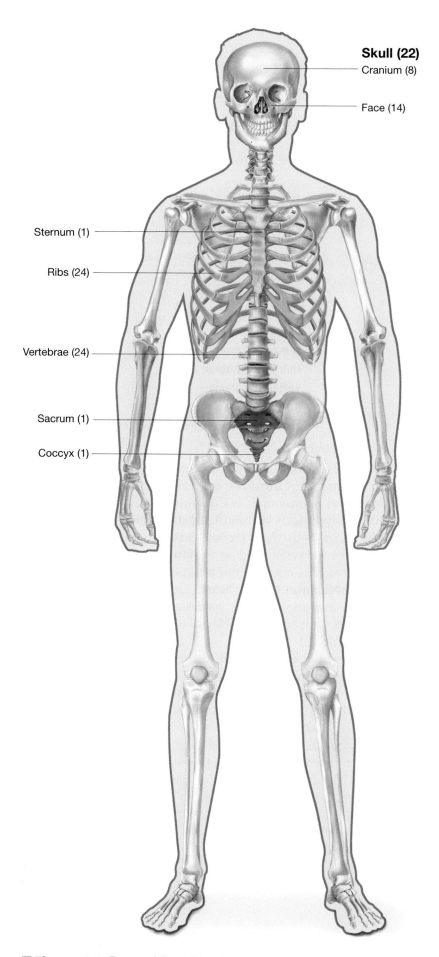

Skull (22)
Cranium (8)

Face (14)

Sternum (1)

Ribs (24)

Vertebrae (24)

Sacrum (1)

Coccyx (1)

■ **Figure 4.4** Bones of the axial skeleton.

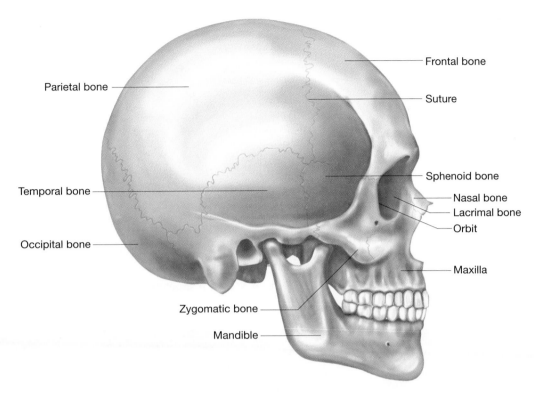

Figure 4.5 Bones of the skull.

Table 4.1	Bones of the Skull	
NAME	**NUMBER**	**DESCRIPTION**
Cranial Bones		
Frontal bone	1	Forehead
Parietal bone	2	Upper sides of cranium and roof of skull
Occipital bone	1	Back and base of skull
Temporal bone	2	Sides and base of cranium
Sphenoid bone	1	Bat-shaped bone that forms part of the base of the skull, floor, and sides of eye orbit
Ethmoid bone	1	Forms part of eye orbit, nose, and floor of cranium
Facial Bones		
Lacrimal bone	2	Inner corner of each eye
Nasal bone	2	Form part of nasal septum and support bridge of nose
Maxilla	1	Upper jaw
Mandible	1	Lower jawbone; only movable bone of the skull
Zygomatic bone	2	Cheekbones
Vomer bone	1	Base of nasal septum
Palatine bone	1	Hard palate (PAH lat) of mouth and floor of the nose

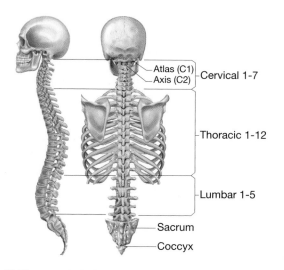

Figure 4.6 Divisions of the vertebral column.

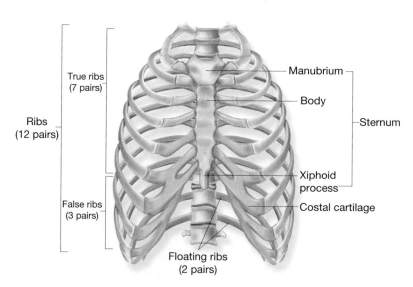

Figure 4.7 The structure of the rib cage.

Table 4.2	Bones of the Vertebral/Spinal Column	
NAME	**NUMBER**	**DESCRIPTION**
Cervical vertebra	7	Vertebrae in the neck region
Thoracic vertebra	12	Vertebrae in the chest region with ribs attached
Lumbar vertebra	5	Vertebrae in the small of the back, about waist level
Sacrum	1	Five vertebrae that become fused into one triangular-shaped flat bone at the base of the vertebral column
Coccyx	1	Three to five very small vertebrae attached to the sacrum, often become fused

Appendicular Skeleton

carpals (CAR-pals)
clavicle (CLAV-ih-kl)
femur (FEE-mer)
fibula (FIB-yoo-lah)
humerus (HYOO-mer-us)
ilium (ILL-ee-um)
innominate bone (ih-NOM-ih-nayt)
ischium (ISS-kee-um)
lower extremities
metacarpals (met-ah-CAR-pals)
metatarsals (met-ah-TAHR-sals)
os coxae (OSS KOK-sigh)

patella (pah-TELL-ah)
pectoral girdle
pelvic girdle
phalanges (fah-LAN-jeez)
pubis (PYOO-bis)
radius (RAY-dee-us)
scapula (SKAP-yoo-lah)
tarsals (TAHR-sals)
tibia (TIB-ee-ah)
ulna (UHL-nah)
upper extremities

Med Term Tip

The term *girdle*, meaning something that encircles or confines, refers to the entire bony structure of the shoulder and the pelvis. If just one bone from these areas is being discussed, like the ilium of the pelvis, it would be named as such. If, however, the entire pelvis is being discussed, it would be called the pelvic girdle.

The appendicular skeleton consists of the **pectoral girdle, upper extremities, pelvic girdle,** and **lower extremities** (see Figure 4.8 ■). These are the bones for our appendages or limbs and along with the muscles attached to them, they are responsible for body movement.

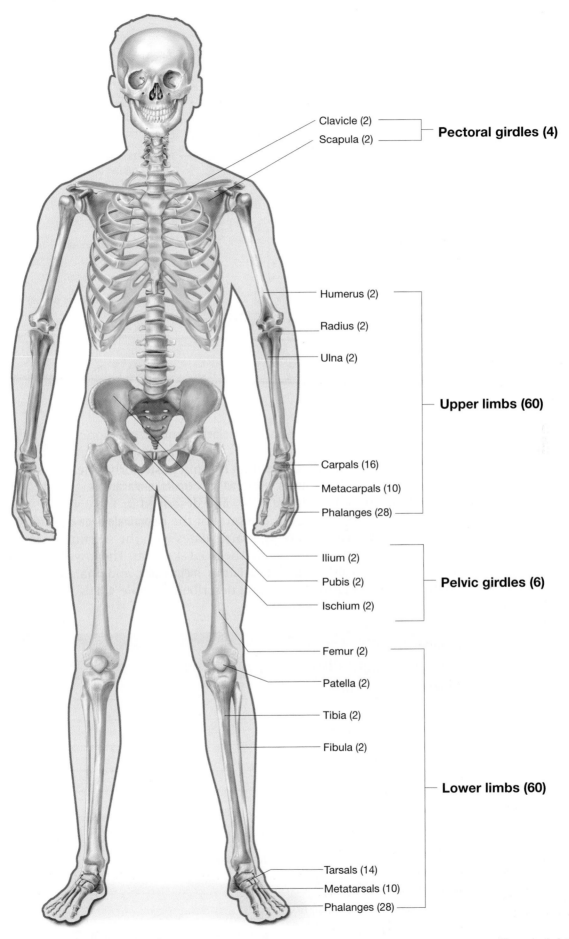

Pectoral girdles (4)
- Clavicle (2)
- Scapula (2)

Upper limbs (60)
- Humerus (2)
- Radius (2)
- Ulna (2)
- Carpals (16)
- Metacarpals (10)
- Phalanges (28)

Pelvic girdles (6)
- Ilium (2)
- Pubis (2)
- Ischium (2)

Lower limbs (60)
- Femur (2)
- Patella (2)
- Tibia (2)
- Fibula (2)
- Tarsals (14)
- Metatarsals (10)
- Phalanges (28)

Figure 4.8 Bones of the appendicular skeleton.

■ **Figure 4.9**
Anatomical and
common names for the
pectoral girdle and
upper extremity.

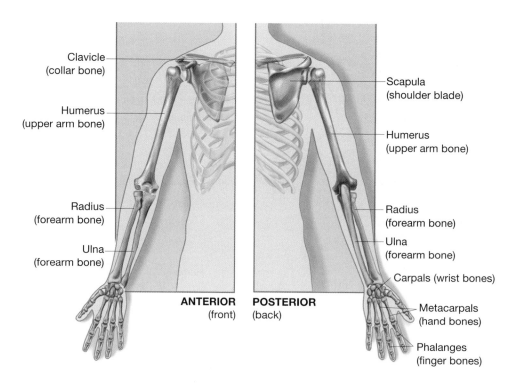

The pectoral girdle consists of the **clavicle** and **scapula** bones. It functions to attach the upper extremity, or arm, to the axial skeleton by articulating with the sternum anteriorly and the vertebral column posteriorly. The bones of the upper extremity include the **humerus, ulna, radius, carpals, metacarpals,** and **phalanges**. These bones are illustrated in Figure 4.9 ■ and described in Table 4.3 ■.

The pelvic girdle is called the **os coxae** or the **innominate bone** or hipbone. It contains the **ilium, ischium,** and **pubis**. It articulates with the sacrum posteriorly to attach the lower extremity, or leg, to the axial skeleton. The lower extremity bones include the **femur, patella, tibia, fibula, tarsals, metatarsals,** and phalanges. These bones are illustrated in Figure 4.10 ■ and described in Table 4.4 ■.

Table 4.3	Bones of the Pectoral Girdle and Upper Extremity	
NAME	**NUMBER**	**DESCRIPTION**
Pectoral Girdle		
Clavicle	2	Collar bone
Scapula	2	Shoulder blade
Upper Extremity		
Humerus	2	Upper arm bone
Radius	2	Forearm bone on thumb side of lower arm
Ulna	2	Forearm bone on little finger side of lower arm
Carpal	16	Bones of wrist
Metacarpals	10	Bones in palm of hand
Phalanges	28	Finger bones; three in each finger and two in each thumb

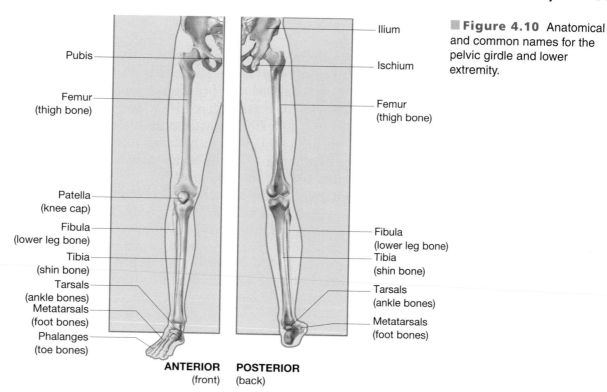

Pubis

Femur
(thigh bone)

Patella
(knee cap)

Fibula
(lower leg bone)

Tibia
(shin bone)

Tarsals
(ankle bones)

Metatarsals
(foot bones)

Phalanges
(toe bones)

Ilium

Ischium

Femur
(thigh bone)

Fibula
(lower leg bone)

Tibia
(shin bone)

Tarsals
(ankle bones)

Metatarsals
(foot bones)

ANTERIOR **POSTERIOR**
(front)   (back)

■ **Figure 4.10** Anatomical and common names for the pelvic girdle and lower extremity.

Joints

articulation (ar-tik-yoo-LAY-shun)

bursa (BER-sah)

cartilaginous joints (car-tih-LAJ-ih-nus)

fibrous joints (FYE-bruss)

joint capsule

synovial fluid

synovial joint (sin-OH-vee-al)

synovial membrane

Joints are formed when two or more bones meet. This is also referred to as an **articulation**. There are three types of joints based on the amount of movement

Table 4.4	Bones of the Pelvic Girdle and Lower Extremity	
NAME	**NUMBER**	**DESCRIPTION**
Pelvic Girdle/Os Coxae		
Ilium	2	Part of the hipbone
Ischium	2	Part of the hipbone
Pubis	2	Part of the hipbone
Lower Extremity		
Femur	2	Upper leg bone; thigh bone
Patella	2	Knee cap
Tibia	2	Shin bone; thicker lower leg bone
Fibula	2	Thinner, long bone in lateral side of lower leg
Tarsals	14	Ankle and heel bones
Metatarsals	10	Forefoot bones
Phalanges	28	Toe bones; three in each toe and two in each great toe

allowed between the bones: **synovial joints**, **cartilaginous joints**, and **fibrous joints** (see Figure 4.11 ■).

Most joints are freely moving synovial joints (see Figure 4.12 ■), which are enclosed by an elastic **joint capsule**. The joint capsule is lined with **synovial membrane**, which secretes **synovial fluid** to lubricate the joint. As noted earlier, the ends of bones in a synovial joint are covered by a layer of articular cartilage. Cartilage is very tough, but still flexible. It withstands high levels of stress to act as a shock absorber for the joint and prevents bone from rubbing against bone. Cartilage is found in several other areas of the body, such as the nasal septum, external ear, eustachian tube, larynx, trachea, bronchi, and intervertebral disks. One example of a synovial joint is the ball-and-socket joint found at the shoulder and hip. The ball rotating in the socket allows for a wide range of motion. Bands of strong connective tissue called ligaments bind bones together at the joint.

Some synovial joints contain a **bursa**, which is a saclike structure composed of connective tissue and lined with synovial membrane. Most commonly found between bones and ligaments or tendons, bursas function to reduce friction. Some common bursa locations are the elbow, knee, and shoulder joints.

Not all joints are freely moving. Fibrous joints allow almost no movement since the ends of the bones are joined by thick fibrous tissue, which may even fuse into solid bone. The sutures of the skull are an example of a fibrous joint. Cartilaginous joints allow for slight movement but hold bones firmly in place by a solid piece of cartilage. An example of this type of joint is the pubic symphysis, the point at which the left and right pubic bones meet in the front of the lower abdomen.

Med Term Tip

Bursitis is an inflammation of the bursa located between bony prominences such as at the shoulder. Housemaid's knee, a term thought to have originated from the damage to the knees that occurred when maids knelt to scrub floors, is a form of bursitis and carries the medical name *prepatellar bursitis*.

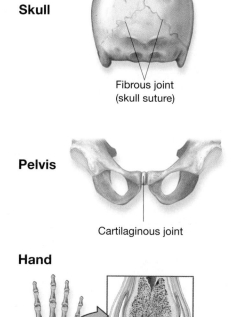

Skull

Fibrous joint
(skull suture)

Pelvis

Cartilaginous joint

Hand

Synovial joint

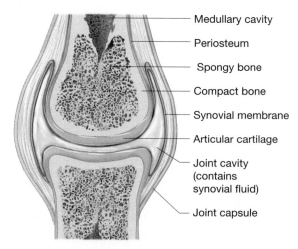

Medullary cavity

Periosteum

Spongy bone

Compact bone

Synovial membrane

Articular cartilage

Joint cavity
(contains
synovial fluid)

Joint capsule

■ **Figure 4.11** Examples of three types of joints found in the body.

■ **Figure 4.12** Structure of a generalized synovial joint.

Word Building

The following list contains examples of medical terms built directly from word parts. The definition for these terms can be determined by a straightforward translation of the word parts.

COMBINING FORM	COMBINED WITH	MEDICAL TERM	DEFINITION
arthr/o	-algia	**arthralgia** (ar-THRAL-jee-ah)	joint pain
	-centesis	**arthrocentesis** (ar-thro-sen-TEE-sis)	puncture to withdraw fluid from a joint
	-clasia	**arthroclasia** (ar-throh-KLAY-see-ah)	surgically breaking a joint
	-desis	**arthrodesis** (ar-throh-DEE-sis)	fusion of a joint
	-gram	**arthrogram** (AR-throh-gram)	record of a joint
	-itis	**arthritis** (ar-THRY-tis)	joint inflammation
	-otomy	**arthrotomy** (ar-THROT-oh-mee)	incision into a joint
	-scope	**arthroscope** (AR-throw-skop)	instrument to view inside a joint
burs/o	-ectomy	**bursectomy** (ber-SEK-toh-mee)	removal of a bursa
	-itis	**bursitis** (ber-SIGH-tis)	inflammation of a bursa
chondr/o	-ectomy	**chondrectomy** (kon-DREK-toh-mee)	removal of cartilage
	-malacia	**chondromalacia** (kon-droh-mah-LAY-she-ah)	cartilage softening
	-oma	**chondroma** (kon-DROH-mah)	cartilage tumor
	-plasty	**chondroplasty** (KON-droh-plas-tee)	surgical repair of cartilage
cortic/o	-al	**cortical** (KOR-ti-kal)	pertaining to the outer portion
crani/o	intra- -al	**intracranial** (in-trah-KRAY-nee-al)	pertaining to inside the skull
	-otomy	**craniotomy** (kray-nee-OTT-oh-mee)	incision into the skull
medull/o	-ary	**medullary** (MED-you-lair-ee)	pertaining to the inner portion
myel/o	-oma	**myeloma** (my-ah-LOH-mah)	bone marrow tumor
oste/o	-algia	**ostealgia** (oss-tee-AL-jee-ah)	bone pain
	chondr/o -oma	**osteochondroma** (oss-tee-oh-kon-DROH-mah)	bone and cartilage tumor
	-clasia	**osteoclasia** (oss-tee-oh-KLAY-see-ah)	to surgically break a bone
	myel/o -itis	**osteomyelitis** (oss-tee-oh-mi-ell-EYE-tis)	inflammation of bone and bone marrow
	-otomy	**osteotomy** (oss-tee-OTT-ah-me)	incision into a bone
	-pathy	**osteopathy** (oss-tee-OPP-ah-thee)	bone disease
	-tome	**osteotome** (OSS-tee-oh-tohm)	instrument to cut bone
synov/o	-itis	**synovitis** (sih-no-VI-tis)	inflammation of synovial membrane
	-ectomy	**synovectomy** (sih-no-VEK-toh-mee)	removal of the synovial membrane
vertebr/o	inter- -al	**intervertebral** (in-ter-VER-teh-bral)	pertaining to between vertebrae

Building Adjective Forms of Bone Names

It is important to learn the names and combining forms of all the bones in medical terminology because they are so frequently used as adjectives to indicate location.

ADJECTIVE SUFFIX	COMBINED WITH	ADJECTIVE FORM	NOUN FORM
-ac	ili/o	**iliac** (ILL-ee-ack)	ilium
-al	carp/o	**carpal** (CAR-pal)	carpus
	cervic/o	**cervical** (CER-vih-kal)	neck
	cost/o	**costal** (COAST-all)	rib
	crani/o	**cranial** (KRAY-nee-all)	cranium
	femor/o	**femoral** (FEM-or-all)	femur
	humer/o	**humeral** (HYOO-mer-all)	humerus
	ischi/o	**ischial** (ISH-ee-all)	ischium
	metacarp/o	**metacarpal** (met-ah-CAR-pal)	metacarpus
	metatars/o	**metatarsal** (met-ah-TAHR-sal)	metatarsus
	radi/o	**radial** (RAY-dee-all)	radius
	sacr/o	**sacral** (SAY-kral)	sacrum
	stern/o	**sternal** (STER-nal)	sternum
	tars/o	**tarsal** (TAHR-sal)	tarsus
	tibi/o	**tibial** (TIB-ee-all)	tibia
-ar	clavicul/o	**clavicular** (cla-VIK-yoo-lar)	clavicle
	fibul/o	**fibular** (FIB-yoo-lar)	fibula
	lumb/o	**lumbar** (LUM-bar)	low back
	mandibul/o	**mandibular** (man-DIB-yoo-lar)	mandible
	patell/o	**patellar** (pa-TELL-ar)	patella
	scapul/o	**scapular** (SKAP-yoo-lar)	scapula
	uln/o	**ulnar** (UHL-nar)	ulna
-ary	maxill/o	**maxillary** (mack-sih-LAIR-ree)	maxilla
-eal	coccyg/o	**coccygeal** (cock-eh-JEE-all)	coccyx
	phalang/o	**phalangeal** (fay-lan-JEE-all)	phalanges
-ic	pelv/o	**pelvic** (PEL-vik)	pelvis
	pub/o	**pubic** (PYOO-bik)	pubis
	thorac/o	**thoracic** (tho-RASS-ik)	thorax

Vocabulary

TERM	DEFINITION
callus (KAL-us)	The mass of bone tissue that forms at a fracture site during its healing.
cast	Application of a solid material to immobilize an extremity or portion of the body as a result of a fracture, dislocation, or severe injury. It may be made of plaster of Paris or fiberglass.
chiropractic (ki-roh-PRAK-tik)	Healthcare profession concerned with diagnosis and treatment of malalignment conditions of the spine and musculoskeletal system with the intention of affecting the nervous system and improving health. Healthcare professional is a *chiropractor*.
crepitation (krep-ih-TAY-shun)	The noise produced by bones or cartilage rubbing together in conditions such as arthritis. Also called *crepitus*.
exostosis (eck-sos-TOH-sis)	A bone spur.
kyphosis (ki-FOH-sis)	Abnormal increase in the outward curvature of the thoracic spine. Also known as *hunchback* or *humpback*. See Figure 4.13 ■ for an illustration of abnormal spine curvatures.

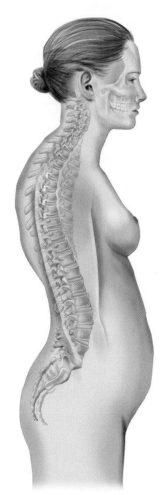 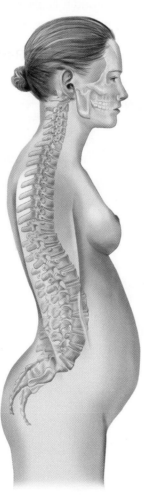 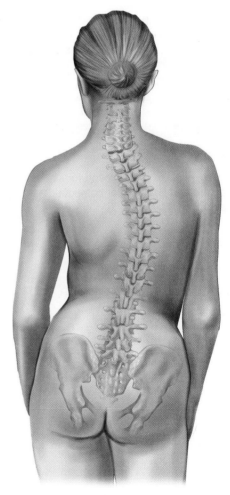

Kyphosis
(excessive posterior thoracic
curvature - hunchback)

Lordosis
(excessive anterior lumbar
curvature - swayback)

Scoliosis
(lateral curvature)

■ **Figure 4.13** Abnormal spinal curvatures: kyphosis, lordosis, and scoliosis.

Vocabulary *(continued)*

TERM	DEFINITION
lordosis (lor-DOH-sis)	Abnormal increase in the forward curvature of the lumbar spine. Also known as *swayback*. See Figure 4.13 for an illustration of abnormal spine curvatures.
orthopedics (or-thoh-PEE-diks)	Branch of medicine specializing in the diagnosis and treatment of conditions of the musculoskeletal system. Also called *orthopedic surgery*. Physician is an *orthopedist* or *orthopedic surgeon*. Name derived from straightening (*orth/o*) deformities in children (*ped/o*).
orthotic (or-THOT-ik)	A brace or splint used to prevent or correct deformities. Person skilled in making and adjusting orthotics is an *orthotist*.
podiatry (po-DYE-ah-tree)	Healthcare profession specializing in diagnosis and treatment of disorders of the feet and lower legs. Healthcare professional is a *podiatrist*.
prosthesis (pross-THEE-sis)	Artificial device that is used as a substitute for a body part that is either congenitally missing or absent as a result of accident or disease. An example would be an artificial leg.
prosthetics (pross-THET-iks)	Healthcare profession specializing in making artificial body parts. Person skilled in making and adjusting prostheses is a *prosthetist*.

Pathology

TERM	DEFINITION
■ *Fractures*	
closed fracture	Fracture in which there is no open skin wound. Also called a *simple fracture*.

■ **Figure 4.14** A) Closed (or simple) fracture and B) open (or compound) fracture.

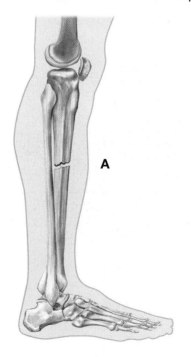
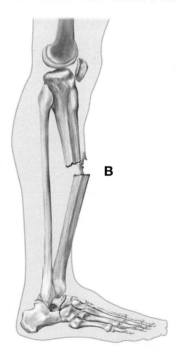

Pathology *(continued)*

TERM	DEFINITION
Colles' (COL-eez) **fracture** ■ **Figure 4.15** Colles' fracture. *(Charles Stewart MD FACEP, FAAEM)*	A common type of wrist fracture. 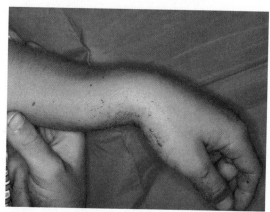
comminuted fracture (kom-ih-NYOOT-ed)	Fracture in which the bone is shattered, splintered, or crushed into many small pieces or fragments.
compound fracture	Fracture in which the skin has been broken through to the fracture. Also called an *open fracture* (see also Figure 4.14B).
compression fracture	Fracture involving loss of height of a vertebral body. It may be the result of trauma, but in older persons, especially women, it may be caused by conditions like osteoporosis.
fracture (FX, Fx)	A broken bone.
greenstick fracture	Fracture in which there is an incomplete break; one side of bone is broken and the other side is bent. This type of fracture is commonly found in children due to their softer and more pliable bone structure.
impacted fracture	Fracture in which bone fragments are pushed into each other.
oblique (oh-BLEEK) **fracture** ■ **Figure 4.16** X-ray showing oblique fracture of the humerus. *(Charles Stewart MD FACEP, FAAEM)*	Fracture at an angle to the bone. 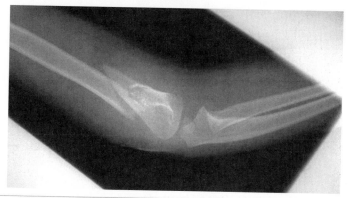
pathologic (path-a-LOJ-ik) **fracture**	Fracture caused by diseased or weakened bone.
spiral fracture	Fracture in which the fracture line spirals around the shaft of the bone. Can be caused by a twisting injury and is often slower to heal than other types of fractures.
stress fracture	A slight fracture caused by repetitive low-impact forces, like running, rather than a single forceful impact.

Pathology *(continued)*

TERM	DEFINITION
transverse fracture	Complete fracture that is straight across the bone at right angles to the long axis of the bone (see Figure 4.17 ■).

■ *Bones*

TERM	DEFINITION
Ewing's sarcoma (YOO-wings sar-KOH-mah)	Malignant growth found in the shaft of long bones that spreads through the periosteum. Removal is treatment of choice, because this tumor will metastasize or spread to other organs.
osteogenic sarcoma (oss-tee-oh-GIN-ik sark-OH-mah)	The most common type of bone cancer. Usually begins in osteocytes found at the ends of long bones.
osteomalacia (oss-tee-oh-mah-LAY-she-ah)	Softening of the bones caused by a deficiency of calcium. It is thought that in children the cause is insufficient sunlight and vitamin D.
osteoporosis (oss-tee-oh-por-ROH-sis)	Decrease in bone mass that results in a thinning and weakening of the bone with resulting fractures. The bone becomes more porous, especially in the spine and pelvis.
Paget's (PAH-jets) **disease**	A fairly common metabolic disease of the bone from unknown causes. It usually attacks middle-aged and elderly people and is characterized by bone destruction and deformity. Named for Sir James Paget, a British surgeon.
rickets (RIK-ets)	Deficiency in calcium and vitamin D found in early childhood that results in bone deformities, especially bowed legs.

■ *Spinal Column*

TERM	DEFINITION
ankylosing spondylitis (ang-kih-LOH-sing spon-dih-LYE-tis)	Inflammatory spinal condition that resembles rheumatoid arthritis. Results in gradual stiffening and fusion of the vertebrae. More common in men than women.
herniated nucleus pulposus (HNP) (HER-nee-ated NOO-klee-us pull-POH-sus)	Herniation or protrusion of an intervertebral disk; also called *herniated disk* or *ruptured disk.* May require surgery (see Figure 4.18 ■).
scoliosis (skoh-lee-OH-sis)	Abnormal lateral curvature of the spine. See Figure 4.13 for an illustration of abnormal spine curvatures.
spina bifida (SPY-nah BIF-ih-dah)	Congenital anomaly that occurs when a vertebra fails to fully form around the spinal cord.
spinal stenosis (ste-NOH-sis)	Narrowing of the spinal canal causing pressure on the cord and nerves.
spondylolisthesis (spon-dih-loh-liss-THEE-sis)	The forward sliding of a lumbar vertebra over the vertebra below it.
spondylosis (spon-dih-LOH-sis)	Specifically refers to ankylosing of the spine, but commonly used in reference to any degenerative condition of the vertebral column.
whiplash	Injury to the bones in the cervical spine as a result of a sudden movement forward and backward of the head and neck. Can occur as a result of a rear-end auto collision.

■ *Joints*

TERM	DEFINITION
bunion (BUN-yun)	Inflammation of the bursa of the first metatarsophalangeal joint (base of the big toe).

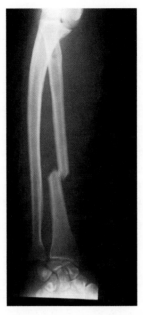

Figure 4.17 X-ray showing transverse fracture of radius. *(James Stevenson/Science Photo Library/ Photo Researchers, Inc.)*

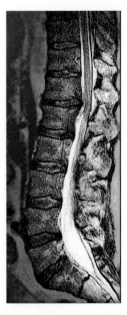

Figure 4.18 Color enhanced magnetic resonance imaging (MRI) image demonstrating a herniated nucleus pulposus putting pressure on the spinal cord (see arrows). *(ISM/Phototake NYC)*

 ## Pathology *(continued)*

TERM	DEFINITION
dislocation	Occurs when the bones in a joint are displaced from their normal alignment and the ends of the bones are no longer in contact.
osteoarthritis (OA) (oss-tee-oh-ar-THRY-tis)	Arthritis resulting in degeneration of the bones and joints, especially those bearing weight. Results in bone rubbing against bone.
rheumatoid arthritis (RA) (ROO-mah-toyd ar-THRY-tis) **Figure 4.19** Patient with typical rheumatoid arthritis contractures.	Chronic form of arthritis with inflammation of the joints, swelling, stiffness, pain, and changes in the cartilage that can result in crippling deformities; considered to be an autoimmune disease. *(Michal Heron/Pearson Education/PH College)*
sprain	Damage to the ligaments surrounding a joint due to overstretching, but no dislocation of the joint or fracture of the bone.
subluxation (sub-LUCKS-a-shun)	An incomplete dislocation, the joint alignment is disrupted, but the ends of the bones remain in contact.
systemic lupus erythematosus (SLE) (sis-TEM-ik LOOP-us air-ih-them-ah-TOH-sis)	Chronic inflammatory autoimmune disease of connective tissue affects many systems that may include joint pain and arthritis. May be mistaken for rheumatoid arthritis.
talipes (TAL-ih-peez)	Congenital deformity causing misalignment of the ankle joint and foot. Also referred to as a *clubfoot*.

Diagnostic Procedures

TERM	DEFINITION
■ *Diagnostic Imaging*	
arthrography (ar-THROG-rah-fee)	Visualization of a joint by radiographic study after injection of a contrast medium into the joint space.
bone scan	A nuclear medicine procedure in which the patient is given a radioactive dye and then scanning equipment is used to visualize bones. It is especially useful in identifying stress fractures, observing progress of treatment for osteomyelitis and locating cancer metastases to the bone.
dual-energy absorptiometry (DXA) (ab-sorp-she-AHM-eh-tree)	Measurement of bone density using low dose x-ray for the purpose of detecting osteoporosis.
myelography (my-eh-LOG-rah-fee)	Study of the spinal column after injecting opaque contrast material; particularly useful in identifying herniated nucleus pulposus pinching a spinal nerve.
radiography	A diagnostic imaging procedure using x-rays to study the internal structure of the body; especially useful for visualizing bones and joints.
■ *Endoscopic Procedures*	
arthroscopy (ar-THROS-koh-pee)	Examination of the interior of a joint by entering the joint with an *arthroscope*. The arthroscope contains a small television camera that allows the physician to view the interior of the joint on a monitor during the procedure. Some joint conditions can be repaired during arthroscopy.

 # Therapeutic Procedures

TERM	DEFINITION
■ *Surgical Procedures*	
amputation (am-pew-TAY-shun)	Partial or complete removal of a limb for a variety of reasons, including tumors, gangrene, intractable pain, crushing injury, or uncontrollable infection.
arthroscopic surgery (ar-throh-SKOP-ic)	Performing a surgical procedure while using an arthroscope to view the internal structure, such as a joint.
bone graft	Piece of bone taken from the patient used to take the place of a removed bone or a bony defect at another site.
bunionectomy (bun-yun-ECK-toh-mee)	Removal of the bursa at the joint of the great toe.
laminectomy (lam-ih-NEK-toh-mee)	Removal of the vertebral posterior arch to correct severe back problems and pain caused by compression of a spinal nerve.
percutaneous diskectomy (per-kyou-TAY-nee-us disk-EK-toh-mee)	A thin catheter tube is inserted into the intervertebral disk through the skin and the herniated or ruptured disk material is sucked out or a laser is used to vaporize it.
spinal fusion	Surgical immobilization of adjacent vertebrae. This may be done for several reasons, including correction for a herniated disk.
total hip arthroplasty (THA) (ar-thro-PLAS-tee)	Surgical reconstruction of a hip by implanting a prosthetic or artificial hip joint. Also called *total hip replacement (THR)* (see Figure 4.20 ■).

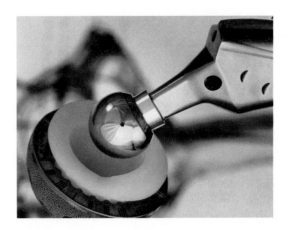

■ Figure 4.20 Prosthetic hip joint.
(Lawrence Livermore National Library/Science Photo Library/Photo Researchers, Inc.)

■ Therapeutic Procedures *(continued)*

TERM	DEFINITION
total knee arthroplasty (TKA) (ar-thro-PLAS-tee)	Surgical reconstruction of a knee joint by implanting a prosthetic knee joint. Also called *total knee replacement (TKR)*.
■ Fracture Care	
fixation	A procedure to stabilize a fractured bone while it heals. *External fixation* includes casts, splints, and pins inserted through the skin. *Internal fixation* includes pins, plates, rods, screws, and wires that are applied during an *open reduction*.
reduction	Correcting a fracture by realigning the bone fragments. *Closed reduction* is doing this manipulation without entering the body. *Open reduction* is the process of making a surgical incision at the site of the fracture to do the reduction. This is necessary when bony fragments need to be removed or *internal fixation* such as plates or pins are required.
traction	Applying a pulling force on a fractured or dislocated limb or the vertebral column in order to restore normal alignment.

■ Pharmacology

CLASSIFICATION	ACTION	GENERIC AND BRAND NAMES
bone reabsorption inhibitors	Conditions that result in weak and fragile bones, such as osteoporosis and Paget's disease, are improved by medications that reduce the reabsorption of bones.	alendronate, Fosamax; ibandronate, Boniva
calcium supplements and Vitamin D therapy	Maintaining high blood levels of calcium in association with vitamin D helps maintain bone density; used to treat osteomalacia, osteoporosis, and rickets.	calcium carbonate, Oystercal, Tums; calcium citrate, Cal-Citrate, Citracal
corticosteroids	A hormone produced by the adrenal cortex that has very strong anti-inflammatory properties. It is particularly useful in treating rheumatoid arthritis.	prednisone; methylprednisolone, Medrol; dexamethasone, Decadron
nonsteroidal anti-inflammatory drugs (NSAIDs)	A large group of drugs that provide mild pain relief and anti-inflammatory benefits for conditions such as arthritis.	ibuprofen, Advil, Motrin; naproxen, Aleve, Naprosyn; salicylates, Aspirin

Abbreviations

AE	above elbow
AK	above knee
BDT	bone density testing
BE	below elbow
BK	below knee
BMD	bone mineral density
C1, C2, etc.	first cervical vertebra, second cervical vertebra, etc.
Ca	calcium
DJD	degenerative joint disease
DXA	dual-energy absorptiometry
FX, Fx	fracture
HNP	herniated nucleus pulposus
JRA	juvenile rheumatoid arthritis
L1, L2, etc.	first lumbar vertebra, second lumbar vertebra, etc.
LE	lower extremity
LLE	left lower extremity
LUE	left upper extremity
NSAID	nonsteroidal anti-inflammatory drug
OA	osteoarthritis
ORIF	open reduction–internal fixation
Orth, ortho	orthopedics
RA	rheumatoid arthritis
RLE	right lower extremity
RUE	right upper extremity
SLE	systemic lupus erythematosus
T1, T2, etc.	first thoracic vertebra, second thoracic vertebra, etc.
THA	total hip arthroplasty
THR	total hip replacement
TKA	total knee arthroplasty
TKR	total knee replacement
UE	upper extremity

Section II: Muscular System at a Glance

Function

Muscles are bundles, sheets, or rings of tissue that produce movement by contracting and pulling on the structures to which they are attached.

Organs

muscles

Combining Forms

fasci/o	fibrous band
fibr/o	fibers
kinesi/o	movement
muscul/o	muscle
my/o	muscle
myocardi/o	heart muscle
myos/o	muscle
plant/o	sole of foot
ten/o	tendon
tend/o	tendon
tendin/o	tendon

Suffixes

-asthenia	weakness
-kinesia	movement
-tonia	tone

Prefixes

ab-	away from
ad-	toward
circum-	around

Muscular System Illustrated

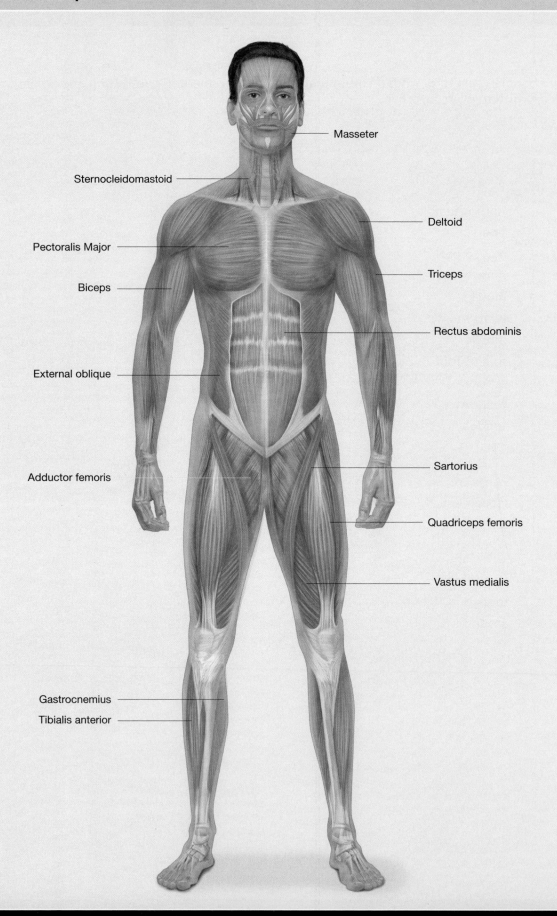

Masseter

Sternocleidomastoid

Deltoid

Pectoralis Major

Triceps

Biceps

Rectus abdominis

External oblique

Sartorius

Adductor femoris

Quadriceps femoris

Vastus medialis

Gastrocnemius

Tibialis anterior

Anatomy and Physiology of the Muscular System

muscle tissue fibers   **muscles**

Muscles are bundles of parallel **muscle tissue fibers**. As these fibers contract (shorten in length) they produce movement of or within the body. The movement may take the form of bringing two bones closer together, pushing food through the digestive system, or pumping blood through blood vessels. In addition to producing movement, muscles also hold the body erect and generate heat.

Types of Muscles

cardiac muscle   **smooth muscle**
involuntary muscles   **voluntary muscles**
skeletal muscle

The three types of muscle tissue are **skeletal muscle**, **smooth muscle**, and **cardiac muscle** (see Figure 4.21 ■). Muscle tissue may be either voluntary or involuntary. **Voluntary muscles** mean that a person consciously chooses which muscles to contract and how long and how hard to contract them. The skeletal muscles of the arm and leg are examples of this type of muscle. **Involuntary muscles** are under the control of the subconscious regions of the brain. The smooth muscles found in internal organs and cardiac muscles are examples of involuntary muscle tissue.

> **Med Term Tip**
>
> The term *muscle* is the diminutive form of the Latin word *mus* or "little mouse." This is thought to describe how the skin ripples when a muscle contracts, like a little mouse running.

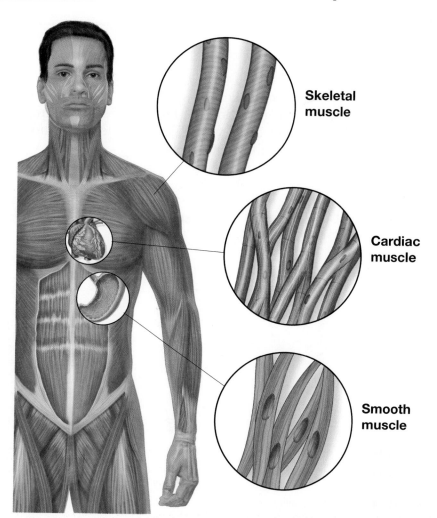

■ **Figure 4.21** The three types of muscles: skeletal, smooth, and cardiac.

Skeletal muscle

Cardiac muscle

Smooth muscle

Skeletal Muscle

fascia (FASH-ee-ah)
motor neurons
myoneural junction (MY-oh-NOO-rall)

striated muscle (stry-a-ted)
tendon (TEN-dun)

Skeletal muscles are directly or indirectly attached to bones and produce voluntary movement of the skeleton. It is also referred to as **striated muscle** because of its striped appearance under the microscope (see Figure 4.22 ■). Each muscle is wrapped in layers of fibrous connective tissue called **fascia**. The fascia tapers at each end of a skeletal muscle to form a very strong **tendon**. The tendon then inserts into the periosteum covering a bone to anchor the muscle to the bone. Skeletal muscles are stimulated by **motor neurons** of the nervous system. The point at which the motor nerve contacts a muscle fiber is called the **myoneural junction**.

Smooth Muscle

visceral muscle (vis-she-ral)

Smooth muscle tissue is found in association with internal organs. For this reason, it is also referred to as **visceral muscle**. The name smooth muscle refers to the muscle's microscopic appearance—it lacks the striations of skeletal muscle (see Figure 4.22). Smooth muscle is found in the walls of the hollow organs, such as the stomach, tube-shaped organs, such as the respiratory airways, and blood vessels. It is responsible for the involuntary muscle action associated with movement of the internal organs, such as churning food, constricting a blood vessel, and uterine contractions.

Cardiac Muscle

myocardium (my-oh-CAR-dee-um)

Cardiac muscle, or **myocardium**, makes up the wall of the heart (see Figure 4.22). With each involuntary contraction the heart squeezes to pump blood out of its chambers and through the blood vessels. This muscle will be more thoroughly described in Chapter 5, Cardiovascular System.

■ **Figure 4.22** Characteristics of the three types of muscles.

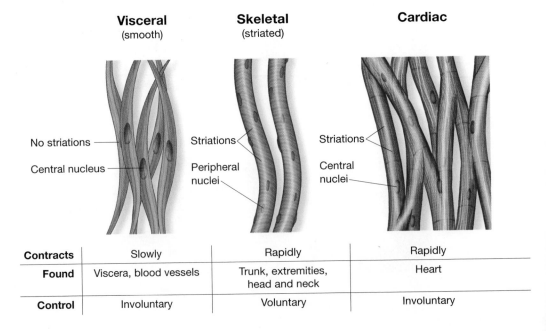

	Visceral (smooth)	Skeletal (striated)	Cardiac
Contracts	Slowly	Rapidly	Rapidly
Found	Viscera, blood vessels	Trunk, extremities, head and neck	Heart
Control	Involuntary	Voluntary	Involuntary

Naming Skeletal Muscles

biceps (BYE-seps)

extensor carpi

external oblique

flexor carpi

gluteus maximus (GLOO-tee-us MACKS-ih-mus)

rectus abdominis (REK-tus ab-DOM-ih-nis)

sternocleidomastoid (STER-noh-KLY-doh-MASS-toid)

The name of a muscle often reflects its location, origin and insertion, size, action, fiber direction, or number of attachment points, as the following examples illustrate.

- **Location:** The term **rectus abdominis** means straight (rectus) abdominal muscle.
- **Origin and insertion:** The **sternocleidomastoid** is named for its two origins (stern/o for sternum and cleid/o for clavicle) and single insertion (mastoid process).
- **Size:** When gluteus, meaning rump area, is combined with maximus, meaning large, we have the term **gluteus maximus**.
- **Action:** The **flexor carpi** and **extensor carpi** muscles are named because they produce flexion and extension at the wrist.
- **Fiber direction:** The **external oblique** muscle is an abdominal muscle whose fibers run at an oblique angle.
- **Number of attachment points:** The term *bi*, meaning two, can form the medical term **biceps**, which refers to the muscle in the upper arm that has two heads or connecting points.

Skeletal Muscle Actions

action

antagonistic pairs

insertion

origin

Skeletal muscles are attached to two different bones and overlap a joint. When a muscle contracts, the two bones move, but not usually equally. The less movable of the two bones is considered to be the starting point of the muscle and is called the **origin**. The more movable bone is considered to be where the muscle ends and is called the **insertion**. The type of movement a muscle produces is called its **action**. Muscles are often arranged around joints in **antagonistic pairs**, meaning they produce opposite actions. For example, one muscle will bend a joint while its antagonist is responsible for straightening the joint. Some common terminology for muscle actions are described in Table 4.5 ■.

Table 4.5   Muscle Actions

ACTION	DESCRIPTION
Grouped by antagonistic pairs	
abduction (ab-DUCK-shun)	Movement away from midline of the body (see Figure 4.23 ■)
adduction (ah-DUCK-shun)	Movement toward midline of the body (see Figure 4.23)
flexion (FLEK-shun)	Act of bending or being bent (see Figure 4.24 ■)
extension (eks-TEN-shun)	Movement that brings limb into or toward a straight condition (see Figure 4.24)
dorsiflexion (dor-see-FLEK-shun)	Backward bending, as of hand or foot (see Figure 4.25A ■)
plantar flexion (PLAN-tar-FLEK-shun)	Bending sole of foot; pointing toes downward (see Figure 4.25B ■)

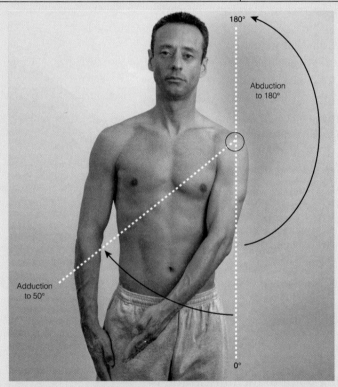

■ **Figure 4.23** Abduction and adduction of the shoulder joint.

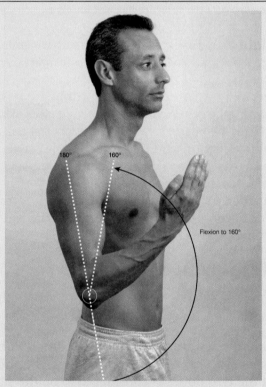

■ **Figure 4.24** Flexion and extension of the elbow joint.

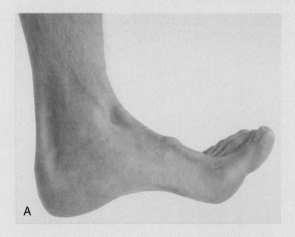

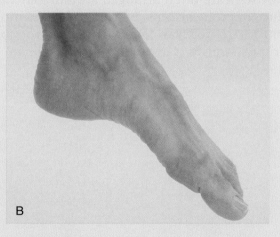

■ **Figure 4.25** Dorsiflexion (a) and plantar flexion (b) of the ankle joint.

Table 4.5	Muscle Actions (continued)
ACTION	**DESCRIPTION**
eversion (ee-VER-zhun)	Turning outward (see Figure 4.26 ■)
inversion (in-VER-zhun)	Turning inward (see Figure 4.26)
pronation (proh-NAY-shun)	To turn downward or backward as with the hand or foot (see Figure 4.27 ■)
supination (soo-pin-NAY-shun)	Turning the palm or foot upward (see Figure 4.27)
elevation	To raise a body part, as in shrugging the shoulders
depression	A downward movement, as in dropping the shoulders
	The circular actions described below are an exception to the antagonistic pair arrangement
circumduction (sir-kum-DUCK-shun)	Movement in a circular direction from a central point. Imagine drawing a large circle in the air
opposition	Moving thumb away from palm; the ability to move the thumb into contact with the other fingers **Med Term Tip** Primates are the only animals with opposable thumbs.
rotation	Moving around a central axis

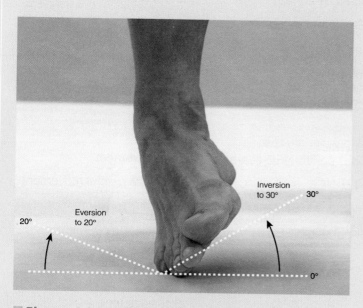

■ **Figure 4.26** Eversion and inversion of the foot.

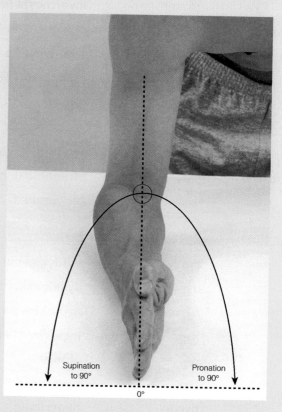

■ **Figure 4.27** Pronation and supination of the forearm.

Word Building

The following list contains examples of medical terms built directly from word parts. The definition for these terms can be determined by a straightforward translation of the word parts.

COMBINING FORM	COMBINED WITH SUFFIX	MEDICAL TERM	DEFINITION
fasci/o	-al	**fascial** (FAS-ee-all)	pertaining to fascia
	-itis	**fasciitis** (fas-ee-EYE-tis)	inflammation of fascia
	-otomy	**fasciotomy** (fas-ee-OT-oh-mee)	incision into fascia
kinesi/o	-logy	**kinesiology** (kih-NEE-see-oh-loh-jee)	study of movement
muscul/o	-ar	**muscular** (MUSS-kew-lar)	pertaining to muscles
my/o	-algia	**myalgia** (my-AL-jee-ah)	muscle pain
	-asthenia	**myasthenia** (my-ass-THEE-nee-ah)	muscle weakness
	electr/o -gram	**electromyogram** (EMG) (ee-lek-troh-MY-oh-gram)	record of muscle electricity
	cardi/o -al	**myocardial** (my-oh-CAR-dee-al)	pertaining to heart muscle
	-pathy	**myopathy** (my-OPP-ah-thee)	muscle disease
	-plasty	**myoplasty** (MY-oh-plas-tee)	surgical repair of muscle
	-rrhaphy	**myorrhaphy** (MY-or-ah-fee)	suture a muscle
	-rrhexis	**myorrhexis** (my-oh-REK-sis)	muscle rupture
myos/o	poly- -itis	**polymyositis** (pol-ee-my-oh-SIGH-tis)	inflammation of many muscles
ten/o	-dynia	**tenodynia** (ten-oh-DIN-ee-ah)	tendon pain
	-plasty	**tenoplasty** (TEN-oh-plas-tee)	surgical repair of a tendon
	-rrhaphy	**tenorrhaphy** (tah-NOR-ah-fee)	suture a tendon
tend/o	-plasty	**tendoplasty** (TEN-doh-plas-tee)	surgical repair of tendon
	-otomy	**tendotomy** (tend-OT-oh-mee)	incision into tendon
tendin/o	-itis	**tendinitis** (ten-dih-NIGH-tis)	inflammation of tendon
	-ous	**tendinous** (TEN-din-us)	pertaining to tendons

SUFFIX	COMBINED WITH PREFIX	MEDICAL TERM	DEFINITION
-kinesia	brady-	**bradykinesia** (brad-ee-kih-NEE-see-ah)	slow movement
	dys-	**dyskinesia** (dis-kih-NEE-see-ah)	difficult or painful movement
	hyper-	**hyperkinesia** (high-per-kih-NEE-see-ah)	excessive movement
	hypo-	**hypokinesia** (HI-poh-kih-NEE-see-ah)	insufficient movement
-tonia	a-	**atonia**	lack of tone
	dys-	**dystonia**	abnormal tone
	hyper-	**hypertonia**	excessive tone
	hypo-	**hypotonia**	insufficient tone
	my/o	**myotonia**	muscle tone

Vocabulary

TERM	DEFINITION
adhesion	Scar tissue forming in the fascia surrounding a muscle, making it difficult to stretch the muscle.
atrophy (AT-rah-fee)	Poor muscle development as a result of muscle disease, nervous system disease, or lack of use; commonly referred to as *muscle wasting.*
contracture (kon-TRACK-chur)	Abnormal shortening of muscle fibers, tendons, or fascia making it difficult to stretch the muscle.
hypertrophy (high-PER-troh-fee)	Increase in muscle bulk as a result of using it, as in lifting weights
intermittent claudication (klaw-dih-KAY-shun)	Attacks of severe pain and lameness caused by ischemia of the muscles, typically the calf muscles; brought on by walking even very short distances.
spasm	Sudden, involuntary, strong muscle contraction.
torticollis (tore-tih-KOLL-iss)	Severe neck spasms pulling the head to one side. Commonly called *wryneck* or a *crick in the neck.*

Pathology

TERM	DEFINITION
■ *Muscles*	
fibromyalgia (figh-broh-my-AL-jee-ah)	Condition with widespread aching and pain in the muscles and soft tissue.
lateral epicondylitis (ep-ih-kon-dih-LYE-tis)	Inflammation of the muscle attachment to the lateral epicondyle of the elbow. Often caused by strongly gripping. Commonly called *tennis elbow.*
muscular dystrophy (MD) (MUSS-kew-ler DIS-troh-fee)	Inherited disease causing a progressive muscle degeneration, weakness, and atrophy.
pseudohypertrophic muscular dystrophy (soo-doh-HIGH-per-troh-fic)	One type of inherited muscular dystrophy in which the muscle tissue is gradually replaced by fatty tissue, making the muscle look strong. Also called *Duchenne's muscular dystrophy.*
■ *Tendons, Muscles, and/or Ligaments*	
carpal tunnel syndrome (CTS)	Repetitive motion disorder with pain caused by compression of the finger flexor tendons and median nerve as they pass through the carpal tunnel of the wrist.
ganglion cyst (GANG-lee-on)	Cyst that forms on tendon sheath, usually on hand, wrist, or ankle.
repetitive motion disorder	Group of chronic disorders involving the tendon, muscle, joint, and nerve damage, resulting from the tissue being subjected to pressure, vibration, or repetitive movements for prolonged periods.
rotator cuff injury	The rotator cuff consists of the joint capsule of the shoulder joint reinforced by the tendons from several shoulder muscles. The high degree of flexibility at the shoulder joint puts the rotator cuff at risk for strain and tearing.
strain	Damage to the muscle, tendons, or ligaments due to overuse or overstretching.

Diagnostic Procedures

TERM	DEFINITION
■ *Clinical Laboratory Test*	
creatine phosphokinase (CPK) (KREE-ah-teen foss-foe-KYE-nase)	Muscle enzyme found in skeletal muscle and cardiac muscle. Blood levels become elevated in disorders such as heart attack, muscular dystrophy, and other skeletal muscle pathologies.
■ *Additional Diagnostic Procedures*	
deep tendon reflexes (DTR)	Muscle contraction in response to a stretch caused by striking the muscle tendon with a reflex hammer. Test used to determine if muscles are responding properly.
electromyography (EMG) (ee-lek-troh-my-OG-rah-fee)	Study and record of the strength and quality of muscle contractions as a result of electrical stimulation.
muscle biopsy (BYE-op-see)	Removal of muscle tissue for pathological examination.

Treatment Procedures

TERM	DEFINITION
■ *Surgical Procedures*	
carpal tunnel release	Surgical cutting of the ligament in the wrist to relieve nerve pressure caused by carpal tunnel syndrome, which can result from repetitive motion such as typing.
tenodesis (ten-oh-DEE-sis)	Surgical procedure to stabilize a joint by anchoring down the tendons of the muscles that move the joint.

Pharmacology

CLASSIFICATION	ACTION	GENERIC AND BRAND NAMES
skeletal muscle relaxants	Medication to relax skeletal muscles in order to reduce muscle spasms. Also called *antispasmodics*.	cyclobenzaprine, Flexeril; carisoprodol, Soma

Abbreviations

CTS	carpal tunnel syndrome	**EMG**	electromyogram
CPK	creatine phosphokinase	**IM**	intramuscular
DTR	deep tendon reflex	**MD**	muscular dystrophy

Chapter Review

Terminology Checklist

 Below are all Anatomy and Physiology key terms, Word Building, Vocabulary, Pathology, Diagnostic, Therapeutic, and Pharmacology terms presented in this chapter. Use this list as a study tool by placing a check in the box in front of each term as you master its meaning.

- ☐ abduction
- ☐ action
- ☐ adduction
- ☐ adhesion
- ☐ amputation
- ☐ ankylosing spondylitis
- ☐ antagonistic pairs
- ☐ appendicular skeleton
- ☐ arthralgia
- ☐ arthritis
- ☐ arthrocentesis
- ☐ arthroclasia
- ☐ arthrodesis
- ☐ arthrogram
- ☐ arthrography
- ☐ arthroscope
- ☐ arthroscopic surgery
- ☐ arthroscopy
- ☐ arthrotomy
- ☐ articular cartilage
- ☐ articulation
- ☐ atonia
- ☐ atrophy
- ☐ axial skeleton
- ☐ biceps
- ☐ bone graft
- ☐ bone marrow
- ☐ bone reabsorption inhibitors
- ☐ bones
- ☐ bone scan
- ☐ bradykinesia
- ☐ bunion
- ☐ bunionectomy
- ☐ bursa
- ☐ bursectomy
- ☐ bursitis
- ☐ calcium supplements
- ☐ callus
- ☐ cancellous bone

- ☐ cardiac muscle
- ☐ carpal
- ☐ carpal tunnel release
- ☐ carpal tunnel syndrome
- ☐ cartilage
- ☐ cartilaginous joints
- ☐ cast
- ☐ cervical
- ☐ cervical vertebrae
- ☐ chiropractic
- ☐ chondrectomy
- ☐ chondroma
- ☐ chondromalacia
- ☐ chondroplasty
- ☐ circumduction
- ☐ clavicle
- ☐ clavicular
- ☐ closed fracture
- ☐ coccygeal
- ☐ coccyx
- ☐ Colles' fracture
- ☐ comminuted fracture
- ☐ compact bone
- ☐ compound fracture
- ☐ compression fracture
- ☐ condyle
- ☐ contracture
- ☐ cortical
- ☐ cortical bone
- ☐ corticosteroids
- ☐ costal
- ☐ cranial
- ☐ craniotomy
- ☐ cranium
- ☐ creatine phosphokinase
- ☐ crepitation
- ☐ deep tendon reflex
- ☐ diaphysis
- ☐ dislocation

- ☐ dorsiflexion
- ☐ dual-energy absorptiometry
- ☐ dyskinesia
- ☐ dystonia
- ☐ electromyogram
- ☐ electromyography
- ☐ elevation
- ☐ epicondyle
- ☐ epiphysis
- ☐ ethmoid bone
- ☐ eversion
- ☐ Ewing's sarcoma
- ☐ exostosis
- ☐ extension
- ☐ extensor carpi
- ☐ external oblique
- ☐ facial bones
- ☐ fascia
- ☐ fascial
- ☐ fasciitis
- ☐ fasciotomy
- ☐ femoral
- ☐ femur
- ☐ fibromyalgia
- ☐ fibrous joints
- ☐ fibula
- ☐ fibular
- ☐ fissure
- ☐ fixation
- ☐ flat bones
- ☐ flexion
- ☐ flexor carpi
- ☐ foramen
- ☐ fossa
- ☐ fracture
- ☐ frontal bone
- ☐ ganglion cyst
- ☐ gluteus maximus
- ☐ greenstick fracture

- head
- herniated nucleus pulposus
- humeral
- humerus
- hyoid bone
- hyperkinesia
- hypertonia
- hypertrophy
- hypokinesia
- hypotonia
- iliac
- ilium
- impacted fracture
- innominate bone
- insertion
- intermittent claudication
- intervertebral
- intervertebral disc
- intracranial
- inversion
- involuntary muscle
- irregular bones
- ischial
- ischium
- joint capsule
- joints
- kinesiology
- kyphosis
- lacrimal bone
- laminectomy
- lateral epicondylitis
- ligaments
- long bones
- lordosis
- lower extremities
- lumbar
- lumbar vertebrae
- mandible
- mandibular
- maxilla
- maxillary
- medullary
- medullary cavity
- metacarpal
- metatarsal

- motor neurons
- muscle biopsy
- muscles
- muscle tissue fibers
- muscular
- muscular dystrophy
- myalgia
- myasthenia
- myelography
- myeloma
- myocardial
- myocardium
- myoneural junction
- myopathy
- myoplasty
- myorrhaphy
- myorrhexis
- myotonia
- nasal bone
- neck
- nonsteroidal anti-inflammatory drugs
- oblique fracture
- occipital bone
- opposition
- origin
- orthopedics
- orthotic
- os coxae
- osseous tissue
- ossification
- ostealgia
- osteoarthritis
- osteoblasts
- osteochondroma
- osteoclasia
- osteocytes
- osteogenic sarcoma
- osteomalacia
- osteomyelitis
- osteopathy
- osteoporosis
- osteotome
- osteotomy
- Paget's disease

- palatine bone
- parietal bone
- patella
- patellar
- pathologic fracture
- pectoral girdle
- pelvic
- pelvic girdle
- percutaneous diskectomy
- periosteum
- phalangeal
- phalanges
- plantar flexion
- podiatry
- polymyositis
- process
- pronation
- prosthesis
- prosthetics
- pseudohypertrophic muscular dystrophy
- pubic
- pubis
- radial
- radiography
- radius
- rectus abdominis
- red bone marrow
- reduction
- repetitive motion disorder
- rheumatoid arthritis
- rib cage
- rickets
- rotation
- rotator cuff injury
- sacral
- sacrum
- scapula
- scapular
- scoliosis
- short bones
- sinus
- skeletal muscle
- skeletal muscle relaxants
- skeleton

☐ smooth muscle	☐ synovial fluid	☐ tibial
☐ spasm	☐ synovial joint	☐ torticollis
☐ sphenoid bone	☐ synovial membrane	☐ total hip arthroplasty
☐ spina bifida	☐ synovitis	☐ total knee arthroplasty
☐ spinal fusion	☐ systemic lupus erythematosus	☐ traction
☐ spinal stenosis	☐ talipes	☐ transverse fracture
☐ spiral fracture	☐ tarsal	☐ trochanter
☐ spondylolisthesis	☐ temporal bone	☐ tubercle
☐ spondylosis	☐ tendinitis	☐ tuberosity
☐ spongy bone	☐ tendinous	☐ ulna
☐ sprain	☐ tendon	☐ ulnar
☐ sternal	☐ tendoplasty	☐ upper extremities
☐ sternocleidomastoid	☐ tendotomy	☐ vertebral column
☐ sternum	☐ tenodesis	☐ visceral muscle
☐ strain	☐ tenodynia	☐ Vitamin D therapy
☐ stress fracture	☐ tenoplasty	☐ voluntary muscle
☐ striated muscle	☐ tenorrhaphy	☐ vomer bone
☐ subluxation	☐ thoracic	☐ whiplash
☐ supination	☐ thoracic vertebrae	☐ yellow bone marrow
☐ synovectomy	☐ tibia	☐ zygomatic bone

Practice Exercises

A. Complete the following statements.

1. The two divisions of the human skeleton are the _____ and _____.

2. Another name for visceral muscle is _____ muscle.

3. The five functions of the skeletal system are to _____, _____,

   _____, _____, and _____.

4. Nerves contact skeletal muscle fibers at the _____ junction.

5. _____ bones are roughly as long as they are wide.

6. The membrane covering bones is called the _____.

7. A Colles' fracture occurs in the _____.

8. Another name for spongy bone is _____ bone.

9. _____ joints are the most common joints in the body.

10. The three types of muscle are _____, _____, and _____.

11. A _____ is a smooth round opening in bones.

12. The _____ is the shaft of a long bone.

B. State the terms described using the combining forms provided.

The combining form *oste/o* refers to bone. Use it to write a term that means:

1. bone cell _____

2. embryonic bone cell _____

3. porous bone _____

4. disease of the bone _____

5. incision of the bone _____

6. instrument to cut bone _____

7. inflammation of the bone and bone marrow _____

8. softening of the bones _____

9. tumor composed of both bone and cartilage _____

The combining form *my/o* refers to muscle. Use it to write a term that means:

10. muscle disease _____

11. surgical repair of muscle _____

12. suture of muscle _____

13. record of muscle electricity _____

14. muscle weakness _____

The combining form *ten/o* refers to tendons. Use it to write a term that means:

15. tendon pain _____

16. tendon suture _____

The combining form *arthr/o* refers to the joints. Use it to write a term that means:

17. surgical fusion of a joint _____

18. surgical repair of a joint _____

19. incision into a joint _____

20. inflammation of a joint _____

21. puncture to withdraw fluid from a joint _____

22. pain in the joints _____

The combining form *chondr/o* refers to cartilage. Use it to write a term that means:

23. cartilage removal _____

24. cartilage tumor _____

25. cartilage softening _____

C. Write the suffix for each expression and provide an example of its use from the chapter.

	Suffix	Musculoskeletal Term
1. fuse	_____	_____
2. weakness	_____	_____
3. slipping	_____	_____
4. to surgically break	_____	_____
5. movement	_____	_____
6. porous	_____	_____

D. Give the adjective form for the following bones.

1. femur _____
2. sternum _____
3. clavicle _____
4. coccyx _____
5. maxilla _____

6. tibia _____
7. patella _____
8. phalanges _____
9. humerus _____
10. pubis _____

E. Define the following combining forms and use them to form musculoskeletal terms.

	Definition	Musculoskeletal Term
1. lamin/o	_____	_____
2. ankyl/o	_____	_____
3. chondr/o	_____	_____
4. spondyl/o	_____	_____
5. my/o	_____	_____
6. orth/o	_____	_____
7. kyph/o	_____	_____
8. tend/o	_____	_____
9. myel/o	_____	_____
10. articul/o	_____	_____

F. Define the following terms.

1. chondroplasty _____

2. bradykinesia _____

3. osteoporosis _____

4. lordosis _____

5. atrophy _____

6. myeloma _____

7. prosthesis _____

8. craniotomy _____

9. arthrocentesis _____

10. bursitis _____

G. Name the five regions of the spinal column and indicate the number of bones in each area.

Name	Number of Bones
1. _____	_____
2. _____	_____
3. _____	_____
4. _____	_____
5. _____	_____

H. Circle the prefix and/or suffix and place a *P* for prefix or an *S* for suffix over these word parts. In the space provided, define the term.

1. arthroscopy _____

2. intervertebral _____

3. chondromalacia _____

4. diskectomy _____

5. intracranial _____

6. subscapular _____

I. Match each term to its definition.

1. _____ abduction   a. backward bending of the foot

2. _____ rotation   b. bending the foot to point toes toward the ground

3. _____ plantar flexion   c. straightening motion

4. _____ extension   d. motion around a central axis

5. _____ dorsiflexion   e. motion away from the body

6. _____ flexion   f. moving the thumb away from the palm

7. _____ adduction   g. motion toward the body

8. _____ opposition   h. bending motion

J. Match each fracture type to its definition.

1. _____ comminuted   a. fracture line is at an angle

2. _____ greenstick   b. fracture line curves around the bone

3. _____ compound   c. bone is splintered or crushed

4. _____ simple   d. bone is pressed into itself

5. _____ impacted   e. fracture line is straight across bone

6. _____ transverse   f. skin has been broken

7. _____ oblique   g. no open wound

8. _____ spiral   h. bone only partially broken

K. Define the following medical specialties and specialists.

1. orthopedics _____

2. chiropractic _____

3. podiatry _____

4. orthotics _____

5. prosthetics _____

L. Write the anatomical name for each of the following common bone names.

1. knee cap _____   6. wrist bones _____

2. ankle bones _____   7. shin bone _____

3. collar bone _____   8. shoulder blade _____

4. thigh bone _____   9. finger bones _____

5. toe bones _____

M. Identify the following abbreviations.

1. DJD _____

2. EMG _____

3. C1 _____

4. T6 _____

5. IM _____

6. DTR _____

7. JRA _____

8. LLE _____

9. ortho _____

10. CTS _____

N. Write the abbreviations for the following terms.

1. intramuscular _____

2. total knee replacement _____

3. herniated nucleus pulposus _____

4. deep tendon reflex _____

5. upper extremity _____

6. fifth lumbar vertebra _____

7. bone density testing _____

8. above the knee _____

9. fracture _____

10. nonsteroidal anti-inflammatory drug _____

O. Use the following terms in the sentences that follow.

carpal tunnel syndrome   rickets   lateral epicondylitis   systemic lupus
scoliosis   osteogenic sarcoma   pseudohypertrophic   erythematosus
herniated nucleus   osteoporosis   muscular dystrophy
   pulposus   spondylolisthesis

1. Mrs. Lewis, age 84, broke her hip. Her physician will be running tests for what potential ailment? _____

2. Jamie, age 6 months, is being given orange juice and vitamin supplements to avoid what condition? _____

3. George has severe elbow pain after playing tennis four days in a row. He may have _____.

4. Marshall's doctor told him that he had a ruptured disk. The medical term for this is? _____

5. Mr. Jefferson's physician has discovered a tumor at the end of his femur. He has been admitted to the hospital for a biopsy

   to rule out what type of bone cancer? _____

6. The school nurse has asked Janelle to bend over so that she may examine her back to see if she is developing a lateral

   curve. What is the nurse looking for? _____

7. Gerald has experienced a gradual loss of muscle strength over the past five years even though his muscles look large and

   healthy. The doctors believe he has an inherited muscle disease. What is that disease? _____

8. Roberta has suddenly developed arthritis in her hands and knees. Rheumatoid arthritis had been ruled out, but what

   other auto-immune disease might Roberta have? _____

9. Mark's x-ray demonstrated forward sliding of a lumbar vertebra; the radiologist diagnosed _____.

10. The orthopedist determined that Marcia's repetitive wrist movements at work caused her to develop _____.

P. Fill in the classification for each drug description, then match the brand name.

	Drug Description	Classification	Brand Name
1.	_____ Treats mild pain and anti-inflammatory	_____	a. Flexeril
2.	_____ Hormone with anti-inflammatory properties	_____	b. Aleve
3.	_____ Reduces muscle spasms	_____	c. Fosamax
4.	_____ Treats conditions of weakened bones	_____	d. Oystercal
5.	_____ Maintains blood calcium levels	_____	e. Medrol

Medical Record Analysis

Below is an item from a patient's medical record. Read it carefully, make sure you understand all the medical terms used, and then answer the questions that follow.

Discharge Summary

Admitting Diagnosis:	Osteoarthritis bilateral knees.
Final Diagnosis:	Osteoarthritis bilateral knees with prosthetic right knee replacement.
History of Present Illness:	Patient is a 68-year-old male. He reports he has experienced occasional knee pain and swelling since he injured his knees playing football in high school. These symptoms became worse while he was in his 50s and working on a concrete surface. The right knee has always been more painful than the left. Arthroscopy twelve years ago revealed a torn lateral meniscus and chondromalacia of the patella on the right. He had an arthroscopic meniscectomy with a 50% improvement in symptoms at that time. He returned to his orthopedic surgeon six months ago because of constant knee pain and swelling severe enough to interfere with sleep and all activities. He required a cane to walk. CT scan indicated severe bilateral osteoarthritis, with complete loss of the joint space on the right. He was referred to a physiatrist who prescribed Motrin; physical therapy for ROM; strengthening exercises; and a low-fat, low-calorie weight loss diet for moderate obesity that greatly added to the strain on his knees. Over the course of the next two months, the left knee improved, but the right knee did not. Due to the failure of conservative treatment, he is admitted to the hospital at this time for prosthetic replacement of the right knee. Patient's other medical history is significant for hypertension and coronary artery disease that is controlled with medication. He has lost weight through diet, which has improved his hypertension, if not his knee pain.
Summary of Hospital Course:	Patient tolerated the surgical procedure well. He began intensive physical therapy for lower extremity ROM and strengthening exercises and gait training with a walker. He received occupational therapy instruction in ADLs, especially dressing and personal care. He was able to transfer himself out of bed by the third post-op day and was able to ambulate 150 ft with a walker and dress himself on the fifth post-op day. His right knee flexion was 90° and he lacked 5° of full extension.
Discharge Plans:	Patient was discharged home with his wife one week post-op. He will continue rehabilitation as an outpatient. Return to office for post-op checkup in one week.

Critical Thinking Questions

1. What is the specialty of a physiatrist? Describe in your own words what the physiatrist ordered for this patient.

_____

_____

2. What surgical procedure did the patient have twelve years ago? What two pathologies were revealed by that procedure? What surgical procedure was performed to correct his problems at that time?

_____

_____

3. The following medical terms are not defined in your text. Based on your reading of this discharge summary, what do you think each term means in general—not the specifics of this patient?

    a. conservative treatment _____

    b. outpatient _____

4. What two types of post-op therapy did this patient receive? Describe the treatment each type of therapy provided for this patient.

_____

_____

5. Describe how much the patient could move his right knee when he was discharged from the hospital.

_____

6. The following medical terms are introduced in a later chapter. Use your text as a dictionary to describe, in your own words, what each term means.

    a. coronary artery disease _____

    b. hypertension _____

Chart Note Transcription

The chart note below contains eleven phrases that can be reworded with a medical term that you learned in this chapter. Each phrase is identified with an underline. Determine the medical term and write your answers in the space provided.

Current Complaint:	An 82-year-old female was transported to the Emergency Room via ambulance with severe left hip pain following a fall on the ice.
Past History:	Patient suffered a <u>wrist broken bone</u> **1** two years earlier that required <u>immobilization by solid material</u>. **2** Following this <u>broken bone</u>, **3** her <u>physician who specializes in treatment of bone conditions</u> **4** diagnosed her with moderate <u>porous bones</u> **5** on the basis of a <u>computer-assisted X-ray</u>. **6**
Signs and Symptoms:	Patient reported severe left hip pain, rating it as 8 on a scale of 1 to 10. She held her hip <u>in a bent position</u> **7** and could not tolerate <u>movement toward a straight position</u>. **8** X-rays of the left hip and leg were taken.
Diagnosis:	<u>Shattered broken bone</u> **9** in the neck of the left <u>thigh bone</u>. **10**
Treatment:	<u>Implantation of an artificial hip joint</u> **11** on the left.

1 _____

2 _____

3 _____

4 _____

5 _____

6 _____

7 _____

8 _____

9 _____

10 _____

11 _____

Labeling Exercise

A. System Review

Write the labels for this figure on the numbered lines provided.

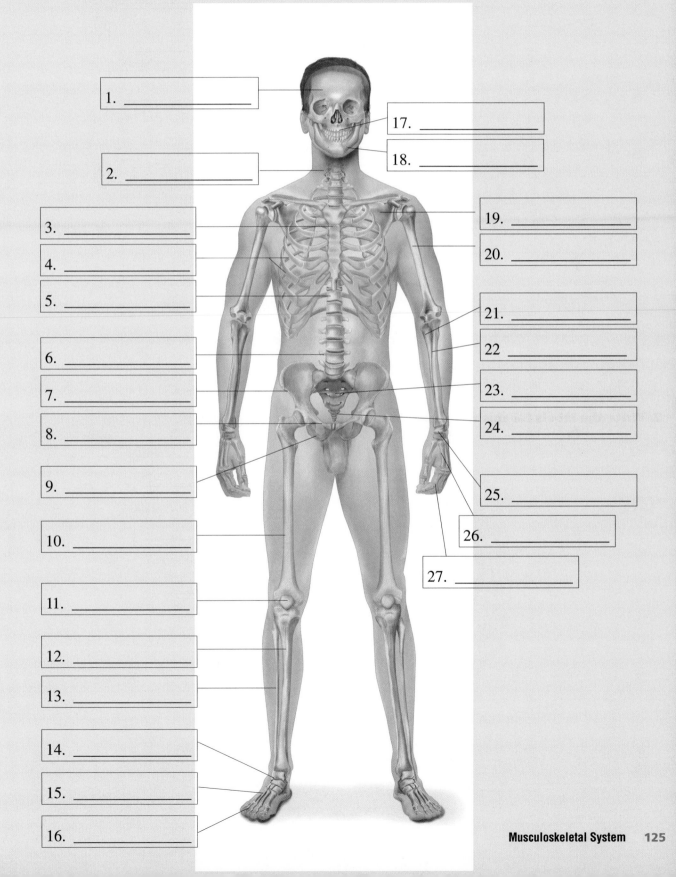

1. _____

2. _____

3. _____

4. _____

5. _____

6. _____

7. _____

8. _____

9. _____

10. _____

11. _____

12. _____

13. _____

14. _____

15. _____

16. _____

17. _____

18. _____

19. _____

20. _____

21. _____

22 _____

23. _____

24. _____

25. _____

26. _____

27. _____

B. Anatomy Challenge

1. Write the labels for this figure on the numbered lines provided.

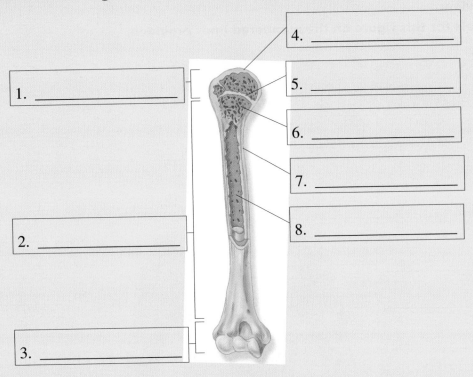

4. _____

1. _____

5. _____

6. _____

7. _____

2. _____

8. _____

3. _____

2. Write the labels for this figure on the numbered lines provided.

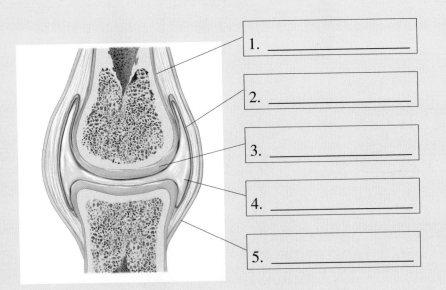

1. _____

2. _____

3. _____

4. _____

5. _____

Multimedia Preview

Additional interactive resources and activities for this chapter can be found on the Companion Website. For videos, games, and pronunciations, please access the accompanying DVD-ROM that comes with this book.

DVD-ROM Highlights

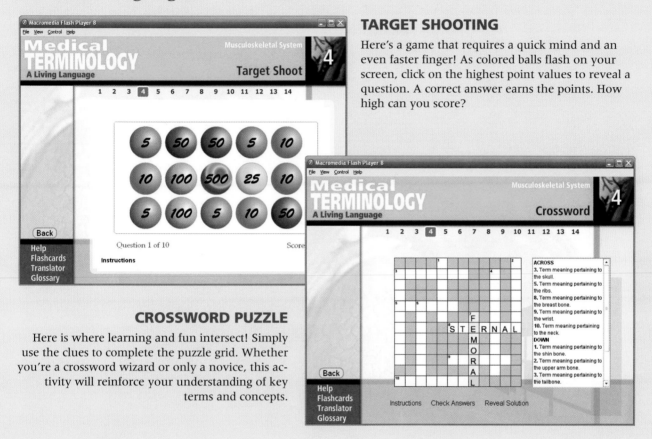

TARGET SHOOTING

Here's a game that requires a quick mind and an even faster finger! As colored balls flash on your screen, click on the highest point values to reveal a question. A correct answer earns the points. How high can you score?

CROSSWORD PUZZLE

Here is where learning and fun intersect! Simply use the clues to complete the puzzle grid. Whether you're a crossword wizard or only a novice, this activity will reinforce your understanding of key terms and concepts.

Website Highlights—www.prenhall.com/fremgen

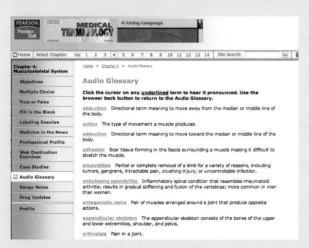

AUDIO GLOSSARY

Click here and take advantage of the free-access on-line study guide that accompanies your textbook. You'll find an audio glossary with definitions and audio pronunciations for every term in the book. By clicking on this URL you'll also access a variety of quizzes with instant feedback, links to download mp3 audio reviews, and current news articles.

5 Cardiovascular System

Learning Objectives

Upon completion of this chapter, you will be able to:

- Identify and define the combining forms and suffixes introduced in this chapter.
- Correctly spell and pronounce medical terms and major anatomical structures relating to the cardiovascular system.
- Describe the major organs of the cardiovascular system and their functions.
- Describe the anatomy of the heart.
- Describe the flow of blood through the heart.
- Explain how the electrical conduction system controls the heartbeat.
- List and describe the characteristics of the three types of blood vessels.
- Define pulse and blood pressure.
- Build and define cardiovascular system medical terms from word parts.
- Identify and define cardiovascular system vocabulary terms.
- Identify and define selected cardiovascular system pathology terms.
- Identify and define selected cardiovascular system diagnostic procedures.
- Identify and define selected cardiovascular system therapeutic procedures.
- Identify and define selected medications relating to the cardiovascular system.
- Define selected abbreviations associated with the cardiovascular system.

Cardiovascular System at a Glance

Function

The cardiovascular system consists of the pump and vessels that distribute blood to all areas of the body. This system allows for the delivery of needed substances to the cells of the body as well as for the removal of wastes.

Organs

blood vessels
- arteries
- capillaries
- veins

heart

Combining Forms

angi/o	vessel	**sphygm/o**	pulse
aort/o	aorta	**steth/o**	chest
arteri/o	artery	**thromb/o**	clot
ather/o	fatty substance	**valv/o**	valve
atri/o	atrium	**valvul/o**	valve
cardi/o	heart	**vascul/o**	blood vessel
coron/o	heart	**vas/o**	vessel, duct
hemangi/o	blood vessel	**ven/o**	vein
phleb/o	vein	**ventricul/o**	ventricle

Suffixes

-manometer	instrument to measure pressure
-ole	small
-tension	pressure
-ule	small

Cardiovascular System Illustrated

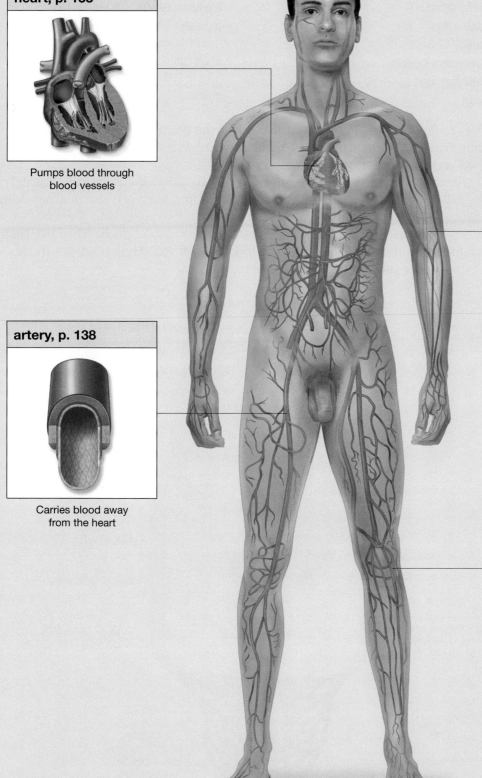

heart, p. 133
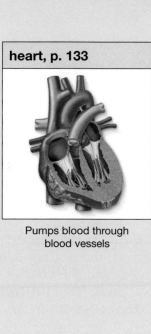
Pumps blood through
blood vessels

artery, p. 138
Carries blood away
from the heart

vein, p. 141
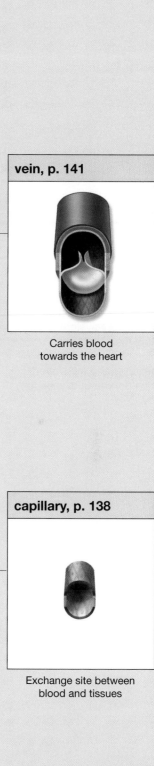
Carries blood
towards the heart

capillary, p. 138
Exchange site between
blood and tissues

Anatomy and Physiology of the Cardiovascular System

arteries	**oxygen**
blood vessels	**oxygenated** (OK-sih-jen-ay-ted)
capillaries	**pulmonary circulation**
carbon dioxide	(PULL-mon-air-ee ser-kew-LAY-shun)
circulatory system	**systemic circulation**
deoxygenated (dee-OK-sih-jen-ay-ted)	(sis-TEM-ik ser-kew-LAY-shun)
heart	**veins**

The cardiovascular (CV) system, also called the **circulatory system,** maintains the distribution of blood throughout the body and is composed of the **heart** and the **blood vessels—arteries, capillaries,** and **veins.**

The circulatory system is composed of two parts: the **pulmonary circulation** and the **systemic circulation.** The pulmonary circulation, between the heart and lungs, transports **deoxygenated** blood to the lungs to get oxygen, and then back to the heart. The systemic circulation carries **oxygenated** blood away from the heart to the tissues and cells, and then back to the heart (see Figure 5.1 ■). In this way all the body's cells receive blood and oxygen.

■ Figure 5.1 A schematic of the circulatory system illustrating the pulmonary circulation picking up oxygen from the lungs and the systemic circulation delivering oxygen to the body.

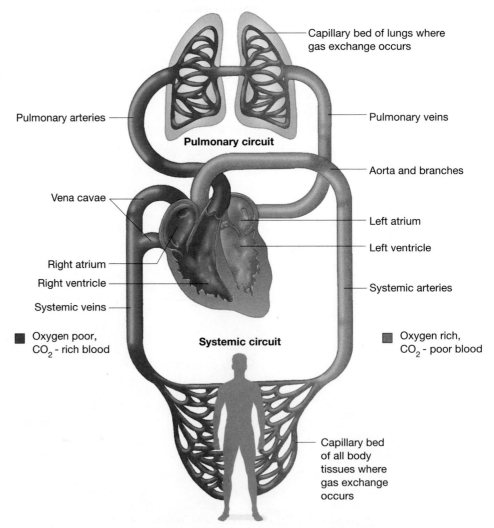

Capillary bed of lungs where gas exchange occurs

Pulmonary arteries

Pulmonary veins

Pulmonary circuit

Aorta and branches

Vena cavae

Left atrium

Left ventricle

Right atrium

Right ventricle

Systemic arteries

Systemic veins

■ Oxygen poor, CO_2 - rich blood

Systemic circuit

■ Oxygen rich, CO_2 - poor blood

Capillary bed of all body tissues where gas exchange occurs

In addition to distributing **oxygen** and other nutrients, such as glucose and amino acids, the cardiovascular system also collects the waste products from the body's cells. **Carbon dioxide** and other waste products produced by metabolic reaction are transported by the cardiovascular system to the lungs, liver, and kidneys where they are eliminated from the body.

Heart

apex (AY-peks)   **cardiac muscle** (CAR-dee-ak)

The heart is a muscular pump made up of **cardiac muscle** fibers that could be considered a muscle rather than an organ. It has four chambers, or cavities, and beats an average of 60 to 100 beats per minute (bpm) or about 100,000 times in one day. Each time the cardiac muscle contracts, blood is ejected from the heart and pushed throughout the body within the blood vessels.

The heart is located in the mediastinum in the center of the chest cavity, however, it is not exactly centered; more of the heart is on the left side of the mediastinum than the right. At about the size of a fist and shaped like an upside-down pear the heart lies directly behind the sternum. The tip of the heart at the lower edge is called the **apex** (see Figure 5.2 ■).

Heart Layers

endocardium (en-doh-CAR-dee-um)   **pericardium** (pair-ih-CAR-dee-um)
epicardium (ep-ih-CAR-dee-um)   **visceral pericardium**
myocardium (my-oh-CAR-dee-um)   (VISS-er-al pair-ih-CAR-dee-um)
parietal pericardium
  (pah-RYE-eh-tal pair-ih-CAR-dee-um)

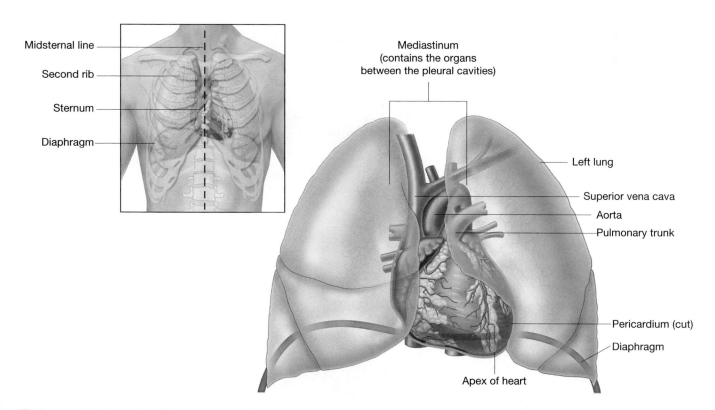

■ **Figure 5.2** Location of the heart within the mediastinum of the thoracic cavity.

Med Term Tip

These layers become important when studying the disease conditions affecting the heart. For instance, when the prefix *endo-* is added to *carditis,* forming *endocarditis,* we know that the inflammation is within the "inner layer of the heart." In discussing the muscular action of the heart the prefix *myo-,* meaning "muscle," is added to *cardium* to form the word *myocardium.* The diagnosis *myocardial infarction* (MI), or heart attack, means that the patient has an infarct or "dead tissue in the muscle of the heart." The prefix *peri-,* meaning "around," when added to the word *cardium* refers to the sac "surrounding the heart." Therefore, *pericarditis* is an "inflammation of the outer sac of the heart."

The wall of the heart is quite thick and composed of three layers (see Figures 5.3 ▬ and 5.4 ▬):

1. The **endocardium** is the inner layer of the heart lining the heart chambers. It is a very smooth, thin layer that serves to reduce friction as the blood passes through the heart chambers.
2. The **myocardium** is the thick muscular middle layer of the heart. Contraction of this muscle layer develops the pressure required to pump blood through the blood vessels.
3. The **epicardium** is the outer layer of the heart. The heart is enclosed within a double-layered pleural sac, called the **pericardium**. The epicardium is the **visceral pericardium,** or inner layer of the sac. The outer layer of the sac is the **parietal pericardium**. Fluid between the two layers of the sac reduces friction as the heart beats.

Heart Chambers

atria (AY-tree-ah)
interatrial septum
     (in-ter-AY-tree-al SEP-tum)

interventricular septum
     (in-ter-ven-TRIK-yoo-lar SEP-tum)
ventricles (VEN-trik-lz)

The heart is divided into four chambers or cavities (see Figures 5.3 and 5.4). There are two **atria**, or upper chambers, and two **ventricles**, or lower chambers. These chambers are divided into right and left sides by walls called the **interatrial septum** and the **interventricular septum**. The atria are the receiving chambers of the heart. Blood returning to the heart via veins first collects in the atria. The ventricles are the pumping chambers. They have a much thicker myocardium and their contraction ejects blood out of the heart and into the great arteries.

Med Term Tip

The term *ventricle* comes from the Latin term *venter,* which means "little belly." Although it originally referred to the abdomen and then the stomach, it came to stand for any hollow region inside an organ.

▬ **Figure 5.3** Internal view of the heart illustrating the heart chambers, heart layers, heart valves, and major blood vessels associated with the heart.

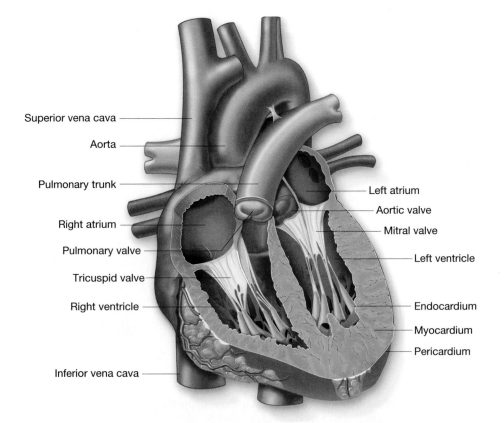

Superior vena cava
Aorta
Pulmonary trunk
Right atrium
Pulmonary valve
Tricuspid valve
Right ventricle
Inferior vena cava
Left atrium
Aortic valve
Mitral valve
Left ventricle
Endocardium
Myocardium
Pericardium

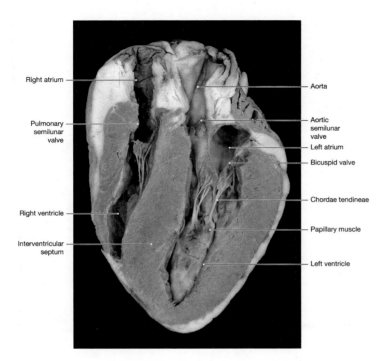

Heart Valves

aortic valve (ay-OR-tik)

atrioventricular valve
   (ay-tree-oh-ven-TRIK-yoo-lar)

bicuspid valve (bye-CUSS-pid)

cusps

mitral valve (MY-tral)

pulmonary valve (PULL-mon-air-ee)

semilunar valve (sem-ih-LOO-nar)

tricuspid valve (try-CUSS-pid)

Four valves act as restraining gates to control the direction of blood flow. They are situated at the entrances and exits to the ventricles (see Figures 5.4 ■ and 5.5 ■). Properly functioning valves allow blood to flow only in the forward direction by blocking it from returning to the previous chamber.

The four valves are as follows:

1. **Tricuspid valve:** an **atrioventricular valve** (AV), meaning that it controls the opening between the right atrium and the right ventricle. Once the blood enters the right ventricle, it cannot go back up into the atrium again. The prefix *tri-*, meaning three, indicates that this valve has three leaflets or **cusps**.

2. **Pulmonary valve:** a **semilunar valve**. The prefix *semi-*, meaning half, and the term **lunar**, meaning moon, indicate that this valve looks like a half moon. Located between the right ventricle and the pulmonary artery, this valve prevents blood that has been ejected into the pulmonary artery from returning to the right ventricle as it relaxes.

3. **Mitral valve:** also called the **bicuspid valve**, indicating that it has two cusps. Blood flows through this atrioventricular valve to the left ventricle and cannot go back up into the left atrium.

4. **Aortic valve:** a semilunar valve located between the left ventricle and the aorta. Blood leaves the left ventricle through this valve and cannot return to the left ventricle.

Med Term Tip

The heart makes two distinct sounds referred to as "lub-dupp." These sounds are produced by the forceful snapping shut of the heart valves. *Lub* is the closing of the atrioventricular valves. *Dupp* is the closing of the semilunar valves.

Blood Flow Through the Heart

aorta (ay-OR-tah)

diastole (dye-ASS-toe-lee)

inferior vena cava (VEE-nah KAY-vah)

pulmonary artery (PULL-mon-air-ee)

pulmonary veins

superior vena cava

systole (SIS-toe-lee)

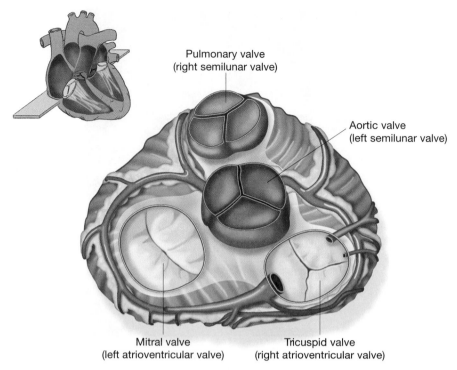

Figure 5.5 Superior view of heart valves illustrating position, size, and shape of each valve.

The flow of blood through the heart is very orderly (see Figure 5.6 ■). It progresses through the heart to the lungs, where it receives oxygen; then goes back to the heart; and then out to the body tissues and parts. The normal process of blood flow is as follows:

1. Deoxygenated blood from all the tissues in the body enters a relaxed right atrium via two large veins called the **superior vena cava** and **inferior vena cava**.
2. The right atrium contracts and blood flows through the tricuspid valve into the relaxed right ventricle.
3. The right ventricle then contracts and blood is pumped through the pulmonary valve into the **pulmonary artery**, which carries it to the lungs for oxygenation.
4. The left atrium receives blood returning to the heart after being oxygenated by the lungs. This blood enters the relaxed left atrium from the four **pulmonary veins**.
5. The left atrium contracts and blood flows through the mitral valve into the relaxed left ventricle.
6. When the left ventricle contracts, the blood is pumped through the aortic valve and into the **aorta**, the largest artery in the body. The aorta carries blood to all parts of the body.

It can be seen that the heart chambers alternate between relaxing in order to fill and contracting to push blood forward. The period of time a chamber is relaxed is **diastole**. The contraction phase is **systole**.

Conduction System of the Heart

atrioventricular bundle

atrioventricular node

autonomic nervous system (aw-toh-NOM-ik NER-vus SIS-tem)

bundle branches

bundle of His

pacemaker

Purkinje fibers (per-KIN-gee)

sinoatrial node (sigh-noh-AY-tree-al)

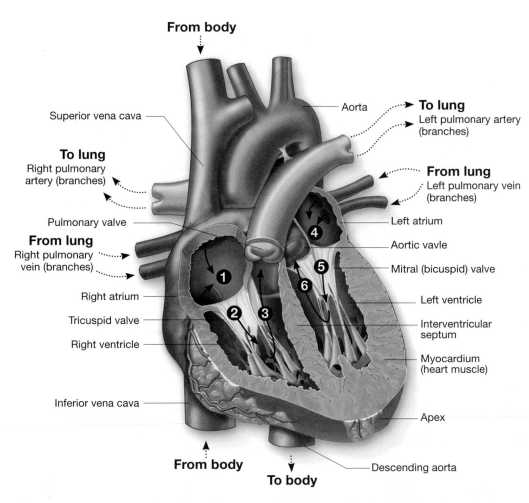

From body

Superior vena cava

To lung
Right pulmonary
artery (branches)

Pulmonary valve

From lung
Right pulmonary
vein (branches)

Right atrium

Tricuspid valve

Right ventricle

Inferior vena cava

From body

To body

Aorta

To lung
Left pulmonary artery
(branches)

From lung
Left pulmonary vein
(branches)

Left atrium

Aortic vavle

Mitral (bicuspid) valve

Left ventricle

Interventricular
septum

Myocardium
(heart muscle)

Apex

Descending aorta

Figure 5.6 The path of blood flow through the chambers of the left and right side of the heart, including the veins delivering blood to the heart and arteries receiving blood ejected from the heart.

The heart rate is regulated by the **autonomic nervous system**; therefore, we have no voluntary control over the beating of our heart. Special tissue within the heart is responsible for conducting an electrical impulse stimulating the different chambers to contract in the correct order.

The path that the impulses travel is as follows (see Figure 5.7 ■):

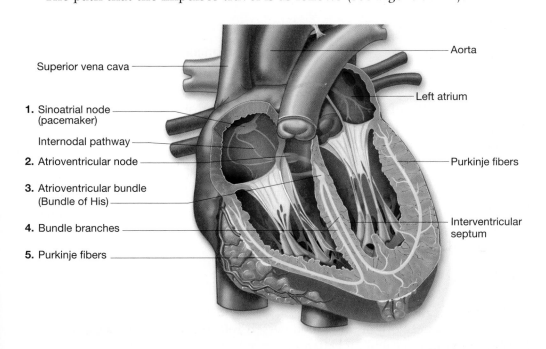

Superior vena cava

1. Sinoatrial node
(pacemaker)

Internodal pathway

2. Atrioventricular node

3. Atrioventricular bundle
(Bundle of His)

4. Bundle branches

5. Purkinje fibers

Aorta

Left atrium

Purkinje fibers

Interventricular
septum

Figure 5.7 The conduction system of the heart; traces the path of the electrical impulse that stimulates the heart chambers to contract in the correct sequence.

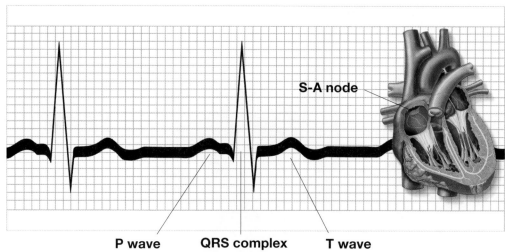

P wave
precedes atrial systole

QRS complex
precedes ventricular systole

T wave
precedes ventricular diastole

S-A node

1. The **sinoatrial (SA) node**, or **pacemaker**, is where the electrical impulses begin. From the sinoatrial node a wave of electricity travels through the atria, causing them to contract, or go into systole.
2. The **atrioventricular node** is stimulated.
3. This node transfers the stimulation wave to the **atrioventricular bundle** (formerly called **bundle of His**).
4. The electrical signal next travels down the **bundle branches** within the interventricular septum.
5. The **Purkinje fibers** out in the ventricular myocardium are stimulated, resulting in ventricular systole.

Blood Vessels

lumen (LOO-men)

There are three types of blood vessels: arteries, capillaries, and veins (see Figure 5.9 ■). These are the pipes that circulate blood through out the body. The **lumen** is the channel within these vessels through which blood flows.

Arteries

arterioles (ar-TEE-ree-ohlz)   **coronary arteries** (KOR-ah-nair-ee
                                                    AR-te-reez)

The arteries are the large, thick-walled vessels that carry the blood away from the heart. The walls of arteries contain a thick layer of smooth muscle that can contract or relax to change the size of the arterial lumen. The pulmonary artery carries deoxygenated blood from the right ventricle to the lungs. The largest artery, the aorta, begins from the left ventricle of the heart and carries oxygenated blood to all the body systems. The **coronary arteries** then branch from the aorta and provide blood to the myocardium (see Figure 5.10 ■). As they travel through the body, the arteries branch into progressively smaller sized arteries. The smallest of the arteries, called **arterioles**, deliver blood to the capillaries. Figure 5.11 ■ illustrates the major systemic arteries.

Capillaries

capillary bed

Capillaries are a network of tiny blood vessels referred to as a **capillary bed**. Arterial blood flows into a capillary bed, and venous blood flows back out (see Figure

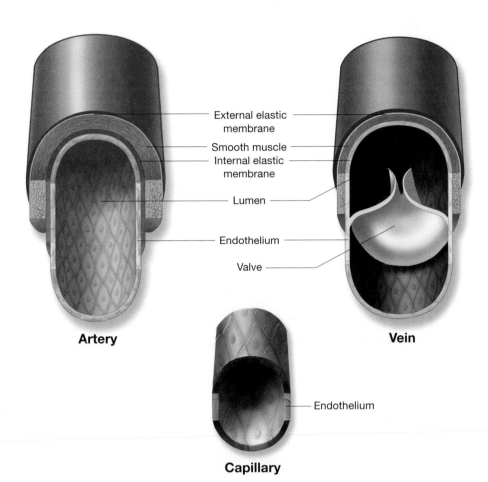

Figure 5.9 Comparative structure of arteries, capillaries, and veins.

External elastic membrane

Smooth muscle

Internal elastic membrane

Lumen

Endothelium

Valve

Artery

Vein

Endothelium

Capillary

5.9). Capillaries are very thin walled, allowing for the diffusion of the oxygen and nutrients from the blood into the body tissues. Likewise, carbon dioxide and waste products are able to diffuse out of the body tissues and into the bloodstream to be carried away. Since the capillaries are so small in diameter, the blood will not flow as quickly through them as it does through the arteries and veins. This means that the blood has time for an exchange of nutrients, oxygen, and waste material to take place. As blood exits a capillary bed, it returns to the heart through a vein.

Figure 5.10 The coronary arteries.

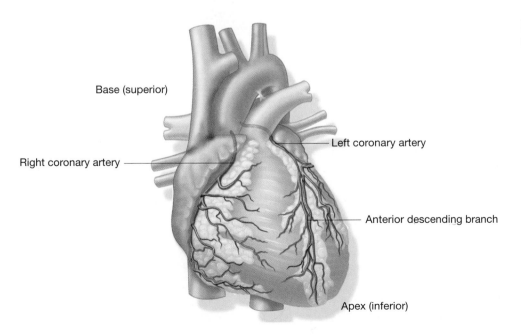

Base (superior)

Left coronary artery

Right coronary artery

Anterior descending branch

Apex (inferior)

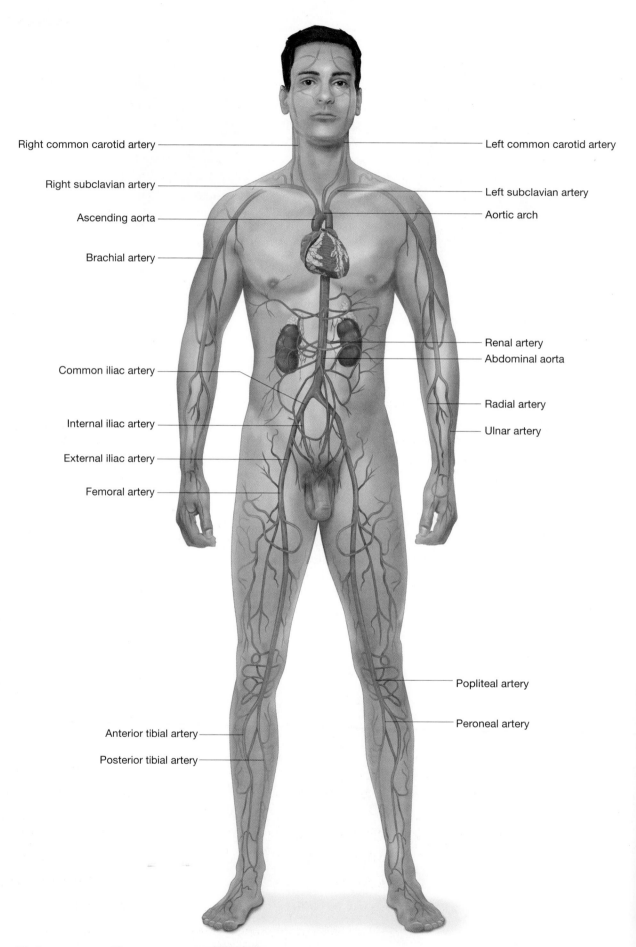

Right common carotid artery

Right subclavian artery

Ascending aorta

Brachial artery

Common iliac artery

Internal iliac artery

External iliac artery

Femoral artery

Anterior tibial artery

Posterior tibial artery

Left common carotid artery

Left subclavian artery

Aortic arch

Renal artery

Abdominal aorta

Radial artery

Ulnar artery

Popliteal artery

Peroneal artery

■ **Figure 5.11** The major arteries of the body.

Veins

venules (VEN-yools)

The veins carry blood back to the heart. Blood leaving capillaries first enters small **venules**, which then merge into larger veins. Veins have much thinner walls than arteries, causing them to collapse easily. The veins also have valves that allow the blood to move only toward the heart. These valves prevent blood from backflowing; ensuring that blood always flows toward the heart (see Figure 5.9). The two large veins that enter the heart are the superior vena cava, which carries blood from the upper body, and the inferior vena cava, which carries blood from the lower body. Blood pressure in the veins is much lower than in the arteries. Muscular action against the veins and skeletal muscle contractions help in the movement of blood. Figure 5.12 ■ illustrates the major systemic veins.

Pulse and Blood Pressure

blood pressure (BP)
diastolic pressure (dye-ah-STOL-ik)

pulse
systolic pressure (sis-TOL-ik)

Blood pressure (BP) is a measurement of the force exerted by blood against the wall of a blood vessel. During ventricular systole, blood is under a lot of pressure from the ventricular contraction, giving the highest blood pressure reading—the **systolic pressure**. The **pulse** felt at the wrist or throat is the surge of blood caused by the heart contraction. This is why pulse rate is normally equal to heart rate. During ventricular diastole, blood is not being pushed by the heart at all and the blood pressure reading drops to its lowest point—the **diastolic pressure**. Therefore, to see the full range of what is occurring with blood pressure, both numbers are required. Blood pressure is also affected by several other characteristics of the blood and the blood vessels. These include the elasticity of the arteries, the diameter of the blood vessels, the viscosity of the blood, the volume of blood flowing through the vessels, and the amount of resistance to blood flow.

> **Med Term Tip**
>
> The instrument used to measure blood pressure is called a *sphygmomanometer*. The combining form *sphygm/o* means "pulse" and the suffix *-manometer* means "instrument to measure pressure." A blood pressure reading is reported as two numbers, for example, 120/80. The 120 is the systolic pressure and the 80 is the diastolic pressure. There is not one "normal" blood pressure number. The normal range for blood pressure in an adult is 90/60 to 140/90.

Word Building

The following list contains examples of medical terms built directly from word parts. The definition for these terms can be determined by a straightforward translation of the word parts.

COMBINING FORM	COMBINED WITH	MEDICAL TERM	DEFINITION
angi/o	-gram	**angiogram** (AN-jee-oh-gram)	record of a vessel
	-itis	**angiitis** (an-jee-EYE-tis)	inflammation of a vessel
	-plasty	**angioplasty** (AN-jee-oh-plas-tee)	surgical repair of a vessel
	-spasm	**angiospasm** (AN-jee-oh-spazm)	involuntary muscle contraction of a vessel
	-stenosis	**angiostenosis** (an-jee-oh-sten-OH-sis)	narrowing of a vessel
aort/o	-ic	**aortic** (ay-OR-tik)	pertaining to the aorta
arteri/o	-al	**arterial** (ar-TEE-ree-al)	pertaining to the artery
	-ole	**arteriole** (ar-TEE-ree-ohl)	small artery
	-rrhexis	**arteriorrhexis** (ar-tee-ree-oh-REK-sis)	ruptured artery
ather/o	-ectomy	**atherectomy** (ath-er-EK-toh-mee)	removal of fatty substance

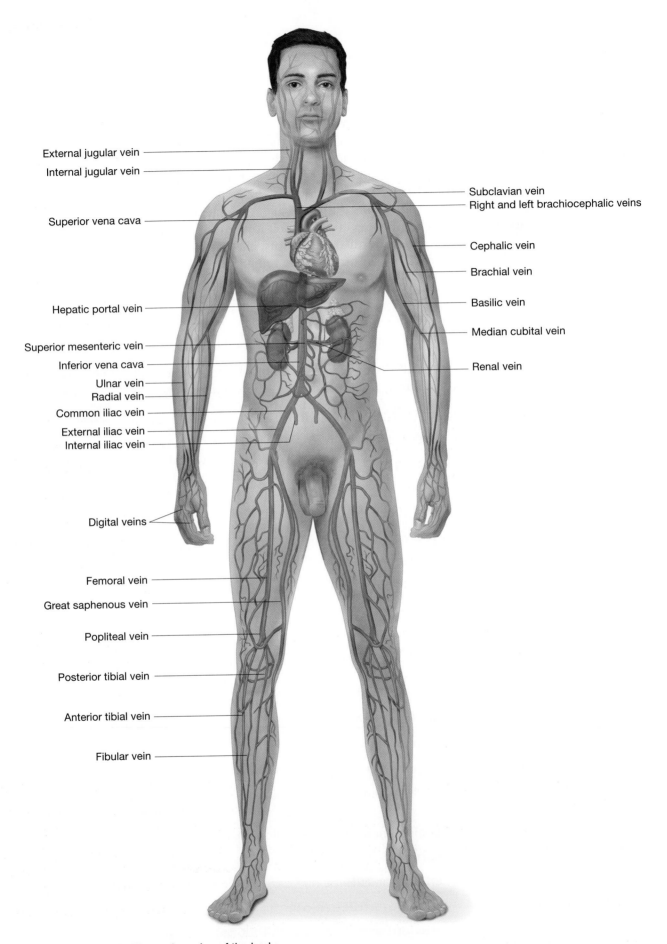

External jugular vein

Internal jugular vein

Superior vena cava

Hepatic portal vein

Superior mesenteric vein

Inferior vena cava

Ulnar vein

Radial vein

Common iliac vein

External iliac vein

Internal iliac vein

Digital veins

Femoral vein

Great saphenous vein

Popliteal vein

Posterior tibial vein

Anterior tibial vein

Fibular vein

Subclavian vein

Right and left brachiocephalic veins

Cephalic vein

Brachial vein

Basilic vein

Median cubital vein

Renal vein

■ **Figure 5.12** The major veins of the body.

Word Building *(continued)*

COMBINING FORM	COMBINED WITH	MEDICAL TERM	DEFINITION
	-oma	**atheroma** (ath-er-OH-mah)	fatty substance tumor/growth
atri/o	-al	**atrial** (AY-tree-al)	pertaining to the atrium
	inter- -al	**interatrial** (in-ter-AY-tree-al)	pertaining to between the atria
cardi/o	-ac	**cardiac** (CAR-dee-ak)	pertaining to the heart
	brady- -ia	**bradycardia** (brad-ee-CAR-dee-ah)	state of slow heart
	electr/o -gram	**electrocardiogram** (ee-lek-tro-CAR-dee-oh-gram)	record of heart electricity
	-megaly	**cardiomegaly** (car-dee-oh-MEG-ah-lee)	enlarged heart
	my/o -al	**myocardial** (my-oh-CAR-dee-al)	pertaining to heart muscle
	-logist	**cardiologist** (car-dee-ALL-oh-jist)	specialist in the heart
	-rrhexis	**cardiorrhexis** (card-dee-oh-REK-sis)	ruptured heart
	tachy- -ia	**tachycardia** (tak-ee-CAR-dee-ah)	state of fast heart
coron/o	-ary	**coronary** (KOR-ah-nair-ee)	pertaining to the heart
phleb/o	-itis	**phlebitis** (fleh-BYE-tis)	inflammation of a vein
valv/o	-plasty	**valvoplasty** (VAL-voh-plas-tee)	surgical repair of a valve
valvul/o	-itis	**valvulitis** (val-view-LYE-tis)	inflammation of a valve
	-ar	**valvular** (VAL-view-lar)	pertaining to a valve
vascul/o	-ar	**vascular** (VAS-kwee-lar)	pertaining to a blood vessel
ven/o	-ous	**venous** (VEE-nus)	pertaining to a vein
	-ule	**venule** (VEN-yool)	small vein
	-gram	**venogram** (VEN-oh-gram)	record of a vein
ventricul/o	-ar	**ventricular** (ven-TRIK-yoo-lar)	pertaining to a ventricle
	inter- -ar	**interventricular** (in-ter-ven-TRIK-yoo-lar)	pertaining to between the ventricles

Vocabulary

TERM	DEFINITION
auscultation (oss-kul-TAY-shun)	The process of listening to the sounds within the body by using a stethoscope.
cardiology (car-dee-ALL-oh-jee)	The branch of medicine involving diagnosis and treatment of conditions and diseases of the cardiovascular system. Physician is a *cardiologist.*
catheter (KATH-eh-ter)	A flexible tube inserted into the body for the purpose of moving fluids into or out of the body. In the cardiovascular system a catheter is used to place dye into blood vessels so they may be visualized on x-rays.
infarct (IN-farkt)	An area of tissue within an organ or part that undergoes necrosis (death) following the loss of its blood supply.
ischemia (is-KEYH-mee-ah)	The localized and temporary deficiency of blood supply due to an obstruction to the circulation.

Vocabulary *(continued)*

TERM	DEFINITION
murmur (MUR-mur)	An abnormal heart sound such as a soft blowing sound or harsh click. It may be quiet and heard only with a stethoscope, or so loud it can be heard several feet away. Also referred to as a *bruit.*
orthostatic hypotension (or-thoh-STAT-ik)	The sudden drop in blood pressure a person experiences when standing up suddenly.
palpitations (pal-pih-TAY-shunz)	Pounding, racing heartbeats.
plaque (plak)	A yellow, fatty deposit of lipids in an artery that are the hallmark of atherosclerosis.
regurgitation (re-ger-gih-TAY-shun)	To flow backwards. In the cardiovascular system this refers to the backflow of blood through a valve.
sphygmomanometer (sfig-moh-mah-NOM-eh-ter)	Instrument for measuring blood pressure. Also referred to as a *blood pressure cuff* (see Figure 5.13 ■).
stent	A stainless steel tube placed within a blood vessel or a duct to widen the lumen (see Figure 5.14 ■).
stethoscope (STETH-oh-scope)	Instrument for listening to body sounds (auscultation), such as the chest, heart, or intestines.

Pathology

TERM	DEFINITION
■ *Heart*	
angina pectoris (an-JYE-nah PECK-tor-is)	Condition in which there is severe pain with a sensation of constriction around the heart. Caused by a deficiency of oxygen to the heart muscle.

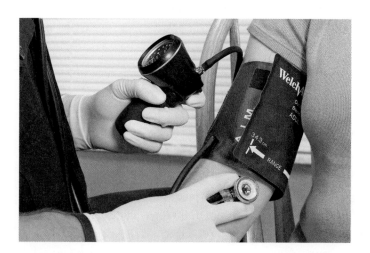

■ **Figure 5.13** Using a sphygmomanometer to measure blood pressure.

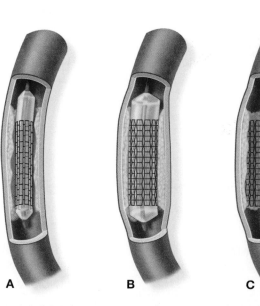

■ **Figure 5.14** The process of placing a stent in a blood vessel. A) A catheter is used to place a collapsed stent next to an atherosclerotic plaque; B) stent is expanded; C) catheter is removed, leaving the expanded stent behind.

Pathology *(continued)*

TERM	DEFINITION
arrhythmia (ah-RITH-mee-ah)	Irregularity in the heartbeat or action. Comes in many different forms; some are not serious, while others are life threatening.
bundle branch block (BBB)	Occurs when the electrical impulse is blocked from traveling down the bundle of His or bundle branches. Results in the ventricles beating at a different rate than the atria. Also called a *heart block*.
cardiac arrest	Complete stopping of heart activity.
cardiomyopathy (car-dee-oh-my-OP-ah-thee)	General term for a disease of the myocardium. Can be caused by alcohol abuse, parasites, viral infection, and congestive heart failure. One of the most common reasons a patient may require a heart transplant.
congenital septal defect (CSD)	A hole, present at birth, in the septum between two heart chambers; results in a mixture of oxygenated and deoxygenated blood. There can be an *atrial septal defect* (ASD) and a *ventricular septal defect* (VSD).
congestive heart failure (CHF) (kon-JESS-tiv)	Pathological condition of the heart in which there is a reduced outflow of blood from the left side of the heart because the left ventricle myocardium has become too weak to efficiently pump blood. Results in weakness, breathlessness, and edema.
coronary artery disease (CAD) (KOR-ah-nair-ee AR-ter-ee dis-EEZ)	Insufficient blood supply to the heart muscle due to an obstruction of one or more coronary arteries. May be caused by atherosclerosis and may cause angina pectoris and myocardial infarction.

Med Term Tip

All types of cardiovascular disease have been the number one killer of Americans since the 19th century. This disease kills more people annually than the next six causes of death combined.

Figure 5.15 Formation of an atherosclerotic plaque within a coronary artery; may lead to coronary artery disease, angina pectoris, and myocardial infarction.

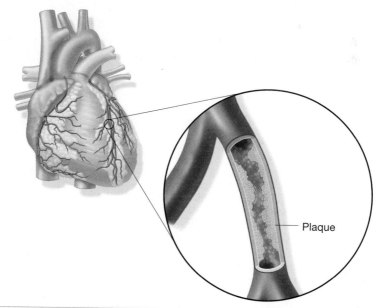

Plaque

endocarditis (en-doh-car-DYE-tis)	Inflammation of the lining membranes of the heart. May be due to bacteria or to an abnormal immunological response. In bacterial endocarditis, the mass of bacteria that forms is referred to as *vegetation*.
fibrillation (fih-brill-AY-shun)	An extremely serious arrhythmia characterized by an abnormal quivering or contraction of heart fibers. When this occurs in the ventricles, cardiac arrest and death can occur. Emergency equipment to defibrillate, or convert the heart to a normal beat, is necessary.

Pathology *(continued)*

TERM	DEFINITION
flutter	An arrhythmia in which the atria beat too rapidly, but in a regular pattern.
heart valve prolapse (PROH-laps)	Condition in which the cusps or flaps of the heart valve are too loose and fail to shut tightly, allowing blood to flow backward through the valve when the heart chamber contracts. Most commonly occurs in the mitral valve, but may affect any of the heart valves.
heart valve stenosis (steh-NOH-sis)	The cusps or flaps of the heart valve are too stiff. Therefore, they are unable to open fully, making it difficult for blood to flow through, or shut tightly, allowing blood to flow backward. This condition may affect any of the heart valves.
myocardial infarction (MI) (my-oh-CAR-dee-al in-FARC-shun)	Condition caused by the partial or complete occlusion or closing of one or more of the coronary arteries. Symptoms include a squeezing pain or heavy pressure in the middle of the chest (angina pectoris). A delay in treatment could result in death. Also referred to as a *heart attack*.

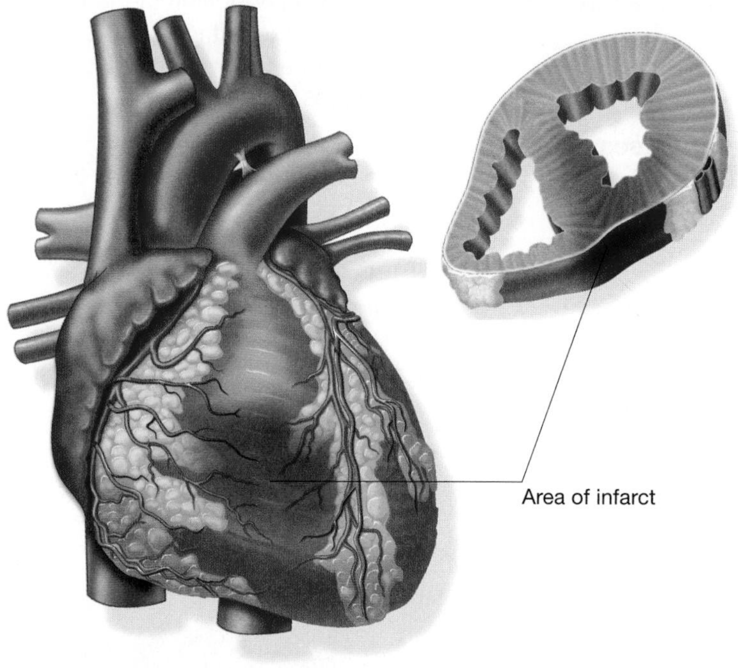

■ **Figure 5.16** External and cross-sectional view of an infarct caused by a myocardial infarction.

Area of infarct

myocarditis (my-oh-car-DYE-tis)	Inflammation of the muscle layer of the heart wall.
pericarditis (pair-ih-car-DYE-tis)	Inflammation of the pericardial sac around the heart.
tetralogy of Fallot (teh-TRALL-oh-jee of fal-LOH)	Combination of four congenital anomalies: pulmonary stenosis, an interventricular septal defect, improper placement of the aorta, and hypertrophy of the right ventricle. Needs immediate surgery to correct.

■ *Blood Vessels*

aneurysm (AN-yoo-rizm)	Weakness in the wall of an artery resulting in localized widening of the artery. Although an aneurysm may develop in any artery, common sites include the aorta in the abdomen and the cerebral arteries in the brain (see Figure 5.17 ■).
arteriosclerosis (ar-tee-ree-oh-skleh-ROH-sis)	Thickening, hardening, and loss of elasticity of the walls of the arteries. Most often due to atherosclerosis.

Pathology *(continued)*

TERM	DEFINITION
atherosclerosis (ath-er-oh-skleh-ROH-sis)	The most common form of arteriosclerosis. Caused by the formation of yellowish plaques of cholesterol on the inner walls of arteries (see Figure 5.18 ■).
coarctation of the aorta (CoA) (koh-ark-TAY-shun)	Severe congenital narrowing of the aorta.
embolus (EM-boh-lus)	The obstruction of a blood vessel by a blood clot that has broken off from a thrombus somewhere else in the body and traveled to the point of obstruction. If it occurs in a coronary artery, it may result in a myocardial infarction (see Figure 5.19 ■).
hemorrhoid (HIM-oh-royd)	Varicose veins in the anal region.

■ Figure 5.17 Illustration of a large aneurysm in the abdominal aorta which has ruptured.

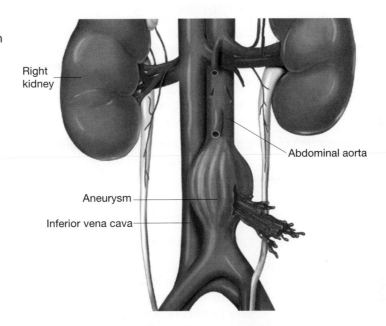

Right kidney

Abdominal aorta

Aneurysm

Inferior vena cava

■ Figure 5.18 Development of an atherosclerotic plaque that progressively narrows the lumen of an artery to the point that a thrombus fully occludes the lumen.

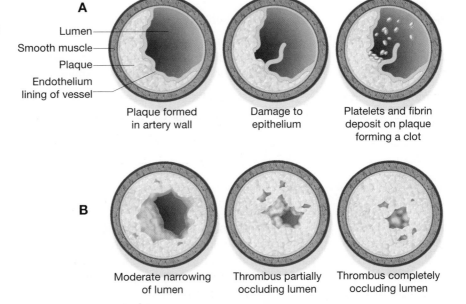

A

Lumen
Smooth muscle
Plaque
Endothelium lining of vessel

Plaque formed in artery wall

Damage to epithelium

Platelets and fibrin deposit on plaque forming a clot

B

Moderate narrowing of lumen

Thrombus partially occluding lumen

Thrombus completely occluding lumen

Figure 5.19 Illustration of an embolus floating in an artery. The embolus will eventually lodge in an artery that is smaller than it is, resulting in occlusion of that artery.

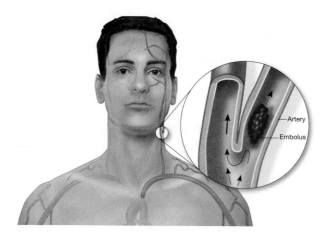

Pathology *(continued)*

TERM	DEFINITION
hypertension (HTN) (high-per-TEN-shun)	Blood pressure above the normal range. *Essential* or *primary hypertension* occurs directly from cardiovascular disease. *Secondary hypertension* refers to high blood pressure resulting from another disease such as kidney disease.
hypotension (high-poh-TEN-shun)	Decrease in blood pressure. Can occur in shock, infection, cancer, anemia, or as death approaches.
patent ductus arteriosus (PDA) (PAY-tent DUCK-tus ar-tee-ree-OH-sis)	Congenital heart anomaly in which the fetal connection between the pulmonary artery and the aorta fails to close at birth. This condition requires surgery.
peripheral vascular disease (PVD)	Any abnormal condition affecting blood vessels outside the heart. Symptoms may include pain, pallor, numbness, and loss of circulation and pulses.
polyarteritis (pol-ee-ar-ter-EYE-tis)	Inflammation of several arteries.
Raynaud's phenomenon (ray-NOZ)	Periodic ischemic attacks affecting the extremities of the body, especially the fingers, toes, ears, and nose. The affected extremities become cyanotic and very painful. These attacks are brought on by arterial constriction due to extreme cold or emotional stress.
thrombophlebitis (throm-boh-fleh-BYE-tis)	Inflammation of a vein resulting in the formation of blood clots within the vein.
thrombus (THROM-bus)	A blood clot forming within a blood vessel (see Figure 5.18). May partially or completely occlude the blood vessel.
varicose veins (VAIR-ih-kohs)	Swollen and distended veins, usually in the legs.

Diagnostic Procedures

TERM	DEFINITION
■ Clinical Laboratory Tests	
cardiac enzymes (CAR-dee-ak EN-zyms)	Blood test to determine the level of enzymes specific to heart muscles in the blood. An increase in the enzymes may indicate heart muscle damage such as a myocardial infarction. These enzymes include creatine phosphokinase (CPK), lactate dehydrogenase (LDH), and glutamic oxaloacetic transaminase (GOT).
serum lipoprotein level (SEE-rum lip-oh-PROH-teen)	Blood test to measure the amount of cholesterol and triglycerides in the blood. An indicator of atherosclerosis risk.

Diagnostic Procedures *(continued)*

TERM	DEFINITION
■ Diagnostic Imaging	
angiography (an-jee-OG-rah-fee)	X-rays taken after the injection of an opaque material into a blood vessel. Can be performed on the aorta as an aortic angiogram, on the heart as an angiocardiogram, and on the brain as a cerebral angiogram.
cardiac scan	Patient is given radioactive thallium intravenously and then scanning equipment is used to visualize the heart. It is especially useful in determining myocardial damage.
Doppler ultrasonography (DOP-ler ul-trah-son-OG-rah-fee)	Measurement of sound-wave echoes as they bounce off tissues and organs to produce an image. In this system, used to measure velocity of blood moving through blood vessels to look for blood clots or deep vein thromboses.
echocardiography (ek-oh-car-dee-OG-rah-fee)	Noninvasive diagnostic method using ultrasound to visualize internal cardiac structures. Cardiac valve activity can be evaluated using this method.
venography (vee-NOG-rah-fee)	X-ray of the veins by tracing the venous pulse. May be used to identify a thrombus. Also called *phlebography*.
■ Cardiac Function Tests	
cardiac catheterization (CAR-dee-ak cath-eh-ter-ih-ZAY-shun)	Passage of a thin tube catheter through a blood vessel leading to the heart. Done to detect abnormalities, to collect cardiac blood samples, and to determine the blood pressure within the heart.
electrocardiography (ECG, EKG) (ee-lek-troh-car-dee-OG-rah-fee)	Process of recording the electrical activity of the heart. Useful in the diagnosis of abnormal cardiac rhythm and heart muscle (myocardium) damage.
Holter monitor	Portable ECG monitor worn by a patient for a period of a few hours to a few days to assess the heart and pulse activity as the person goes through the activities of daily living. Used to assess a patient who experiences chest pain and unusual heart activity during exercise and normal activities.
stress testing	Method for evaluating cardiovascular fitness. The patient is placed on a treadmill or a bicycle and then subjected to steadily increasing levels of work. An EKG and oxygen levels are taken while the patient exercises. The test is stopped if abnormalities occur on the EKG. Also called an *exercise test* or a *treadmill test*

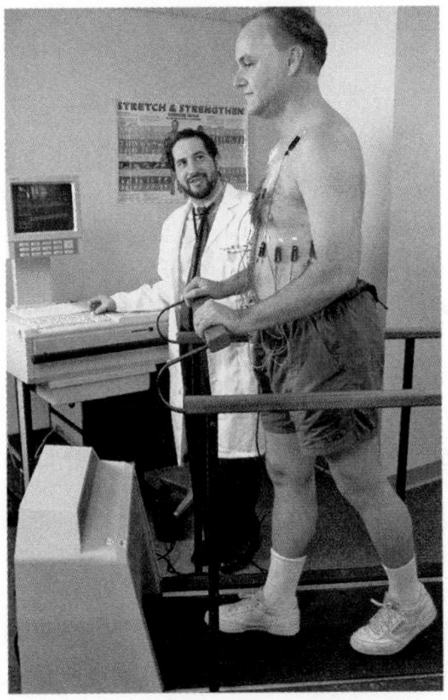

■ **Figure 5.20** Man undergoing a stress test on a treadmill while physician monitors his condition. *(Jonathan Nourok/PhotoEdit Inc.)*

Therapeutic Procedures

TERM	DEFINITION
Medical Procedures	
cardiopulmonary resuscitation (CPR) (car-dee-oh-PULL-mon-air-ee ree-suss-ih-TAY-shun)	Procedure to restore cardiac output and oxygenated air to the lungs for a person in cardiac arrest. A combination of chest compressions (to push blood out of the heart) and artificial respiration (to blow air into the lungs) performed by one or two CPR-trained rescuers.
defibrillation (dee-fib-rih-LAY-shun)	A procedure that converts serious irregular heartbeats, such as fibrillation, by giving electric shocks to the heart using an instrument called a defibrillator. Also called *cardioversion*.
■ **Figure 5.21** An emergency medical technician positions defibrillator paddles on the chest of a supine male patient.	
extracorporeal circulation (ECC) (EX-tra-core-poor-EE-al)	During open-heart surgery, the routing of blood to a heart-lung machine so it can be oxygenated and pumped to the rest of the body.
implantable cardioverter-defibrillator (CAR-dee-oh-ver-ter de-FIB-rih-lay-tor)	A device implanted in the heart that delivers an electrical shock to restore a normal heart rhythm. Particularly useful for persons who experience ventricular fibrillation.
pacemaker implantation	Electrical device that substitutes for the natural pacemaker of the heart. It controls the beating of the heart by a series of rhythmic electrical impulses. An external pacemaker has the electrodes on the outside of the body. An internal pacemaker has the electrodes surgically implanted within the chest wall (see Figure 5.22 ■).
thrombolytic therapy (throm-boh-LIT-ik THAIR-ah-pee)	Process in which drugs, such as streptokinase (SK) or tissue-type plasminogen activator (tPA), are injected into a blood vessel to dissolve clots and restore blood flow.
Surgical Procedures	
aneurysmectomy (an-yoo-riz-MEK-toh-mee)	The surgical removal of the sac of an aneurysm.
arterial anastomosis (ar-TEE-ree-all ah-nas-toe-MOE-sis)	The surgical joining together of two arteries. Performed if an artery is severed or if a damaged section of an artery is removed.
coronary artery bypass graft (CABG) (KOR-ah-nair-ee)	Open-heart surgery in which a blood vessel from another location in the body (often a leg vein) is grafted to route blood around a blocked coronary artery.
embolectomy (em-boh-LEK-toh-mee)	The removal of an embolus or clot from a blood vessel.
endarterectomy (end-ar-teh-REK-toh-mee)	Removal of the diseased or damaged inner lining of an artery. Usually performed to remove atherosclerotic plaques.

Therapeutic Procedures *(continued)*

TERM	DEFINITION
heart transplantation	Replacement of a diseased or malfunctioning heart with a donor's heart.
intracoronary artery stent (in-trah-KOR-ah-nair-ee AR-ter-ee)	Placing of a stent within a coronary artery to treat coronary ischemia due to atherosclerosis (see Figure 5.14).
ligation and stripping (lye-GAY-shun)	Surgical treatment for varicose veins. The damaged vein is tied off (ligation) and removed (stripping).
percutaneous transluminal coronary angioplasty (PTCA) (per-kyoo-TAY-nee-us trans-LOO-mih-nal KOR-ah-nair-ee AN-jee-oh-plas-tee)	The method for treating localized coronary artery narrowing. A balloon catheter is inserted through the skin into the coronary artery and inflated to dilate the narrow blood vessel (see Figure 5.23 ■).
valve replacement	Removal of a diseased heart valve and replacement with an artificial valve.

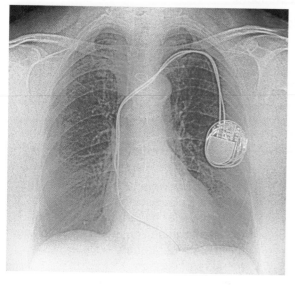

■ **Figure 5.22** Color enhanced X-ray showing a pacemaker implanted in the left side of the chest and the electrode wires running to the heart muscle. *(UHB Trust/Getty Images Inc.—Stone Allstock)*

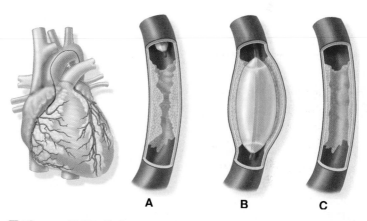

A   B   C

■ **Figure 5.23** Balloon angioplasty: A) deflated balloon catheter is approaching an atherosclerotic plaque; B) plaque is compressed by inflated balloon; C) plaque remains compressed after balloon catheter is removed.

Pharmacology

CLASSIFICATION	ACTION	GENERIC AND BRAND NAMES
ACE inhibitor drugs	Produce vasodilation and decrease blood pressure.	benazepril, Lotensin; catopril, Capoten
antiarrhythmic (an-tye-a-RHYTH-mik)	Reduces or prevents cardiac arrhythmias.	flecainide, Tambocor; ibutilide, Corvert
anticoagulant (an-tye-koh-AG-you-lant)	Prevent blood clot formation.	warfarin sodium, Coumadin, Warfarin
antilipidemic (an-tye-lip-ih-DEM-ik)	Reduces amount of cholesterol and lipids in the bloodstream; treats hyperlipidemia.	atorvastatin, Lipitor; simvastatin, Zocor

Pharmacology (continued)

CLASSIFICATION	ACTION	GENERIC AND BRAND NAMES
beta-blocker drugs	Treats hypertension and angina pectoris by lowering the heart rate.	metoprolol, Lopressor; propranolol, Inderal
calcium channel blocker drugs	Treats hypertension, angina pectoris, and congestive heart failure by causing the heart to beat less forcefully and less often.	diltiazem, Cardizem; nifedipine, Procardia
cardiotonic (card-ee-oh-TAHN-ik)	Increases the force of cardiac muscle contraction; treats congestive heart failure.	digoxin, Lanoxin
diuretic (dye-you-RET-ik)	Increases urine production by the kidneys, which works to reduce plasma and therefore blood volume, resulting in lower blood pressure.	furosemide, Lasix
thrombolytic (throm-boh-LIT-ik)	Dissolves existing blood clots.	clopidogrel, Plavix; alteplase, Activase
vasoconstrictor (vaz-oh-kon-STRICK-tor)	Contracts smooth muscle in walls of blood vessels; raises blood pressure.	metaraminol, Aramine
vasodilator (vaz-oh-DYE-late-or)	Relaxes the smooth muscle in the walls of arteries, thereby increasing diameter of the blood vessel. Used for two main purposes: increasing circulation to an ischemic area; reducing blood pressure.	nitroglycerine, Nitro-Dur; isoxsuprine, Vasodilan

Abbreviations

AF	atrial fibrillation	**IV**	intravenous
AMI	acute myocardial infarction	**LDH**	lactate dehydrogenase
AS	arteriosclerosis	**LVAD**	left ventricular assist device
ASD	atrial septal defect	**LVH**	left ventricular hypertrophy
ASHD	arteriosclerotic heart disease	**MI**	myocardial infarction, mitral insufficiency
AV, A-V	atrioventricular	**mm Hg**	millimeters of mercury
BBB	bundle branch block (L for left; R for right)	**MR**	mitral regurgitation
BP	blood pressure	**MS**	mitral stenosis
bpm	beats per minute		
CABG	coronary artery bypass graft		
CAD	coronary artery disease		
cath	catheterization		

Med Term Tip

Word alert – be careful using the abbreviation *MS* which can mean either "mitral stenosis" or "multiple sclerosis."

CC	cardiac catheterization, chief complaint	**MVP**	mitral valve prolapse
CCU	coronary care unit	**P**	pulse
CHF	congestive heart failure	**PAC**	premature atrial contraction
CoA	coarctation of the aorta	**PDA**	patent ductus arteriosus
CP	chest pain	**PTCA**	percutaneous transluminal coronary angioplasty
CPK	creatine phosphokinase		
CPR	cardiopulmonary resuscitation	**PVC**	premature ventricular contraction
CSD	congenital septal defect	**S1**	first heart sound
CV	cardiovascular	**S2**	second heart sound
DVT	deep vein thrombosis	**SA, S-A**	sinoatrial
ECC	extracorporeal circulation	**SGOT**	serum glutamic oxaloacetic transaminase
ECG, EKG	electrocardiogram	**SK**	streptokinase
ECHO	echocardiogram	**tPA**	tissue-type plasminogen activator
GOT	glutamic oxaloacetic transaminase	**Vfib**	ventricular fibrillation
HTN	hypertension	**VSD**	ventricular septal defect
ICU	intensive care unit	**VT**	ventricular tachycardia

Chapter Review

Terminology Checklist

Below are all Anatomy and Physiology key terms, Word Building, Vocabulary, Pathology, Diagnostic, Therapeutic, and Pharmacology terms presented in this chapter. Use this list as a study tool by placing a check in the box in front of each term as you master its meaning.

- ☐ ACE inhibitor drugs
- ☐ aneurysm
- ☐ aneurysmectomy
- ☐ angiitis
- ☐ angina pectoris
- ☐ angiogram
- ☐ angiography
- ☐ angioplasty
- ☐ angiospasm
- ☐ angiostenosis
- ☐ antiarrhythmic
- ☐ anticoagulant
- ☐ antilipidemic
- ☐ aorta
- ☐ aortic
- ☐ aortic valve
- ☐ apex
- ☐ arrhythmia
- ☐ arterial
- ☐ arterial anastomosis
- ☐ arteries
- ☐ arterioles
- ☐ arteriorrhexis
- ☐ arteriosclerosis
- ☐ atherectomy
- ☐ atheroma
- ☐ atherosclerosis
- ☐ atria
- ☐ atrial
- ☐ atrioventricular bundle
- ☐ atrioventricular node
- ☐ atrioventricular valve
- ☐ auscultation
- ☐ autonomic nervous system
- ☐ beta blocker drugs
- ☐ bicuspid valve
- ☐ blood pressure
- ☐ blood vessels

- ☐ bradycardia
- ☐ bundle branch block
- ☐ bundle branches
- ☐ bundle of His
- ☐ calcium channel blocker drugs
- ☐ capillaries
- ☐ capillary bed
- ☐ carbon dioxide
- ☐ cardiac
- ☐ cardiac arrest
- ☐ cardiac catheterization
- ☐ cardiac enzymes
- ☐ cardiac muscle
- ☐ cardiac scan
- ☐ cardiologist
- ☐ cardiology
- ☐ cardiomegaly
- ☐ cardiomyopathy
- ☐ cardiopulmonary resuscitation
- ☐ cardiorrhexis
- ☐ cardiotonic
- ☐ catheter
- ☐ circulatory system
- ☐ coarctation of the aorta
- ☐ congenital septal defect
- ☐ congestive heart failure
- ☐ coronary
- ☐ coronary arteries
- ☐ coronary artery bypass graft
- ☐ coronary artery disease
- ☐ cusps
- ☐ defibrillation
- ☐ deoxygenated
- ☐ diastole
- ☐ diastolic pressure
- ☐ diuretic
- ☐ Doppler ultrasonography
- ☐ echocardiography

- ☐ electrocardiogram
- ☐ electrocardiography
- ☐ embolectomy
- ☐ embolus
- ☐ endarterectomy
- ☐ endocarditis
- ☐ endocardium
- ☐ epicardium
- ☐ extracorporeal circulation
- ☐ fibrillation
- ☐ flutter
- ☐ heart
- ☐ heart transplantation
- ☐ heart valve prolapse
- ☐ heart valve stenosis
- ☐ hemorrhoid
- ☐ Holter monitor
- ☐ hypertension
- ☐ hypotension
- ☐ implantable cardioverter-defibrillator
- ☐ infarct
- ☐ inferior vena cava
- ☐ interatrial
- ☐ interatrial septum
- ☐ interventricular
- ☐ interventricular septum
- ☐ intracoronary artery stent
- ☐ ischemia
- ☐ ligation and stripping
- ☐ lumen
- ☐ mitral valve
- ☐ murmur
- ☐ myocardial
- ☐ myocardial infarction
- ☐ myocarditis
- ☐ myocardium
- ☐ orthostatic hypotension

- oxygen
- oxygenated
- pacemaker
- pacemaker implantation
- palpitations
- parietal pericardium
- patent ductus arteriosus
- percutaneous transluminal coronary angioplasty
- pericarditis
- pericardium
- peripheral vascular disease
- phlebitis
- phlebogram
- plaque
- polyarteritis
- pulmonary artery
- pulmonary circulation
- pulmonary valve
- pulmonary vein
- pulse
- Purkinje fibers
- Raynaud's phenomenon
- regurgitation
- semilunar valves
- serum lipoprotein
- sinoatrial node
- sphygmomanometer
- stent
- stethoscope
- stress testing
- superior vena cava
- systemic circulation
- systole
- systolic pressure
- tachycardia
- tetralogy of Fallot
- thrombolytic
- thrombolytic therapy
- thrombophlebitis
- thrombus
- tricuspid valve
- valve replacement
- valvoplasty
- valvular
- valvulitis
- varicose veins
- vascular
- vasoconstrictor
- vasodilator
- veins
- venography
- venous
- ventricles
- ventricular
- venules
- visceral pericardium

Practice Exercises

A. Complete the following statements.

1. The study of the heart is called _____.

2. The three layers of the heart are _____, _____, and _____.

3. The impulse for the heartbeat (the pacemaker) originates in the _____.

4. Arteries carry blood _____ the heart.

5. The four heart valves are _____, _____, _____, and _____.

6. The _____ are the receiving chambers of the heart and the _____ are the pumping chambers.

7. The _____ circulation carries blood to and from the lungs.

8. The pointed tip of the heart is called the _____.

9. The _____ divides the heart into left and right halves.

10. _____ is the contraction phase of the heart beat and _____ is the relaxation phase.

B. State the terms described using the combining forms provided.

The combining form *cardi/o* refers to the heart. Use it to write a term that means:

1. pertaining to the heart _____

2. disease of the heart muscle _____

3. enlargement of the heart _____

4. abnormally fast heart rate _____

5. abnormally slow heart rate _____

6. rupture of the heart _____

The combining form *angi/o* refers to the vessel. Use it to write a term that means:

7. vessel narrowing _____

8. vessel inflammation _____

9. involuntary muscle contraction of a vessel _____

The combining form *arteri/o* refers to the artery. Use it to write a term that means:

10. pertaining to an artery _____

11. hardening of an artery _____

12. small artery _____

C. Add a prefix to *-carditis* to form the term for:

1. inflammation of the inner lining of the heart _____

2. inflammation of the outer layer of the heart _____

3. inflammation of the muscle of the heart _____

D. Define the following combining forms and use them to form cardiovascular terms.

	Definition	Cardiovascular Term
1. cardi/o		
2. valvul/o		
3. steth/o		
4. arteri/o		
5. phleb/o		
6. angi/o		
7. ventricul/o		

8. thromb/o _____ _____

9. atri/o _____ _____

10. ather/o _____ _____

E. Write medical terms for the following definitions.

1. pertaining to a vein _____

2. study of the heart _____

3. record of a vein _____

4. process of recording electrical activity of heart _____

5. high blood pressure _____

6. low blood pressure _____

7. surgical repair of valve _____

8. pertaining to between ventricles _____

9. removal of fatty substance _____

10. narrowing of the arteries _____

F. Write the suffix for each expression and provide an example of its use.

	Suffix	Example
1. pressure	_____	_____
2. abnormal narrowing	_____	_____
3. instrument to measure pressure	_____	_____
4. small	_____	_____
5. hardening	_____	_____

G. Identify the following abbreviations.

1. BP _____

2. CHF _____

3. MI _____

4. CCU _____

5. PVC _____

6. CPR _____

7. CAD _____

8. CP _____

9. EKG _____

10. S1 _____

H. Write the abbreviations for the following terms.

1. mitral valve prolapse _____   6. lactate dehydrogenase _____

2. ventricular septal defect _____   7. coarctation of the aorta _____

3. percutaneous transluminal coronary angioplasty _____   8. tissue-type plasminogen activator _____

   _____   _____

4. ventricular fibrillation _____   9. cardiovascular _____

5. deep vein thrombosis _____   10. extracorporeal circulation _____

I. Match each term to its definition.

1. _____ arrhythmia   a. swollen, distended veins

2. _____ thrombus   b. inflammation of vein

3. _____ bradycardia   c. serious congenital anomaly

4. _____ murmur   d. slow heart rate

5. _____ phlebitis   e. insertion of thin tubing

6. _____ hypotension   f. irregular heartbeat

7. _____ varicose vein   g. an abnormal heart sound

8. _____ tetralogy of Fallot h. clot in blood vessel

9. _____ catheterization   i. low blood pressure

10. _____ sphygmomanometer   j. blood pressure cuff

J. Define the following terms.

1. catheter _____

2. infarct _____

3. thrombus _____

4. palpitation _____

5. regurgitation _____

6. aneurysm _____

7. cardiac arrest _____

8. fibrillation _____

9. myocardial infarction _____

10. hemorrhoid _____

K. Match each procedure to its definition.

1. _____ cardiac enzymes

2. _____ Doppler ultrasound

3. _____ Holter monitor

4. _____ cardiac scan

5. _____ stress testing

6. _____ echocardiography

7. _____ extracorporeal circulation

8. _____ ligation and stripping

9. _____ thrombolytic therapy

10. _____ PTAC

a. visualizes heart after patient is given radioactive thallium

b. uses ultrasound to visualize heart beating

c. blood test that indicates heart muscle damage

d. uses treadmill to evaluate cardiac fitness

e. removes varicose veins

f. clot dissolving drugs

g. measures velocity of blood moving through blood vessels

h. balloon angioplasty

i. use of a heart-lung machine

j. portable EKG monitor

L. Fill in the classification for each drug description, then match the brand name.

Drug Description	Classification	Brand Name
1. _____ prevents arrhthymia	_____	a. Plavix
2. _____ reduces cholesterol	_____	b. Coumadin
3. _____ increases force of heart contraction	_____	c. Cardizem
4. _____ increases urine production	_____	d. Nitro-Dur
5. _____ prevents blood clots	_____	e. Tambocor
6. _____ dissolves blood clots	_____	f. Lanoxin
7. _____ relaxes smooth muscle in artery wall	_____	g. Lipitor
8. _____ cause heart to beat less forcefully	_____	h. Lasix

M. Use the following terms in the sentences that follow.

angiography	murmur	varicose veins	echocardiogram	pacemaker	CHF
defibrillation	angina pectoris	Holter monitor	hypertension	MI	CCU

1. Tiffany was born with a congenital condition resulting in an abnormal heart sound called a(n) _____.

2. Joseph suffered an arrhythmia resulting in a cardiac arrest. The emergency team used an instrument to give electric shocks to the heart to create a normal heart rhythm. This procedure is called _____.

3. Marguerite has been placed on a low-sodium diet and medication to bring her blood pressure down to a normal range. She suffers from _____.

4. Tony has had an artificial device called a(n) _____ inserted to control the beating of his heart by producing rhythmic electrical impulses.

5. Derrick's physician determined that he had _____ after examining his legs and finding swollen, tortuous veins.

6. Laura has persistent chest pains that require medication. The term for the pain is _____.

7. La Tonya will be admitted to what hospital unit after surgery to correct her heart condition? _____

8. Stephen is going to have a coronary artery bypass graft to correct the blockage in his coronary arteries. He recently suffered a heart attack as a result of this occlusion. His attack is called a(n) _____.

9. Stephen's physician scheduled a(n) _____, an X-ray to determine the extent of his blood vessel damage.

10. A patient scheduled to have a diagnostic procedure that uses ultrasound to produce an image of the heart valves is going to have a(n) _____.

11. Eric must wear a device for 24 hours that will keep track of his heart activity as he performs his normal daily routine. This device is called a(n) _____.

12. Lydia is 82 years old and is suffering from a heart condition that causes weakness, edema, and breathlessness. Her heart failure is the cause of her lung congestion. This condition is called _____.

Medical Record Analysis

Below is an item from a patient's medical record. Read it carefully, make sure you understand all the medical terms used, and then answer the questions that follow.

Discharge Summary

Admitting Diagnosis:	Difficulty breathing, hypertension, tachycardia
Final Diagnosis:	CHF secondary to mitral valve prolapse
History of Present Illness:	Patient was brought to the Emergency Room by her family because of SOB, tachycardia, and anxiety. Patient reports that she has experienced these symptoms for the past six months, brought on by exertion. The current episode began while she was cleaning house and is more severe than any previous episode. Upon admission in the ER, HR was 120 beats per minute and blood pressure was 180/110. The patient was cyanotic around the lips and nail beds and had severe edema in feet and lower legs. The results of an EKG and cardiac enzyme blood tests were normal. Medication improved the symptoms, but she was admitted for observation and a complete cardiac workup for tachycardia, hypertension.
Summary of Hospital Course:	Patient underwent a full battery of cardiac diagnostic tests. A prolapsed mitral valve was observed on an echocardiogram. A treadmill test had to be stopped early due to onset of severe difficulty in breathing and cyanosis of the lips. Arterial blood gases showed low oxygen, and supplemental oxygen per nasal canula was required to resolve cyanosis. Angiocardiography failed to demonstrate significant coronary artery thrombosis. Blood pressure, tachycardia, anxiety, and pitting edema were controlled with medications. Patient took Lopressor to control blood pressure, Norpace to slow heart rate, Valium for the anxiety, and Lasix to reduce edema. At discharge, HR was 88 beats per minute, blood pressure was 165/98, and there was no evidence of edema unless she was on her feet too long.
Discharge Plans:	There was no evidence of a myocardial infarction and with lack of significant coronary thrombosis, angioplasty is not indicated for this patient. Patient was placed on a low-salt and low-cholesterol diet. She received instructions on beginning a carefully graded exercise program. She is to continue Lasix, Norpace, Valium, and Lopressor. If symptoms are not controlled by these measures, a mitral valve replacement will be considered.

Critical Thinking Questions

1. List the four medications this patient was given in the hospital and describe in your own words what condition each medication treats.

   a. _____

   b. _____

   c. _____

   d. _____

2. Two diagnostic tests conducted in the Emergency Room were normal. List them and describe each test in your own words. Because the results from these two tests were normal, a very serious heart condition could be ruled out. This is noted in the discharge plans. Identify the serious heart condition and describe it in your own words.

_____

_____

_____

3. Explain in your own words why the treadmill test had to be stopped. _____

_____

_____

4. Which of the following is NOT one of the admitting diagnoses?
   a. high blood pressure
   b. dizziness
   c. difficulty breathing
   d. fast heartbeat

5. The physician has two treatment options for this patient: medication and surgery. If the medication fails to control her condition, then describe what surgery will be considered. _____

_____

_____

6. Compare and contrast valve stenosis and valve prolapse. _____

_____

_____

Chart Note Transcription

The chart note below contains eleven phrases that can be reworded with a medical term that you learned in this chapter. Each phrase is identified with an underline. Determine the medical term and write your answers in the space provided.

Current Complaint: A 56-year-old male was admitted to the Cardiac Care Unit from the Emergency Room with left arm pain, severe pain around the heart, ❶ an abnormally slow heartbeat, ❷ nausea, and vomiting.

Past History: Patient reports no heart problems prior to this episode. He has taken medication for high blood pressure ❸ for the past five years. His family history is significant for a father and brother who both died in their 50s from death of heart muscle. ❹

Signs and Symptoms: Patient reports severe pain around the heart that radiates into his left jaw and arm. A record of the heart's electrical activity ❺ and a blood test to determine the amount of heart damage ❻ were abnormal.

Diagnosis: An acute death of heart muscle ❹ resulting from insufficient blood flow to heart muscle due to obstruction of coronary artery. ❼

Treatment: First, provide supportive care during the acute phase. Second, evaluate heart damage by passing a thin tube through a blood vessel into the heart to detect abnormalities ❽ and evaluate heart fitness by having patient exercise on a treadmill. ❾ Finally, perform surgical intervention by either inflating a balloon catheter to dilate a narrow vessel ❿ or by open heart surgery to create a shunt around a blocked vessel. ⓫

❶ _____

❷ _____

❸ _____

❹ _____

❺ _____

❻ _____

❼ _____

❽ _____

❾ _____

❿ _____

⓫ _____

Labeling Exercise

A. System Review

Write the labels for this figure on the numbered lines provided.

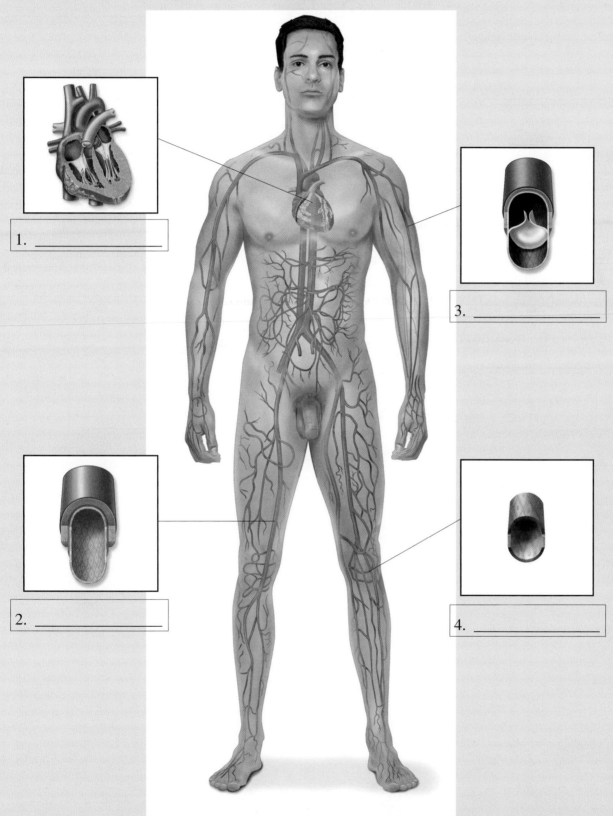

1. _____

2. _____

3. _____

4. _____

B. Anatomy Challenge

1. Write the labels for this figure on the numbered lines provided.

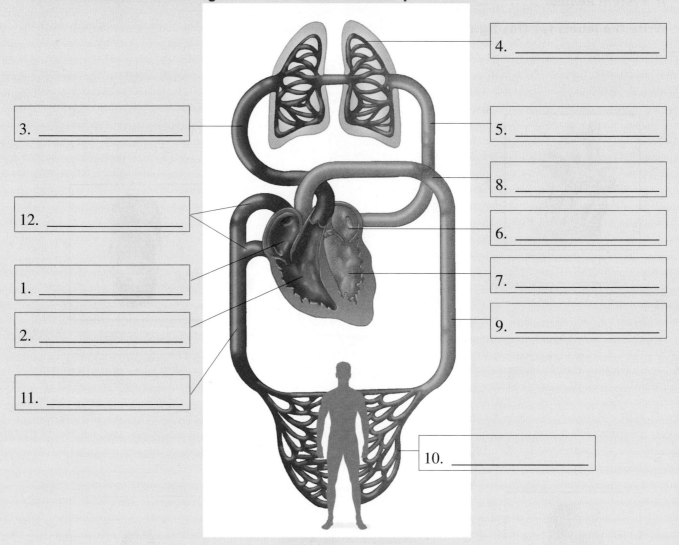

3. _____

12. _____

1. _____

2. _____

11. _____

4. _____

5. _____

8. _____

6. _____

7. _____

9. _____

10. _____

2. Write the labels for this figure on the numbered lines provided.

13. _____

12. _____

5. _____

4. _____

1. _____

2. _____

3. _____

14. _____

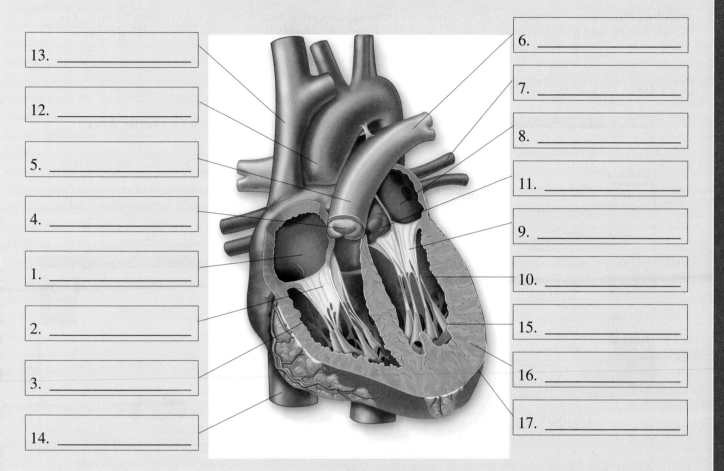

6. _____

7. _____

8. _____

11. _____

9. _____

10. _____

15. _____

16. _____

17. _____

Multimedia Preview

Additional interactive resources and activities for this chapter can be found on the Companion Website. For videos, games, and pronunciations, please access the accompanying DVD-ROM that comes with this book.

DVD-ROM Highlights

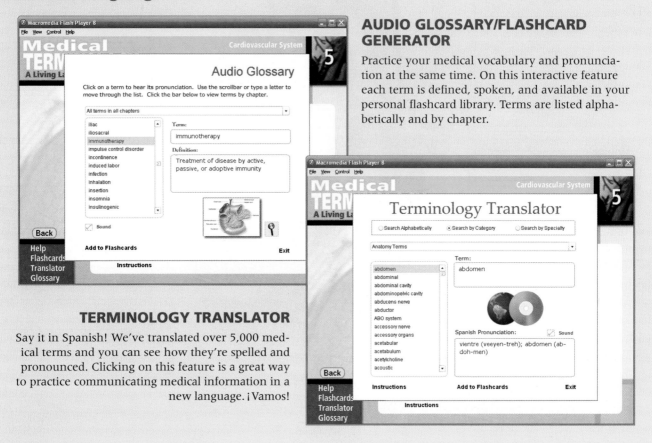

AUDIO GLOSSARY/FLASHCARD GENERATOR

Practice your medical vocabulary and pronunciation at the same time. On this interactive feature each term is defined, spoken, and available in your personal flashcard library. Terms are listed alphabetically and by chapter.

TERMINOLOGY TRANSLATOR

Say it in Spanish! We've translated over 5,000 medical terms and you can see how they're spelled and pronounced. Clicking on this feature is a great way to practice communicating medical information in a new language. ¡Vamos!

Website Highlights — www.prenhall.com/fremgen

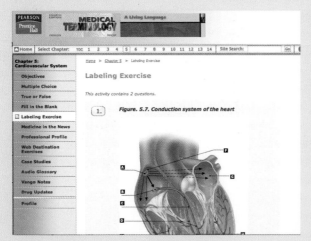

LABELING EXERCISE

Click here and take advantage of the free-access on-line study guide that accompanies your textbook. You'll find a figure labeling quiz that corresponds to this chapter. By clicking on this URL you'll also access links to download mp3 audio reviews, current news articles, and an audio glossary.

6

Blood and the Lymphatic and Immune Systems

Learning Objectives

Upon completion of this chapter, you will be able to:

- Recognize the combining forms and suffixes introduced in this chapter.
- Gain the ability to pronounce medical terms and major anatomical structures.
- List the major components, structures, and organs of the blood and lymphatic and immune systems and their functions.
- Describe the blood typing systems.
- Discuss immunity, the immune response, and standard precautions.
- Build blood and lymphatic and immune system medical terms from word parts.
- Define vocabulary, pathology, diagnostic, and therapeutic medical terms relating to the blood and lymphatic and immune system.
- Recognize types of medication associated with blood and the lymphatic and immune systems.
- Interpret abbreviations associated with blood and the lymphatic and immune systems.

Section I: Blood at a Glance

Function

Blood transports to all areas of the body gases, nutrients, and wastes either attached to red blood cells or dissolved in the plasma. White blood cells fight infection and disease, and platelets initiate the blood clotting process.

Components

formed elements
- **erythrocytes**
- **platelets**
- **leukocytes**

plasma

Combining Forms

agglutin/o	clumping		**hem/o**	blood
bas/o	base		**hemat/o**	blood
chrom/o	color		**leuk/o**	white
coagul/o	clotting		**morph/o**	shape
eosin/o	rosy red		**neutr/o**	neutral
erythr/o	red		**phag/o**	eat, swallow
fibrin/o	fibers, fibrous		**sanguin/o**	blood
granul/o	granules		**thromb/o**	clot

Suffixes

-apheresis	removal, carry away
-cytosis	more than the normal number of cells
-emia	blood condition
-globin	protein
-penia	abnormal decrease, too few
-phil	attracted to
-poiesis	formation
-stasis	standing still

Blood Illustrated

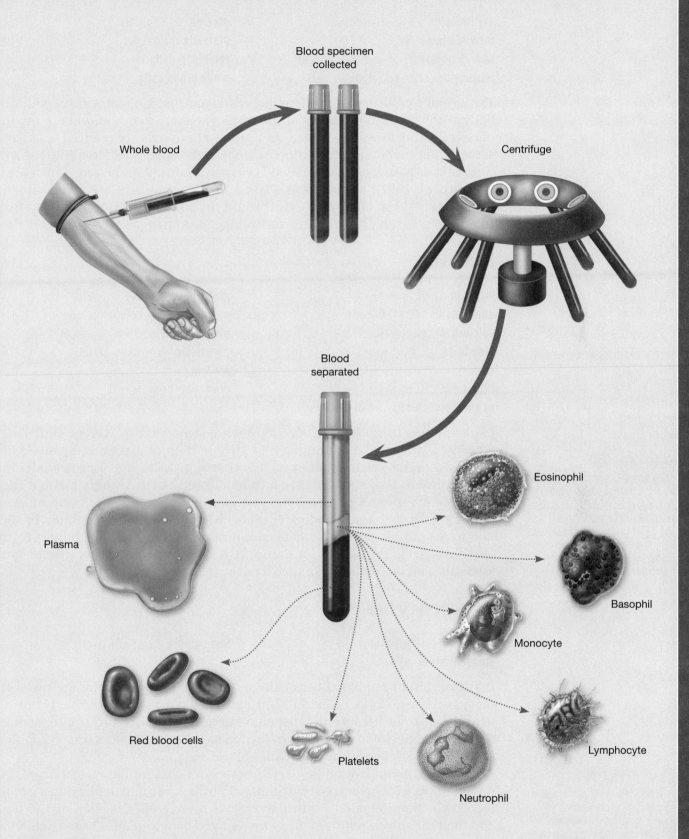

Whole blood

Blood specimen collected

Centrifuge

Blood separated

Plasma

Eosinophil

Basophil

Monocyte

Red blood cells

Platelets

Neutrophil

Lymphocyte

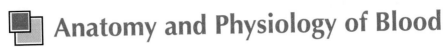 Anatomy and Physiology of Blood

erythrocytes (eh-RITH-roh-sights)
formed elements
hematopoiesis (hee-mah-toh-poy-EE-sis)
leukocytes (LOO-koh-sights)

plasma (PLAZ-mah)
platelets (PLAYT lets)
red blood cells
white blood cells

The average adult has about five liters of blood that circulates throughout the body within the blood vessels of the cardiovascular system. Blood is a mixture of cells floating in watery **plasma**. As a group, these cells are referred to as **formed elements**, but there are three different kinds: **erythrocytes** or **red blood cells**, **leukocytes** or **white blood cells**, and **platelets**. Blood cells are produced in the red bone marrow by a process called **hematopoiesis**. Plasma and erythrocytes are responsible for transporting substances, leukocytes protect the body from invading microorganisms, and platelets play a role in controlling bleeding.

Plasma

albumin (al-BEW-min)
amino acids (ah-MEE-noh)
calcium (KAL-see-um)
creatinine (kree-AT-in-in)
fats
fibrinogen (fye-BRIN-oh-jen)
gamma globulin (GAM-ah GLOB-yoo-lin)

globulins (GLOB-yew-lenz)
glucose (GLOO-kohs)
plasma proteins
potassium (poh-TASS-ee-um)
sodium
urea (yoo-REE-ah)

Med Term Tip

Word watch—plasma and *serum* are not interchangeable words. Serum is plasma, but with fibrinogen removed or inactivated. This way it can be handled and tested without it clotting. The term *serum* is also sometimes used to mean antiserum or antitoxin.

Liquid plasma composes about 55% of whole blood in the average adult and is 90 to 92% water. The remaining 8 to 10% portion of plasma is dissolved substances, especially **plasma proteins** such as **albumin**, **globulins**, and **fibrinogen**. Albumin helps transport fatty substances that cannot dissolve in the watery plasma. There are three main types of globulins. The most commonly known one of these, **gamma globulin**, acts as antibodies. Fibrinogen is a blood-clotting protein. In addition to the plasma proteins, smaller amounts of other important substances are also dissolved in the plasma for transport: **calcium**, **potassium**, **sodium**, **glucose**, **amino acids**, **fats**, and waste products such as **urea** and **creatinine**.

Erythrocytes

bilirubin (bil-ly-ROO-bin)
enucleated (ee-NEW-klee-ate-ed)

hemoglobin (hee-moh-GLOH-bin)

Erythrocytes, or red blood cells (RBCs), are biconcave disks that are **enucleated**, meaning they no longer contain a nucleus (see Figure 6.1 ■). Red blood cells appear red in color because they contain **hemoglobin**, which is an iron-containing pigment. Hemoglobin is the part of the red blood cell that picks up oxygen from the lungs and delivers it to the tissues of the body.

There are about five million erythrocytes per cubic millimeter of blood. The total number in an average-sized adult is 35 trillion, with males having more red blood cells than females. Erythrocytes have an average life span of 120 days, and then the spleen removes the worn-out and damaged ones from circulation. Much of the red blood cell, such as the iron, can be reused, but one portion, **bilirubin**, is a waste product disposed of by the liver.

Med Term Tip

Your body makes about 2 million erythrocytes every second. Of course, it must then destroy 2 million every second to maintain a relatively constant 30 trillion red blood cells.

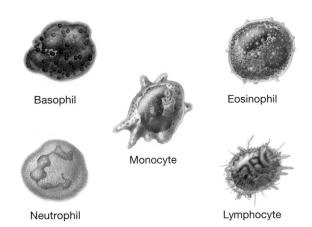

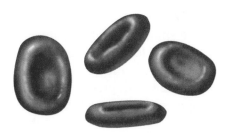

■ **Figure 6.1** The biconcave disk shape of erythrocytes (red blood cells).

■ **Figure 6.2** The five different types of leukocytes (white blood cells).

Leukocytes

agranulocytes (ah-GRAN-yew-loh-sights)

granulocytes (GRAN-yew-loh-sights)

pathogens (PATH-oh-ginz)

Leukocytes, also referred to as white blood cells (WBCs), provide protection against the invasion of **pathogens** such as bacteria, viruses, and other foreign material. In general, white blood cells have a spherical shape with a large nucleus, and there are about 8,000 per cubic millimeter of blood (see Figure 6.2 ■). There are five different types of white blood cells, each with its own strategy for protecting the body. The five can be subdivided into two categories: **granulocytes** (with granules in the cytoplasm) and **agranulocytes** (without granules in the cytoplasm). The name and function of each type is presented in Table 6.1 ■.

Med Term Tip

A **phagocyte** is a cell that has the ability to ingest (eat) and digest bacteria and other foreign particles. This process, **phagocytosis**, is critical for the control of bacteria within the body.

Table 6.1	Leukocyte Classification	
LEUKOCYTE	**FUNCTION**
Granulocytes	
Basophils (basos) (BAY-soh-fillz)	Release histamine and heparin to damaged tissues
Eosinophils (eosins) (ee-oh-SIN-oh-fillz)	Destroy parasites and increase during allergic reactions
Neutrophils (NOO-troh-fillz)	Important for phagocytosis; most numerous of the leukocytes
Agranulocytes	
Monocytes (monos) (MON-oh-sights)	Important for phagocytosis
Lymphocytes (lymphs) (LIM-foh-sights)	Plays several different roles in immune response

Platelets

agglutinate (ah-GLOO-tih-nayt)

fibrin (FYE-brin)

hemostasis (hee-moh-STAY-sis)

prothrombin (proh-THROM-bin)

thrombin (THROM-bin)

thrombocyte (THROM-boh-sight)

thromboplastin (throm-boh-PLAS-tin)

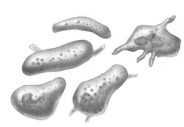

■**Figure 6.3** Platelet structure.

Platelet, the modern term for **thrombocyte,** refers to the smallest of all the formed blood elements. Platelets are not whole cells, but rather are formed when the cytoplasm of a large precursor cell shatters into small plate-like fragments (see Figure 6.3 ■). There are between 200,000 and 300,000 per cubic millimeter in the body.

Platelets play a critical part in the blood-clotting process or **hemostasis.** They **agglutinate** or clump together into small clusters when a blood vessel is cut or damaged. Platelets also release a substance called **thromboplastin**, which, in the presence of calcium, reacts with **prothrombin**, a clotting protein in the blood, to form **thrombin**. Then thrombin, in turn, works to convert fibrinogen to **fibrin**, which eventually becomes the meshlike blood clot.

Blood Typing

ABO system

blood typing

Rh factor

Each person's blood is different due to the presence of antigens or markers on the surface of erythrocytes. Before a person receives a blood transfusion, it is important to do **blood typing.** This laboratory test determines if the donated blood is compatible with the recipient's blood. There are many different subgroups of blood markers, but the two most important ones are the **ABO system** and **Rh factor.**

ABO System

type A

type AB

type B

type O

universal donor

universal recipient

In the ABO blood system there are two possible red blood cell markers, A and B. A marker is one method by which cells identify themselves. A person with an A marker is said to have **type A** blood. Type A blood produces anti-B antibodies that will attack type B blood. The presence of a B marker gives **type B** blood and anti-A antibodies (that will attack type A blood). If both markers are present, the blood is **type AB** and does not contain any antibodies. Therefore, type AB blood will not attack any other blood type. The absence of either an A or a B marker results in **type O** blood, which contains both anti-A and anti-B antibodies. Type O blood will attack all other blood types, A, B, and AB. For further information on antibodies, refer to the lymphatic section later in this chapter.

Because type O blood does not have either marker A or B, it will not react with anti-A or anti-B antibodies. For this reason, a person with type O blood is referred to as a **universal donor.** In extreme cases, type O blood may be given to a person with any of the other blood types. Similarly, type AB blood is the **universal recipient**. A person with type AB blood has no antibodies against the other blood types and, therefore, in extreme cases, can receive any type of blood.

Rh Factor

Rh-negative

Rh-positive

Rh factor is not as difficult to understand as the ABO system. A person with the Rh factor on his or her red blood cells is said to be **Rh-positive** (Rh+). Since this person has the factor, he or she will not make anti-Rh antibodies. A person without the Rh factor is **Rh-negative** (Rh−) and will produce anti-Rh antibodies. Therefore, an Rh+ person may receive both an Rh+ and an Rh− transfusion, but an Rh− person can receive only Rh− blood.

 ## Word Building

The following list contains examples of medical terms built directly from word parts. Their definitions can be determined by a straightforward translation of the word parts.

COMBINING FORM	COMBINED WITH	MEDICAL TERM	DEFINITION
fibrin/o	-gen	**fibrinogen** (fye-BRIN-oh-jen)	fiber producing
	-lysis	**fibrinolysis** (fye-brin-oh-LYE-sis)	destruction of fibers
	-ous	**fibrinous** (fye-brin-us)	pertaining to fibers
hem/o	-globin	**hemoglobin** (hee-moh-GLOH-bin)	blood protein
	-lysis	**hemolysis** (hee-MALL-ih-sis)	blood destruction
	-lytic	**hemolytic** (hee-moh-LIH-tik)	blood destruction
	-rrhage	**hemorrhage** (HEM-er-rij)	rapid flow of blood
hemat/o	-logist	**hematologist** (hee-mah-TALL-oh-jist)	blood specialist
	-ic	**hematic** (hee-MAT-ik)	pertaining to blood
sanguin/o	-ous	**sanguinous** (SANG-gwih-nus)	pertaining to blood

SUFFIX	COMBINED WITH	MEDICAL TERM	DEFINITION
-cyte	erythr/o	**erythrocyte** (eh-RITH-roh-sight)	red cell
	leuk/o	**leukocyte** (LOO-koh-sight)	white cell
	thromb/o	**thrombocyte** (THROM-boh-sight)	clotting cell
	granul/o	**granulocyte** (GRAN-yew-loh-sight)	granular cell
	a- granul/o	**agranulocyte** (ah-GRAN-yew-loh-sight)	nongranular cell
-cytosis	erythr/o	**erythrocytosis** (ee-RITH-row-sigh-toe-sis)	too many red cells
	leuk/o	**leukocytosis** (LOO-koh-sigh-toh-sis)	too many white cells
	thromb/o	**thrombocytosis** (throm-boh-sigh-TOH-sis)	too many clotting cells
-penia	erythr/o	**erythropenia** (ee-RITH-row-pen-ee-ah)	too few red (cells)
	leuk/o	**leukopenia** (LOO-koh-pen-ee-ah)	too few white (cells)
	thromb/o	**thrombopenia** (THROM-boh-pen-ee-ah)	too few clotting (cells)
	pan- cyt/o	**pancytopenia** (pan-sigh-toe-PEN-ee-ah)	too few of all cells
-poiesis	erythr/o	**erythropoiesis** (eh-rith-roh-poy-EE-sis)	red (cell) producing
	hemat/o	**hematopoiesis** (hee-mah-toh-poy-EE-sis)	blood producing
	leuk/o	**leukopoiesis** (loo-koh-poy-EE-sis)	white (cell) producing
	thromb/o	**thrombopoiesis** (throm-boh-poy-EE-sis)	clotting (cell) producing

Vocabulary

TERM	DEFINITION
blood clot	The hard collection of fibrin, blood cells, and tissue debris that is the end result of hemostasis or the blood-clotting process.

■ **Figure 6.4** Electronmicrograph showing a blood clot. It is composed of fibrin, red blood cells, and tissue debris.

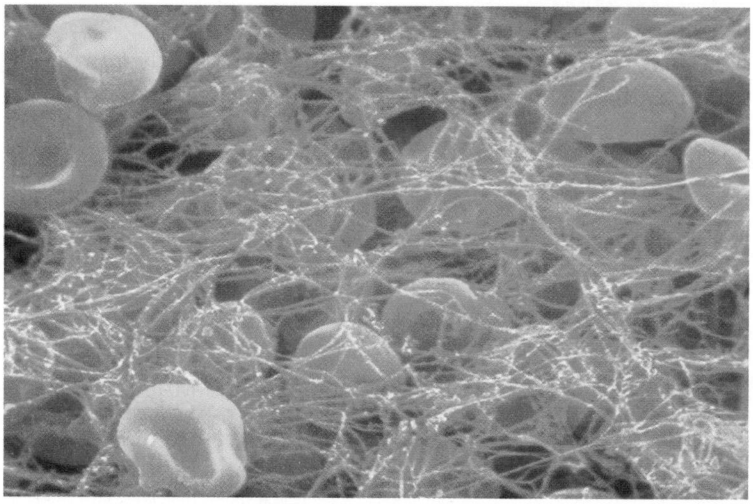

(CNRI/Photo Researchers, Inc.)

TERM	DEFINITION
coagulate (koh-ag-YOO-late)	To convert from a liquid to a gel or solid, as in blood coagulation.
dyscrasia (dis-CRAZ-ee-ah)	A general term indicating the presence of a disease affecting blood.
hematology (hee-mah-TALL-oh-jee)	The branch of medicine that specializes in treating diseases and conditions of the blood. Physician is a *hematologist*.
hematoma (hee-mah-TOH-mah)	The collection of blood under the skin as the result of blood escaping into the tissue from damaged blood vessels. Commonly referred to as a *bruise*. **Med Term Tip** Word watch—the term *hematoma* is confusing. Its simple translation is "blood tumor." However, it is used to refer to blood that has leaked out of a blood vessel and pooled in the tissues.
hemostasis (hee-moh-STAY-sis)	To stop bleeding or the stagnation of blood flow through the tissues.
packed cells	A transfusion of only the formed elements and without plasma.
whole blood	Refers to the mixture of both plasma and formed elements.

Pathology

TERM	DEFINITION
■ *Blood*	
hemophilia (hee-moh-FILL-ee-ah)	Hereditary blood disease in which blood-clotting time is prolonged due to a lack of one vital clotting factor. It is transmitted by a sex-linked trait from females to males, appearing almost exclusively in males.
hyperlipidemia (HYE-per-lip-id-ee-mee-ah)	Condition of having too high a level of lipids such as cholesterol in the bloodstream. A risk factor for developing atherosclerosis and coronary artery disease.

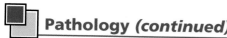

Pathology *(continued)*

TERM	DEFINITION
septicemia (sep-tih-SEE-mee-ah)	Having bacteria or their toxins in the bloodstream. *Sepsis* is a term that means putrefaction. Commonly referred to as *blood poisoning*.

■ *Erythrocytes*

TERM	DEFINITION
anemia (an-NEE-mee-ah)	A large group of conditions characterized by a reduction in the number of red blood cells or the amount of hemoglobin in the blood; results in less oxygen reaching the tissues.
aplastic anemia (a-PLAS-tik an-NEE-mee-ah)	Severe form of anemia that develops as a consequence of loss of functioning red bone marrow. Results in a decrease in the number of all the formed elements. Treatment may eventually require a bone marrow transplant.
hemolytic anemia (hee-moh-LIT-ik an-NEE-mee-ah)	An anemia that develops as the result of the excessive loss of erythrocytes.
hemolytic reaction (hee-moh-LIT-ik)	The destruction of a patient's erythrocytes that occurs when receiving a transfusion of an incompatible blood type. Also called a *transfusion reaction*.
hypochromic anemia (hi-poe-CHROME-ik an-NEE-mee-ah)	Anemia resulting from having insufficient hemoglobin in the erythrocytes. Named because the hemoglobin molecule is responsible for the dark red color of the erythrocytes.
iron-deficiency anemia	Anemia that results from having insufficient iron to manufacture hemoglobin.
pernicious anemia (PA) (per-NISH-us an-NEE-mee-ah)	Anemia associated with insufficient absorption of vitamin B_{12} by the digestive system. Vitamin B_{12} is necessary for erythrocyte production.
polycythemia vera (pol-ee-sigh-THEE-mee-ah VAIR-rah)	Production of too many red blood cells by the bone marrow. Blood becomes too thick to easily flow through the blood vessels.
sickle cell anemia	A genetic disorder in which erythrocytes take on an abnormal curved or "sickle" shape. These cells are fragile and are easily damaged, leading to a hemolytic anemia.

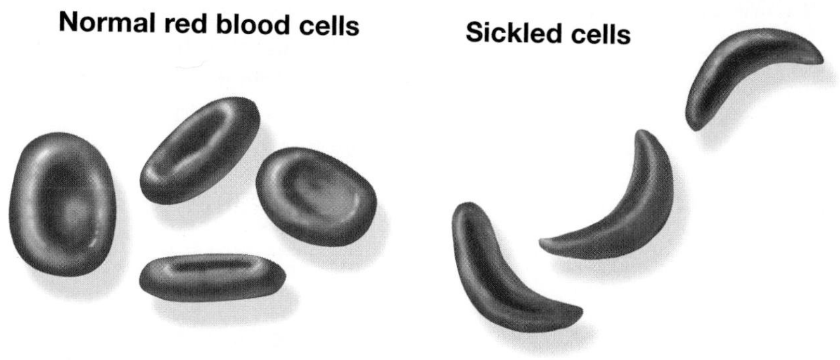

■ **Figure 6.5** Comparison of normal-shaped erythrocytes and the abnormal sickle shape noted in patients with sickle cell anemia.

Normal red blood cells   **Sickled cells**

TERM	DEFINITION
thalassemia (thal-ah-SEE-mee-ah)	A genetic disorder in which the body is unable to make functioning hemoglobin, resulting in anemia.

■ *Leukocytes*

TERM	DEFINITION
leukemia (loo-KEE-mee-ah)	Cancer of the white blood cell-forming red bone marrow resulting in a large number of abnormal and immature white blood cells circulating in the blood.

Diagnostic Procedures

TERM	DEFINITION
■ *Clinical Laboratory Tests*	
blood culture and sensitivity (C&S)	Sample of blood is incubated in the laboratory to check for bacterial growth. If bacteria are present, they are identified and tested to determine which antibiotics they are sensitive to.
complete blood count (CBC)	Combination of blood tests including: red blood cell count (RBC), white blood cell count (WBC), hemoglobin (Hgb), hematocrit (Hct), white blood cell differential, and platelet count.
erythrocyte sedimentation rate (ESR, sed rate) (eh-RITH-roh-sight sed-ih-men-TAY-shun)	Blood test to determine the rate at which mature red blood cells settle out of the blood after the addition of an anticoagulant. This is an indicator of the presence of an inflammatory disease.
hematocrit (HCT, Hct, crit) (hee-MAT-oh-krit)	Blood test to measure the volume of red blood cells (erythrocytes) within the total volume of blood.
hemoglobin (Hgb, hb) (hee-moh-GLOH-bin)	A blood test to measure the amount of hemoglobin present in a given volume of blood.
platelet count (PLAYT-let)	Blood test to determine the number of platelets in a given volume of blood.
prothrombin time (Pro time, PT) (proh-THROM-bin)	A measure of the blood's coagulation abilities by measuring how long it takes for a clot to form after prothrombin has been activated.
red blood cell count (RBC)	Blood test to determine the number of erythrocytes in a volume of blood. A decrease in red blood cells may indicate anemia; an increase may indicate polycythemia.
red blood cell morphology	Examination of a specimen of blood for abnormalities in the shape (morphology) of the erythrocytes. Used to determine diseases like sickle cell anemia.
sequential multiple analyzer computer (SMAC)	Machine for doing multiple blood chemistry tests automatically.
white blood cell count (WBC)	Blood test to measure the number of leukocytes in a volume of blood. An increase may indicate the presence of infection or a disease such as leukemia. A decrease in white blood cells may be caused by radiation therapy or chemotherapy.
white blood cell differential (diff) (diff-er-EN-shal)	Blood test to determine the number of each variety of leukocytes.
■ *Medical Procedures*	
bone marrow aspiration (as-pih-RAY-shun)	Sample of bone marrow is removed by aspiration with a needle and examined for diseases such as leukemia or aplastic anemia.

Diagnostic Procedures *(continued)*

TERM	DEFINITION
phlebotomy (fleh-BOT-oh-me)	Incision into a vein in order to remove blood for a diagnostic test. Also called *venipuncture*.

■ **Figure 6.6** Phlebotomist using a needle to withdraw blood.

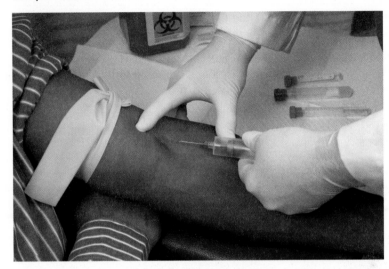

Therapeutic Procedures

TERM	DEFINITION
■ *Medical Procedures*	
autologous transfusion (aw-TALL-oh-gus trans-FYOO-zhun)	Procedure for collecting and storing a patient's own blood several weeks prior to the actual need. It can then be used to replace blood lost during a surgical procedure.
blood transfusion (trans-FYOO-zhun)	Artificial transfer of blood into the bloodstream. **Med Term Tip** Before a patient receives a blood transfusion, the laboratory performs a ***type and crossmatch***. This test first double checks the blood type of both the donor's and recipient's blood. Then a crossmatch is performed. This process mixes together small samples of both bloods and observes the mixture for adverse reactions.
bone marrow transplant (BMT)	Patient receives red bone marrow from a donor after the patient's own bone marrow has been destroyed by radiation or chemotherapy.
homologous transfusion (hoh-MALL-oh-gus trans-FYOO-zhun)	Replacement of blood by transfusion of blood received from another person.
plasmapheresis (plaz-mah-fah-REE-sis)	Method of removing plasma from the body without depleting the formed elements. Whole blood is removed and the cells and plasma are separated. The cells are returned to the patient along with a donor plasma transfusion.

Pharmacology

CLASSIFICATION	ACTION	GENERIC AND BRAND NAMES
anticoagulant (an-tih-koh-AG-yoo-lant)	Substance that prevents blood clot formation. Commonly referred to as *blood thinners*.	heparin, HepLock; warfarin, coumadin
antihemorrhagic (an-tih-hem-er-RAJ-ik)	Substance that prevents or stops hemorrhaging; a *hemostatic agent*.	aminocaproic acid, Amicar; vitamin K
antiplatelet agents (an-tih-PLATE-let)	Substance that interferes with the action of platelets. Prolongs bleeding time. Used to prevent heart attacks and strokes.	clopidogrel, Plavix; ticlopidine, Ticlid
hematinic (hee-mah-TIN-ik)	Substance that increases the number of erythrocytes or the amount of hemoglobin in the blood.	epoetin alfa, Procrit; darbepoetin alfa, Aranesp
thrombolytic (throm-boh-LIT-ik)	Term meaning able to dissolve existing blood clots.	alteplase, Activase; streptokinase, Streptase

Abbreviations

ALL	acute lymphocytic leukemia	**lymphs**	lymphocytes
AML	acute myelogenous leukemia	**monos**	monocytes
basos	basophils	**PA**	pernicious anemia
BMT	bone marrow transplant	**PCV**	packed cell volume
CBC	complete blood count	**PMN, polys**	polymorphonuclear neutrophil
CLL	chronic lymphocytic leukemia	**PT, pro-time**	prothrombin time
CML	chronic myelogenous leukemia	**RBC**	red blood cell
diff	differential	**Rh+**	Rh-positive
eosins, eos	eosinophils	**Rh−**	Rh-negative
ESR, SR, sed rate	erythrocyte sedimentation rate	**segs**	segmented neutrophils
HCT, Hct, crit	hematocrit	**SMAC**	sequential multiple analyzer computer
Hgb, Hb, HGB	hemoglobin	**WBC**	white blood cell

Section II: The Lymphatic and Immune Systems at a Glance

Function

The lymphatic system consists of a network of lymph vessels that pick up excess tissue fluid, cleanse it, and return it to the circulatory system. It also picks up fats that have been absorbed by the digestive system. The immune system fights disease and infections.

Organs

lymph nodes
lymphatic vessels
spleen
thymus gland
tonsils

Combining Forms

adenoid/o	adenoids
immun/o	protection
lymph/o	lymph
lymphaden/o	lymph node
lymphangi/o	lymph vessel
path/o	disease
splen/o	spleen
thym/o	thymus
tonsill/o	tonsils
tox/o	poison

Suffixes Relating

-globulin	protein

The Lymphatic and Immune Systems Illustrated

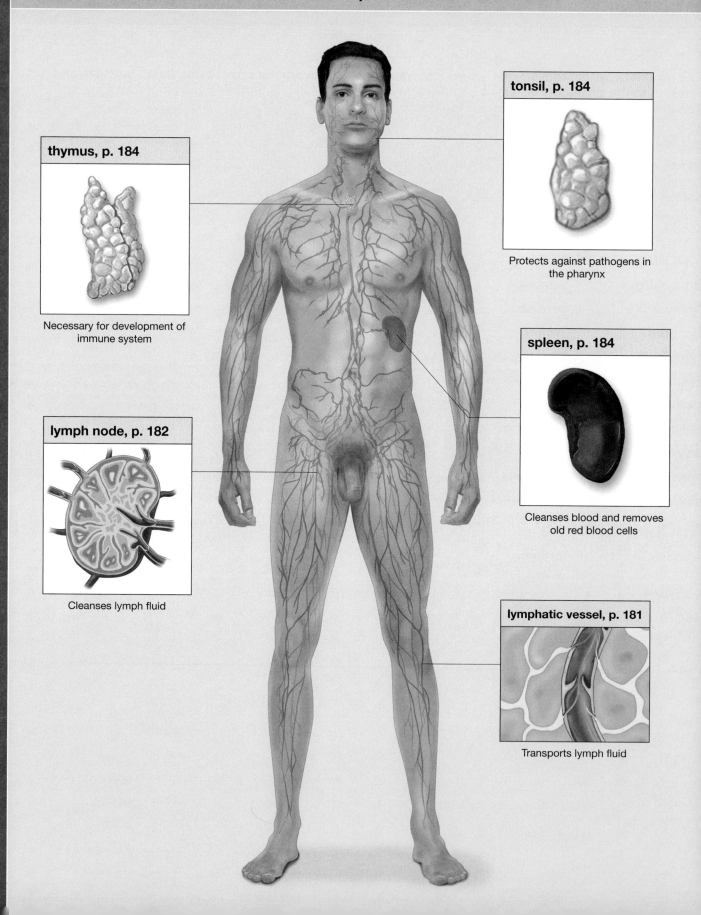

thymus, p. 184

Necessary for development of immune system

tonsil, p. 184

Protects against pathogens in the pharynx

spleen, p. 184

Cleanses blood and removes old red blood cells

lymph node, p. 182

Cleanses lymph fluid

lymphatic vessel, p. 181

Transports lymph fluid

Anatomy and Physiology of the Lymphatic and Immune Systems

lacteals (lack-TEE-als)
lymph (LIMF)
lymph nodes
lymphatic vessels (lim-FAT-ik)

spleen
thymus gland (THIGH-mus)
tonsils (TON-sulls)

The lymphatic system consists of a network of **lymphatic vessels**, **lymph nodes**, the **spleen**, the **thymus gland**, and the **tonsils**. These organs perform several quite diverse functions for the body. First, they collect excess tissue fluid throughout the body and return it to the circulatory system. The fluid, once it is inside a lymphatic vessel, is referred to as **lymph**. Lymph vessels around the small intestines, called **lacteals**, are able to pick up absorbed fats for transport. Additionally, the lymphatic system works with the immune system to form the groups of cells, tissues, organs, and molecules that serve as the body's primary defense against the invasion of pathogens. These systems work together defending the body against foreign invaders and substances, as well as removing our own cells that have become diseased.

Lymphatic Vessels

lymphatic capillaries (CAP-ih-lair-eez)
lymphatic ducts
right lymphatic duct

thoracic duct
valves

The lymphatic vessels form an extensive network of vessels throughout the entire body. However, unlike the circulatory system, these vessels are not in a closed loop. Instead, they serve as one-way pipes conducting lymph from the tissues toward the thoracic cavity (see Figure 6.7 ■). These vessels begin as very

■ Figure 6.7 Lymphatic vessels (green) pick up excess tissue fluid, purify it in lymph nodes, and return it to the circulatory system.

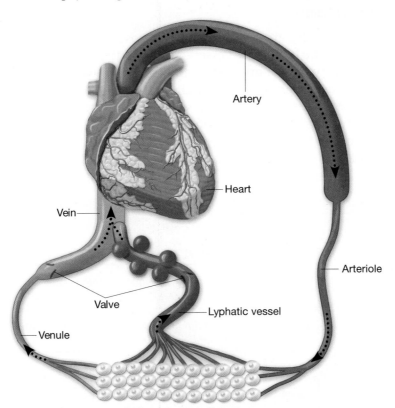

Artery

Heart

Vein

Valve

Arteriole

Venule

Lyphatic vessel

Cells in the body tissues

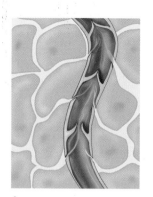
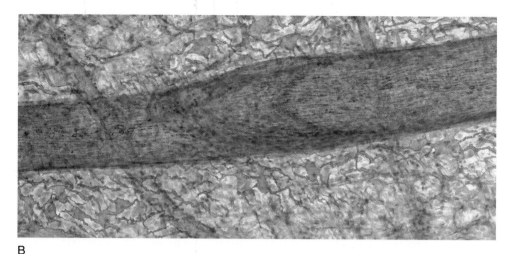

A   B

■ **Figure 6.8** A) Lymphatic vessel with valves within tissue cells; B) Photomicrograph of lymphatic vessel with valve clearly visible. *(Michael Abbey/Photo Researchers, Inc.)*

small **lymphatic capillaries** in the tissues. Excessive tissue fluid enters these capillaries to begin the trip back to the circulatory system. The capillaries merge into larger lymphatic vessels. This is a very low pressure system, so these vessels have **valves** along their length to ensure that lymph can only move forward toward the thoracic cavity (see Figure 6.8 ■). These vessels finally drain into one of two large **lymphatic ducts**, the **right lymphatic duct** or the **thoracic duct**. The smaller right lymphatic duct drains the right arm and the right side of the neck and chest. This duct empties lymph into the right subclavian vein. The larger thoracic duct drains lymph from the rest of the body and empties into the left subclavian vein (see Figure 6.9 ■).

Lymph Nodes

lymph glands

Lymph nodes are small organs composed of lymphatic tissue located along the route of the lymphatic vessels. These nodes, also referred to as **lymph glands**, house lymphocytes and antibodies and therefore work to remove pathogens and cell debris as lymph passes through them on its way back to the thoracic cavity (see Figure 6.10 ■). Lymph nodes also serve to trap and destroy cells from cancerous tumors. Although found throughout the body, lymph nodes are particularly concentrated in several regions. For example, lymph nodes concentrated in the neck region drain lymph from the head. See Table 6.2 ■ and Figure 6.9 for a description of some of the most important sites for lymph nodes.

Table 6.2	**Sites for Lymph Nodes**	
NAME	**LOCATION**	**FUNCTION**
Axillary (AK-sih-lair-ee)	Armpits	Drain arms and shoulder region; cancer cells from breasts may be present
Cervical (SER-vih-kal)	Neck	Drain head and neck; may be enlarged during upper respiratory infections
Inguinal (ING-gwih-nal)	Groin	Drain legs and lower pelvis
Mediastinal (mee-dee-ass-TYE-nal)	Chest	Drain chest cavity

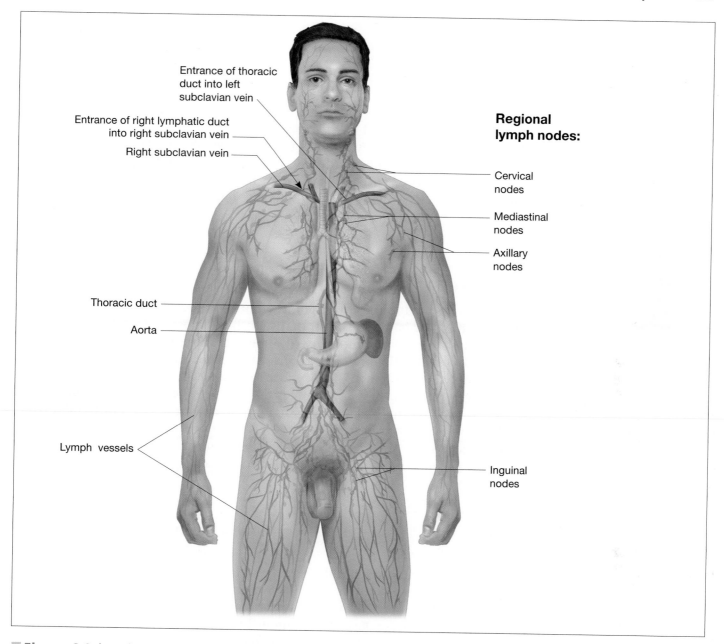

Entrance of thoracic
duct into left
subclavian vein

Entrance of right lymphatic duct
into right subclavian vein

Right subclavian vein

**Regional
lymph nodes:**

Cervical
nodes

Mediastinal
nodes

Axillary
nodes

Thoracic duct

Aorta

Lymph vessels

Inguinal
nodes

■ **Figure 6.9** Location of lymph vessels, lymphatic ducts, and areas of lymph node concentrations.

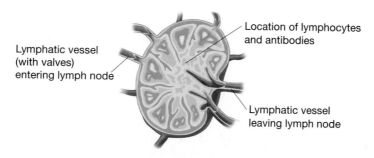

Location of lymphocytes
and antibodies

Lymphatic vessel
(with valves)
entering lymph node

Lymphatic vessel
leaving lymph node

■ **Figure 6.10** Structure of a lymph node.

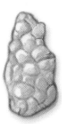

Figure 6.11 The shape of a tonsil.

Tonsils

adenoids (ADD-eh-noydz)
lingual tonsils (LING-gwal)
palatine tonsils (PAL-ah-tyne)

pharyngeal tonsils (fair-IN-jee-al)
pharynx (FAIR-inks)

The tonsils are collections of lymphatic tissue located on each side of the throat or **pharynx** (see Figure 6.11 ■). There are three sets of tonsils: **palatine tonsils**; **pharyngeal tonsils**, commonly referred to as the **adenoids**; and **lingual tonsils**. All tonsils contain a large number of leukocytes and act as filters to protect the body from the invasion of pathogens through the digestive or respiratory systems. Tonsils are not vital organs and can safely be removed if they become a continuous site of infection.

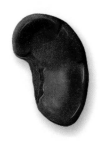

Figure 6.12 The shape of the spleen.

Spleen

blood sinuses

macrophages (MACK-roh-fayj-ez)

The spleen, located in the upper left quadrant of the abdomen, consists of lymphatic tissue that is highly infiltrated with blood vessels (see Figure 6.12 ■). These vessels spread out into slow-moving **blood sinuses**. The spleen filters out and destroys old red blood cells, recycles the iron, and also stores some of the blood supply for the body. Phagocytic **macrophages** line the blood sinuses in the spleen to engulf and remove pathogens. Because the blood is moving through the organ slowly, the macrophages have time to carefully identify pathogens and worn-out red blood cells. The spleen is also not a vital organ and can be removed due to injury or disease. However, without the spleen, a person's susceptibility to a bloodstream infection may be increased.

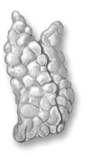

Figure 6.13 The shape of the thymus gland.

Thymus Gland

T cells
T lymphocytes

thymosin (thigh-MOH-sin)

The thymus gland, located in the upper portion of the mediastinum, is essential for the proper development of the immune system (see Figure 6.13 ■). It assists the body with the immune function and the development of antibodies. This organ's hormone, **thymosin**, changes lymphocytes to **T lymphocytes** (simply called **T cells**), which play an important role in the immune response. The thymus is active in the unborn child and throughout childhood until adolescence, when it begins to shrink in size.

Immunity

acquired immunity
active acquired immunity
bacteria (bak-TEE-ree-ah)
cancerous tumors
fungi (FUN-jee)
immune response
immunity (im-YOO-nih-tee)

immunizations (im-yoo-nih-ZAY-shuns)
natural immunity
passive acquired immunity
protozoans (proh-toh-ZOH-anz)
toxins
vaccinations (vak-sih-NAY-shuns)
viruses

Immunity is the body's ability to defend itself against pathogens, such as **bacteria**, **viruses**, **fungi**, **protozoans**, **toxins**, and **cancerous tumors**. Immunity comes in two forms: **natural immunity** and **acquired immunity**. Natural immunity, also called *innate immunity*, is not specific to a particular disease and does not require prior exposure to the pathogenic agent. A good example of natural immunity is the macrophage. These leukocytes are present throughout all the tissues of the body, but are concentrated in areas of high exposure to invading bacteria, like the lungs and digestive system. They are very active phagocytic cells, ingesting and digesting any pathogen they encounter (see Figure 6.14 ■).

Acquired immunity is the body's response to a specific pathogen and may be established either passively or actively. **Passive acquired immunity** results when a person receives protective substances produced by another human or animal. This may take the form of maternal antibodies crossing the placenta to a baby or an antitoxin or gamma globulin injection. **Active acquired immunity** develops following direct exposure to the pathogenic agent. The agent stimulates the body's **immune response**, a series of different mechanisms all geared to neutralize the agent. For example, a person typically can catch chickenpox only once because once the body has successfully fought the virus, it will be able to more quickly recognize and kill it in the future. **Immunizations** or **vaccinations** are special types of active acquired immunity. Instead of actually being exposed to the infectious agent and having the disease, a person is exposed to a modified or weakened pathogen that is still capable of stimulating the immune response but not actually causing the disease.

Immune Response

antibody (AN-tih-bod-ee)	**cell-mediated immunity**
antibody-mediated immunity	**cellular immunity**
antigen–antibody complex	**cytotoxic** (sigh-toh-TOK-sik)
antigens (AN-tih-jens)	**humoral immunity** (HYOO-mor-al)
B cells	**natural killer (NK) cells**
B lymphocytes	

Disease-causing agents are recognized as being foreign because they display proteins that are different from a person's own natural proteins. Those foreign proteins, called **antigens**, stimulate the immune response. The immune response consists of two distinct and different processes: **humoral immunity** (also called **antibody-mediated immunity**) and **cellular immunity** (also called **cell-mediated immunity**).

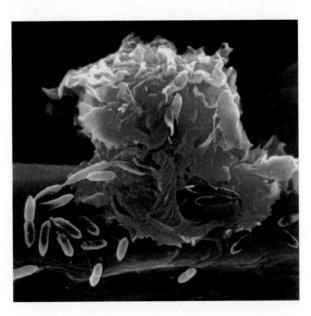

■ **Figure 6.14** Color enhanced photomicrograph showing a macrophage (purple) attacking *Escherichia coli* (yellow), a type of bacteria.
(Dennis Kunkel/Phototake NYC)

Humoral immunity refers to the production of **B lymphocytes**, also called **B cells**, which respond to antigens by producing a protective protein, an **antibody**. Antibodies combine with the antigen to form an **antigen–antibody complex**. This complex either targets the foreign substance for phagocytosis or prevents the infectious agent from damaging healthy cells.

Cellular immunity involves the production of T cells and **natural killer** (NK) **cells**. These defense cells are **cytotoxic**, meaning that they physically attack and destroy pathogenic cells.

Standard Precautions

cross infection	reinfection
nosocomial infection (no-so-KOH-mee-all)	self-inoculation
Occupational Safety and Health Administration (OSHA)	

Hospital and other healthcare settings contain a large number of infective pathogens. Patients and healthcare workers are exposed to each other's pathogens and sometimes become infected. An infection acquired in this manner, as a result of hospital exposure, is referred to as a **nosocomial infection**. Nosocomial infections can spread in several ways. **Cross infection** occurs when a person, either a patient or healthcare worker, acquires a pathogen from another patient or healthcare worker. **Reinfection** takes place when a patient becomes infected again with the same pathogen that originally brought him or her to the hospital. **Self-inoculation** occurs when a person becomes infected in a different part of the body by a pathogen from another part of his or her own body—such as intestinal bacteria spreading to the urethra.

With the appearance of the human immunodeficiency virus (HIV) and the hepatitis B virus (HBV) in the mid-1980s, the fight against spreading infections took on even greater significance. In 1987 the **Occupational Safety and Health Administration** (OSHA) issued mandatory guidelines to ensure that all employees at risk of exposure to body fluids are provided with personal protective equipment. These guidelines state that all human blood, tissue, and body fluids must be treated as if they were infected with HIV, HBV, or other bloodborne pathogens. These guidelines were expanded in 1992 and 1996 to encourage the fight against not just bloodborne pathogens, but all nosocomial infections spread by contact with blood, mucous membranes, nonintact skin, and all body fluids (including amniotic fluid, vaginal secretions, pleural fluid, cerebrospinal fluid, peritoneal fluid, pericardial fluid, and semen). These guidelines are commonly referred to as the Standard Precautions:

1. Wash hands before putting on and after removing gloves and before and after working with each patient or patient equipment.
2. Wear gloves when in contact with any body fluid, mucous membrane, or nonintact skin or if you have chapped hands, a rash, or open sores.
3. Wear a nonpermeable gown or apron during procedures that are likely to expose you to any body fluid, mucous membrane, or nonintact skin.
4. Wear a mask and protective equipment or a face shield when patients are coughing often or if body fluid droplets or splashes are likely.
5. Wear a facemask and eyewear that seal close to the face during procedures that cause body tissues to be vaporized.
6. Remove for proper cleaning any shared equipment—such as a thermometer, stethoscope, or blood pressure cuff—that has come into contact with body fluids, mucous membrane, or nonintact skin.

Word Building

The following list contains examples of medical terms built directly from word parts. The definition for these terms can be determined by a straightforward translation of the word parts.

COMBINING FORM	COMBINED WITH	MEDICAL TERM	DEFINITION
adenoid/o	-ectomy	**adenoidectomy** (add-eh-noyd-EK-toh-mee)	removal of the adenoids
	-itis	**adenoiditis** (add-eh-noyd-EYE-tis)	inflammation of the adenoids
immun/o	-logist	**immunologist** (im-yoo-NALL-oh-jist)	immunity specialist
lymph/o	aden/o –ectomy	**lymphadenectomy** (lim-fad-eh-NEK-toh-mee)	removal of lymph gland
	aden/o –pathy	**lymphadenopathy** (lim-fad-eh-NOP-ah-thee)	lymph gland disease
	angi/o –gram	**lymphangiogram** (lim-FAN-jee-oh-gram)	record of lymph vessels
	angi/o -oma	**lymphangioma** (lim-fan-jee-OH-mah)	lymph vessel tumor
	-oma	**lymphoma** (lim-FOH-mah)	lymph tumor
	-tic	**lymphatic** (lim-FAT-ik)	pertaining to lymph
path/o	-genic	**pathogenic** (path-oh-JEN-ik)	disease producing
	-logy	**pathology** (path-OL-oh-gee)	study of disease
splen/o	-ectomy	**splenectomy** (splee-NEK-toh-mee)	removal of spleen
	-megaly	**splenomegaly** (splee-noh-MEG-ah-lee)	enlarged spleen
thym/o	-ectomy	**thymectomy** (thigh-MEK-toh-mee)	removal of the thymus
	-oma	**thymoma** (thigh-MOH-mah)	thymus tumor
tonsill/o	-ar	**tonsillar** (ton-sih-lar)	pertaining to tonsils
	-ectomy	**tonsillectomy** (ton-sih-LEK-toh-mee)	removal of the tonsils
	-itis	**tonsillitis** (ton-sil-EYE-tis)	inflammation of the tonsils

Vocabulary

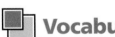

TERM	DEFINITION
allergen (AL-er-jin)	An antigen that causes an allergic reaction.
allergist (AL-er-jist)	A physician who specializes in testing for and treating allergies.
allergy (AL-er-jee)	Hypersensitivity to a common substance in the environment or to a medication.
autoimmune disease	A disease resulting from the body's immune system attacking its own cells as if they were pathogens. Examples include systemic lupus erythematosus, rheumatoid arthritis, and multiple sclerosis.
hives	Appearance of wheals as part of an allergic reaction.

Vocabulary *(continued)*

TERM	DEFINITION
human immunodeficiency virus (HIV) (im-yoo-noh-dee-FIH-shen-see)	Virus that causes AIDS; also known as a **retrovirus.**

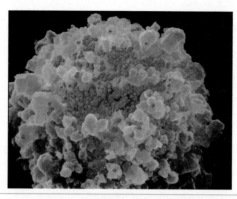

 Figure 6.15 Color enhanced scanning electron micrograph of HIV virus (red) infecting T-helper cells (green). *(NIBSC/Science Photo Library/Photo Researchers, Inc.)*

TERM	DEFINITION
immunocompromised (im-you-noh-KOM-pro-mized)	Having an immune system that is unable to respond properly to pathogens. Also called *immunodeficiency disorder*.
immunoglobulins (im-yoo-noh-GLOB-yoo-linz)	Antibodies secreted by the B cells. All antibodies are immunoglobulins and assist in protecting the body and its surfaces from the invasion of bacteria. For example, the immunoglobulin IgA in colostrum, the first milk from the mother, helps to protect the newborn from infection.
immunology (im-yoo-NALL-oh-jee)	A branch of medicine concerned with diagnosis and treatment of infectious diseases and other disorders of the immune system. Physician is an *immunologist*.
inflammation (in-flah-MA-shun)	The tissues' response to injury from pathogens or physical agents. Characterized by redness, pain, swelling, and feeling hot to touch.

Med Term Tip

Word watch—the terms *inflammation* and *inflammatory* are spelled with two "m"s, while *inflame* and *inflamed* each have only one "m." These may be the most commonly misspelled terms by medical terminology students.

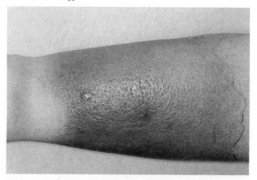

 Figure 6.16 Inflammation as illustrated by cellulitis of the arm. Note that the area is red and swollen. It is also painful and hot to touch.

TERM	DEFINITION
lymphedema (limf-eh-DEE-mah)	Edema appearing in the extremities due to an obstruction of the lymph flow through the lymphatic vessels.
opportunistic infections	Infectious diseases associated with patients who have compromised immune systems and therefore a lowered resistance to infections and parasites. May be the result of HIV infection.
urticaria (er-tih-KAY-ree-ah)	Severe itching associated with hives, usually linked to food allergy, stress, or drug reactions.

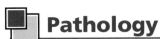

Pathology

TERM	DEFINITION

■ Allergic Reactions

TERM	DEFINITION
anaphylactic shock (an-ah-fih-LAK-tik)	Life-threatening condition resulting from a severe allergic reaction. Examples of instances that may trigger this reaction include bee stings, medications, or the ingestion of foods. Circulatory and respiratory problems occur, including respiratory distress, hypotension, edema, tachycardia, and convulsions. Also called **anaphylaxis**.

■ Lymphatic System

TERM	DEFINITION
elephantiasis (el-eh-fan-TYE-ah-sis)	Inflammation, obstruction, and destruction of the lymph vessels resulting in enlarged tissues due to edema.
Hodgkin's disease (HD) (HOJ-kins dih-ZEEZ)	Also called *Hodgkin's lymphoma*. Cancer of the lymphatic cells found in concentration in the lymph nodes. Named after Thomas Hodgkin, a British physician, who first described it.
lymphadenitis (lim-fad-en-EYE-tis)	Inflammation of the lymph nodes. Referred to as *swollen glands*.
mononucleosis (mono) (mon-oh-nook-lee-OH-sis)	Acute infectious disease with a large number of abnormal lymphocytes. Caused by the Epstein–Barr virus. Abnormal liver function may occur.
non-Hodgkin's lymphoma (NHL)	Cancer of the lymphatic tissues other than Hodgkin's lymphoma.

■ **Figure 6.17** Late-stage Hodgkin's disease with tumor eroding skin above cancerous lymph node.

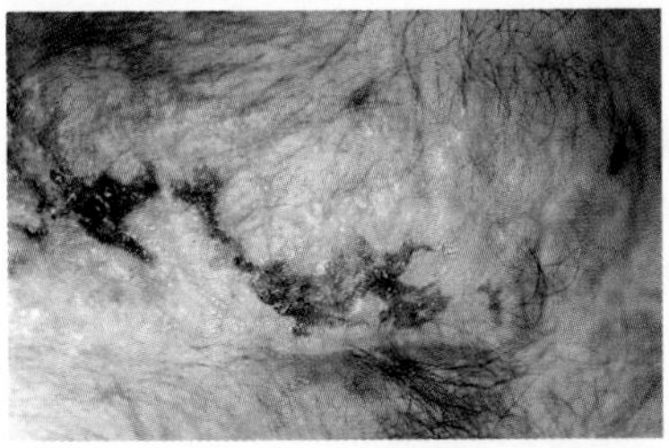

■ Immune System

TERM	DEFINITION
acquired immunodeficiency syndrome (AIDS) (ac-quired im-you-noh-dee-FIH-shen-see SIN-drohm)	Disease involving a defect in the cell-mediated immunity system. A syndrome of opportunistic infections occurring in the final stages of infection with the human immunodeficiency virus (HIV). This virus attacks T4 lymphocytes and destroys them, reducing the person's ability to fight infection.
AIDS-related complex (ARC)	Early stage of AIDS. There is a positive test for the virus, but only mild symptoms of weight loss, fatigue, skin rash, and anorexia.
graft vs. host disease (GVHD)	Serious complication of bone marrow transplant (graft). Immune cells from the donor bone marrow attack the recipient's (host's) tissues.
Kaposi's sarcoma (KS) (KAP-oh-seez sar-KOH-mah)	Form of skin cancer frequently seen in patients with AIDS. It consists of brownish-purple papules that spread from the skin and metastasize to internal organs. Named for Moritz Kaposi, an Austrian dermatologist.
Pneumocystis carinii **pneumonia** (PCP) (noo-moh-SIS-tis kah-RYE-nee-eye new-MOH-nee-ah)	Pneumonia common in patients with AIDS that is caused by infection with an opportunistic parasite.
sarcoidosis (sar-koyd-OH-sis)	Disease of unknown cause that forms fibrous lesions commonly appearing in the lymph nodes, liver, skin, lungs, spleen, eyes, and small bones of the hands and feet.
severe combined immunodeficiency syndrome (SCIDS)	Disease seen in children born with a nonfunctioning immune system. Often these children are forced to live in sealed sterile rooms.

Diagnostic Procedures

TERM	DEFINITION
■ *Clinical Laboratory Tests*	
enzyme-linked immunosorbent assay (ELISA) (EN-zym LINK'T im-yoo-noh-sor-bent ASS-say)	A blood test for an antibody to the AIDS virus. A positive test means that the person has been exposed to the virus. There may be a false-positive reading, and then the Western blot test would be used to verify the results.
Western blot	Test used as a backup to the ELISA blood test to detect the presence of the antibody to HIV (AIDS virus) in the blood.
■ *Diagnostic Imaging*	
lymphangiography (lim-FAN-jee-oh-graf-ee)	X-ray taken of the lymph vessels after the injection of dye into the foot. The lymph flow through the chest is traced.
■ *Additional Diagnostic Procedures*	
Monospot	Test for infectious mononucleosis.
scratch test	Form of allergy testing in which the body is exposed to an allergen through a light scratch in the skin.

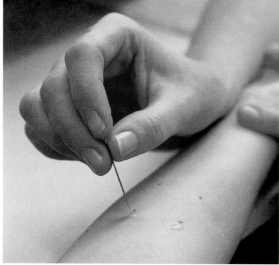

A.

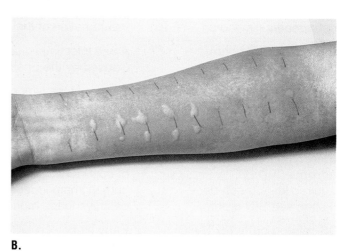

B.

■ **Figure 6.18** A) Scratch test; patient is exposed to allergens through light scratch in the skin. B) Positive scratch test results. Inflammation indicates person is allergic to that substance. *(James King-Holmes/Science Photo Library/Photo Researchers, Inc.)*

Therapeutic Procedures

TERM	DEFINITION
Medical Procedures	
immunotherapy (IM-yoo-noh-thair-ah-pee)	Giving a patient an injection of immunoglobulins or antibodies in order to treat a disease. The antibodies may be produced by another person or animal, for example, antivenom for snake bites. More recent developments include treatments to boost the activity of the immune system, especially to treat cancer and AIDS.
vaccination (vak-sih-NAY-shun)	Exposure to a weakened pathogen that stimulates the immune response and antibody production in order to confer protection against the full-blown disease. Also called *immunization*.
Surgical Procedures	
lymphadenectomy (lim-fad-eh-NEK-toh-mee)	Removal of a lymph node. This is usually done to test for malignancy.

Pharmacology

CLASSIFICATION	ACTION	GENERIC AND BRAND NAMES
antihistamine (an-tih-HIST-ah-meen)	Blocks the effects of histamine released by the body during an allergic reaction.	cetirizine, Zyrtec; diphenhydramine, Benadryl
corticosteroids (core-tih-koh-STARE-royds)	A hormone produced by the adrenal cortex that has very strong anti-inflammatory properties. Particularly useful in treating autoimmune diseases.	prednisone; methylprednisolone, Solu-Medrol
immunosuppressants (im-yoo-noh-sue-PRESS-antz)	Blocks certain actions of the immune system. Required to prevent rejection of a transplanted organ.	mycophenolate mofetil, CellCept; cyclosporine, Neoral
protease inhibitor drugs (PROH-tee-ace)	Inhibits protease, an enzyme viruses need to reproduce.	indinavir, Crixivan; saquinavir, Fortovase
reverse transcriptase inhibitor drugs (trans-KRIP-tays)	Inhibits reverse transcriptase, an enzyme needed by viruses to reproduce.	lamivudine, Epivir; zidovudine, Retrovir

Abbreviations

AIDS	acquired immunodeficiency syndrome	**KS**	Kaposi's sarcoma
ARC	AIDS-related complex	**mono**	mononucleosis
ELISA	enzyme-linked immunosorbent assay	**NHL**	non-Hodgkin's lymphoma
GVHD	graft vs. host disease	**NK**	natural killer cells
HD	Hodgkin's disease	**PCP**	*Pneumocystis carinii* pneumonia
HIV	human immunodeficiency virus	**SCIDS**	severe combined immunodeficiency
Ig	immunoglobulins (IgA, IgD, IgE, IgG, IgM)		syndrome

Chapter Review

Terminology Checklist

Below are all Anatomy and Physiology key terms, Word Building, Vocabulary, Pathology, Diagnostic, Therapeutic, and Pharmacology terms presented in this chapter. Use this list as a study tool by placing a check in the box in front of each term as you master its meaning.

- ☐ ABO system
- ☐ acquired immunity
- ☐ acquired immunodeficiency syndrome
- ☐ active acquired immunity
- ☐ adenoidectomy
- ☐ adenoiditis
- ☐ adenoids
- ☐ agglutinate
- ☐ agranulocytes
- ☐ AIDS-related complex
- ☐ albumin
- ☐ allergen
- ☐ allergist
- ☐ allergy
- ☐ amino acids
- ☐ anaphylactic shock
- ☐ anaphylaxis
- ☐ anemia
- ☐ antibody
- ☐ antibody-mediated immunity
- ☐ anticoagulant
- ☐ antigen
- ☐ antigen–antibody complex
- ☐ antihemorrhagic
- ☐ antihistamine
- ☐ antiplatelet agent
- ☐ aplastic anemia
- ☐ autoimmune disease
- ☐ autologous transfusion
- ☐ axillary
- ☐ bacteria
- ☐ basophils
- ☐ B cells
- ☐ bilirubin
- ☐ blood clot
- ☐ blood culture and sensitivity
- ☐ blood sinuses

- ☐ blood transfusion
- ☐ blood typing
- ☐ B lymphocytes
- ☐ bone marrow aspiration
- ☐ bone marrow transplant
- ☐ calcium
- ☐ cancerous tumors
- ☐ cell-mediated immunity
- ☐ cellular immunity
- ☐ cervical
- ☐ coagulate
- ☐ complete blood count
- ☐ corticosteroids
- ☐ creatinine
- ☐ cross infection
- ☐ cytotoxic
- ☐ dyscrasia
- ☐ elephantiasis
- ☐ enucleated
- ☐ enzyme-linked immunosorbent assay (ELISA)
- ☐ eosinophils
- ☐ erythrocytes
- ☐ erythrocyte sedimentation rate
- ☐ erythrocytosis
- ☐ erythropenia
- ☐ erythropoiesis
- ☐ fats
- ☐ fibrin
- ☐ fibrinogen
- ☐ fibrinolysis
- ☐ fibrinous
- ☐ formed elements
- ☐ fungi
- ☐ gamma globulin
- ☐ globulins
- ☐ glucose
- ☐ graft vs. host disease

- ☐ granulocyte
- ☐ hematic
- ☐ hematinic
- ☐ hematocrit
- ☐ hematologist
- ☐ hematology
- ☐ hematoma
- ☐ hematopoiesis
- ☐ hemoglobin
- ☐ hemolysis
- ☐ hemolytic
- ☐ hemolytic anemia
- ☐ hemolytic reaction
- ☐ hemophilia
- ☐ hemorrhage
- ☐ hemostasis
- ☐ hives
- ☐ Hodgkin's disease
- ☐ homologous transfusion
- ☐ human immunodeficiency virus
- ☐ humoral immunity
- ☐ hyperlipidemia
- ☐ hypochromic anemia
- ☐ immune response
- ☐ immunity
- ☐ immunization
- ☐ immunocompromised
- ☐ immunoglobulins
- ☐ immunologist
- ☐ immunology
- ☐ immunosuppressants
- ☐ immunotherapy
- ☐ inflammation
- ☐ inguinal
- ☐ iron-deficiency anemia
- ☐ Kaposi's sarcoma
- ☐ lacteals
- ☐ leukemia

- [ ] leukocytes
- [ ] leukocytosis
- [ ] leukopenia
- [ ] leukopoiesis
- [ ] lingual tonsils
- [ ] lymph
- [ ] lymphadenectomy
- [ ] lymphadenitis
- [ ] lymphadenopathy
- [ ] lymphangiogram
- [ ] lymphangiography
- [ ] lymphangioma
- [ ] lymphatic
- [ ] lymphatic capillaries
- [ ] lymphatic ducts
- [ ] lymphatic vessels
- [ ] lymphedema
- [ ] lymph glands
- [ ] lymph nodes
- [ ] lymphocytes
- [ ] lymphoma
- [ ] macrophage
- [ ] mediastinal
- [ ] metastasize
- [ ] monocytes
- [ ] mononucleosis
- [ ] Monospot
- [ ] natural immunity
- [ ] natural killer cells
- [ ] neutrophils
- [ ] non-Hodgkin's lymphoma
- [ ] nosocomial infection
- [ ] Occupational Safety and Health Administration
- [ ] opportunistic infections
- [ ] packed cells
- [ ] palatine tonsils
- [ ] pancytopenia
- [ ] passive acquired immunity
- [ ] pathogenic
- [ ] pathogens

- [ ] pathology
- [ ] pernicious anemia
- [ ] phagocyte
- [ ] phagocytosis
- [ ] pharyngeal tonsils
- [ ] pharynx
- [ ] phlebotomy
- [ ] plasma
- [ ] plasmapheresis
- [ ] plasma proteins
- [ ] platelet count
- [ ] platelets
- [ ] *Pneumocystis carinii* pneumonia
- [ ] polycythemia vera
- [ ] potassium
- [ ] protease inhibitor drugs
- [ ] prothrombin
- [ ] prothrombin time
- [ ] protozoans
- [ ] red blood cell count
- [ ] red blood cell morphology
- [ ] red blood cells
- [ ] reinfection
- [ ] reverse transcriptase inhibitor drugs
- [ ] Rh factor
- [ ] Rh-negative
- [ ] Rh-positive
- [ ] right lymphatic duct
- [ ] sanguinous
- [ ] sarcoidosis
- [ ] scratch test
- [ ] self-inoculation
- [ ] septicemia
- [ ] sequential multiple analyzer computer
- [ ] serum
- [ ] severe combined immunodeficiency syndrome
- [ ] sickle cell anemia
- [ ] sodium

- [ ] spleen
- [ ] splenectomy
- [ ] splenomegaly
- [ ] T cells
- [ ] thalassemia
- [ ] thoracic duct
- [ ] thrombin
- [ ] thrombocyte
- [ ] thrombocytosis
- [ ] thrombolytic
- [ ] thrombopenia
- [ ] thromboplastin
- [ ] thrombopoiesis
- [ ] thymectomy
- [ ] thymoma
- [ ] thymosin
- [ ] thymus gland
- [ ] T lymphocytes
- [ ] tonsillar
- [ ] tonsillectomy
- [ ] tonsillitis
- [ ] tonsils
- [ ] toxins
- [ ] type A
- [ ] type AB
- [ ] type and crossmatch
- [ ] type B
- [ ] type O
- [ ] universal donor
- [ ] universal recipient
- [ ] urea
- [ ] urticaria
- [ ] vaccination
- [ ] valves
- [ ] viruses
- [ ] Western blot
- [ ] white blood cell count
- [ ] white blood cell differential
- [ ] white blood cells
- [ ] whole blood

Practice Exercises

A. Complete the following statements.

1. The study of the blood is called _____.

2. The organs of the lymphatic system other than lymphatic vessels and lymph nodes are the _____, _____, and _____.

3. The two lymph ducts are the _____ and _____.

4. The primary concentrations of lymph nodes are the _____, _____, and _____ regions.

5. The process whereby cells ingest and destroy bacteria within the body is _____.

6. The formed elements of blood are the, _____, _____, and _____.

7. The fluid portion of blood is called _____.

8. _____ immunity develops following direct exposure to a pathogen.

9. Humoral immunity is also referred to as _____ immunity.

10. The medical term for blood clotting is _____.

B. State the terms described using the combining forms provided.

The combining form *splen/o* refers to the spleen. Use it to write a term that means:

1. enlargement of the spleen _____

2. surgical removal of the spleen _____

3. incision into the spleen _____

The combining form *lymph/o* refers to the lymph. Use it to write a term that means:

4. lymph cells _____

5. tumor of the lymph system _____

The combining form *lymphaden/o* refers to the lymph glands. Use it to write a term that means:

6. disease of a lymph gland _____

7. tumor of a lymph gland _____

8. inflammation of a lymph gland _____

The combining form *immun/o* refers to the immune system. Use it to write a term that means:

9. specialist in the study of the immune system _____

10. immune protein _____

11. study of the immune system _____

The combining form *hemat/o* refers to blood. Use it to write a term that means:

12. relating to the blood _____

13. blood tumor or mass _____

14. blood formation _____

The combining form *hem/o* refers to blood. Use it to write a term that means:

15. blood destruction _____

16. blood protein _____

C. Use the following suffixes to create medical terms for the following definitions.

-penia   -globin   -cytosis   -cyte   -globulin

1. too few white (cells) _____

2. too few red (cells) _____

3. too few clotting (cells) _____

4. too few of all cells _____

5. increase in white cells _____

6. increase in red cells _____

7. increase in clotting cells _____

8. blood protein _____

9. immunity protein _____

10. red cell _____

11. white cell _____

12. lymph cell _____

D. Write the combining form for each definition and then use it to form a medical term.

	Combining Form	Medical Term
1. lymph node	_____	_____
2. clot	_____	_____
3. blood	_____	_____
4. tonsil	_____	_____
5. poison	_____	_____
6. eat/swallow	_____	_____

7. lymph vessel _____   _____

8. disease _____   _____

9. spleen _____   _____

10. lymph _____   _____

E. Identify the following abbreviations.

1. basos _____

2. CBC _____

3. Hgb _____

4. PT _____

5. GVHD _____

6. RBC _____

7. PCV _____

8. ESR _____

9. diff _____

10. lymphs _____

F. Write the abbreviations for the following terms.

1. acquired immunodeficiency
   syndrome _____

2. AIDS-related complex _____

3. human immunodeficiency
   virus _____

4. acute lymphocytic leukemia _____

5. bone marrow transplant _____

6. mononucleosis _____

7. Kaposi's sarcoma _____

8. eosinophils _____

9. immunoglobulin _____

10. severe combined immunodeficiency
    syndrome _____

G. Match each blood term to its definition.

1. _____ thalassemia

2. _____ lacteals

3. _____ A, B, AB, O

4. _____ plasma

5. _____ dyscrasia

a. fluid portion of blood

b. disease in which blood does not clot

c. conditions with reduced number of RBCs

d. mass of blood

e. blood type

6. _____ hematoma

7. _____ anemia

8. _____ serum

9. _____ hemophilia

10. _____ fibrinogen

f. blood clotting protein

g. type of anemia

h. general term for blood disorders

i. lymph vessels around intestine

j. plasma with inactivated fibrinogen

H. Match each lymphatic and immune system term to its definition.

1. _____ allergy

2. _____ nosocomial

3. _____ phagocytosis

4. _____ hives

5. _____ antibody

6. _____ antigen

7. _____ Hodgkin's disease

8. _____ sarcoidosis

9. _____ vaccination

10. _____ ELISA

a. seen in an allergic reaction

b. substance that stimulates antibody formation

c. a hypersensitivity reaction

d. engulfing

e. protective blood protein

f. a type of cancer

g. autoimmune disease

h. infection acquired in the hospital

i. blood test for AIDS

j. immunization

I. Match each blood test to its definition.

1. _____ culture and sensitivity

2. _____ hematocrit

3. _____ complete blood count

4. _____ erythrocyte sedimentation rate

5. _____ prothrombin time

6. _____ white cell differential

7. _____ red cell morphology

a. measure of blood's clotting ability

b. counts number of each type of blood cell

c. examines cells for abnormal shape

d. checks blood for bacterial growth and best antibiotic to use

e. determines number of each type of white blood cell

f. measures percent of whole blood that is red blood cells

g. an indicator of the presence of an inflammatory condition

J. Fill in the classification for each drug description, then match the brand name.

Drug Description	Classification	Brand Name
1. _____ inhibits enzyme needed for viral reproduction	_____	a. HepLock
2. _____ prevents blood clot formation	_____	b. Activase
3. _____ stops bleeding	_____	c. Solu-Medrol
4. _____ blocks effects of histamine	_____	d. Amicar
5. _____ prevents rejection of a transplanted organ	_____	e. Epivir
6. _____ dissolves existing blood clots	_____	f. CellCept
7. _____ increases number of erythrocytes	_____	g. Procrit
8. _____ strong anti-inflammatory properties	_____	h. Zyrtec
9. _____ interferes with action of platelets	_____	i. Plavix

K. Use the following terms in the sentences below.

Kaposi's sarcoma	mononucleosis	Hodgkin's disease	aplastic
polycythemia vera	anaphylactic shock	AIDS	pernicious
Pneumocystis carinii	HIV		

1. The condition characterized by the production of too many red blood cells is called _____.

2. The Epstein–Barr virus is thought to be responsible for what infectious disease? _____

3. A life-threatening allergic reaction is _____.

4. The virus responsible for causing AIDS is _____.

5. A cancer that is seen frequently in AIDS patients is _____.

6. An ELISA is used to test for _____.

7. Malignant tumors concentrate in lymph nodes with this disease: _____.

8. A type of pneumonia seen in AIDS patients is _____ pneumonia.

9. _____ anemia is a severe form of anemia caused by nonfunctioning red bone marrow.

10. _____ anemia is the result of a vitamin B_{12} deficiency

Medical Record Analysis

Below is an item from a patient's medical record. Read it carefully, make sure you understand all the medical terms used, and then answer the questions that follow.

Discharge Summary

Admitting Diagnosis:	Splenomegaly, weight loss, diarrhea, fatigue, chronic cough
Final Diagnosis:	Non-Hodgkin's lymphoma, primary site spleen; splenectomy
History of Present Illness:	Patient is a 36-year-old businessman who was first seen in the office with complaints of feeling generally "run down," intermittent diarrhea, weight loss, and, more recently, a dry cough. He states he has been aware of these symptoms for approximately six months, but admits it may have been "coming on" for closer to one year. A screening test for mononucleosis was negative. A chest x-ray was negative for pneumonia or bronchitis, but did reveal suspicious nodules in the left thoracic cavity. In spite of a 35-pound weight loss, he has abdominal swelling and splenomegaly detected with abdominal palpation. He was admitted to the hospital for further evaluation and treatment.
Summary of Hospital Course:	Blood tests were negative for the Epstein–Barr virus and hepatitis B. Abdominal ultrasound confirmed generalized splenomegaly and located a 3-cm encapsulated tumor. A lymphangiogram identified the thoracic nodules to be enlarged lymph glands. Biopsies taken from the spleen tumor and thoracic lymph glands confirmed the diagnosis of non-Hodgkin's lymphoma. A full body MRI failed to demonstrate any additional metastases in the liver or brain. The patient underwent splenectomy for removal of the primary tumor.
Discharge Plans:	Patient was discharged home following recovery from the splenectomy. The abdominal swelling and diarrhea were resolved, but the dry cough persisted. He was referred to an oncologist for evaluation and establishment of a chemotherapy and radiation therapy protocol to treat the metastatic thoracic lymphadenomas and ongoing surveillance for additional metastases.

Critical Thinking Questions

1. What complaints caused the patient to go to the doctor? _____

_____

2. Explain in your own words what negative, as in "chest x-ray was negative for pneumonia," means.

_____

_____

_____

3. This discharge summary contains four medical terms that have not been introduced yet. Describe each of these terms in your own words. Use your text as a dictionary.

a. primary site _____

b. encapsulated _____

c. ascites _____

d. metastases _____

4. What is the name of a diagnostic procedure that produces an image from high-frequency sound waves? The

   procedure is _____.

5. Which of the following pathological conditions was discovered using this procedure?

a. inflammatory liver disease
b. an acute infection with a large number of lymphocytes
c. a malignant tumor of the thymus gland
d. an enlarged spleen

6. What diagnostic test failed to find any cancer in other organs of the body? Which organs are free of cancer?

   _____

   _____

7. When the patient was discharged from the hospital, which symptoms were resolved and which persisted?

   Resolved: _____

   Persisted: _____

Chart Note Transcription

The chart note below contains ten phrases that can be reworded with a medical term that you learned in this chapter. Each phrase is identified with an underline. Determine the medical term and write your answers in the space provided.

Current Complaint: Patient is a 22-year-old female referred to the <u>specialist in treating blood disorders</u> ❶ by her internist. Her complaints include fatigue, weight loss, and easy bruising.

Past History: Patient had normal childhood diseases. She is a college student and was feeling well until symptoms gradually appeared starting approximately three months ago.

Signs and Symptoms: An <u>immunoassay test for AIDS</u> ❷ was normal. The <u>measure of the blood's coagulation abilities</u> ❸ indicated that the blood took too long to form a clot. A <u>blood test to count all the blood cells</u> ❹ reported <u>too few red blood cells</u> ❺ and <u>too few clotting cells.</u> ❻ There were <u>too many white blood cells,</u> ❼ but they were immature and abnormal. A <u>sample of bone marrow obtained for microscopic examination</u> ❽ found an excessive number of immature white blood cells.

Diagnosis: <u>Cancer of the white blood cell forming bone marrow.</u> ❾

Treatment: Aggressive chemotherapy for the <u>cancer of the white blood cell forming bone marrow</u> ❾ and <u>replacement blood from another person</u> ❿ to replace the erythrocytes and platelets.

❶ _____

❷ _____

❸ _____

❹ _____

❺ _____

❻ _____

❼ _____

❽ _____

❾ _____

❿ _____

Labeling Exercise

A. System Review

Write the labels for this figure on the numbered lines provided.

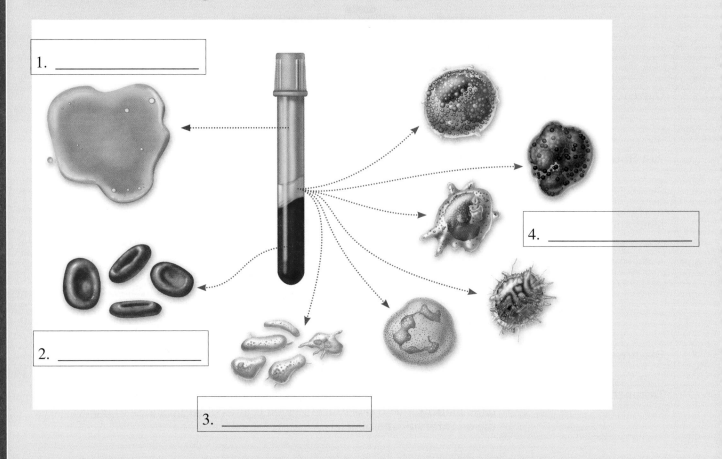

1. _____

2. _____

3. _____

4. _____

B. Anatomy Challenge

1. Write the labels for this figure on the numbered lines provided.

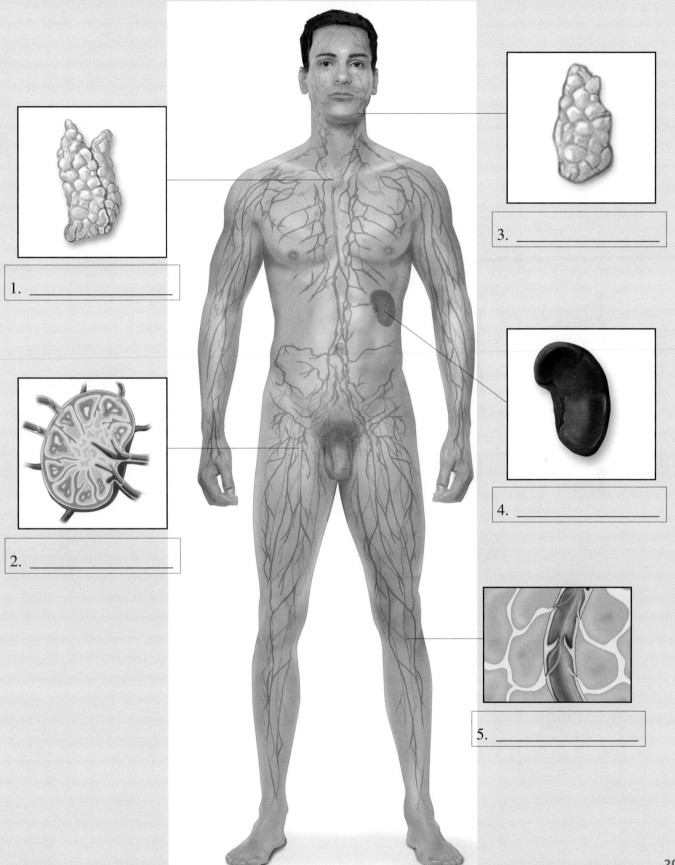

1. _____

2. _____

3. _____

4. _____

5. _____

2. Write the labels for this figure on the numbered lines provided.

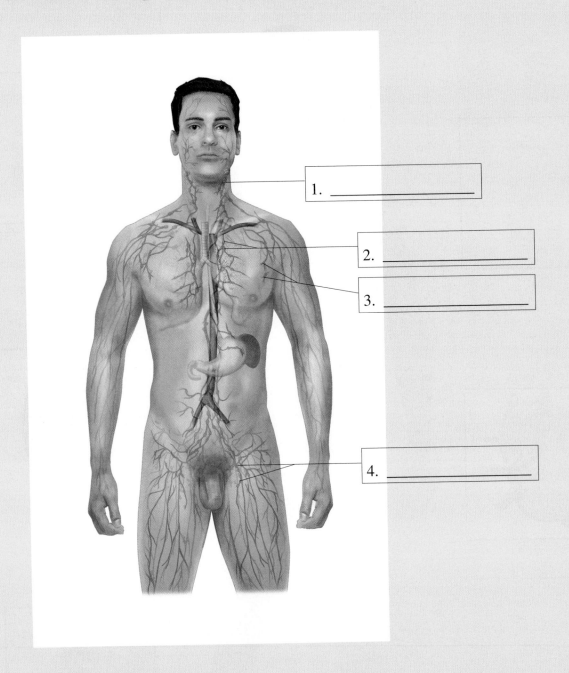

1. _____

2. _____

3. _____

4. _____

Multimedia Preview

Additional interactive resources and activities for this chapter can be found on the Companion Website. For videos, games, and pronunciations, please access the accompanying DVD-ROM that comes with this book.

DVD-ROM Highlights

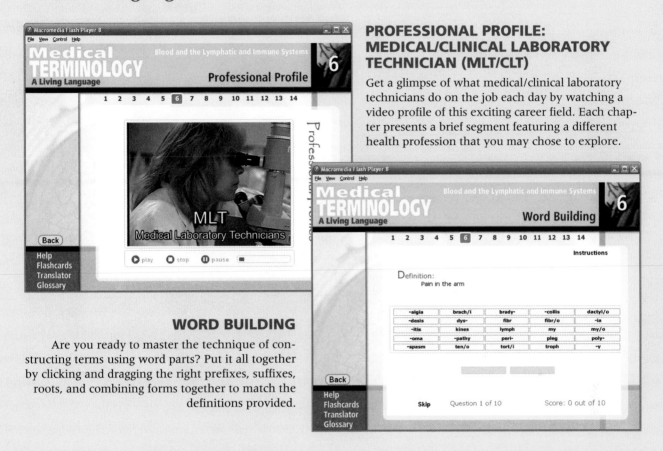

PROFESSIONAL PROFILE: MEDICAL/CLINICAL LABORATORY TECHNICIAN (MLT/CLT)

Get a glimpse of what medical/clinical laboratory technicians do on the job each day by watching a video profile of this exciting career field. Each chapter presents a brief segment featuring a different health profession that you may chose to explore.

WORD BUILDING

Are you ready to master the technique of constructing terms using word parts? Put it all together by clicking and dragging the right prefixes, suffixes, roots, and combining forms together to match the definitions provided.

Website Highlights—www.prenhall.com/fremgen

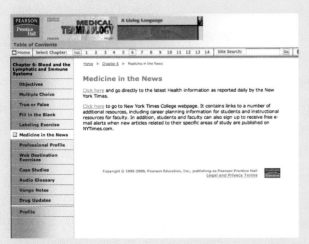

MEDICINE IN THE NEWS

Click here and take advantage of the free-access on-line study guide that accompanies your textbook. You'll be able to stay current with a link to medical news articles updated daily by *The New York Times*. By clicking on this URL you'll also access a variety of quizzes with instant feedback, links to download mp3 audio reviews, and an audio glossary.

7

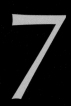

Respiratory System

Learning Objectives

Upon completion of this chapter, you will be able to:

- Identify and define the combining forms and suffixes introduced in this chapter.
- Correctly spell and pronounce medical terms and major anatomical structures relating to the respiratory system.
- Locate and describe the major organs of the respiratory system and their functions.
- List and describe the lung volumes and capacities.
- Describe the process of respiration.
- Build and define respiratory system medical terms from word parts.
- Identify and define respiratory system vocabulary terms.
- Identify and define selected respiratory system pathology terms.
- Identify and define selected respiratory system diagnostic procedures.
- Identify and define selected respiratory system therapeutic procedures.
- Identify and define selected medications relating to the respiratory system.
- Define selected abbreviations associated with the respiratory system.

Respiratory System at a Glance

Function

The organs of the respiratory system are responsible for bringing fresh air into the lungs, exchanging oxygen for carbon dioxide between the air sacs of the lungs and the blood stream, and exhaling the stale air.

Organs

nasal cavity
pharynx
larynx
trachea
bronchial tubes
lungs

Combining Forms

alveol/o	alveolus; air sac	**orth/o**	straight, upright
anthrac/o	coal	**ox/o, ox/i**	oxygen
atel/o	incomplete	**pharyng/o**	pharynx
bronch/o	bronchus	**pleur/o**	pleura
bronchi/o	bronchus	**pneum/o**	lung, air
bronchiol/o	bronchiole	**pneumon/o**	lung, air
coni/o	dust	**pulmon/o**	lung
diaphragmat/o	diaphragm	**rhin/o**	nose
epiglott/o	epiglottis	**sinus/o**	sinus, cavity
laryng/o	larynx	**spir/o**	breathing
lob/o	lobe	**trache/o**	trachea, windpipe
nas/o	nose		

Suffixes

-capnia	carbon dioxide
-ectasis	dilated, expansion
-osmia	smell
-phonia	voice
-pnea	breathing
-ptysis	spitting
-thorax	chest

Respiratory System Illustrated

nasal cavity, p. 210

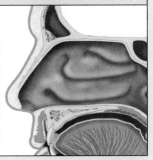

Cleanses, warms, and humidifies inhaled air

pharynx & larynx, pp. 211, 212

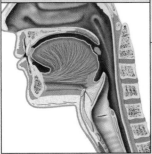

Carries air to the trachea and produces sound

trachea, p. 212

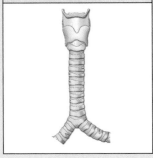

Transports air to and from lungs

bronchial tubes, p. 212

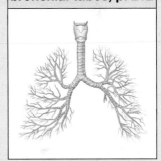

Air passageways inside the lung

lungs, p. 214

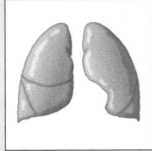

Site of gas exchange between air and blood

Anatomy and Physiology of the Respiratory System

bronchial tubes (BRONG-key-all)

carbon dioxide

exhalation (eks-hah-LAY-shun)

external respiration

inhalation (in-hah-LAY-shun)

internal respiration

larynx (LAIR-inks)

lungs

nasal cavity (NAY-zl)

oxygen (OK-sih-jen)

pharynx (FAIR-inks)

trachea (TRAY-kee-ah)

ventilation

The organs of the respiratory system include the **nasal cavity, pharynx, larynx, trachea, bronchial tubes**, and **lungs**—that function together to perform the mechanical and, for the most part, unconscious mechanism of respiration. The cells of the body require the continuous delivery of oxygen and removal of carbon dioxide. The respiratory system works in conjunction with the cardiovascular system to deliver oxygen to all the cells of the body. The process of respiration must be continuous; interruption for even a few minutes can result in brain damage and/or death.

The process of respiration can be subdivided into three distinct parts: **ventilation, external respiration**, and **internal respiration**. Ventilation is the flow of air between the outside environment and the lungs. **Inhalation** is the flow of air into the lungs, and **exhalation** is the flow of air out of the lungs. Inhalation brings fresh **oxygen** (O_2) into the air sacs, while exhalation removes **carbon dioxide** (CO_2) from the body.

External respiration refers to the exchange of oxygen and carbon dioxide that takes place in the lungs. These gases diffuse in opposite directions between the air sacs of the lungs and the bloodstream. Oxygen enters the bloodstream from the air sacs to be delivered throughout the body. Carbon dioxide leaves the bloodstream and enters the air sacs to be exhaled from the body.

Internal respiration is the process of oxygen and carbon dioxide exchange at the cellular level when oxygen leaves the bloodstream and is delivered to the tissues. Oxygen is needed for the body cells' metabolism, all the physical and chemical changes within the body that are necessary for life. The by-product of metabolism is the formation of a waste product, carbon dioxide. The carbon dioxide enters the bloodstream from the tissues and is transported back to the lungs for disposal.

Nasal Cavity

cilia (SIL-ee-ah)

mucous membrane

mucus (MYOO-kus)

nares (NAIR-eez)

nasal septum

palate (PAL-at)

paranasal sinuses (pair-ah-NAY-zl)

The process of ventilation begins with the nasal cavity. Air enters through two external openings in the nose called the **nares**. The nasal cavity is divided down the middle by the **nasal septum**, a cartilaginous plate. The **palate** in the roof of the mouth separates the nasal cavity above from the mouth below. The walls of the nasal cavity and the nasal septum are made up of flexible cartilage covered with **mucous membrane** (see Figure 7.1 ■). In fact, much of the respiratory tract is covered with mucous membrane, which secretes a sticky fluid, **mucus** (MYOO kus), which helps cleanse the air by trapping dust and bacteria. Since this membrane is also wet, it moisturizes inhaled air as it passes by the surface of the cavity. Very small hairs or **cilia** line the opening to the nose (as well as much of the airways), and filter out large dirt particles before they can enter the lungs. Capillaries in the mucous membranes warm inhaled air as it passes through the airways. In addition, several **paranasal sinuses** or air-filled cavities are located within

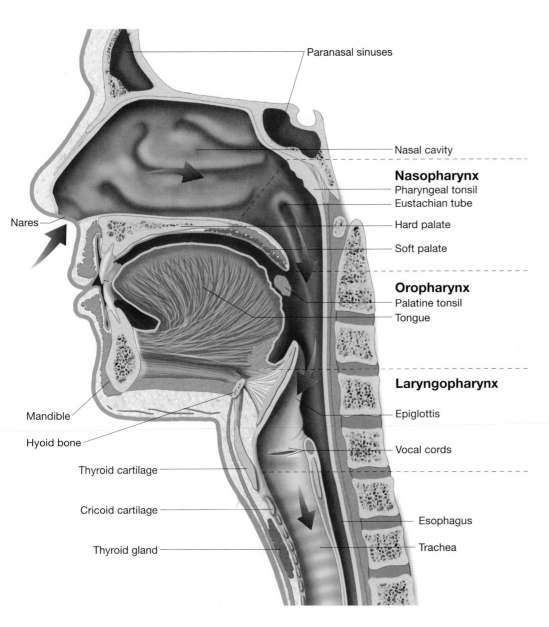

Paranasal sinuses

Nasal cavity

Nasopharynx
Pharyngeal tonsil
Eustachian tube

Hard palate

Soft palate

Oropharynx
Palatine tonsil
Tongue

Laryngopharynx

Epiglottis

Vocal cords

Nares

Mandible

Hyoid bone

Thyroid cartilage

Cricoid cartilage

Thyroid gland

Esophagus

Trachea

the facial bones. The sinuses act as an echo chamber during sound production and give resonance to the voice.

Pharynx

adenoids (ADD-eh-noydz)
auditory tube
eustachian tube (yoo-STAY-she-en)
laryngopharynx (lair-ring-goh-FAIR-inks)
lingual tonsils (LING-gwal)

nasopharynx (nay-zoh-FAIR-inks)
oropharynx (or-oh-FAIR-inks)
palatine tonsils (PAL-ah-tine)
pharyngeal tonsils (fair-IN-jee-al)

Air next enters the pharynx, also called the *throat*, which is used by both the respiratory and digestive systems. At the end of the pharynx, air enters the trachea while food and liquids are shunted into the esophagus.

The pharynx is roughly a 5-inch-long tube consisting of three parts: the upper **nasopharynx**, middle **oropharynx**, and lower **laryngopharynx** (see Figure 7.1). Three pairs of tonsils, collections of lymphatic tissue, are located in the pharynx. Tonsils are strategically placed to help keep pathogens from entering the body through either the air breathed or food and liquid swallowed. The nasopharynx, behind the nose, contains the **adenoids** or **pharyngeal tonsils**. The oropharynx, behind the mouth, contains the **palatine tonsils** and the **lingual tonsils**. Tonsils are considered a part of the lymphatic system and were discussed in Chapter 6.

The opening of the **eustachian** or **auditory tube** is also found in the nasopharynx. The other end of this tube is in the middle ear. Each time you swallow, this tube opens to equalize air pressure between the middle ear and the outside atmosphere.

Larynx

epiglottis (ep-ih-GLOT-iss)
glottis (GLOT-iss)
thyroid cartilage (THIGH-royd CAR-tih-lij)
vocal cords

The larynx or *voice box* is a muscular structure located between the pharynx and the trachea and contains the **vocal cords** (see Figures 7.1 and 7.2 ■). The vocal cords are not actually cordlike in structure, but rather they are folds of membranous tissue that produce sound by vibrating as air passes through the **glottis**, the opening between the two vocal cords.

A flap of cartilaginous tissue, the **epiglottis**, sits above the glottis and provides protection against food and liquid being inhaled into the lungs. The epiglottis covers the larynx and trachea during swallowing and shunts food and liquid from the pharynx into the esophagus. The walls of the larynx are composed of several cartilage plates held together with ligaments and muscles. One of these cartilages, the **thyroid cartilage**, forms what is known as the *Adam's apple*. The thyroid cartilage is generally larger in males than in females and helps to produce the deeper male voice.

Trachea

The trachea, also called the *windpipe*, is the passageway for air that extends from the pharynx and larynx down to the main bronchi (see Figure 7.3 ■). Measuring approximately 4 inches in length, it is composed of smooth muscle and cartilage rings and is lined by mucous membrane and cilia. Therefore, it also assists in cleansing, warming, and moisturizing air as it travels to the lungs.

Bronchial Tubes

alveoli (al-VEE-oh-lye)
bronchioles (BRONG-key-ohlz)
bronchus (BRONG-kus)
pulmonary capillaries
respiratory membrane

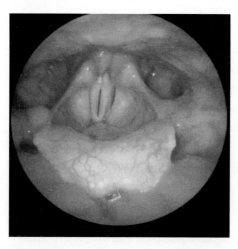

■ **Figure 7.2** The vocal cords within the larynx, superior view from the pharynx.
(CNRI/Phototake NYC)

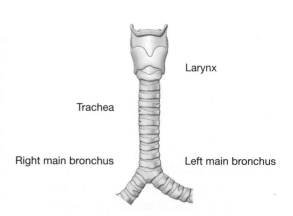

Larynx

Trachea

Right main bronchus

Left main bronchus

■ **Figure 7.3** Structure of the trachea which extends from the larynx above to the primary bronchi below.

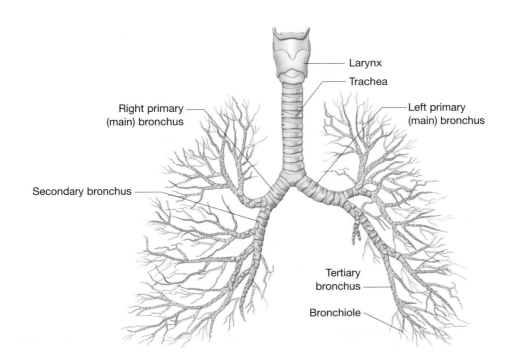

The distal end of the trachea divides to form the left and right primary (main) bronchi. Each **bronchus** enters one of the lungs and branches repeatedly to form secondary and tertiary bronchi. Each branch becomes narrower until the narrowest branches, the **bronchioles**, are formed (see Figure 7.4 ■). Each bronchiole terminates in a small group of air sacs, called **alveoli**. Each lung has approximately 150 million alveoli. The walls of alveoli are elastic, giving them the ability to expand to hold air and then recoil to their original size. A network of **pulmonary capillaries** from the pulmonary blood vessels tightly encases each alveolus (see Figure 7.5 ■). In fact, the walls of the alveoli and capillaries are so tightly associated with each other they are referred to as a single unit, the **respiratory membrane**. The exchange of oxygen and carbon dioxide between the air within the alveolus and the blood inside the capillaries takes place across the respiratory membrane.

Med Term Tip

The respiratory system can be thought of as an upside-down tree and its branches. The trunk of the tree consists of the pharynx, larynx, and trachea. The trachea then divides into two branches, the bronchi. Each bronchus divides into smaller and smaller branches. In fact, this branching system of tubes is referred to as the *bronchial tree*.

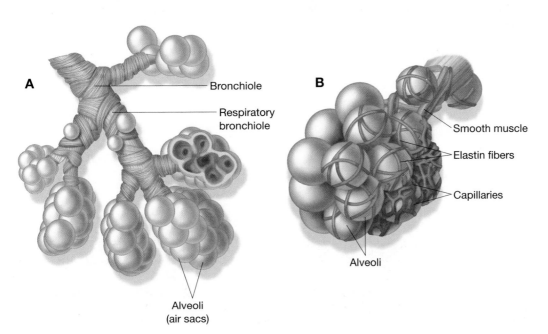

■ **Figure 7.5** A) Each bronchiole terminates in an alveolar sac, a group of alveoli. B) Alveoli encased by network capillaries, forming the respiratory membrane.

Lungs

apex	**parietal pleura** (pah-RYE-eh-tal)
base	**pleura** (PLOO-rah)
hilum (HYE-lum)	**pleural cavity**
lobes	**serous fluid** (SEER-us)
mediastinum (mee-dee-ass-TYE-num)	**visceral pleura** (VISS-er-al)

Med Term Tip

Some of the abnormal lung sounds heard with a stethoscope, such as crackling and rubbing, are made when the parietal and/or visceral pleura become inflamed and rub against one another.

Each lung is the total collection of the bronchi, bronchioles, and alveoli. They are spongy to the touch because they contain air. The lungs are protected by a double membrane called the **pleura**. The pleura's outer membrane is the **parietal pleura**, which also lines the wall of the chest cavity. The inner membrane or **visceral pleura** adheres to the surface of the lungs. The pleural membrane is folded in such a way that it forms a sac around each lung referred to as the **pleural cavity.** There is normally slippery, watery **serous fluid** between the two layers of the pleura that reduces friction when the two layers rub together as the lungs repeatedly expand and contract.

The lungs contain divisions or **lobes.** There are three lobes in the larger right lung and two in the left lung. The pointed superior portion of each lung is the **apex**, while the broader lower area is the **base.** Entry of structures like the bronchi, pulmonary blood vessels, and nerves into each lung occurs along its medial border in an area called the **hilum**. The lungs within the thoracic cavity are protected from puncture and damage by the ribs. The area between the right and left lung is called the **mediastinum** and contains the heart, aorta, esophagus, thymus gland, and trachea. See Figure 7.6 ■ for an illustration of the lungs within the chest cavity.

Lung Volumes and Capacities

pulmonary function test   **respiratory therapist**

For some types of medical conditions, like emphysema, it is important to measure the volume of air flowing in and out of the lungs to determine lung capac-

■ Figure 7.6 Position of the lungs within the thoracic cavity, anterior view illustrating regions of the lungs and their relationship to other thoracic organs.

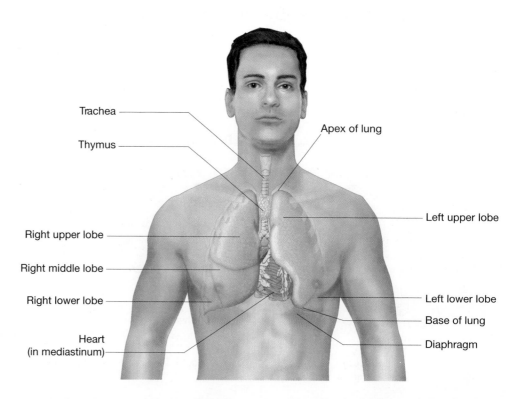

Trachea

Thymus

Apex of lung

Right upper lobe

Left upper lobe

Right middle lobe

Right lower lobe

Left lower lobe

Base of lung

Heart
(in mediastinum)

Diaphragm

ity. Lung volumes are measured by **respiratory therapists** to aid in determining the functioning level of the respiratory system. Collectively, these measurements are called **pulmonary function tests**. Table 7.1 ■ lists and defines the four lung volumes and four lung capacities.

Respiratory Muscles

diaphragm   **intercostal muscles** (in-ter-COS-tal)

Air moves in and out of the lungs due to the difference between the atmospheric pressure and the pressure within the chest cavity. This difference in pressure is produced by the **diaphragm**, which is the muscle separating the abdomen from the thoracic cavity. To do this, the diaphragm contracts and moves downward. This increase in thoracic cavity volume causes a decrease in pressure, or negative thoracic pressure, within the chest cavity. Air then flows into the lungs, inhalation, to equalize the pressure. The **intercostal muscles** between the ribs assist in inhalation by raising the rib cage to further enlarge the thoracic cavity. See Figure 7.7 ■ for an illustration of the role of the diaphragm in inhalation. Similarly, when the diaphragm and intercostal muscles relax, the thoracic cavity becomes smaller. This produces an increase in pressure within the cavity, or positive thoracic pressure, and air flows out of the lungs, resulting in exhalation. Therefore, a quiet, unforced exhalation is a passive process since it does not require any muscle contraction. When a forceful inhalation or exhalation is required, additional chest and neck muscles become active to create larger changes in thoracic pressure.

Med Term Tip

Diaphragmatic breathing is taught to singers and public speakers. You can practice this type of breathing by allowing your abdomen to expand during inhalation and contract during exhalation while your shoulders remain motionless.

Respiratory Rate

vital signs

Respiratory rate (measured in breaths per minute) is one of our **vital signs** (VS), along with heart rate, temperature, and blood pressure. Normally, respiratory rate

Table 7.1	Lung Volumes and Capacities
TERM	**DEFINITION**
Tidal volume (TV)	The amount of air that enters the lungs in a single inhalation or leaves the lungs in a single exhalation of quiet breathing. In an adult this is normally 500 mL.*
Inspiratory reserve volume (IRV)	The air that can be forcibly inhaled after a normal respiration has taken place. Also called *complemental air*; generally measures around 3,000 mL.*
Expiratory reserve volume (ERV)	The amount of air that can be forcibly exhaled after a normal quiet respiration. This is also called *supplemental air*; approximately 1,000 mL.*
Residual volume (RV)	The air remaining in the lungs after a forced exhalation; about 1,500 mL* in the adult.
Inspiratory capacity (IC)	The volume of air inhaled after a normal exhale.
Functional residual capacity (FRC)	The air that remains in the lungs after a normal exhalation has taken place.
Vital capacity (VC)	The total volume of air that can be exhaled after a maximum inhalation. This amount will be equal to the sum of TV, IRV, and ERV.
Total lung capacity (TLC)	The volume of air in the lungs after a maximal inhalation.

*There is a normal range for measurements of the volume of air exchanged. The numbers given are for the average measurement.

Figure 7.7 A) Bell jar apparatus demonstrating how downward movement of the diaphragm results in air flowing into the lungs. B) Action of the intercostal muscles lift the ribs to assist the diaphragm in enlarging the volume of the thoracic cavity.

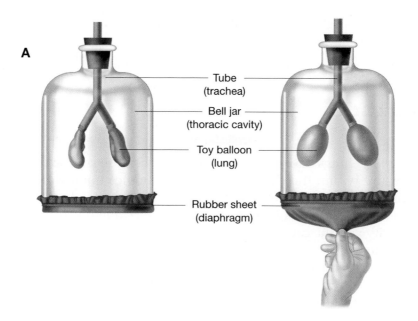

A

Tube
(trachea)

Bell jar
(thoracic cavity)

Toy balloon
(lung)

Rubber sheet
(diaphragm)

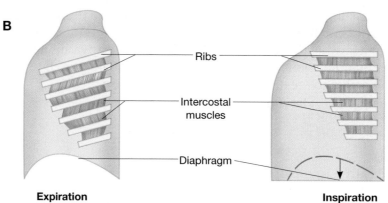

B

Ribs

Intercostal
muscles

Diaphragm

Expiration   Inspiration

Med Term Tip

When divers wish to hold their breath longer, they first hyperventilate (breath faster and deeper) in order to get rid of as much CO_2 as possible. This will hold off the urge to breathe longer, allowing a diver to stay submerged longer.

is regulated by the level of CO_2 in the blood. When the CO_2 level is high, we breathe more rapidly to expel the excess. Then, when CO_2 levels drop, our respiratory rate will also drop.

When the respiratory rate falls outside the range of normal, it may indicate an illness or medical condition. For example, when a patient is running an elevated temperature and has shortness of breath (SOB) due to pneumonia, the respiratory rate may increase dramatically. Or a brain injury or some medications, such as those for pain, can cause a decrease in the respiratory rate. See Table 7.2 ■ for normal respiratory rate ranges for different age groups.

Table 7.2	Respiratory Rates for Different Age Groups
AGE	**RESPIRATIONS PER MINUTE**
Newborn	30–60
1-year-old	18–30
16-year-old	16–20
Adult	12–20

Word Building

The following list contains examples of medical terms built directly from word parts. The definition for these terms can be determined by a straightforward translation of the word parts.

COMBINING FORM	COMBINED WITH	MEDICAL TERM	DEFINITION
bronch/o	-gram	**bronchogram** (BRONG-koh-gram)	record of the bronchus
	-itis	**bronchitis** (brong-KIGH-tis)	inflammation of a bronchus
	-plasty	**bronchoplasty** (BRONG-koh-plas-tee)	surgical repair of a bronchus
	-genic	**bronchogenic** (brong-koh-JEN-ik)	produced by the bronchus
	-scope	**bronchoscope** (BRONG-koh-scope)	instrument to view inside of bronchus
	-spasm	**bronchospasm** (BRONG-koh-spazm)	involuntary muscle spasm of bronchus
	-ial	**bronchial** (BRONG-ee-all)	pertaining to a bronchus
bronchi/o	-ectasis	**bronchiectasis** (brong-key-EK-tah-sis)	dilated bronchus
diaphragmat/o	-ic	**diaphragmatic** (dye-ah-frag-MAT-ik)	pertaining to the diaphragm
laryng/o	-ectomy	**laryngectomy** (lair-in-JEK-toh-mee)	removal of the voice box
	-itis	**laryngitis** (lair-in-JYE-tis)	inflammation of the voice box
	-plasty	**laryngoplasty** (lair-RING-goh-plas-tee)	surgical repair of the voice box
	-scope	**laryngoscope** (lair-RING-go-scope)	instrument to view voice box
	-eal	**laryngeal** (lair-in-GEE-all)	pertaining to the voice box
	-plegia	**laryngoplegia** (lair-RING-goh-plee-gee-ah)	paralysis of the voice box
lob/o	-ectomy	**lobectomy** (loh-BEK-toh-mee)	removal of a (lung) lobe
ox/i	-meter	**oximeter** (ox-IM-eh-ter)	instrument to measure oxygen
ox/o	an- -ia	**anoxia** (ah-NOK-see-ah)	condition of no oxygen
	hypo- -emia	**hypoxemia** (high-pox-EE-mee-ah)	insufficient oxygen in the blood
	hypo- -ia	**hypoxia** (high-POX-ee-ah)	insufficient oxygen condition
pleur/o	-centesis	**pleurocentesis** (ploor-oh-sen-TEE-sis)	puncture of the pleura to withdraw fluid
	-ectomy	**pleurectomy** (ploor-EK-toh-mee)	removal of the pleura
	-dynia	**pleurodynia** (ploor-oh-DIN-ee-ah)	pleural pain
pharyng/o	-itis	**pharyngitis** (fair-in-JYE-tis)	throat inflammation (*i.e., sore throat*)
	-eal	**pharyngeal** (fair-in-GEE-all)	pertaining to the throat
	nas/o -itis	**nasopharyngitis** (nay-zoh-fair-in-JYE-tis)	nose and throat inflammation (*i.e., common cold*)
pulmon/o	-logist	**pulmonologist** (pul-mon-ALL-oh-jist)	lung specialist
	-ary	**pulmonary** (PULL-mon-air-ee)	pertaining to the lung
rhin/o	-itis	**rhinitis** (rye-NYE-tis)	inflammation of the nose
	myc/o -osis	**rhinomycosis** (rye-noh-my-KOH-sis)	abnormal condition of nose fungus
	-plasty	**rhinoplasty** (RYE-noh-plas-tee)	surgical repair of the nose

Word Building *(continued)*

COMBINING FORM	COMBINED WITH	MEDICAL TERM	DEFINITION
	-rrhagia	**rhinorrhagia** (rye-noh-RAH-jee-ah)	rapid flow (of blood) from the nose
	-rrhea	**rhinorrhea** (rye-noh-REE-ah)	nose discharge (*i.e., runny nose*)
sinus/o	pan- -itis	**pansinusitis** (pan-sigh-nus-EYE-tis)	inflammation of all the sinuses
thorac/o	-algia	**thoracalgia** (thor-ah-KAL-jee-ah)	chest pain
	-ic	**thoracic** (tho-RASS-ik)	pertaining to the chest
	-otomy	**thoracotomy** (thor-ah-KOT-oh-mee)	incision into the chest
trache/o	endo- -al	**endotracheal** (en-doh-TRAY-kee-al)	pertaining to inside the trachea
	-otomy	**tracheotomy** (tray-kee-OTT-oh-mee)	incision into the trachea
	-stenosis	**tracheostenosis** (tray-kee-oh-steh-NOH-sis)	narrowing of the trachea

SUFFIX	COMBINED WITH	MEDICAL TERM	DEFINITION
-phonia	a-	**aphonia** (a-FOH-nee-ah)	no voice
	dys-	**dysphonia** (dis-FOH-nee-ah)	abnormal voice
-capnia	a-	**acapnia** (a-CAP-nee-ah)	lack of carbon dioxide
	hyper-	**hypercapnia** (high-per-CAP-nee-ah)	excessive carbon dioxide
-osmia	an-	**anosmia** (ah-NOZ-mee-ah)	lack of (sense of) smell
-pnea	a-	**apnea** (AP-nee-ah)	not breathing
	brady-	**bradypnea** (bray-DIP-nee-ah)	slow breathing
	dys-	**dyspnea** (DISP-nee-ah)	difficult, labored breathing
	eu-	**eupnea** (yoop-NEE-ah)	normal breathing
	hyper-	**hyperpnea** (high-per-NEE-ah)	excessive (deep) breathing
	hypo-	**hypopnea** (high-POP-nee-ah)	insufficient (shallow) breathing
	ortho-	**orthopnea** (or-THOP-nee-ah)	(sitting) straight breathing
	tachy-	**tachypnea** (tak-ip-NEE-ah)	rapid breathing
-thorax	hem/o	**hemothorax** (hee-moh-THOH-raks)	blood in the chest
	py/o	**pyothorax** (pye-oh-THOH-raks)	pus in the chest
	pneum/o	**pneumothorax** (new-moh-THOH-raks)	air in the chest

 Vocabulary

TERM	DEFINITION
asphyxia (as-FIK-see-ah)	Lack of oxygen that can lead to unconsciousness and death if not corrected immediately; also called *asphyxiation* or *suffocation*. Some common causes include drowning, foreign body in the respiratory tract, poisoning, and electric shock.

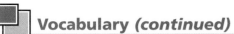

Vocabulary *(continued)*

TERM	DEFINITION
aspiration (as-peer-RAY-shun)	Refers to withdrawing fluid from a body cavity using suction. For example, using a long needle and syringe to withdraw fluid from the pleural cavity or using a vacuum pump to remove phlegm from a patient's airways. In addition, it also refers to inhaling food, liquid, or a foreign object into the airways which may lead to the development of pneumonia.
Cheyne–Stokes respiration (CHAIN STOHKS res-pir-AY-shun)	Abnormal breathing pattern in which there are long periods (10 to 60 seconds) of apnea followed by deeper, more rapid breathing. Named for John Cheyne, a Scottish physician, and Sir William Stokes, an Irish surgeon.
clubbing	The abnormal widening and thickening of the ends of the fingers and toes associated with chronic oxygen deficiency. Seen in patients with chronic respiratory conditions or circulatory problems.
cyanosis (sigh-ah-NO-sis)	Refers to the bluish tint of skin that is receiving an insufficient amount of oxygen or circulation.
epistaxis (ep-ih-STAKS-is)	Nosebleed.
hemoptysis (hee-MOP-tih-sis)	To cough up blood or blood-stained sputum.
hyperventilation (HYE-per-vent-ill-a-shun)	To breathe both too fast (tachypnea) and too deep (hyperpnea).
hypoventilation (HYE-poh-vent-ill-a-shun)	To breathe both too slow (bradypnea) and too shallow (hypopnea).
internal medicine	Branch of medicine involving the diagnosis and treatment of diseases and conditions of internal organs such as the respiratory system. The physician is an *internist*.
nasal cannula (CAN-you-lah)	Two-pronged plastic device for delivering oxygen into the nose; one prong is inserted into each naris.
orthopnea (or-THOP-nee-ah)	A term to describe dyspnea that is worsened by lying flat. In other words, the patient is able to breath easier when sitting straight up.
otorhinolaryngology (ENT) (oh-toh-rye-noh-lair-in-GOL-oh-jee)	Branch of medicine involving the diagnosis and treatment of conditions and diseases of the ear, nose, and throat region. The physician is an *otorhinolaryngologist*. This medical specialty may also be referred to *otolaryngology*.
patent (PAY-tent)	Open or unblocked, such as a patent airway.
percussion (per-KUH-shun)	Use of the fingertips to tap on a surface to determine the condition beneath the surface. Determined in part by the feel of the surface as it is tapped and the sound generated.
phlegm (FLEM)	Thick mucus secreted by the membranes that line the respiratory tract. When phlegm is coughed through the mouth, it is called *sputum*. Phlegm is examined for color, odor, and consistency.
pleural rub (PLOO-ral)	Grating sound made when the two layers of the pleura rub together during respiration. It is caused when one of the surfaces becomes thicker as a result of inflammation or other disease conditions. This rub can be felt through the fingertips when they are placed on the chest wall or heard through the stethoscope.

Vocabulary *(continued)*

TERM	DEFINITION
pulmonology (pull-mon-ALL-oh-jee)	Branch of medicine involved in diagnosis and treatment of diseases and disorders of the respiratory system. Physician is a *pulmonologist*.
rales (RALZ)	Abnormal crackling sound made during inspiration. Usually indicates the presence of fluid or mucus in the airways.
respiratory therapy	Allied health specialty that assists patients with respiratory and cardiopulmonary disorders. Duties of a *respiratory therapist* include conducting pulmonary function tests, monitoring oxygen and carbon dioxide levels in the blood, administering breathing treatments, and ventilator management.
rhonchi (RONG-kigh)	Somewhat musical sound during expiration, often found in asthma or infection. Caused by spasms of the bronchial tubes. Also called *wheezing*.
shortness of breath (SOB)	Term used to indicate that a patient is having some difficulty breathing; also called *dyspnea*. The causes can range from mild SOB after exercise to SOB associated with heart disease.
sputum (SPEW-tum)	Mucus or phlegm that is coughed up from the lining of the respiratory tract.
	Med Term Tip
	The term *sputum,* from the Latin word meaning "to spit," now refers to the material coughed up and spit out from the respiratory system.
stridor (STRIGH-dor)	Harsh, high-pitched, noisy breathing sound made when there is an obstruction of the bronchus or larynx. Found in conditions such as croup in children.
thoracic surgery (tho-RASS-ik)	Branch of medicine involving diagnosis and treatment of conditions and diseases of the respiratory system by surgical means. Physician is a *thoracic surgeon*.

Pathology

TERM	DEFINITION
■ *Upper Respiratory System*	
croup (KROOP)	Acute respiratory condition found in infants and children that is characterized by a barking type of cough or stridor.
diphtheria (dif-THEAR-ee-ah)	Bacterial upper respiratory infection characterized by the formation of a thick membranous film across the throat and a high mortality rate. Rare now due to the DPT (diphtheria, pertussis, tetanus) vaccine.
pertussis (per-TUH-is)	Commonly called *whooping cough*, due to the whoop sound made when coughing. An infectious bacterial disease of the upper respiratory system that children receive immunization against as part of their DPT shots.
■ *Bronchial Tubes*	
asthma (AZ-mah)	Disease caused by various conditions, like allergens, and resulting in constriction of the bronchial airways, dyspnea, coughing, and wheezing. Can cause violent spasms of the bronchi (bronchospasms) but is generally not a life-threatening condition. Medication can be very effective.
	Med Term Tip
	The term *asthma,* from the Greek word meaning "panting," describes the breathing pattern of a person having an asthma attack.

Pathology *(continued)*

TERM	DEFINITION
bronchiectasis (brong-key-EK-tah-sis)	The abnormal enlargement of bronchi; may be the result of a lung infection. This condition can be irreversible and result in destruction of the bronchial walls. Major symptoms include coughing up a large amount of purulent sputum, rales, and hemoptysis.
bronchogenic carcinoma (brong-koh-JEN-ik car-sin-OH-mah)	Malignant tumor originating in the bronchi. Usually associated with a history of cigarette smoking.

■ **Figure 7.8** Color enchanced X-ray of large malignant tumor in right lower lung. *(ISM/Phototake NYC)*

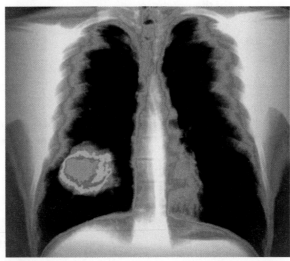

■ *Lungs*

adult respiratory distress syndrome (ARDS)	Acute respiratory failure in adults characterized by tachypnea, dyspnea, cyanosis, tachycardia, and hypoxemia. May follow trauma, pneumonia, or septic infections. Also called *acute respiratory distress syndrome*.
anthracosis (an-thra-KOH-sis)	A type of pneumoconiosis that develops from the collection of coal dust in the lung. Also called *black lung* or *miner's lung*.
asbestosis (az-bes-TOH-sis)	A type of pneumoconiosis that develops from collection of asbestos fibers in the lungs. May lead to the development of lung cancer.
atelectasis (at-eh-LEK-tah-sis)	Condition in which the alveoli in a portion of the lung collapse, preventing the respiratory exchange of oxygen and carbon dioxide. Can be caused by a variety of conditions, including pressure on the lung from a tumor or other object. Term also used to describe the failure of a newborn's lungs to expand.
chronic obstructive pulmonary disease (COPD) (PULL-mon-air-ee)	Progressive, chronic, and usually irreversible group of conditions, like emphysema, in which the lungs have a diminished capacity for inspiration (inhalation) and expiration (exhalation). The person may have dyspnea upon exertion and a cough.
cystic fibrosis (CF) (SIS-tik fye-BROH-sis)	Hereditary condition causing the exocrine glands to malfunction. The patient produces very thick mucus that causes severe congestion within the lungs and digestive system. Through more advanced treatment, many children are now living into adulthood with this disease.
emphysema (em-fih-SEE-mah)	Pulmonary condition characterized by the destruction of the walls of the alveoli, resulting in fewer overexpanded air sacs. Can occur as a result of long-term heavy smoking. Air pollution also worsens this disease. The patient may not be able to breathe except in a sitting or standing position.

Pathology *(continued)*

TERM	DEFINITION
histoplasmosis (his-toh-plaz-MOH-sis)	Pulmonary infection caused by the fungus *Histoplasma capsulatum*, found in dust and in the droppings of pigeons and chickens.
infant respiratory distress syndrome (IRDS)	A lung condition most commonly found in premature infants that is characterized by tachypnea and respiratory grunting. The condition is caused by a lack of surfactant necessary to keep the lungs inflated. Also called *hyaline membrane disease* (HMD) and *respiratory distress syndrome of the newborn.*
influenza (in-floo-EN-za)	Viral infection of the respiratory system characterized by chills, fever, body aches, and fatigue. Commonly called the *flu.*
Legionnaire's disease (lee-jen-AYRZ)	Severe, often fatal bacterial infection characterized by pneumonia and liver and kidney damage. Named after people who came down with it at an American Legion convention in 1976.
***Mycoplasma* pneumonia** (MY-koh-plaz-em)	A less severe but longer lasting form of pneumonia caused by the *Mycoplasma pneumoniae* bacteria. Also called *walking pneumonia.*
pneumoconiosis (noo-moh-koh-nee-OH-sis)	Condition that is the result of inhaling environmental particles that become toxic. Can be the result of inhaling coal dust (anthracosis) or asbestos (asbestosis).
***Pneumocystis carinii* pneumonia** (PCP) (noo-moh-SIS-tis kah-RYE-nee-eye new-MOH-nee-ah)	Pneumonia with a nonproductive cough, very little fever, and dyspnea caused by the fungus *Pneumocystis carinii*. An opportunistic infection often seen in those with weakened immune systems, such as AIDS patients.
pneumonia (new-MOH-nee-ah)	Inflammatory condition of the lung that can be caused by bacterial and viral infections, diseases, and chemicals. Results in the filling of the alveoli and air spaces with fluid.
pulmonary edema (PULL-mon-air-ee eh-DEE-mah)	Condition in which lung tissue retains an excessive amount of fluid, especially in the alveoli. Results in dyspnea.
pulmonary embolism (PULL-mon-air-ee EM-boh-lizm)	Blood clot or air bubble in the pulmonary artery or one of its branches. May cause an infarct in the lung tissue.
pulmonary fibrosis (fi-BROH-sis)	Formation of fibrous scar tissue in the lungs that leads to decreased ability to expand the lungs. May be caused by infections, pneumoconiosis, autoimmune diseases, and toxin exposure.
severe acute respiratory syndrome (SARS)	Acute viral respiratory infection that begins like the flu but quickly progresses to severe dyspnea; high fatality rate. First appeared in China in 2003.
silicosis (sil-ih-KOH-sis)	A type of pneumoconiosis that develops from the inhalation of silica (quartz) dust found in quarrying, glass works, sandblasting, and ceramics.
sleep apnea (AP-nee-ah)	Condition in which breathing stops repeatedly during sleep long enough to cause a drop in oxygen levels in the blood.
sudden infant death syndrome (SIDS)	Unexpected and unexplained death of an apparently well infant under one year of age. The child suddenly stops breathing for unknown reasons.
tuberculosis (TB) (too-ber-kyoo-LOH-sis)	Infectious disease caused by the bacteria *Mycobacterium tuberculosis*. Most commonly affects the respiratory system and causes inflammation and calcification in the lungs. Tuberculosis incidence is on the increase and is seen in many patients with weakened immune systems. Multidrug resistant tuberculosis is a particularly dangerous form of the disease because some bacteria have developed a resistance to the standard drug therapy.

Pathology *(continued)*

TERM	DEFINITION
■ *Pleural Cavity*	
empyema (em-pye-EE-mah)	Pus within the pleural space usually associated with a bacterial infection. Also called *pyothorax*.
pleural effusion (PLOO-ral eh-FYOO-zhun)	Abnormal accumulation of fluid in the pleural cavity preventing the lungs from fully expanding. Physicians can detect the presence of fluid by tapping the chest (percussion) or listening with a stethoscope (auscultation).
pleurisy (PLOOR-ih-see)	Inflammation of the pleura characterized by sharp chest pain with each breath. Also called *pleuritis*.
pneumothorax (new-moh-THOH-raks)	Collection of air or gas in the pleural cavity, which may result in collapse of the lung.

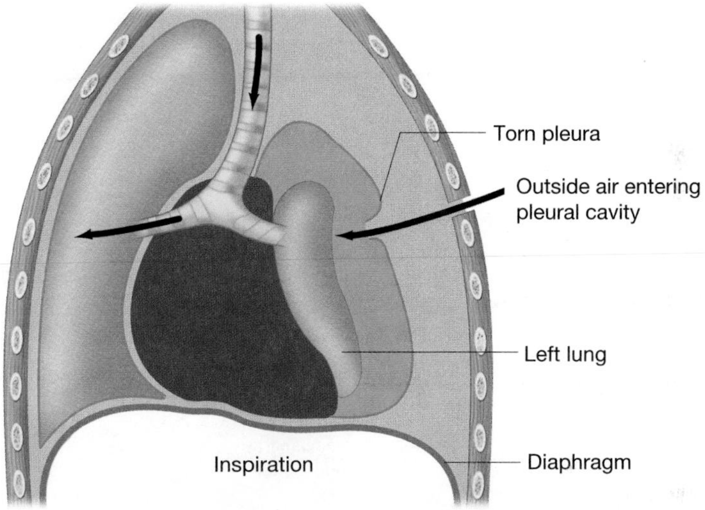

■ **Figure 7.9** Pneumothorax. Figure illustrates how puncture of thoracic wall and tearing of pleural membrane allows air into lung and results in a collapsed lung.

Torn pleura

Outside air entering pleural cavity

Left lung

Inspiration

Diaphragm

Diagnostic Procedures

TERM	DEFINITION
■ *Clinical Laboratory Tests*	
arterial blood gases (ABGs) (ar-TEE-ree-al)	Testing for the gases present in the blood. Generally used to assist in determining the levels of oxygen (O_2) and carbon dioxide (CO_2) in the blood.
sputum culture and sensitivity (C&S) (SPEW-tum)	Testing sputum by placing it on a culture medium and observing any bacterial growth. The specimen is then tested to determine antibiotic effectiveness.
sputum cytology (SPEW-tum sigh-TALL-oh-jee)	Examining sputum for malignant cells.
■ *Diagnostic Imaging*	
bronchography (brong-KOG-rah-fee)	X-ray of the lung after a radiopaque substance has been inserted into the trachea or bronchial tube. Resulting x-ray is called a *bronchogram*.
chest x-ray (CXR)	Taking a radiographic picture of the lungs and heart from the back and sides.

Diagnostic Procedures *(continued)*

TERM	DEFINITION
pulmonary angiography (PULL-mon-air-ee an-jee-OG-rah-fee)	Injecting dye into a blood vessel for the purpose of taking an x-ray of the arteries and veins of the lungs.
ventilation-perfusion scan (per-FUSE-shun)	A nuclear medicine diagnostic test that is especially useful in identifying pulmonary emboli. Radioactive air is inhaled for the ventilation portion to determine if air is filling the entire lung. Radioactive intravenous injection shows whether blood is flowing to all parts of the lung.

■ *Endoscopic Procedures*

TERM	DEFINITION
bronchoscopy (Bronch) (brong-KOSS-koh-pee) ■ **Figure 7.10** Bronchoscopy. Figure illustrates physician using a bronchoscope to inspect the patient's bronchial tubes. Advances in technology include using a videoscope which projects the internal view of the bronchus onto a video screen.	Visual examination of the inside of the bronchi; uses an instrument called a *bronchoscope*.

Cross Section of Scope

Eye piece

Viewing channel

Light source

Biopsy forceps and instrument channel

Flexible bronchoscopic tube

TERM	DEFINITION
laryngoscopy (lair-in-GOSS-koh-pee)	Examination of the interior of the larynx with a lighted instrument called a *laryngoscope*.

■ *Pulmonary Function Tests*

TERM	DEFINITION
oximetry (ox-IM-eh-tree)	Measures the oxygen level in the blood using a device, an *oximeter*, placed on the patient's fingertip or ear lobe.
pulmonary function test (PFT) (PULL-mon-air-ee)	A group of diagnostic tests that give information regarding air flow in and out of the lungs, lung volumes, and gas exchange between the lungs and bloodstream.
spirometry (spy-ROM-eh-tree)	Procedure to measure lung capacity using a **spirometer**.

■ *Additional Diagnostic Procedures*

TERM	DEFINITION
polysomnography (polly-som-NOG-rah-fee)	Monitoring a patient while sleeping to identify sleep apnea. Also called *sleep apnea study*.
sweat test	A test for cystic fibrosis. Patients with this disease have an abnormally large amount of salt in their sweat.
tuberculin skin tests (TB test) (too-BER-kyoo-lin)	Applying the tuberculin purified protein derivative (PPD) under the surface of the skin to determine if the patient has been exposed to tuberculosis. Also called a *Tine* or *Mantoux test*.

Therapeutic Procedures

TERM	DEFINITION
■ *Respiratory Therapy*	
aerosol therapy (AIR-oh-sol)	Medication suspended in a mist that is intended to be inhaled. Delivered by a *nebulizer*, which delivers the mist for a period of time while the patient breathes, or a *metered dose inhaler* (MDI), which delivers a single puff of mist.
endotracheal intubation (en-doh-TRAY-kee-al in-too-BAY-shun)	Placing a tube through the mouth, through the glottis, and into the trachea to create a patent airway.

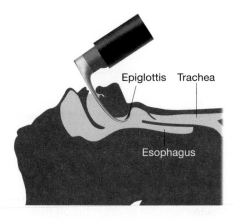 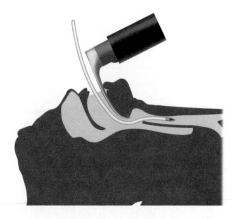 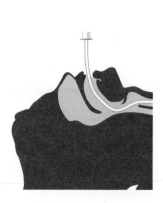

Epiglottis   Trachea

Esophagus

■ Figure 7.11 Endotracheal intubation. First, a lighted scope is used to identify the trachea from the esophagus. Next, the tube is placed through the pharynx and into the trachea. Finally, the scope is removed, leaving the tube in place.

TERM	DEFINITION
intermittent positive pressure breathing (IPPB)	Method for assisting patients in breathing using a mask that is connected to a machine that produces an increased positive thoracic pressure.
postural drainage	Drainage of secretions from the bronchi by placing the patient in a position that uses gravity to promote drainage. Used for the treatment of cystic fibrosis and bronchiectasis.
supplemental oxygen therapy	Providing a patient with additional concentration of oxygen to improve oxygen levels in the bloodstream. Oxygen may be provided by a mask or nasal cannula.
ventilator (VENT-ih-later)	A machine that provides artificial ventilation for a patient unable to breathe on his or her own. Also called a *respirator*.

■ Figure 7.12 Patient with tracheostomy tube in place receiving oxygen through mask placed over the tracheostomy opening and attached to a ventilator. *(Ansell Horn/Phototake NYC)*

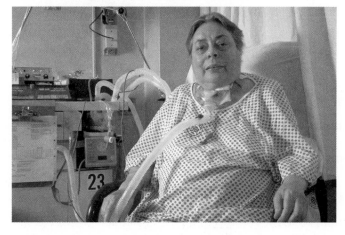

Therapeutic Procedures *(continued)*

TERM	DEFINITION

■ *Surgical Procedures*

thoracentesis
(thor-ah-sen-TEE-sis)

■ **Figure 7.13** Thoracentesis. The needle is inserted between the ribs to withdraw fluid from the pleural sac at the base of the left lung.

Surgical puncture of the chest wall for the removal of fluids. Also called *thoracocentesis*.

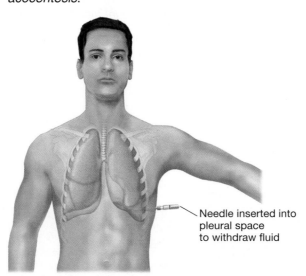

Needle inserted into pleural space to withdraw fluid

---

thoracostomy
(thor-ah-KOS-toh-mee)

Insertion of a tube into the chest for the purpose of draining off fluid or air. Also called *chest tube*.

---

tracheostomy
(tray-kee-OSS-toh-mee)

A surgical procedure often performed in an emergency that creates an opening directly into the trachea to allow the patient to breathe easier; also called *tracheotomy*.

■ **Figure 7.14** A tracheostomy tube in place, inserted through an opening in the front of the neck and anchored within the trachea.

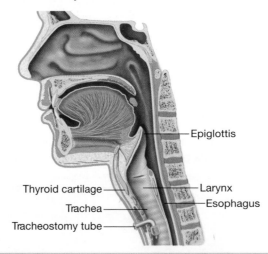

Epiglottis

Thyroid cartilage
Trachea
Tracheostomy tube

Larynx
Esophagus

■ *Additional Procedures*

cardiopulmonary resuscitation
(CPR)
(car-dee-oh-PULL-mon-air-ee ree-suss-ih-TAY-shun)

Emergency treatment provided by persons trained in CPR and given to patients when their respirations and heart stop. CPR provides oxygen to the brain, heart, and other vital organs until medical treatment can restore a normal heart and pulmonary function.

Heimlich maneuver (HYME-lik)

Technique for removing a foreign body from the trachea or pharynx by exerting diaphragmatic pressure. Named for Harry Heimlich, a U.S. thoracic surgeon.

Pharmacology

CLASSIFICATION	ACTION	GENERIC AND BRAND NAMES
antibiotic (an-tih-bye-AW-tic)	Kills bacteria causing respiratory infections.	ampicillin; amoxicillin, Amoxil; ciprofloxacin, Cipro
antihistamine (an-tih-HIST-ah-meen)	Blocks the effects of histamine that has been released by the body during an allergy attack.	fexofenadine, Allegra; loratadine, Claritan; diphenhydramine, Benadryl
antitussive (an-tih-TUSS-ive)	Relieves urge to cough.	hydrocodon, Hycodan; dextromethorphan, Vicks Formula 44
bronchodilator (BRONG-koh-dye-late-or)	Relaxes muscle spasms in bronchial tubes. Used to treat asthma.	albuterol, Proventil, Ventolin; salmetrol, Serevent; theophyllin, Theo-Dur
corticosteroids (core-tih-koh-STAIR-ryods)	Reduces inflammation and swelling in the respiratory tract.	fluticasone, Flonase; mometasone, Nasonex; triamcinolone, Azmacort
decongestant (dee-kon-JES-tant)	Reduces stuffiness and congestion throughout the respiratory system.	oxymetazoline, Afrin, Dristan, Sinex; pseudoephedrine, Drixoral, Sudafed
expectorant (ek-SPEK-toh-rant)	Improves the ability to cough up mucus from the respiratory tract.	guaifenesin, Robitussin, Mucinex
mucolytic (myoo-koh-LIT-ik)	Liquefies mucus so it is easier to cough and clear it from the respiratory tract.	N-acetyl-cysteine, Mucomyst

Abbreviations

ABGs	arterial blood gases	**O$_2$**	oxygen
ARDS	adult (or acute) respiratory distress syndrome	**PCP**	*Pneumocystis carinii* pneumonia
Bronch	bronchoscopy	**PFT**	pulmonary function test
CO$_2$	carbon dioxide	**PPD**	purified protein derivative
COPD	chronic obstructive pulmonary disease	**R**	respiration
CPR	cardiopulmonary resuscitation	**RA**	room air
C&S	culture and sensitivity	**RDS**	respiratory distress syndrome
CTA	clear to auscultation	**RLL**	right lower lobe
CXR	chest x-ray	**RML**	right middle lobe
DOE	dyspnea on exertion	**RRT**	registered respiratory therapist
DPT	diphtheria, pertussis, tetanus injection	**RV**	reserve volume
ENT	ear, nose, and throat	**RUL**	right upper lobe
ERV	expiratory reserve volume	**SARS**	severe acute respiratory syndrome
FRC	functional residual capacity	**SIDS**	sudden infant death syndrome
HMD	hyaline membrane disease	**SOB**	shortness of breath
IC	inspiratory capacity	**TB**	tuberculosis
IPPB	intermittent positive pressure breathing	**TLC**	total lung capacity
IRDS	infant respiratory distress syndrome	**TPR**	temperature, pulse, and respiration
IRV	inspiratory reserve volume	**TV**	tidal volume
LLL	left lower lobe	**URI**	upper respiratory infection
LUL	left upper lobe	**VC**	vital capacity
MDI	metered dose inhaler		

Chapter Review

Terminology Checklist

Below are all Anatomy and Physiology key terms, Word Building, Vocabulary, Pathology, Diagnostic, Therapeutic, and Pharmacology terms presented in this chapter. Use this list as a study tool by placing a check in the box in front of each term as you master its meaning.

- acapnia
- adenoids
- adult respiratory distress syndrome
- aerosol therapy
- alveoli
- anosmia
- anoxia
- anthracosis
- antibiotic
- antihistamine
- antitussive
- apex
- aphonia
- apnea
- arterial blood gases
- asbestosis
- asphyxia
- aspiration
- asthma
- atelectasis
- auditory tube
- base
- bradypnea
- bronchial
- bronchial tube
- bronchiectasis
- bronchioles
- bronchitis
- bronchodilator
- bronchogenic
- bronchogenic carcinoma
- bronchogram
- bronchography
- bronchoplasty
- bronchoscope
- bronchoscopy
- bronchospasm

- bronchus
- carbon dioxide
- cardiopulmonary resuscitation
- chest x-ray
- Cheyne–Stokes respiration
- chronic obstructive pulmonary disease
- cilia
- clubbing
- corticosteroids
- croup
- cyanosis
- cystic fibrosis
- decongestant
- diaphragm
- diaphragmatic
- diphtheria
- dysphonia
- dyspnea
- emphysema
- empyema
- endotracheal
- endotracheal intubation
- epiglottis
- epistaxis
- eupnea
- eustachian tube
- exhalation
- expectorant
- expiratory reserve volume
- external respiration
- functional residual capacity
- glottis
- Heimlich maneuver
- hemoptysis
- hemothorax
- hilum
- histoplasmosis
- hypercapnia

- hyperpnea
- hyperventilation
- hypopnea
- hypoventilation
- hypoxemia
- hypoxia
- infant respiratory distress syndrome
- influenza
- inhalation
- inspiratory capacity
- inspiratory reserve volume
- intercostal muscles
- intermittent positive pressure breathing
- internal medicine
- internal respiration
- laryngeal
- laryngectomy
- laryngitis
- laryngopharynx
- laryngoplasty
- laryngoplegia
- laryngoscope
- laryngoscopy
- larynx
- Legionnaire's disease
- lingual tonsils
- lobectomy
- lobes
- lungs
- mediastinum
- mucolytic
- mucous membrane
- mucus
- *Mycoplasma* pneumonia
- nares
- nasal cannula
- nasal cavity

- nasal septum
- nasopharyngitis
- nasopharynx
- oropharynx
- orthopnea
- otorhinolaryngology
- oximeter
- oximetry
- oxygen
- palate
- palatine tonsils
- pansinusitis
- paranasal sinuses
- parietal pleura
- patent
- percussion
- pertussis
- pharyngeal
- pharyngeal tonsils
- pharyngitis
- pharynx
- phlegm
- pleura
- pleural cavity
- pleural effusion
- pleural rub
- pleurectomy
- pleurisy
- pleurocentesis
- pleurodynia
- pneumoconiosis
- *Pneumocystis carinii* pneumonia
- pneumonia
- pneumothorax
- polysomnography
- postural drainage
- pulmonary
- pulmonary angiography
- pulmonary capillaries
- pulmonary edema
- pulmonary embolism
- pulmonary fibrosis
- pulmonary function test
- pulmonologist
- pulmonology
- pyothorax
- rales
- residual volume
- respiratory membrane
- respiratory therapist
- respiratory therapy
- rhinitis
- rhinomycosis
- rhinoplasty
- rhinorrhagia
- rhinorrhea
- rhonchi
- serous fluid
- severe acute respiratory syndrome
- shortness of breath
- silicosis
- sleep apnea
- spirometer
- spirometry
- sputum
- sputum culture and sensitivity
- sputum cytology
- stridor
- sudden infant death syndrome
- supplemental oxygen therapy
- sweat test
- tachypnea
- thoracalgia
- thoracentesis
- thoracic
- thoracic surgery
- thoracostomy
- thoracotomy
- thyroid cartilage
- tidal volume
- total lung capacity
- trachea
- tracheostenosis
- tracheostomy
- tracheotomy
- tuberculin skin tests
- tuberculosis
- ventilation
- ventilation-perfusion scan
- ventilator
- visceral pleura
- vital capacity
- vital signs
- vocal cords

Practice Exercises

A. Complete the following statements.

1. The primary function of the respiratory system is _____.

2. The movement of air in and out of the lungs is called _____.

3. Define external respiration: _____.

4. Define internal respiration: _____.

5. The organs of the respiratory system are _____, _____, _____, _____, _____, and _____.

6. The passageway for food, liquids, and air is the _____.

7. The _____ helps to keep food out of the respiratory tract.

8. The function of the cilia in the nose is to _____.

9. The muscle that divides the thoracic cavity from the abdominal cavity is the _____.

10. The respiratory rate for an adult is _____ to _____ respirations per minute.

11. The respiratory rate for a newborn is _____ to _____ respirations per minute.

12. The right lung has _____ lobes; the left lung has _____ lobes.

13. The air sacs at the ends of the bronchial tree are called _____.

14. The term for the double membrane around the lungs is _____.

15. The nasal cavity is separated from the mouth by the _____.

16. The small branches of the bronchi are the _____.

B. State the terms described using the combining forms provided.

The combining form *rhin/o* refers to the nose. Use it to write a term that means:

1. inflammation of the nose _____

2. rapid flow from the nose _____

3. discharge from the nose _____

4. surgical repair of the nose _____

The combining form *laryng/o* refers to the larynx or voice box. Use it to write a term that means:

5. inflammation of the larynx _____

6. spasm of the larynx _____

7. visual examination of the larynx _____

8. pertaining to the larynx _____

9. incision of the larynx _____

10. removal of the larynx _____

11. surgical repair of the larynx _____

12. paralysis of the larynx _____

The combining form *bronch/o* refers to the bronchus. Use it to write a term that means:

13. pertaining to bronchus _____

14. inflammation of the bronchus _____

15. visually examine the interior of the bronchus _____

16. produced by bronchus _____

17. spasm of the bronchus _____

The combining form *thorac/o* refers to the chest. Use it to write a term that means:

18. surgical repair of the chest _____

19. incision into the chest _____

20. chest pain _____

21. pertaining to chest _____

The combining form *trache/o* refers to the trachea. Use it to write a term that means:

22. cutting into the trachea _____

23. surgical repair of the trachea _____

24. narrowing of the trachea _____

25. pertaining to inside trachea _____

26. inflammation of the trachea _____

27. forming an artificial opening into the trachea _____

C. Define the following combining forms and use them to form respiratory terms.

	Definition	Respiratory Term
1. trache/o	_____	_____
2. laryng/o	_____	_____
3. bronch/o	_____	_____
4. spir/o	_____	_____
5. pneum/o	_____	_____
6. rhin/o	_____	_____
7. coni/o	_____	_____
8. pleur/o	_____	_____
9. epiglott/o	_____	_____
10. alveol/o	_____	_____
11. pulmon/o	_____	_____
12. ox/o	_____	_____

13. sinus/o _____   _____

14. lob/o _____   _____

15. nas/o _____   _____

D. Define each suffix and use it to form a term from the respiratory system.

	Meaning	Respiratory Term

1. -ectasis _____   _____

2. -capnia _____   _____

3. -phonia _____   _____

4. -thorax _____   _____

5. -pnea _____   _____

6. -ptysis _____   _____

7. -osmia _____   _____

E. The suffix *-pnea* means breathing. Use this suffix to write a medical term that means:

1. normal breathing _____

2. difficult or labored breathing _____

3. rapid breathing _____

4. can breathe only in an upright position _____

5. lack of breathing _____

F. Define the following terms.

1. total lung capacity _____

2. tidal volume _____

3. residual volume _____

G. Write the medical term for each definition.

1. the process of breathing in _____

2. spitting up of blood _____

3. blood clot in the pulmonary artery _____

4. inflammation of a sinus _____

5. sore throat _____

6. air in the pleural cavity _____

7. whooping cough _____

8. incision into the pleura _____

9. pain in the pleural region _____

10. common cold _____

H. Write the abbreviations for the following terms.

1. upper respiratory infection_____

2. pulmonary function test _____

3. left lower lobe _____

4. oxygen _____

5. carbon dioxide _____

6. intermittent positive pressure breathing _____

7. chronic obstructive pulmonary disease _____

8. bronchoscopy _____

9. total lung capacity _____

10. tuberculosis _____

11. infant respiratory distress syndrome _____

I. Identify the following abbreviations.

1. CXR _____

2. TV _____

3. TPR _____

4. ABGs _____

5. DOE _____

6. RUL _____

7. SIDS _____

8. TLC _____

9. ARDS _____

10. MDI _____

11. CTA _____

12. SARS _____

J. Match each term to its definition.

1. _____ inhaling environmental particles   a. polysomnography

2. _____ whooping cough   b. Tine test

3. _____ may result in collapsed lung   c. oximetry

4. _____ test to identify sleep apnea   d. epistaxis

5. _____ respiratory tract mucus   e. pneumoconiosis

6. _____ sweat test   f. emphysema

7. _____ measures oxygen levels in blood   g. walking pneumonia

8. _____ *Mycoplasma* pneumonia   h. pneumothorax

9. _____ disease with overexpanded air sacs   i. empyema

10. _____ tuberculin test   j. phlegm

11. _____ nose bleed   k. pertussis

12. _____ pus in the pleural space   l. test for cystic fibrosis

K. Use the following terms in the sentences below.

anthracosis   thoracentesis   supplemental oxygen   sputum cytology

respirator   hyperventilation   cardiopulmonary resuscitation   ventilation-perfusion scan

patent   rhonchi

1. When the patient's breathing and heart stopped, the paramedics began _____.

2. The physician performed a _____ to remove fluid from the chest.

3. A _____ is also called a ventilator.

4. The patient received _____ through a nasal cannula.

5. An endotracheal intubation was performed to establish a _____ airway.

6. A _____ is a particularly useful test to identify a pulmonary embolus.

7. The result of the _____ was negative for cancer.

8. _____ involves tachypnea and hyperpnea.

9. _____ are wheezing lung sounds.

10. Miners are at risk of developing _____.

L. Fill in the classification for each drug description, then match the brand name.

Drug Description	Classification	Brand Name
1. _____ Reduces stuffiness and congestion	_____	a. Hycodan
2. _____ Relieves the urge to cough	_____	b. Flonase
3. _____ Kills bacteria	_____	c. Cipro
4. _____ Improves ability to cough up mucus	_____	d. Ventolin
5. _____ Liquefies mucus	_____	e. Allegra
6. _____ Relaxes bronchial muscle spasms	_____	f. Afrin
7. _____ Blocks allergy attack	_____	g. Robitussin
8. _____ Reduces inflammation and swelling	_____	h. Mucomyst

Medical Record Analysis

Below is an item from a patient's medical record. Read it carefully, make sure you understand all the medical terms used, and then answer the questions that follow.

Pulmonology Consultation Report

Reason for Consultation: Evaluation of increasingly severe asthma.

History of Present Illness: Patient is a 10-year-old male who first presented to the Emergency Room with dyspnea, coughing, and wheezing at 7 years of age. Paroxysmal attacks are increasing in frequency, and there do not appear to be any precipitating factors such as exercise. No other family members are asthmatics.

Results of Physical Examination: Patient is currently in the ER with a paroxysmal attack with marked dyspnea, cyanosis around the lips, prolonged expiration, and a hacking cough producing thick, nonpurulent phlegm. Thoracic auscultation with stethoscope revealed rhonchi throughout bilateral lung fields. Chest x-ray shows poor pulmonary expansion, with hypoxemia indicated by ABG. A STAT pulmonary function test reveals moderately severe airway obstruction during expiration. This patient responded to oxygen therapy and IV Alupent and steroids, and he is beginning to cough less and breathe with less effort.

Assessment: Acute asthma attack with severe airway obstruction. There is no evidence of pulmonary infection. In view of increasing severity and frequency of attacks, all his medications should be reevaluated for effectiveness and all attempts to identify precipitating factors should be made.

Recommendations: Patient is to continue to use Alupent for relief of bronchospasms and steroids to reduce general inflammation. Instructions for taking medications and controlling severity of asthma attacks were carefully reviewed with the patient and his family. A referral to an allergist was made to evaluate this young man for presence of environmental allergies.

Critical Thinking Questions

1. What does the medical term *paroxysmal* mean? _____
_____

2. What do the following abbreviations stand for?
   a. IV _____
   b. STAT _____
   c. ABG _____

3. The patient was discharged and sent home with two medications. Explain in your own words the purpose of each of these medications. _____
_____

4. What important information regarding this young man's asthma is unknown to the physician? What does this consulting physician recommend to address this problem? _____
_____

5. Describe the characteristics related to this patient's cough in your own words. _____
_____

6. Which of the following is not one of the symptoms seen in the emergency room?
   a. crackling lung sounds
   b. bluish skin
   c. difficulty breathing
   d. extended breathing out time

Chart Note Transcription

The chart note below contains eleven phrases that can be reworded with a medical term that you learned in this chapter. Each phrase is identified with an underline. Determine the medical term and write your answers in the space provided.

Current Complaint: A 43-year-old female was brought to the Emergency Room by her family. She complained of <u>painful and labored breathing</u>, ❶ <u>rapid breathing</u>, ❷ and fever. Symptoms began three days ago, but have become much worse during the past 12 hours.

Past History: Patient is a mother of three and a business executive. She has had no surgeries or previous serious illnesses.

Signs and Symptoms: Temperature is 103°F, respiratory rate is 20 breaths/minute, blood pressure is 165/98, and heart rate is 90 bpm. <u>A blood test to measure the levels of oxygen in the blood</u> ❸ indicates a marked <u>low level of oxygen in the blood</u>. ❹ The <u>process of listening to body sounds</u> ❺ of the lungs revealed <u>abnormal crackling sounds</u> ❻ over the left lower chest. She is producing large amounts of <u>pus-filled</u> ❼ <u>mucus coughed up from the respiratory tract</u> ❽ and a <u>chest x-ray</u> ❾ shows a large cloudy patch in the lower lobe of the left lung.

Diagnosis: Left lower lobe <u>inflammatory condition of the lungs caused by bacterial infection</u>. ❿

Treatment: Patient was started on intravenous antibiotics. She also required a <u>tube placed through the mouth to create an airway</u> ⓫ for 3 days.

❶ _____

❷ _____

❸ _____

❹ _____

❺ _____

❻ _____

❼ _____

❽ _____

❾ _____

❿ _____

⓫ _____

Labeling Exercise

A. System Review
Write the labels for this figure on the numbered lines provided.

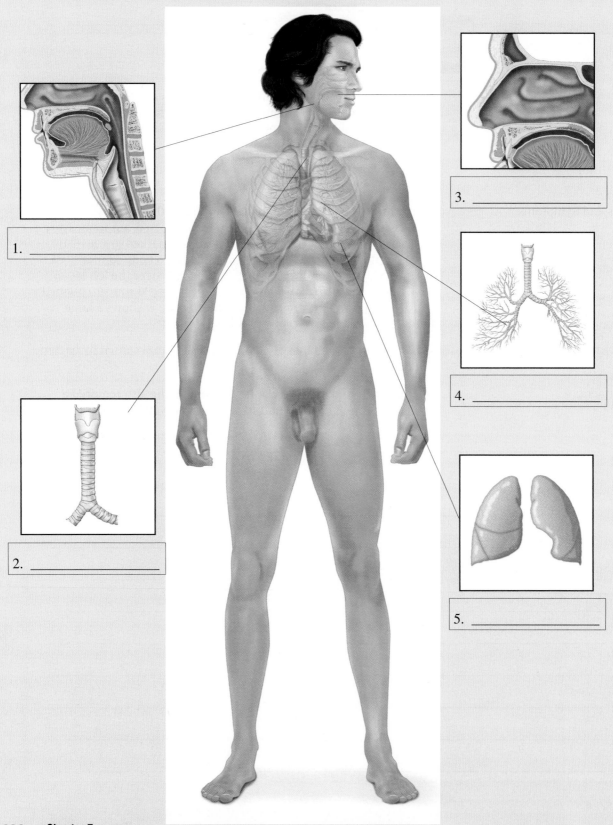

1. _____

2. _____

3. _____

4. _____

5. _____

B. Anatomy Challenge

1. Write the labels for this figure on the numbered lines provided.

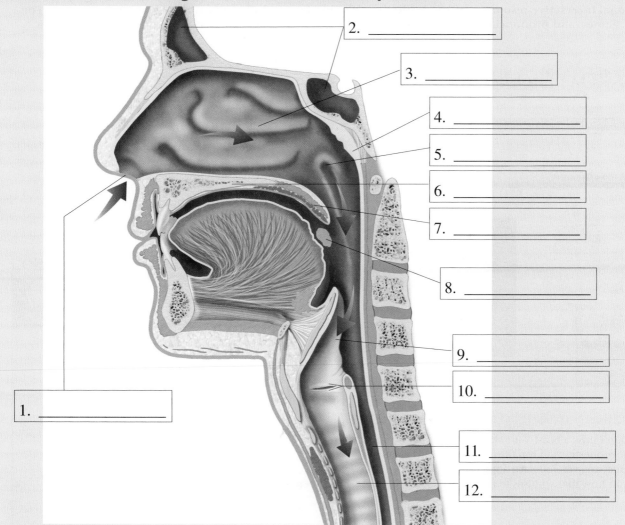

2. _____

3. _____

4. _____

5. _____

6. _____

7. _____

8. _____

9. _____

10. _____

11. _____

12. _____

1. _____

2. Write the labels for this figure on the numbered lines provided.

1. _____

2. _____

3. _____

4. _____

5. _____

6. _____

7. _____

8. _____

Multimedia Preview

Additional interactive resources and activities for this chapter can be found on the Companion Website. For videos, games, and pronunciations, please access the accompanying DVD-ROM that comes with this book.

DVD-ROM Highlights

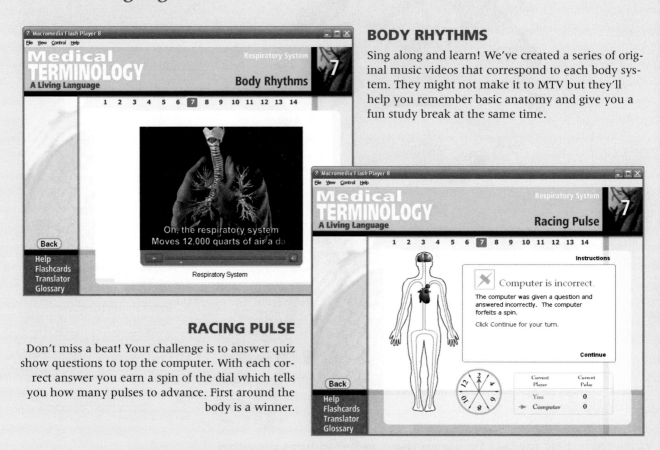

BODY RHYTHMS

Sing along and learn! We've created a series of original music videos that correspond to each body system. They might not make it to MTV but they'll help you remember basic anatomy and give you a fun study break at the same time.

RACING PULSE

Don't miss a beat! Your challenge is to answer quiz show questions to top the computer. With each correct answer you earn a spin of the dial which tells you how many pulses to advance. First around the body is a winner.

Website Highlights—www.prenhall.com/fremgen

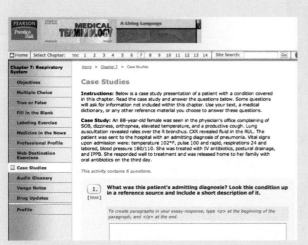

CASE STUDY

Put your understanding of medical terms to the test within a real-world scenario. Here you'll be presented with a clinical case followed by a series of questions that quiz your grasp of the situation.

8 Digestive System

Learning Objectives

Upon completion of this chapter, you will be able to:

- Identify and define the combining forms and suffixes introduced in this chapter.
- Correctly spell and pronounce medical terms and major anatomical structures relating to the digestive system.
- Locate and describe the major organs of the digestive system and their functions.
- Describe the function of the accessory organs of the digestive system.
- Identify the shape and function of each type of tooth.
- Build and define digestive system medical terms from word parts.
- Identify and define digestive system vocabulary terms.
- Identify and define selected digestive system pathology terms.
- Identify and define selected digestive system diagnostic procedures.
- Identify and define selected digestive system therapeutic procedures.
- Identify and define selected medications relating to the digestive system.
- Define selected abbreviations associated with the digestive system.

Digestive System at a Glance

Function

The digestive system begins breaking down food through mechanical and chemical digestion. After being digested, nutrient molecules are absorbed into the body and enter the blood stream. Any food not digested or absorbed is eliminated as solid waste.

Organs

colon
esophagus
gallbladder (GB)
liver
oral cavity
pancreas
pharynx
salivary glands
small intestine
stomach

Combining Forms

an/o	anus	gloss/o	tongue
append/o	appendix	hepat/o	liver
appendic/o	appendix	ile/o	ileum
bar/o	weight	jejun/o	jejunum
bucc/o	cheek	labi/o	lip
cec/o	cecum	lapar/o	abdomen
chol/e	bile, gall	lingu/o	tongue
cholangi/o	bile duct	lith/o	stone
cholecyst/o	gallbladder	odont/o	tooth
choledoch/o	common bile duct	or/o	mouth
col/o	colon	palat/o	palate
colon/o	colon	pancreat/o	pancreas
dent/o	tooth	pharyng/o	throat, pharynx
duoden/o	duodenum	proct/o	anus and rectum
enter/o	small intestine	pylor/o	pylorus
esophag/o	esophagus	rect/o	rectum
gastr/o	stomach	sialaden/o	salivary gland
gingiv/o	gums	sigmoid/o	sigmoid colon

Suffixes

-emesis	vomit	-phagia	eat, swallow
-lithiasis	condition of stones	-prandial	pertaining to a meal
-orexia	appetite	-tripsy	surgical crushing
-pepsia	digestion		

Digestive System Illustrated

salivary glands, p. 250

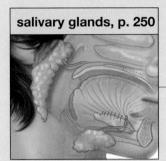

Produces saliva

oral cavity, p. 244

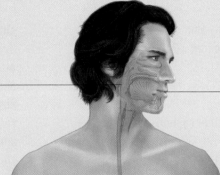

Ingests, chews, and swallows food

esophagus, p. 247

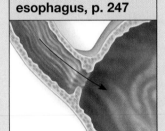

Transports food to the stomach

stomach, p. 248

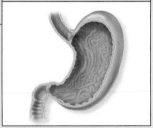

Secretes acid and mixes food to start digestion

pancreas, p. 251

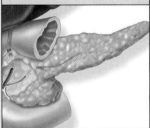

Secretes digestive enzymes and buffers

liver & gallbladder, pp. 250, 251

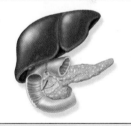

Produces and stores bile

small intestine, p. 248

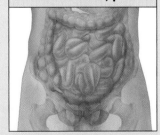

Digests and absorbs nutrients

colon, p. 249

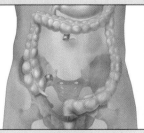

Reabsorbs water and stores feces

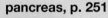
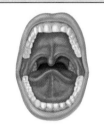

Anatomy and Physiology of the Digestive System

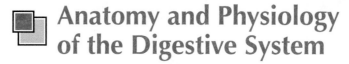

accessory organs

alimentary canal (al-ih-MEN-tar-ree)

colon (COH-lon)

esophagus (eh-SOFF-ah-gus)

gallbladder

gastrointestinal system
(gas-troh-in-TESS-tih-nal)

gastrointestinal tract

gut

liver

oral cavity

pancreas (PAN-kree-ass)

pharynx (FAIR-inks)

salivary glands (SAL-ih-vair-ee)

small intestine

stomach (STUM-ak)

Med Term Tip

The term *alimentary* comes from the Latin term *alimentum* meaning "nourishment."

The digestive system, also known as the **gastrointestinal (GI) system,** includes approximately 30 feet of a continuous muscular tube, called the **gut, alimentary canal,** or **gastrointestinal tract** that stretches between the mouth and the anus. Most of the organs in this system are actually different sections of this tube. In order, beginning at the mouth and continuing to the anus, these organs are the **oral cavity, pharynx, esophagus, stomach, small intestine,** and **colon.** The **accessory organs** of digestion are organs that participate in the digestion process, but are not part of the continuous alimentary canal. These organs, which are connected to the gut by a duct, are the **liver, pancreas, gallbladder,** and **salivary glands.**

The digestive system has three main functions: digesting food, absorbing nutrients, and eliminating waste. Digestion includes the physical and chemical breakdown of large food particles into simple nutrient molecules like glucose, triglycerides, and amino acids. These simple nutrient molecules are absorbed from the intestines and circulated throughout the body by the cardiovascular system. They are used for growth and repair of organs and tissues. Any food that cannot be digested or absorbed by the body is eliminated from the gastrointestinal system as a solid waste.

Oral Cavity

cheeks

gingiva (JIN-jih-veh)

gums

lips

palate (PAL-at)

saliva (suh-LYE-vah)

taste buds

teeth

tongue

uvula (YU-vyu-lah)

Digestion begins when food enters the mouth and is mechanically broken up by the chewing movements of the **teeth.** The muscular **tongue** moves the food within the mouth and mixes it with **saliva** (see Figure 8.1 ■). Saliva contains digestive enzymes to break down carbohydrates and slippery lubricants to make food easier to swallow. **Taste buds,** found on the surface of the tongue, can distinguish the bitter, sweet, sour, and salty flavors in our food. The roof of the oral cavity is known as the **palate** and is subdivided into the hard palate, the bony anterior portion, and the soft palate, the flexible posterior portion. Hanging down from the posterior edge of the soft palate is the **uvula.** The uvula serves two important functions. First, it has a role in speech production. Second, it is the location of the gag reflex. This reflex is stimulated when food enters the throat without swallowing (for example, laughing with food in your mouth). It is important because swallowing also results in the epiglottis covering the larynx to prevent food from entering the lungs (see Figure 8.2 ■). The **cheeks** form the lateral walls of this cavity and the **lips** are the anterior opening. The entire oral cavity is lined

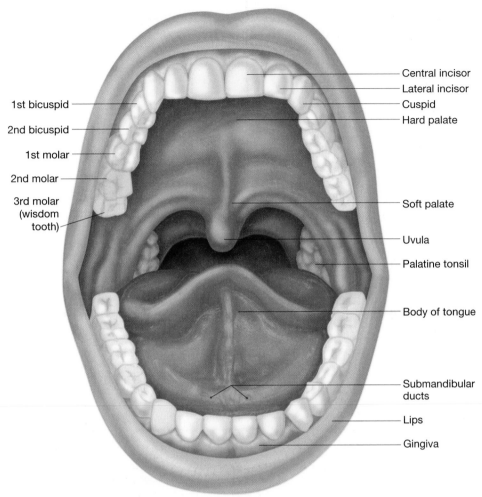

■ **Figure 8.1** Anatomy of structures of the oral cavity.

Central incisor

Lateral incisor

1st bicuspid

Cuspid

2nd bicuspid

Hard palate

1st molar

2nd molar

3rd molar (wisdom tooth)

Soft palate

Uvula

Palatine tonsil

Body of tongue

Submandibular ducts

Lips

Gingiva

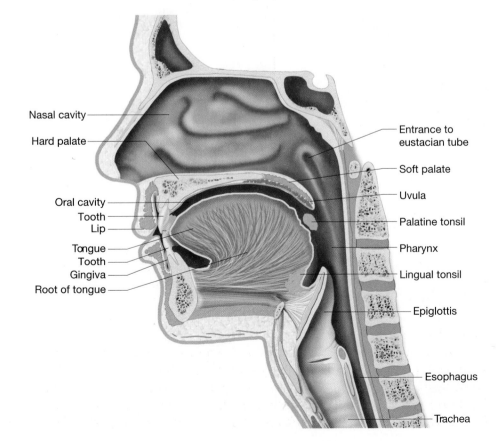

■ **Figure 8.2** Sagittal view of the head and neck, illustrating structures of the oral cavity, and pharynx, and esophagus.

Nasal cavity

Hard palate

Entrance to eustacian tube

Soft palate

Uvula

Oral cavity

Tooth

Lip

Palatine tonsil

Tongue

Pharynx

Tooth

Gingiva

Lingual tonsil

Root of tongue

Epiglottis

Esophagus

Trachea

with mucous membrane. A portion of this mucous membrane forms the **gums**, or **gingiva**, which combine with connective tissue to cover the jaw bone and seal off the teeth in their bony sockets.

Teeth

bicuspids (bye-CUSS-pids)
canines (KAY-nines)
cementum (see-MEN-tum)
crown
cuspids (CUSS-pids)
deciduous teeth (dee-SID-yoo-us)
dentin (DEN-tin)
enamel

incisors (in-SIGH-zors)
molars (MOH-lars)
periodontal ligaments (pair-ee-on-DON-tal)
permanent teeth
premolars (pree-MOH-lars)
pulp cavity
root
root canal

Teeth are an important part of the first stage of digestion. The teeth in the front of the mouth bite, tear, or cut food into small pieces. These cutting teeth include the **incisors** and the **cuspids** or **canines** (see Figure 8.3 ■). The remaining posterior teeth grind and crush food into even finer pieces. These grinding teeth include the **bicuspids**, or **premolars**, and the **molars**. A tooth can be subdivided into the **crown** and the **root**. The crown is that part of the tooth visible above the gum line; the

■ **Figure 8.3** A) The name and shape of the adult teeth. These teeth represent those found in the right side of the mouth. Those of the left side would be a mirror image. The incisors and cuspids are cutting teeth. The bicuspids and molars are grinding teeth. B) Color enhanced x-ray of all teeth. Note the four wisdom teeth (3rd molars) that have not erupted. *(Science Photo Library/Photo Researchers, Inc.)*

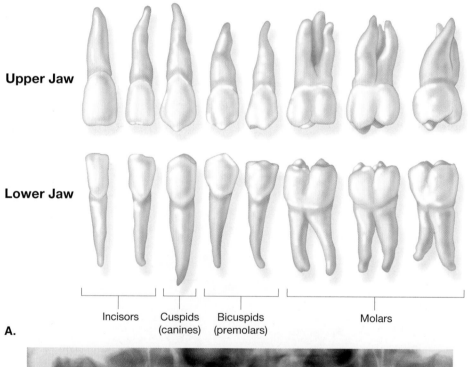

Upper Jaw

Lower Jaw

Incisors   Cuspids (canines)   Bicuspids (premolars)   Molars

A.

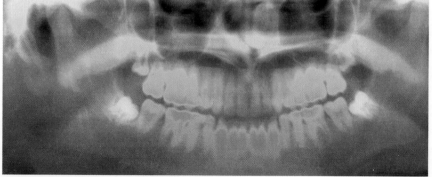

B.

root is below the gum line. The root is anchored in the bony socket of the jaw by **cementum** and tiny **periodontal ligaments**. The crown of the tooth is covered by a layer of **enamel**, the hardest substance in the body. Under the enamel layer is **dentin**, the substance that makes up the main bulk of the tooth. The hollow interior of a tooth is called the **pulp cavity** in the crown and the **root canal** in the root. These cavities contain soft tissue made up of blood vessels, nerves, and lymph vessels (see Figure 8.4 ▉).

Humans have two sets of teeth. The first set, often referred to as baby teeth, are **deciduous teeth.** There are 20 teeth in this set that erupt through the gums between the ages of 6 and 28 months. At approximately 6 years of age, these teeth begin to fall out and are replaced by the 32 **permanent teeth**. This replacement process continues until about 18 to 20 years of age.

Pharynx

epiglottis (ep-ih-GLOT-iss)   **oropharynx**
laryngopharynx

When food is swallowed, it enters the **oropharynx** and then the **laryngopharynx** (see Figure 8.2). Remember from your study of the respiratory system in Chapter 7 that air is also traveling through these portions of the pharynx. The **epiglottis** is a cartilaginous flap that folds down to cover the larynx and trachea so that food is prevented from entering the respiratory tract and instead continues into the esophagus.

Esophagus

peristalsis (pair-ih-STALL-sis)

The esophagus is a muscular tube of about 10 inches long in adults. Food entering the esophagus is carried through the thoracic cavity and diaphragm and into the abdominal cavity where it enters the stomach (see Figure 8.5 ▉). Food is

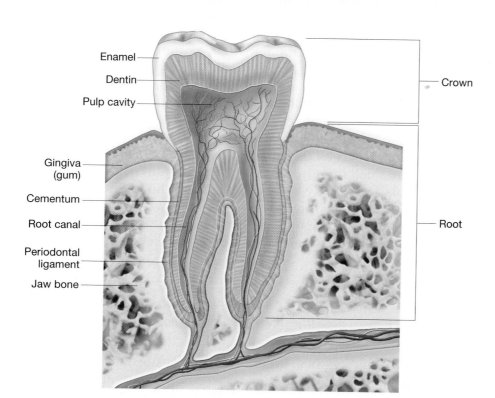

Enamel
Dentin
Pulp cavity
Gingiva (gum)
Cementum
Root canal
Periodontal ligament
Jaw bone
Crown
Root

▉ **Figure 8.4** An adult tooth, longitudinal view showing internal structures of the crown and root.

Figure 8.5 The stomach, longitudinal view showing regions and internal structures.

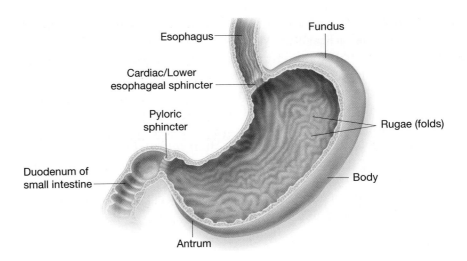

Esophagus

Fundus

Cardiac/Lower esophageal sphincter

Pyloric sphincter

Rugae (folds)

Duodenum of small intestine

Body

Antrum

Med Term Tip

It takes about 10 seconds for swallowed food to reach the stomach.

propelled along the esophagus by wavelike muscular contractions called **peristalsis**. In fact, peristalsis works to push food through the entire gastrointestinal tract.

Stomach

antrum (AN-trum)

body

cardiac sphincter

chyme (KIGHM)

fundus (FUN-dus)

hydrochloric acid

lower esophageal sphincter
(eh-soff-ah-JEE-al SFINGK-ter)

pyloric sphincter (pigh-LOR-ik SFINGK-ter)

rugae (ROO-gay)

sphincters (SFINGK-ters)

The stomach, a J-shaped muscular organ that acts as a bag or sac to collect and churn food with digestive juices, is composed of three parts: the **fundus** or upper region, the **body** or main portion, and the **antrum** or lower region (see Figure 8.5). The folds in the lining of the stomach are called **rugae**. When the stomach fills with food, the rugae stretch out and disappear. **Hydrochloric acid** (HCl) is secreted by glands in the mucous membrane lining of the stomach. Food mixes with hydrochloric acid and other gastric juices to form a liquid mixture called **chyme**, which then passes through the remaining portion of the digestive system.

Entry into and exit from the stomach is controlled by muscular valves called **sphincters**. These valves open and close to ensure that food can only move forward down the gut tube. The **cardiac sphincter**, named for its proximity to the heart, is located between the esophagus and the fundus. Also called the **lower esophageal sphincter** (LES), it keeps food from flowing backward into the esophagus.

The antrum tapers off into the **pyloric sphincter**, which regulates the passage of food into the small intestine. Only a small amount of the chyme is allowed to enter the small intestine with each opening of the sphincter for two important reasons. First, the small intestine is much narrower than the stomach and cannot hold as much as the stomach can. Second, the chyme is highly acidic and must be thoroughly neutralized as it leaves the stomach.

Med Term Tip

It is easier to remember the function of the pyloric sphincter when you note that *pylor/o* means "gate-keeper." This gatekeeper controls the forward movement of food. Sphincters are rings of muscle that can be opened and closed to control entry and exit from hollow organs like the stomach, colon, and bladder.

Small Intestine

duodenum
(doo-oh-DEE-num / doo-OD-eh-num)

ileocecal valve (ill-ee-oh-SEE-kal)

ileum (ILL-ee-um)

jejunum (jee-JOO-num)

The small intestine, or small bowel, is the major site of digestion and absorption of nutrients from food. It is located between the pyloric sphincter and the colon (see Figure 8.6 ■). Because the small intestine is concerned with absorption of food products, an abnormality in this organ can cause malnutrition. The small intestine, with an average length of 20 feet, is the longest portion of the alimentary canal and has three sections: the **duodenum**, the **jejunum**, and the **ileum**.

- The duodenum, which extends from the pyloric sphincter to the jejunum, is about 10 to 12 inches long. Digestion is completed in the duodenum after the liquid chyme from the stomach is mixed with digestive juices from the pancreas and gallbladder.
- The jejunum, or middle portion, extends from the duodenum to the ileum and is about 8 feet long.
- The ileum is the last portion of the small intestine and extends from the jejunum to the colon. At 12 feet in length, it is the longest portion of the small intestine. The ileum connects to the colon with a sphincter called the **ileocecal valve**.

Colon

anal sphincter (AY-nal SFINGK-ter)	**feces** (FEE-seez)
anus (AY-nus)	**rectum** (REK-tum)
ascending colon	**sigmoid colon** (SIG-moyd)
cecum (SEE-kum)	**transverse colon**
defecation	**vermiform appendix**
descending colon	(VER-mih-form ah-PEN-diks)

Fluid that remains after the complete digestion and absorption of nutrients in the small intestine enters the colon or large intestine (see Figure 8.7 ■). Most of this fluid is water that is reabsorbed into the body. The material that remains after absorption is solid waste called **feces** (or stool). This is the product evacuated in bowel movements (BM).

The colon is approximately 5 feet long and extends from the ileocecal valve of the small intestine to the **anus**. The **cecum** is a pouch or saclike area in the first two to three inches at the beginning of the colon. The **vermiform appendix** is a small worm-shaped outgrowth at the end of the cecum. The remaining colon consists of the **ascending colon**, **transverse colon**, **descending colon**, and **sigmoid colon**. The ascend-

---

Med Term Tip

Word watch—Be careful not to confuse the word root *ile/o* meaning "ileum," a portion of the small intestines, and *ili/o* meaning "ilium," a pelvic bone.

Med Term Tip

We can survive without a portion of the small intestine. For example, in cases of cancer, much of the small intestine and/or colon may have to be removed. The surgeon then creates an opening between the remaining intestine and the abdominal wall. The combining form for the section of intestine connected to the abdominal wall and the suffix *-ostomy* are used to describe this procedure. For example, if a person has a *jejunostomy*, the jejunum is connected to the abdominal wall and the ileum (and remainder of the gut tube) has been removed.

Med Term Tip

The term *colon* refers to the large intestine. However, you should be aware that many people use it incorrectly as a general term referring to the entire intestinal system, both small and large intestines.

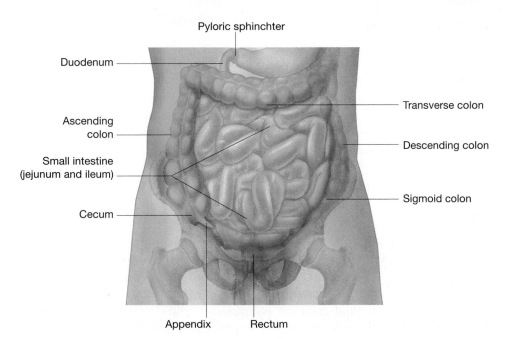

■ **Figure 8.6** The small intestine. Anterior view of the abdominopelvic cavity illustrating how the three sections of small intestine—duodenum, jejunum, ileum—begin at the pyloric sphincter and end at the colon, but are not arranged in a orderly fashion.

Pyloric sphinchter

Duodenum

Ascending colon

Small intestine (jejunum and ileum)

Cecum

Transverse colon

Descending colon

Sigmoid colon

Appendix   Rectum

■ **Figure 8.7** The regions
of the colon beginning with
the cecum and ending at the
anus.

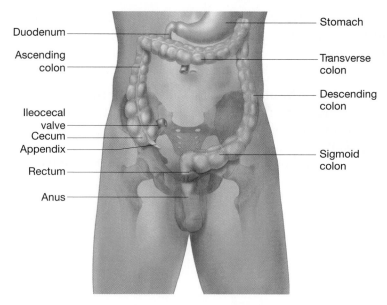

ing colon on the right side extends from the cecum to the lower border of the
liver. The transverse colon begins where the ascending colon leaves off and
moves horizontally across the upper abdomen toward the spleen. The descending colon then travels down the left side of the body to where the sigmoid colon
begins. The sigmoid colon curves in an S-shape back to the midline of the body
and ends at the **rectum**. The rectum, where feces is stored, leads into the anus,
which contains the **anal sphincter**. This sphincter consists of rings of voluntary and
involuntary muscles to control the evacuation of feces or **defecation**.

Accessory Organs of the Digestive System

As described earlier, the accessory organs of the digestive system are the salivary glands, the liver, the pancreas, and the gallbladder. In general, these organs
function by producing much of the digestive fluids and enzymes necessary for
the chemical breakdown of food. Each is attached to the gut tube by a duct.

Salivary Glands

amylase (AM-ill-ace)

bolus

parotid glands (pah-ROT-id)

sublingual glands (sub-LING-gwal)

submandibular glands (sub-man-DIB-yoo-lar)

Salivary glands in the oral cavity produce saliva. This very watery and slick fluid
allows food to be swallowed with less danger of choking. Saliva mixed with food
in the mouth forms a **bolus**, chewed food that is ready to swallow. Saliva also contains the digestive enzyme **amylase** that begins the digestion of carbohydrates.
There are three pairs of salivary glands. The **parotid glands** are in front of the ears,
and the **submandibular glands** and **sublingual glands** are in the floor of the mouth (see
Figure 8.8 ■).

Liver

bile (BYE-al)

emulsification (ee-mull-sih-fih-KAY-shun)

The liver, a large organ located in the right upper quadrant of the abdomen, has
several functions, including processing the nutrients absorbed by the intestines,
detoxifying harmful substances in the body, and producing **bile** (see Figure 8.9 ■).
Bile is important for the digestion of fats and lipids because it breaks up large fat
globules into much smaller droplets, making them easier to digest in the watery
environment inside the intestines. The process is called **emulsification**.

Med Term Tip

In anatomy the term *accessory*
generally means that the structure
is auxiliary to a more important
structure. This is not true for these
organs. Digestion would not be
possible without the digestive
juices produced by these organs.

Med Term Tip

The liver weighs about 4 pounds
and has so many important functions that people cannot live without it. It has become a major
transplant organ. The liver is also
able to regenerate itself. You can
lose more than half of your liver,
and it will regrow.

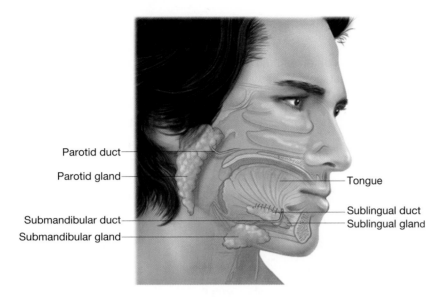

Gallbladder

common bile duct

cystic duct (SIS-tik)

hepatic duct (hep-PAT-tik)

Bile produced by the liver is stored in the gallbladder (GB). As the liver produces bile, it travels down the **hepatic duct** and up the **cystic duct** into the gallbladder (see Figure 8.9). In response to the presence of fat in the chyme, the muscular wall of the gallbladder contracts and sends bile back down the cystic duct and into the **common bile duct** (CBD), which carries bile to the duodenum where it is able to emulsify the fat in chyme.

Pancreas

buffers

pancreatic duct (pan-kree-AT-ik)

pancreatic enzymes
(pan-kree-AT-ik EN-zimes)

The pancreas, connected to the duodenum by the **pancreatic duct,** produces two important secretions for digestion—**buffers** and **pancreatic enzymes** (see Figure 8.9). Buffers neutralize acidic chyme that has just left the stomach, and pancreatic enzymes chemically digest carbohydrates, fats, and proteins. The pancreas is also an endocrine gland that produces the hormones insulin and glucagon, which play a role in regulating the level of glucose in the blood and are discussed in further detail in Chapter 11.

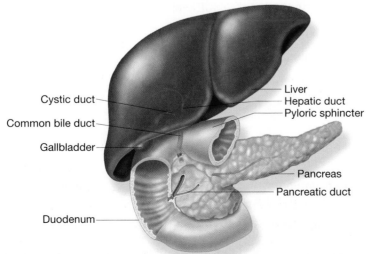

Figure 8.9 The accessory organs of the digestive system: the liver, gallbladder, and pancreas. Image shows the relationship of these three organs and their ducts to the duodenum.

Word Building

The following list contains examples of medical terms built directly from word parts. The definitions for these terms can be determined by a straightforward translation of the word parts.

COMBINING FORM	COMBINED WITH	MEDICAL TERM	DEFINITION
an/o	-al	**anal**	pertaining to the anus

> **Med Term Tip**
>
> Word watch—Be careful when using the combining form *an/o* meaning "anus" and the prefix *an* meaning "none."

COMBINING FORM	COMBINED WITH	MEDICAL TERM	DEFINITION
append/o	-ectomy	**appendectomy** (ap-en-DEK-toh-mee)	removal of the appendix
appendic/o	-itis	**appendicitis** (ah-pen-dih-SIGH-tis)	inflammation of the appendix
bucc/o	-al	**buccal** (BYOO-kal)	pertaining to cheeks
	labi/o -al	**buccolabial** (BYOO-koh-labe-ee-all)	pertaining to cheeks and lips
cholecyst/o	-ectomy	**cholecystectomy** (koh-lee-sis-TEK-toh-mee)	removal of the gallbladder
	-gram	**cholecystogram** (koh-lee-SIS-toh-gram)	record of the gallbladder
	-ic	**cholecystic** (koh-lee-SIS-tik)	pertaining to the gallbladder
	-algia	**cholecystalgia** (koh-lee-sis-TAL-jee-ah)	gallbladder pain
col/o	-ectomy	**colectomy** (koh-LEK-toh-mee)	removal of the colon
	-ostomy	**colostomy** (koh-LOSS-toh-mee)	create an opening in the colon
	rect/o -al	**colorectal** (kohl-oh-REK-tall)	pertaining to the colon and rectum
colon/o	-scope	**colonoscope** (koh-LON-oh-scope)	instrument to view colon
	-ic	**colonic** (koh-LON-ik)	pertaining to the colon
dent/o	-al	**dental** (DENT-al)	pertaining to teeth
	-algia	**dentalgia** (dent-AL-gee-ah)	tooth pain
duoden/o	-al	**duodenal** (duo-DEN-all / do-ODD-in-all)	pertaining to the duodenum
enter/o	-ic	**enteric** (en-TARE-ik)	pertaining to the small intestine
	-itis	**enteritis** (en-ter-EYE-tis)	small intestine inflammation
esophag/o	-eal	**esophageal** (eh-soff-ah-JEE-al)	pertaining to the esophagus
	-ectasis	**esophagectasis** (eh-soff-ah-JEK-tah-sis)	dilated esophagus
gastr/o	-algia	**gastralgia** (gas-TRAL-jee-ah)	stomach pain
	-ic	**gastric** (GAS-trik)	pertaining to the stomach
	enter/o -itis	**gastroenteritis** (gas-troh-en-ter-EYE-tis)	inflammation of stomach and small intestine
	enter/o -ologist	**gastroenterologist** (gas-troh-en-ter-ALL-oh-jist)	specialist in the stomach and small intestine
	-malacia	**gastromalacia** (gas-troh-mah-LAY-she-ah)	softening of the stomach
	nas/o -ic	**nasogastric** (nay-zoh-GAS-trik)	pertaining to the nose and stomach
	-ostomy	**gastrostomy** (gas-TROSS-toh-mee)	create an opening in the stomach

Word Building *(continued)*

COMBINING FORM	COMBINED WITH	MEDICAL TERM	DEFINITION
	-scope	**gastroscope** (GAS-troh-scope)	instrument to view inside the stomach
	-itis	**gastritis** (gas-TRY-tis)	stomach inflammation
	-ectomy	**gastrectomy** (gas-TREK-toh-mee)	removal of the stomach
gingiv/o	-al	**gingival** (JIN-jih-vul)	pertaining to the gums
	-itis	**gingivitis** (jin-jih-VIGH-tis)	inflammation of the gums
gloss/o	-al	**glossal** (GLOSS-all)	pertaining to the tongue
	hypo- -al	**hypoglossal** (high-poe-GLOSS-all)	pertaining to under the tongue
hepat/o	-itis	**hepatitis** (hep-ah-TYE-tis)	inflammation of the liver
	-oma	**hepatoma** (hep-ah-TOH-mah)	liver tumor
	-ic	**hepatic** (hep-AT-ik)	pertaining to the liver
ile/o	-al	**ileal** (ILL-ee-all)	pertaining to the ileum
	-ostomy	**ileostomy** (ill-ee-OSS-toh-mee)	create an opening in the ileum
jejun/o	-al	**jejunal** (jih-JUNE-all)	pertaining to the jejunum
lapar/o	-otomy	**laparotomy** (lap-ah-ROT-oh-mee)	incision into the abdomen
	-scope	**laparoscope** (LAP-ah-roh-scope)	instrument to view inside the abdomen
lingu/o	sub- -al	**sublingual** (sub-LING-gwal)	pertaining to under the tongue
odont/o	orth/o -ic	**orthodontic** (or-thoh-DON-tik)	pertaining to straight teeth
	peri- -ic	**periodontic** (pair-ee-oh-DON-tik)	pertaining to around the teeth
or/o	-al	**oral** (OR-ral)	pertaining to the mouth
palat/o	-plasty	**palatoplasty** (pa-LOT-toh-plas-tee)	surgical repair of the palate
pancreat/o	-itis	**pancreatitis** (pan-kree-ah-TYE-tis)	inflammation of the pancreas
	-ic	**pancreatic** (pan-kree-AT-ik)	pertaining to the pancreas
pharyng/o	-eal	**pharyngeal** (fair-in-JEE-all)	pertaining to the throat
	-plegia	**pharyngoplegia** (fair-in-goh-PLEE-jee-ah)	paralysis of the throat
	-plasty	**pharyngoplasty** (fair-ING-oh-plas-tee)	surgical repair of the throat
proct/o	-ptosis	**proctoptosis** (prok-top-TOH-sis)	drooping rectum and anus
	-logist	**proctologist** (prok-TOL-oh-jist)	specialist in the rectum and anus
	-pexy	**proctopexy** (PROK-toh-pek-see)	surgical fixation of the rectum and anus
pylor/o	-ic	**pyloric** (pie-LORE-ik)	pertaining to the pylorus
rect/o	-al	**rectal** (RECK-tall)	pertaining to the rectum
sialaden/o	-itis	**sialadenitis** (sigh-al-add-eh-NIGH-tis)	inflammation of a salivary gland
sigmoid/o	-scope	**sigmoidoscope** (sig-MOYD-oh-scope)	instrument to view inside the sigmoid colon
	-al	**sigmoidal** (sig-MOYD-all)	pertaining to the sigmoid colon

Word Building *(continued)*

SUFFIX	COMBINED WITH	MEDICAL TERM	DEFINITION
-emesis	hemat/o	**hematemesis** (hee-mah-TEM-eh-sis)	vomiting blood
	hyper-	**hyperemesis** (high-per-EM-eh-sis)	excessive vomiting
-orexia	an-	**anorexia** (an-oh-REK-see-ah)	absence of an appetite
	dys-	**dysorexia** (dis-oh-REKS-ee-ah)	abnormal appetite
-pepsia	brady-	**bradypepsia** (brad-ee-PEP-see-ah)	slow digestion
	dys-	**dyspepsia** (dis-PEP-see-ah)	difficult digestion
-phagia	a-	**aphagia** (ah-FAY-jee-ah)	unable to swallow/eat
	dys-	**dysphagia** (dis-FAY-jee-ah)	difficulty swallowing/eating
	poly-	**polyphagia** (pall-ee-FAY-jee-ah)	many (excessive) eating
-prandial	post-	**postprandial** (post-PRAN-dee-all)	after a meal

Vocabulary

TERM	DEFINITION
anorexia (an-oh-REK-see-ah)	A general term meaning loss of appetite that may accompany other conditions. Also used to refer to *anorexia nervosa*, which is a personality disorder involving refusal to eat.
ascites (ah-SIGH-teez)	Collection or accumulation of fluid in the peritoneal cavity.
bowel incontinence (in-CON-tih-nence)	Inability to control defecation.
bridge	Dental appliance that is attached to adjacent teeth for support to replace missing teeth.
cachexia (ka-KEK-see-ah)	Loss of weight and generalized wasting that occurs during a chronic disease.
constipation (kon-stih-PAY-shun)	Experiencing difficulty in defecation or infrequent defecation.
crown	Artificial covering for the tooth created to replace the original crown.
dental caries (KAIR-eez)	Gradual decay and disintegration of teeth caused by bacteria; may lead to abscessed teeth. Commonly called a *tooth cavity*.
dentistry	Branch of healthcare involved with the prevention, diagnosis, and treatment of conditions involving the teeth, jaw, and mouth. Dentistry is practiced by a *dentist* or *oral surgeon*.
denture (DEN-chur)	Partial or complete set of artificial teeth that are set in plastic materials. Acts as a substitute for the natural teeth and related structures.
diarrhea (dye-ah-REE-ah)	Passing of frequent, watery bowel movements. Usually accompanies gastrointestinal (GI) disorders.

Vocabulary *(continued)*

TERM	DEFINITION
emesis (EM-eh-sis)	Vomiting.
gastroenterology (gas-troh-en-ter-ALL-oh-jee)	Branch of medicine involved in diagnosis and treatment of diseases and disorders of the digestive system. Physician is a *gastroenterologist*.
hematochezia (he-mat-oh-KEY-zee-ah)	Passing bright red blood in the stools.
implant (IM-plant)	Prosthetic device placed in the jaw to which a tooth or denture may be anchored.
internal medicine	Branch of medicine involving the diagnosis and treatment of diseases and conditions of internal organs such as the digestive system. The physician is an *internist*.
jaundice (JAWN-diss)	Yellow cast to the skin, mucous membranes, and the whites of the eyes caused by the deposit of bile pigment from too much bilirubin in the blood. Bilirubin is a waste product produced when worn-out red blood cells are broken down. May be a symptom of a disorder such as gallstones blocking the common bile duct or carcinoma of the liver.
melena (me-LEE-nah)	Passage of dark tarry stools. Color is the result of digestive enzymes working on blood in the gastrointestinal tract.
nausea (NAW-see-ah)	The urge to vomit. **Med Term Tip** The term *nausea* comes from the Greek word for "seasickness."
obesity	Body weight that is above a healthy level. A person whose weight interferes with normal activity and body function has *morbid obesity*.
orthodontics (or-thoh-DON-tiks)	Branch of dentistry concerned with correction of problems with tooth alignment. A specialist is an *orthodontist*.
periodontics (pair-ee-oh-DON-tiks)	Branch of dentistry concerned with treating conditions involving the gums and tissues surrounding the teeth. A specialist is a *periodontist*.
polyp (POLL-ip)	Small tumor with a pedicle or stem attachment. Commonly found on mucous membranes such as those lining the colon or nasal cavity. Colon polyps may be precancerous.
proctology (prok-TOL-oh-jee)	Branch of medicine involved in diagnosis and treatment of diseases and disorders of the anus and rectum. Physician is a *proctologist*.
pyrosis (pie-ROW-sis)	Pain and burning sensation usually caused by stomach acid splashing up into the esophagus. Commonly called *heartburn*.
regurgitation (ree-gur-jih-TAY-shun)	Return of fluids and solids from the stomach into the mouth.

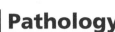
Pathology

TERM	DEFINITION
■ Oral Cavity	
aphthous ulcers (AF-thus)	Painful ulcers in the mouth of unknown cause. Commonly called *canker sores*.
cleft lip (CLEFT)	Congenital anomaly in which the upper lip and jaw bone fail to fuse in the midline leaving an open gap. Often seen along with a cleft palate. Corrected with surgery.
cleft palate (CLEFT-PAL-at)	Congenital anomaly in which the roof of the mouth has a split or fissure. Corrected with surgery.
herpes labialis (HER-peez lay-bee-AL-iz)	Infection of the lip by the herpes simplex virus type 1 (HSV-1). Also called *fever blisters* or *cold sores*.
periodontal disease (pair-ee-oh-DON-tal dih-ZEEZ)	Disease of the supporting structures of the teeth, including the gums and bones; the most common cause of tooth loss.
■ Esophagus	
esophageal varices (eh-soff-ah-JEE-al VAIR-ih-seez)	Enlarged and swollen varicose veins in the lower end of the esophagus. If these rupture, serious hemorrhage results; often related to liver disease.
gastroesophageal reflux disease (GERD) (gas-troh-ee-sof-ah-GEE-all REE-fluks)	Acid from the stomach flows backward up into the esophagus causing inflammation and pain.
■ Stomach	
gastric carcinoma (GAS-trik car-si-NOH-mah)	Cancerous tumor in the stomach.
hiatal hernia (high-AY-tal HER-nee-ah)	Protrusion of the stomach through the diaphragm (also called a *diaphragmatocele*) and extending into the thoracic cavity; gastroesophageal reflux disease is a common symptom.

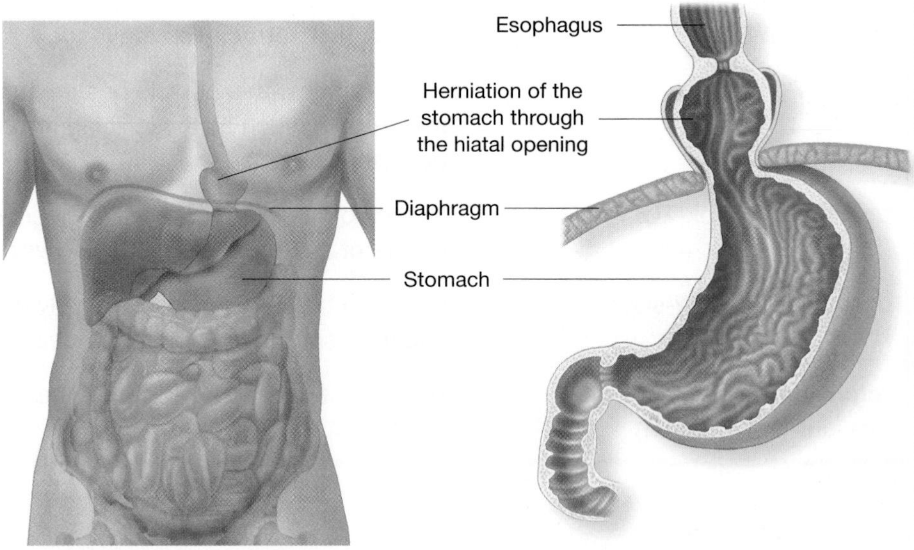

■ **Figure 8.10** A hiatal hernia or diaphragmatocele. A portion of the stomach protrudes through the diaphragm into the thoracic cavity.

Esophagus

Herniation of the stomach through the hiatal opening

Diaphragm

Stomach

Pathology (continued)

TERM	DEFINITION
peptic ulcer disease (PUD) (PEP-tik ULL-sir)	Ulcer occurring in the lower portion of the esophagus, stomach, and/or duodenum; thought to be caused by the acid of gastric juices. Initial damage to the protective lining of the stomach may be caused by a *Helicobacter pylori* (*H. pylori*) bacterial infection. If the ulcer extends all the way through the wall of the stomach, it is called a *perforated ulcer* which requires immediate surgery to repair.

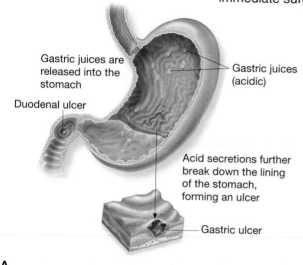

Gastric juices are released into the stomach

Gastric juices (acidic)

Duodenal ulcer

Acid secretions further break down the lining of the stomach, forming an ulcer

Gastric ulcer

A.

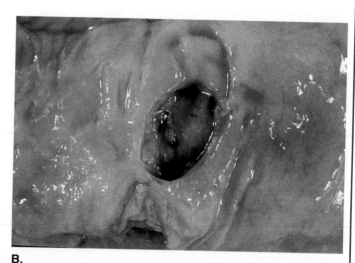

B.

Figure 8.11 A) Figure illustrating the location and appearance of a peptic ulcer in both the stomach and the duodenum. B) Photomicrograph illustrating a gastric ulcer. *(Dr. E. Walker/Science Photo Library/Photo Researchers, Inc.)*

Small Intestine and Colon

anal fistula (FIH-styoo-lah)	Abnormal tubelike passage from the surface around the anal opening directly into the rectum.
colorectal carcinoma (kohl-oh-REK-tall car-ci-NOH-mah)	Cancerous tumor along the length of the colon and rectum.
Crohn's disease (KROHNZ dih-ZEEZ)	Form of chronic inflammatory bowel disease affecting primarily the ileum and/or colon. Also called *regional ileitis.* This autoimmune condition affects all the layers of the bowel wall and results in scarring and thickening of the gut wall.
diverticulitis (dye-ver-tik-yoo-LYE-tis)	Inflammation of a *diverticulum* (an outpouching off the gut), especially in the colon. Inflammation often results when food becomes trapped within the pouch.

Figure 8.12 Diverticulosis. Figure illustrates external and internal appearance of diverticula.

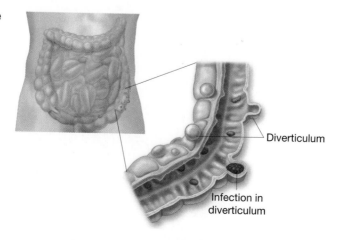

Diverticulum

Infection in diverticulum

Pathology *(continued)*

TERM	DEFINITION
diverticulosis (dye-ver-tik-yoo-LOW-sis)	Condition of having diverticula (outpouches off the gut). May lead to *diverticulitis* if one becomes inflamed.
dysentery (dis-in-TARE-ee)	Disease characterized by diarrhea, often with mucus and blood, severe abdominal pain, fever, and dehydration. Caused by ingesting food or water contaminated by chemicals, bacteria, protozoans, or parasites.
hemorrhoids (HEM-oh-roydz)	Varicose veins in the rectum.
ileus (ILL-ee-us)	Severe abdominal pain, inability to pass stools, vomiting, and abdominal distension as a result of an intestinal blockage. May require surgery to reverse the blockage.
inguinal hernia (ING-gwih-nal HER-nee-ah)	Hernia or protrusion of a loop of small intestines into the inguinal (groin) region through a weak spot in the abdominal muscle wall that develops into a hole. May become *incarcerated* or *strangulated* if the muscle tightens down around the loop of intestines and cuts off its blood flow.

■ **Figure 8.13** An inguinal hernia. A portion of the small intestine is protruding through the abdominal muscles into the groin region.

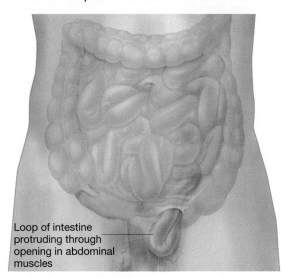

Loop of intestine protruding through opening in abdominal muscles

intussusception (in-tuh-suh-SEP-shun)	Result of the intestine slipping or telescoping into another section of intestine just below it. More common in children.

■ **Figure 8.14** Intussusception. A short length of small intestine has telescoped into itself.

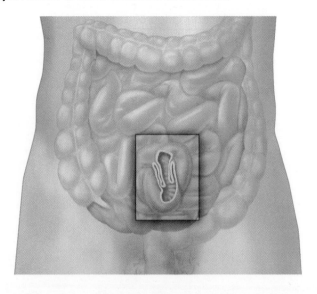

Pathology *(continued)*

TERM	DEFINITION
irritable bowel syndrome (IBS)	Disturbance in the functions of the intestine from unknown causes. Symptoms generally include abdominal discomfort and an alteration in bowel activity. Also called *spastic colon* or *functional bowel syndrome*.
polyposis (pall-ee-POH-sis)	Small tumors that contain a pedicle or stemlike attachment in the mucous membranes of the large intestine (colon); may be precancerous.

■ **Figure 8.15** Photograph showing a polyp in the colon. Note the mushroom-like shape, an enlarged top growing at the end of a stem.
(ISM/Phototake NYC)

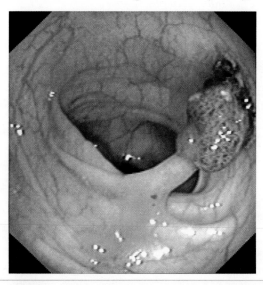

TERM	DEFINITION
ulcerative colitis (ULL-sir-ah-tiv koh-LYE-tis)	Chronic inflammatory condition that produces numerous ulcers to form on the mucous membrane lining of the colon; the cause is unknown. Also known as *inflammatory bowel disease* (IBD).
volvulus (VOL-vyoo-lus)	Condition in which the bowel twists upon itself and causes an obstruction. Painful and requires immediate surgery.

■ **Figure 8.16** Volvulus. A length of small intestine has twisted around itself, cutting off blood circulation to the twisted loop.

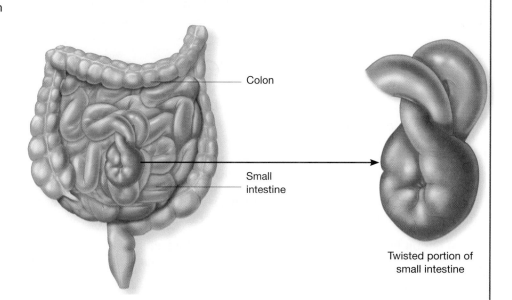

Colon

Small intestine

Twisted portion of small intestine

Pathology *(continued)*

TERM	DEFINITION
■ *Accessory Organs*	
cholecystitis (koh-lee-sis-TYE-tis)	Inflammation of the gallbladder; most commonly caused by gallstones in the gallbladder or common bile duct that block the flow of bile.
cholelithiasis (koh-lee-lih-THIGH-ah-sis)	Presence of gallstones; may or may not cause symptoms such as *cholecystalgia*.

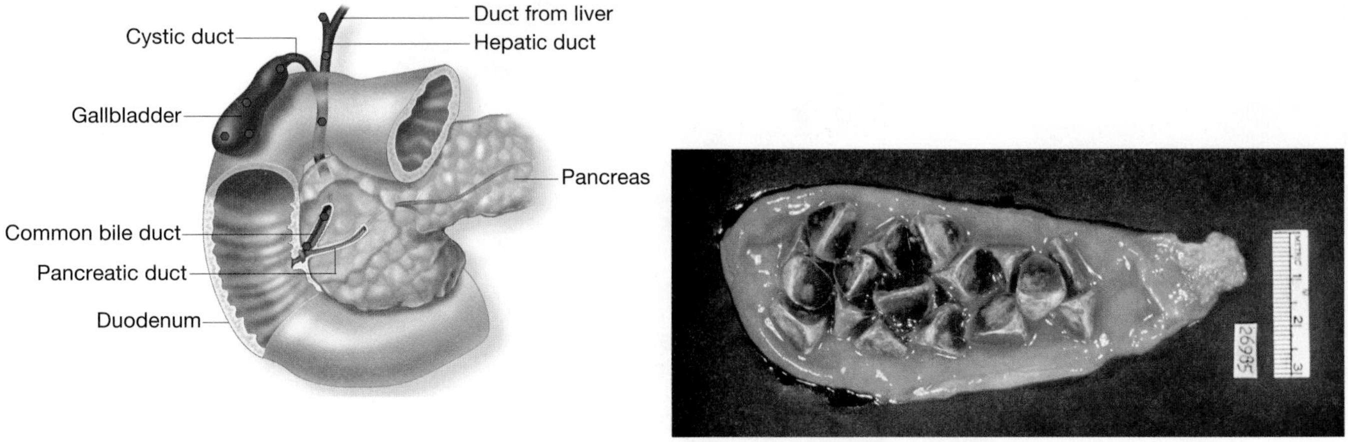

Cystic duct — Duct from liver — Hepatic duct

Gallbladder —

— Pancreas

Common bile duct —
Pancreatic duct —
Duodenum —

A.   B.

■ Figure 8.17 A) Cholelithiasis, red circles indicate common sites for gallstones including the gallbladder, cystic duct, hepatic duct, and common bile duct. B) Photograph of a gallbladder specimen with multiple gallstones. *(Martin Rotker/Phototake NYC)*

cirrhosis (sih-ROH-sis)	Chronic disease of the liver associated with failure of the liver to function properly.
hepatitis (hep-ah-TYE-tis)	Inflammation of the liver, usually due to a viral infection. Different viruses are transmitted by different routes, such as sexual contact or from exposure to blood or fecally contaminated water or food.

Diagnostic Procedures

TERM	DEFINITION
■ *Clinical Laboratory Tests*	
alanine transaminase (ALT) (AL-ah-neen trans-AM-in-nase)	Enzyme normally present in the blood. Blood levels are increased in persons with liver disease.
aspartate transaminase (AST) (ass-PAR-tate trans-AM-in-nase)	Enzyme normally present in the blood. Blood levels are increased in persons with liver disease.
fecal occult blood test (FOBT) (uh-CULT)	Laboratory test on the feces to determine if microscopic amounts of blood are present. Also called *hemoccult* or *stool guaiac*.
ova and parasites (O&P) (OH-vah and PAR-ah-sights)	Laboratory examination of feces with a microscope for the presence of parasites or their eggs.
serum bilirubin (SEE-rum BILLY-rubin)	Blood test to determine the amount of the waste product bilirubin in the bloodstream. Elevated levels indicate liver disease.

Diagnostic Procedures *(continued)*

TERM	DEFINITION
stool culture	Laboratory test of feces to determine if any pathogenic bacteria are present.

■ *Diagnostic Imaging*

bite-wing x-ray	X-ray taken with a part of the film holder held between the teeth and parallel to the teeth.
intravenous cholecystography (in-trah-VEE-nus koh-lee-sis-TOG-rah-fee)	Dye is administered intravenously to the patient, which allows for x-ray visualization of the gallbladder and bile ducts.
lower gastrointestinal series (lower GI series)	X-ray image of the colon and rectum is taken after the administration of barium (a radiopaque dye) by enema. Also called a *barium enema (BE)*.

■ **Figure 8.18** Color enhanced x-ray of the colon taken during a barium enema. *(CNRI/Science Photo Library/Photo Researchers, Inc.)*

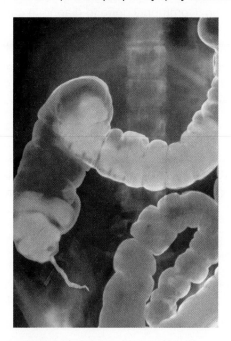

percutaneous transhepatic cholangiography (PTC) (per-kyoo-TAY-nee-us trans-heh-PAT-ik koh-lan-jee-OG-rah-fee)	Procedure in which contrast medium is injected directly into the liver to visualize the bile ducts. Used to detect obstructions.
upper gastrointestinal (UGI) **series**	Administering of a barium contrast material orally and then taking an x-ray to visualize the esophagus, stomach, and duodenum. Also called a *barium swallow*.

■ *Endoscopic Procedures*

colonoscopy (koh-lon-OSS-koh-pee)	Flexible fiberscope called a *colonoscope* is passed through the anus, rectum, and colon; used to examine the upper portion of the colon. Polyps and small growths can be removed during this procedure (see Figure 8.15).
endoscopic retrograde cholangiopancreatography (ERCP) (en-doh-SKOP-ik RET-roh-grayd koh-lan-jee-oh-pan-kree-ah-TOG-rah-fee)	Procedure using an endoscope to visually examine the hepatic duct, common bile duct, and pancreatic duct. Retrograde means to go in the backwards direction. In this case the endoscope is inserted through the anus and worked backwards to the area where the pancreatic and common bile ducts empty into the duodenum.

Diagnostic Procedures *(continued)*

TERM	DEFINITION
esophagogastroduodenoscopy (EGD) (eh-soff-ah-go-gas-troh-duo-den-OS-koh-pee)	Use of a flexible fiberoptic endoscope to visually examine the esophagus, stomach, and beginning of the duodenum.
gastroscopy (gas-TROS-koh-pee)	Procedure in which a flexible *gastroscope* is passed through the mouth and down the esophagus in order to visualize inside the stomach. Used to diagnose peptic ulcers and gastric carcinoma.
laparoscopy (lap-ar-OSS-koh-pee)	*Laparoscope* is passed into the abdominal wall through a small incision. The abdominal cavity is then visually examined for tumors and other conditions with this lighted instrument. Also called *peritoneoscopy*.
sigmoidoscopy (sig-moid-OS-koh-pee)	Procedure using a flexible *sigmoidoscope* to visually examine the sigmoid colon. Commonly done to diagnose cancer and polyps.
■ *Additional Diagnostic Procedures*	
paracentesis (pair-ah-sin-TEE-sis)	Insertion of a needle into the abdominal cavity to withdraw fluid. Tests to diagnose diseases may be conducted on the fluid.

Therapeutic Procedures

TERM	DEFINITION
■ *Dental Procedures*	
extraction	Removing or "pulling" of teeth.
root canal	Dental treatment involving the pulp cavity of the root of a tooth. Procedure is used to save a tooth that is badly infected or abscessed.
■ *Medical Procedures*	
gavage	Using a nasogastric (NG) tube to place liquid nourishment directly into the stomach.
lavage	Using a nasogastric (NG) tube to wash out the stomach. For example, after ingestion of dangerous substances.
nasogastric intubation (NG tube) (NAY-zo-gas-trik in-two-BAY-shun)	Flexible catheter is inserted into the nose and down the esophagus to the stomach. May be used for feeding or to suction out stomach fluids.
total parenteral nutrition (TPN) (pair-in-TARE-all)	Providing 100% of a patient's nutrition intravenously. Used when a patient is unable to eat.
■ *Surgical Procedures*	
anastomosis (ah-nas-toh-MOH-sis)	To surgically create a connection between two organs or vessels. For example, joining together two cut ends of the intestines after a section is removed.

Therapeutic Procedures *(continued)*

TERM	DEFINITION
bariatric surgery (bear-ee-AT-rik)	A group of surgical procedures such as stomach stapling and restrictive banding to reduce the size of the stomach. A treatment for morbid (extreme) obesity.
choledocholithotripsy (koh-led-oh-koh-LITH-oh-trip-see)	Crushing of a gallstone in the common bile duct.
colostomy (koh-LOSS-toh-mee)	Surgical creation of an opening of some portion of the colon through the abdominal wall to the outside surface. Fecal material (stool) drains into a bag worn on the abdomen.

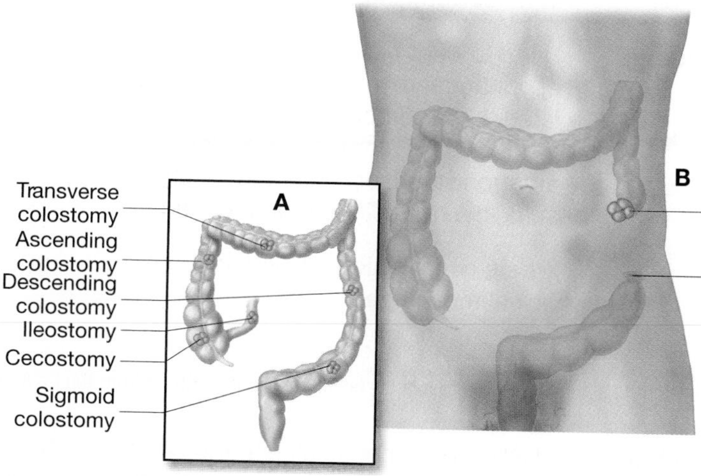

■ **Figure 8.19** A) The colon illustrating various ostomy sites. B) Colostomy in the descending colon, illustrating functioning stoma and nonfunctioning distal sigmoid colon and rectum.

Transverse colostomy
Ascending colostomy
Descending colostomy
Ileostomy
Cecostomy
Sigmoid colostomy

A

B

Functioning stoma

Non-functioning remaining colon

diverticulectomy (dye-ver-tik-yoo-LEK-toh-mee)	Surgical removal of a diverticulum.
exploratory laparotomy (ek-SPLOR-ah-tor-ee lap-ah-ROT-oh-mee)	Abdominal operation for the purpose of examining the abdominal organs and tissues for signs of disease or other abnormalities.
fistulectomy (fis-tyoo-LEK-toh-mee)	Removal of a fistula.
gastric stapling	Procedure that closes off a large section of the stomach with rows of staples. Results in a much smaller stomach to assist very obese patients to lose weight.
hemorrhoidectomy (hem-oh-royd-EK-toh-mee)	Surgical removal of hemorrhoids from the anorectal area.
hernioplasty (her-nee-oh-PLAS-tee)	Surgical repair of a hernia. Also called *herniorrhaphy*.
laparoscopic cholecystectomy (lap-ar-oh-SKOP-ik koh-lee-sis-TEK-toh-mee)	Surgical removal of the gallbladder through a very small abdominal incision with the assistance of a laparoscope.
liver transplant	Transplant of a liver from a donor.

Pharmacology

CLASSIFICATION	ACTION	GENERIC AND BRAND NAMES
anorexiant (an-oh-REKS-ee-ant)	Treats obesity by suppressing appetite.	phendimetrazine, Adipost, Obezine; phentermine, Zantryl, Adipex
antacid	Used to neutralize stomach acids.	calcium carbonate, Tums; aluminum hydroxide and magnesium hydroxide, Maalox, Mylanta
antidiarrheal	Used to control diarrhea.	loperamide, Imodium; diphenoxylate, Lomotil; kaolin/pectin, Kaopectate
antiemetic (an-tye-ee-MEH-tik)	Treats nausea, vomiting, and motion sickness.	prochlorperazine, Compazine; promethazine, Phenergan
emetic (ee-MEH-tik)	Induces vomiting.	Ipecac syrup
H_2-receptor antagonist	Used to treat peptic ulcers and gastroesophageal reflux disease. When stimulated, H_2-receptors increase the production of stomach acid. Using an antagonist to block these receptors results in a low acid level in the stomach.	ranitidine, Zantac; cimetidine, Tagamet; famotidine, Pepcid
laxative	Treats constipation by stimulating a bowel movement.	senosides, Senokot; psyllium, Metamucil

Med Term Tip

The term *laxative* that refers to a medication to stimulate a bowel movement comes from the Latin term meaning "to relax."

CLASSIFICATION	ACTION	GENERIC AND BRAND NAMES
proton pump inhibitors	Used to treat peptic ulcers and gastroesophageal reflux disease. Blocks the stomach's ability to secrete acid.	esomeprazole, Nexium; omeprazole, Prilosec

Abbreviations

ac	before meals	**HCV**	hepatitis C virus
ALT	alanine transaminase	**HDV**	hepatitis D virus
AST	aspartate transaminase	**HEV**	hepatitis E virus
Ba	barium	**HSV-1**	herpes simplex virus type 1
BE	barium enema	**IBD**	inflammatory bowel disease
BM	bowel movement	**IBS**	irritable bowel syndrome
BS	bowel sounds	**IVC**	intravenous cholangiography
CBD	common bile duct	**NG**	nasogastric (tube)
EGD	esophagogastroduodenoscopy	**NPO**	nothing by mouth
ERCP	endoscopic retrograde cholangio-pancreatography	**n&v**	nausea and vomiting
		O&P	ova and parasites
FOBT	fecal occult blood test	**pc**	after meals
GB	gallbladder	**PO**	by mouth
GERD	gastroesophageal reflux disease	**pp**	postprandial
GI	gastrointestinal	**PTC**	percutaneous transhepatic cholangiography
HAV	hepatitis A virus	**PUD**	peptic ulcer disease
HBV	hepatitis B virus	**TPN**	total parenteral nutrition
HCl	hydrochloric acid	**UGI**	upper gastrointestinal series

Chapter Review

Terminology Checklist

Below are all Anatomy and Physiology key terms, Word Building, Vocabulary, Pathology, Diagnostic, Therapeutic, and Pharmacology terms presented in this chapter. Use this list as a study tool by placing a check in the box in front of each term as you master its meaning.

- [ ] accessory organs
- [ ] alanine transaminase
- [ ] alimentary canal
- [ ] amylase
- [ ] anal
- [ ] anal fistula
- [ ] anal sphincter
- [ ] anastomosis
- [ ] anorexia
- [ ] anorexiant
- [ ] antacid
- [ ] antidiarrheal
- [ ] antiemetic
- [ ] antrum
- [ ] anus
- [ ] aphagia
- [ ] aphthous ulcers
- [ ] appendectomy
- [ ] appendicitis
- [ ] ascending colon
- [ ] ascites
- [ ] aspartate transaminase
- [ ] bariatric surgery
- [ ] bicuspids
- [ ] bile
- [ ] bite-wing x-ray
- [ ] body
- [ ] bolus
- [ ] bowel incontinence
- [ ] bradypepsia
- [ ] bridge
- [ ] buccal
- [ ] buccolabial
- [ ] buffers
- [ ] cachexia
- [ ] canines
- [ ] cardiac sphincter
- [ ] cecum
- [ ] cementum

- [ ] cheeks
- [ ] cholecystalgia
- [ ] cholecystectomy
- [ ] cholecystic
- [ ] cholecystitis
- [ ] cholecystogram
- [ ] choledocholithotripsy
- [ ] cholelithiasis
- [ ] chyme
- [ ] cirrhosis
- [ ] cleft lip
- [ ] cleft palate
- [ ] colectomy
- [ ] colon
- [ ] colonic
- [ ] colonoscope
- [ ] colonoscopy
- [ ] colorectal
- [ ] colorectal carcinoma
- [ ] colostomy
- [ ] common bile duct
- [ ] constipation
- [ ] Crohn's disease
- [ ] crown
- [ ] cuspids
- [ ] cystic duct
- [ ] deciduous teeth
- [ ] defecation
- [ ] dental
- [ ] dental caries
- [ ] dentalgia
- [ ] dentin
- [ ] dentistry
- [ ] denture
- [ ] descending colon
- [ ] diarrhea
- [ ] diverticulectomy
- [ ] diverticulitis
- [ ] diverticulosis

- [ ] duodenal
- [ ] duodenum
- [ ] dysentery
- [ ] dysorexia
- [ ] dyspepsia
- [ ] dysphagia
- [ ] emesis
- [ ] emetic
- [ ] emulsification
- [ ] enamel
- [ ] endoscopic retrograde cholangiopancreatography
- [ ] enteric
- [ ] enteritis
- [ ] epiglottis
- [ ] esophageal
- [ ] esophageal varices
- [ ] esophagectasis
- [ ] esophagogastroduodenoscopy
- [ ] esophagus
- [ ] exploratory laparotomy
- [ ] extraction
- [ ] fecal occult blood test
- [ ] feces
- [ ] fistulectomy
- [ ] fundus
- [ ] gallbladder
- [ ] gastralgia
- [ ] gastrectomy
- [ ] gastric
- [ ] gastric carcinoma
- [ ] gastric stapling
- [ ] gastritis
- [ ] gastroenteritis
- [ ] gastroenterologist
- [ ] gastroenterology
- [ ] gastroesophageal reflux disease
- [ ] gastrointestinal system

- [ ] gastrointestinal tract
- [ ] gastromalacia
- [ ] gastroscope
- [ ] gastroscopy
- [ ] gastrostomy
- [ ] gavage
- [ ] gingiva
- [ ] gingival
- [ ] gingivitis
- [ ] glossal
- [ ] gums
- [ ] gut
- [ ] H$_2$-receptor antagonist
- [ ] hematemesis
- [ ] hematochezia
- [ ] hemorrhoidectomy
- [ ] hemorrhoids
- [ ] hepatic
- [ ] hepatic duct
- [ ] hepatitis
- [ ] hepatoma
- [ ] hernioplasty
- [ ] herpes labialis
- [ ] hiatal hernia
- [ ] hydrochloric acid
- [ ] hyperemesis
- [ ] hypoglossal
- [ ] ileal
- [ ] ileocecal valve
- [ ] ileostomy
- [ ] ileum
- [ ] ileus
- [ ] implant
- [ ] incisors
- [ ] inguinal hernia
- [ ] internal medicine
- [ ] intravenous cholecystography
- [ ] intussusception
- [ ] irritable bowel syndrome
- [ ] jaundice
- [ ] jejunal
- [ ] jejunum
- [ ] laparoscope
- [ ] laparoscopic cholecystectomy
- [ ] laparoscopy

- [ ] laparotomy
- [ ] laryngopharynx
- [ ] lavage
- [ ] laxative
- [ ] lips
- [ ] liver
- [ ] liver transplant
- [ ] lower esophageal sphincter
- [ ] lower gastrointestinal series
- [ ] melena
- [ ] molars
- [ ] nasogastric
- [ ] nasogastric intubation
- [ ] nausea
- [ ] obesity
- [ ] oral
- [ ] oral cavity
- [ ] oropharynx
- [ ] orthodontic
- [ ] orthodontics
- [ ] ova and parasites
- [ ] palate
- [ ] palatoplasty
- [ ] pancreas
- [ ] pancreatic
- [ ] pancreatic duct
- [ ] pancreatic enzymes
- [ ] pancreatitis
- [ ] paracentesis
- [ ] parotid glands
- [ ] peptic ulcer disease
- [ ] percutaneous transhepatic cholangiography
- [ ] periodontal disease
- [ ] periodontal ligaments
- [ ] periodontic
- [ ] periodontics
- [ ] peristalsis
- [ ] permanent teeth
- [ ] pharyngeal
- [ ] pharyngoplasty
- [ ] pharyngoplegia
- [ ] pharynx
- [ ] polyp

- [ ] polyphagia
- [ ] polyposis
- [ ] postprandial
- [ ] premolar
- [ ] proctologist
- [ ] proctology
- [ ] proctopexy
- [ ] proctoptosis
- [ ] proton pump inhibitor
- [ ] pulp cavity
- [ ] pyloric
- [ ] pyloric sphincter
- [ ] pyrosis
- [ ] rectal
- [ ] rectum
- [ ] regurgitation
- [ ] root
- [ ] root canal
- [ ] rugae
- [ ] saliva
- [ ] salivary glands
- [ ] serum bilirubin
- [ ] sialadenitis
- [ ] sigmoidal
- [ ] sigmoid colon
- [ ] sigmoidoscope
- [ ] sigmoidoscopy
- [ ] small intestine
- [ ] sphincter
- [ ] stomach
- [ ] stool culture
- [ ] sublingual
- [ ] sublingual glands
- [ ] submandibular glands
- [ ] taste buds
- [ ] teeth
- [ ] tongue
- [ ] total parenteral nutrition
- [ ] transverse colon
- [ ] ulcerative colitis
- [ ] upper gastrointestinal series
- [ ] uvula
- [ ] vermiform appendix
- [ ] volvulus

Practice Exercises

A. Complete the following statements.

1. The digestive system is also known as the _____ system.

2. The continuous muscular tube of the digestive system is called the _____ or _____ and stretches between the _____ and _____.

3. The accessory organs of the digestive system are the _____, _____, _____, and _____.

4. The three main functions of the digestive system are: _____, _____, and _____.

5. The incisors are examples of _____ teeth and the molars are examples of _____ teeth.

6. Food is propelled through the gut by wavelike muscular contractions called _____.

7. Food in the stomach is mixed with _____ and other gastric juices to form a watery mixture called _____.

8. The three sections of small intestine in order are the _____, _____, and _____.

9. The S-shaped section of colon that curves back towards the rectum is called the _____ colon.

10. _____ produced by the liver is responsible for the _____ of fats. It is stored in the _____.

B. Define the following combining forms and use them to form digestive terms.

	Definition	Digestive Term
1. esophag/o	_____	_____
2. hepat/o	_____	_____
3. ile/o	_____	_____
4. proct/o	_____	_____
5. gloss/o	_____	_____
6. labi/o	_____	_____
7. jejun/o	_____	_____
8. sigmoid/o	_____	_____
9. rect/o	_____	_____
10. gingiv/o	_____	_____

11. cholecyst/o _____ _____

12. duoden/o _____ _____

13. an/o _____ _____

14. enter/o _____ _____

15. dent/o _____ _____

C. State the terms described using the combining forms provided.

The combining form *gastr/o* refers to the stomach. Use it to write a term that means:

1. inflammation of the stomach _____

2. study of the stomach and small intestines _____

3. removal of the stomach _____

4. visual exam of the stomach _____

5. stomach pain _____

6. enlargement of the stomach _____

7. incision into the stomach _____

The combining form *esophag/o* refers to the esophagus. Use it to write a term that means:

8. inflammation of the esophagus _____

9. visual examination of the esophagus _____

10. surgical repair of the esophagus _____

11. pertaining to the esophagus _____

12. stretched out esophagus _____

The combining form *proct/o* refers to the rectum and anus. Use it to write a term that means:

13. surgical fixation of the rectum and anus _____

14. drooping of the rectum and anus _____

15. inflammation of the rectum and anus _____

16. specialist in the study of the rectum and anus _____

The combining form *cholecyst/o* refers to the gallbladder. Use it to write a term that means:

17. removal of the gallbladder _____

18. condition of having gallbladder stones _____

19. gallbladder stone surgical crushing _____

20. gallbladder inflammation _____

The combining form *laparo* refers to the abdomen. Use it to write a term that means:

21. instrument to view inside the abdomen _____

22. incision into the abdomen _____

23. visual examination of the abdomen _____

The combining form *hepato* refers to the liver. Use it to write a term that means:

24. liver tumor _____

25. enlargement of the liver _____

26. pertaining to the liver _____

27. inflammation of the liver _____

The combining form *pancreato* refers to the pancreas. Use it to write a term that means:

28. inflammation of the pancreas _____

29. pertaining to the pancreas _____

The combining form *colo* refers to the colon. Use it to write a term that means:

30. create an opening in the colon _____

31. inflammation of the colon _____

D. Use the following suffixes to create a medical term for each definition relating to the digestive system.

-orexia   -phagia   -pepsia   -prandial

-emesis   -lithiasis

1. taken after meals _____

2. gallstones _____

3. no appetite _____

4. difficulty swallowing _____

5. vomiting blood _____

6. slow digestion _____

E. Identify the following abbreviations.

1. BM _____

2. UGI _____

3. BE _____

4. BS _____

5. n & v _____

6. O & P _____

7. PO _____

8. CBD _____

9. NPO _____

10. pp _____

F. Write the abbreviation for the following terms.

1. nasogastric _____

2. gastrointestinal _____

3. hepatitis B virus _____

4. fecal occult blood test _____

5. inflammatory bowel disease _____

6. herpes simplex virus type 1 _____

7. aspartate transaminase _____

8. after meals _____

9. peptic ulcer disease _____

10. gastroesophageal reflux disease _____

G. Define the following terms.

1. colonoscopy _____

2. bite-wing x-ray _____

3. hematochezia _____

4. serum bilirubin _____

5. cachexia _____

6. lavage _____

7. hernioplasty _____

8. extraction _____

9. choledocholithotripsy _____

10. anastomosis _____

H. Match each term to its definition.

1. _____ dentures

2. _____ anorexia

3. _____ hematemesis

4. _____ pyrosis

5. _____ obesity

a. excess body weight

b. chronic liver disease

c. heart burn

d. small colon tumors

e. fluid accumulation in abdominal cavity

6. _____ constipation   f. vomit blood

7. _____ melena   g. bowel twists on self

8. _____ ascites   h. set of artificial teeth

9. _____ cirrhosis   i. loss of appetite

10. _____ spastic colon   j. difficulty having BM

11. _____ polyposis   k. irritable bowel syndrome

12. _____ volvulus   l. black tarry stool

13. _____ hiatal hernia   m. yellow skin color

14. _____ ulcerative colitis   n. bloody diarrhea

15. _____ dysentery   o. diaphragmatocele

16. _____ jaundice   p. inflammatory bowel disease

I. Use the following terms in the sentences below.

colonoscopy	barium swallow	lower GI series
gastric stapling	colostomy	colectomy
total parenteral nutrition	choledocholithotripsy	liver biopsy
ileostomy	fecal occult blood test	intravenous cholecystography

1. Excising a small piece of hepatic tissue for microscopic examination is called a(n) _____ .

2. When a surgeon performs a total or partial colectomy for cancer, she may have to create an opening on the surface of the skin for fecal matter to leave the body. This procedure is called a(n) _____ .

3. Another name for an upper GI series is a(n) _____ .

4. Mr. White has had a radiopaque material placed into his large bowel by means of an enema for the purpose of viewing his colon. This procedure is called a(n) _____ .

5. A(n) _____ is the surgical removal of the colon.

6. Jessica has been on a red-meat-free diet in preparation for a test of her feces for the presence of hidden blood. This test is called a(n) _____ .

7. Dr. Mendez uses equipment to crush gallstones in the common bile duct. This procedure is called a(n)

_____ .

8. Mrs. Alcazar required _____ because she could not eat following her intestinal surgery.

9. Mr. Bright had a _____ to treat his morbid obesity.

10. Visualizing the gallbladder and bile ducts by injecting a dye into the patient's arm is called an _____ .

11. Passing an instrument into the anus and rectum in order to see the colon is called a(n) _____ .

12. Ms. Fayne suffers from Crohn's disease, which has necessitated the removal of much of her small intestine. She has had a

surgical passage created for the external disposal of waste material from the ileum. This is called a(n) _____ .

J. Match each term to its definition.

1. _____ dentures

2. _____ cementum

3. _____ root canal

4. _____ crown

5. _____ bridge

6. _____ implant

7. _____ gingivitis

8. _____ dental caries

a. tooth decay

b. prosthetic device used to anchor a tooth

c. inflammation of the gums

d. full set of artificial teeth

e. portion of the tooth covered by enamel

f. replacement for missing teeth

g. anchors root in bony socket of jaw

h. surgery on the tooth pulp

K. Fill in the classification for each drug description, then match the brand name.

Drug Description	Classification	Brand Name
1. _____ Controls diarrhea	_____	a. Pepcid
2. _____ Blocks stomach's ability to secrete acid	_____	b. Obezine
3. _____ Induces vomiting	_____	c. Metamucil
4. _____ Treats motion sickness	_____	d. Compazine
5. _____ Blocks acid-producing receptors	_____	e. Maalox
6. _____ Suppresses appetite	_____	f. Ipecac syrup
7. _____ Stimulates a bowel movement	_____	g. Imodium
8. _____ Neutralizes stomach acid	_____	h. Nexium

Medical Record Analysis

Below is an item from a patient's medical record. Read it carefully, make sure you understand all the medical terms used, and then answer the questions that follow.

Gastroenterology Consultation Report

Reason for Consultation:	Evaluation of recurrent epigastric and LUQ pain with anemia.
History of Present Illness:	Patient is a 56-year-old male. He reports a long history of mild dyspepsia characterized by burning epigastric pain, especially when his stomach is empty. This pain has been relieved by over-the-counter antacids. Approximately two weeks ago, the pain became significantly worse; he is also nauseated and has vomited several times.
Past Medical History:	Patient's history is not significant for other digestive system disorders. He had a tonsillectomy at age 8. He sustained a compound fracture of the left ankle in a bicycle accident at age 11 that required surgical fixation. More recently he has been diagnosed with an enlarged prostate gland, and surgery has been recommended. However, he would like to resolve this epigastric pain before going forward with the TUR.
Results of Physical Examination:	CBC indicates anemia, and a fecal occult blood test is positive for blood in the feces. A blood test for *Helicobacter pylori* is positive. Erosion in the gastric lining was visualized on an upper GI. Follow-up gastroscopy found evidence of mild reflux esophagitis and an ulcerated lesion in the lining of the pyloric section of the stomach. This ulcer is 1.5 cm in diameter and deep. There is evidence of active bleeding from the ulcer. Multiple biopsies were taken, and they were negative for gastric cancer. IV Tagamet relieved the painful symptoms in two days.
Assessment:	Peptic ulcer. Gastric cancer has been ruled out in light of the negative biopsies.
Recommendations:	A gastrectomy to remove the ulcerated portion of stomach is indicated because the ulcer is already bleeding. Patient should continue on Tagamet to reduce stomach acid. Two medications will be added: Keflex to treat the bacterial infection and iron pills to reverse the anemia. Patient was instructed to eat frequent small meals and avoid alcohol and irritating foods.

Critical Thinking Questions

1. This patient reports LUQ pain. What does LUQ stand for and what organs do you find there? _____
_____

2. This patient had two diagnostic tests that indicated he was losing blood. Name these two tests and then describe them in your own words. _____
_____
_____

3. This patient had a procedure to visually examine the ulcer. Name the procedure and then describe in your own words what the physician observed. _____
_____
_____

4. Name the serious pathological condition that was ruled out. _____

5. Which of the following is NOT a recommendation of the consulting physician?
   a. medication to reduce stomach acid
   b. surgical removal of a portion of the stomach
   c. an antibiotic
   d. blood transfusion

6. Briefly describe this patient's past medical history in your own words. _____
_____

Chart Note Transcription

The chart note below contains twelve phrases that can be reworded with a medical term that you learned in this chapter. Each phrase is identified with an underline. Determine the medical term and write your answers in the space provided.

Current Complaint: Patient is a 74-year-old female seen by a <u>physician who specializes in the treatment of the gastrointestinal tract</u> ❶ with complaints of severe lower abdominal pain and extreme <u>difficulty with having a bowel movement</u>. ❷

Past History: Patient has a history of the <u>presence of gallstones</u> ❸, requiring a <u>surgical removal of the gallbladder</u> ❹ ten years ago and chronic <u>acid backing up from the stomach into the esophagus.</u> ❺

Signs and Symptoms: The patient's abdomen is distended with <u>fluid collecting in the abdominal cavity.</u> ❻ <u>X-ray of the colon after inserting barium dye with an enema</u> ❼ revealed <u>the presence of multiple small tumors growing on a stalk</u> ❽ throughout the colon. <u>Visual examination of the colon by a scope inserted through the rectum</u>❾ was performed, and biopsies taken for microscopic examination located a tumor.

Diagnosis: Carcinoma of the section of colon between <u>the descending colon and the rectum.</u> ❿

Treatment: <u>Surgical removal of the colon</u> ⓫ between the descending colon and the rectum with <u>the surgical creation of an opening of the colon through the abdominal wall.</u> ⓬

❶ _____

❷ _____

❸ _____

❹ _____

❺ _____

❻ _____

❼ _____

❽ _____

❾ _____

❿ _____

⓫ _____

⓬ _____

Labeling Exercise

A. System Review
Write the labels for this figure on the numbered lines provided.

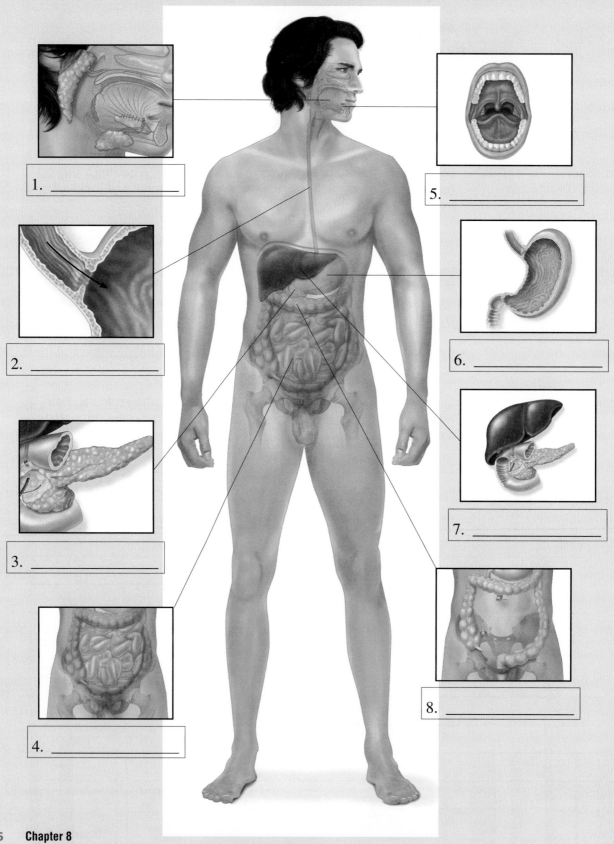

1. _____

2. _____

3. _____

4. _____

5. _____

6. _____

7. _____

8. _____

B. Anatomy Challenge

1. Write the labels for this figure on the numbered lines provided.

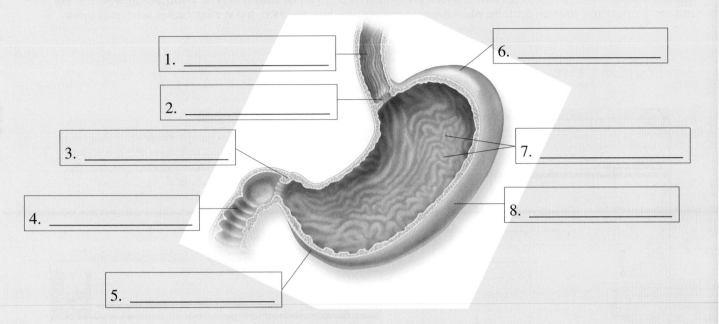

1. _____

2. _____

3. _____

4. _____

5. _____

6. _____

7. _____

8. _____

2. Write the labels for this figure on the numbered lines provided.

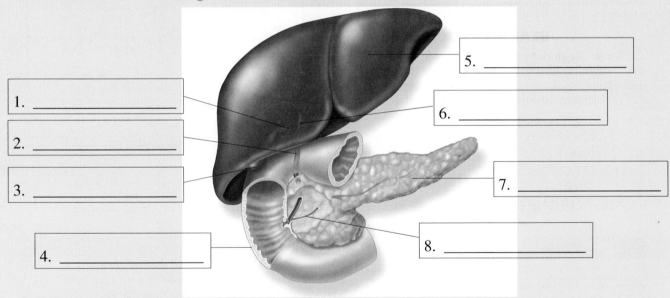

1. _____

2. _____

3. _____

4. _____

5. _____

6. _____

7. _____

8. _____

Multimedia Preview

Additional interactive resources and activities for this chapter can be found on the Companion Website. For videos, games, and pronunciations, please access the accompanying DVD-ROM that comes with this book.

DVD-ROM Highlights

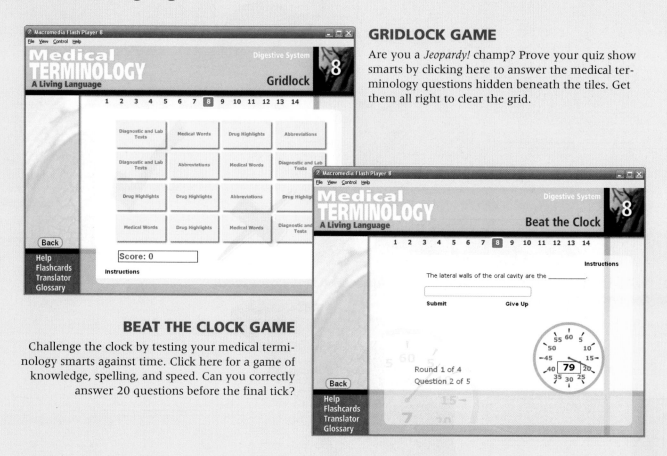

GRIDLOCK GAME

Are you a *Jeopardy!* champ? Prove your quiz show smarts by clicking here to answer the medical terminology questions hidden beneath the tiles. Get them all right to clear the grid.

BEAT THE CLOCK GAME

Challenge the clock by testing your medical terminology smarts against time. Click here for a game of knowledge, spelling, and speed. Can you correctly answer 20 questions before the final tick?

Website Highlights—www.prenhall.com/fremgen

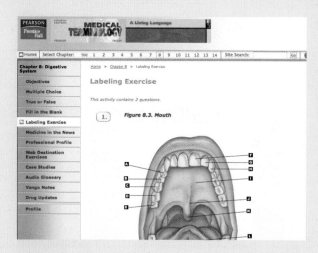

LABELING EXERCISE

Click here and take advantage of the free-access on-line study guide that accompanies your textbook. You'll find a figure labeling quiz that corresponds to this chapter. By clicking on this URL you'll also access links to download mp3 audio reviews, current news articles, and an audio glossary.

9 Urinary System

Learning Objectives

Upon completion of this chapter, you will be able to:

- Identify and define the combining forms and suffixes introduced in this chapter.
- Correctly spell and pronounce medical terms and major anatomical structures relating to the urinary system.
- Locate and describe the major organs of the urinary system and their functions.
- Describe the nephron and the mechanisms of urine production.
- Identify the characteristics of urine and a urinalysis.
- Build and define urinary system medical terms from word parts.
- Identify and define urinary system vocabulary terms.
- Identify and define selected urinary system pathology terms.
- Identify and define selected urinary system diagnostic procedures.
- Identify and define selected urinary system therapeutic procedures.
- Identify and define selected medications relating to the urinary system.
- Define selected abbreviations associated with the urinary system.

Urinary System at a Glance

Function

The urinary system is responsible for maintaining a stable internal environment for the body. In order to achieve this state, the urinary system removes waste products, adjusts water and electrolyte levels, and maintains the correct pH.

Organs

kidneys
ureters
urethra
urinary bladder

Combining Forms

azot/o	nitrogenous waste	**noct/i**	night
bacteri/o	bacteria	**olig/o**	scanty
cyst/o	urinary bladder	**pyel/o**	renal pelvis
glomerul/o	glomerulus	**ren/o**	kidney
glycos/o	sugar, glucose	**ur/o**	urine
keton/o	ketones	**ureter/o**	ureter
lith/o	stone	**urethr/o**	urethra
meat/o	meatus	**urin/o**	urine
nephr/o	kidney		

Suffixes

-lith	stone
-lithiasis	condition of stones
-ptosis	drooping
-tripsy	surgical crushing
-uria	condition of the urine

Urinary System Illustrated

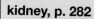

kidney, p. 282

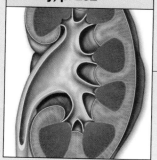

Filters blood and
produces urine

urinary bladder, p. 284

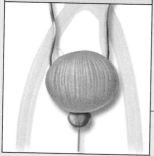

Stores urine

female urethra, p. 285

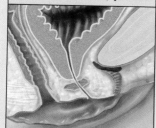

Transports urine to exterior

ureter, p. 283

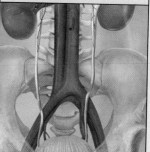

Transports urine to the bladder

male urethra, p. 285

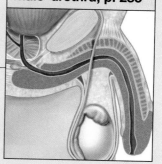

Transports urine to exterior

Anatomy and Physiology of the Urinary System

genitourinary system
  (jen-ih-toh-YOO-rih-nair-ee)

kidneys

nephrons (NEF-ronz)

uremia (yoo-REE-mee-ah)

ureters (yoo-REE-ters)

urethra (yoo-REE-thrah)

urinary bladder (YOO-rih-nair-ee)

urine (YOO-rin)

Think of the urinary system, sometimes referred to as the **genitourinary (GU) system**, as similar to a water filtration plant. Its main function is to filter and remove waste products from the blood. These waste materials result in the production and excretion of **urine** from the body.

The urinary system is one of the hardest working systems of the body. All the body's metabolic processes result in the production of waste products. These waste products are a natural part of life but quickly become toxic if they are allowed to build up in the blood, resulting in a condition called **uremia**. Waste products in the body are removed through a very complicated system of blood vessels and kidney tubules. The actual filtration of wastes from the blood takes place in millions of **nephrons**, which make up each of your two **kidneys**. As urine drains from each kidney, the **ureters** transport it to the **urinary bladder**. We are constantly producing urine, and our bladders can hold about one quart of this liquid. When the urinary bladder empties, urine moves from the bladder down the **urethra** to the outside of the body.

Kidneys

calyx (KAY-liks)

cortex (KOR-teks)

hilum (HIGH-lum)

medulla (meh-DULL-ah)

renal artery

renal papilla (pah-PILL-ah)

renal pelvis

renal pyramids

renal vein

retroperitoneal (ret-roh-pair-ih-toh-NEE-al)

The two kidneys are located in the lumbar region of the back above the waist on either side of the vertebral column. They are not inside the peritoneal sac, a location referred to as **retroperitoneal**. Each kidney has a concave or indented area on the edge toward the center that gives the kidney its bean shape. The center of this concave area is called the **hilum**. The hilum is where the **renal artery** enters and the **renal vein** leaves the kidney (see Figure 9.1 ■). The renal artery delivers the blood that is full of waste products to the kidney and the renal vein returns the now cleansed blood to the general circulation. The ureters also leave the kidneys at the hilum. The ureters are narrow tubes that lead from the kidneys to the bladder.

When a surgeon cuts into a kidney, several structures or areas are visible. The outer portion, called the **cortex**, is much like a shell for the kidney. The inner area is called the **medulla**. Within the medulla are a dozen or so triangular-shaped areas, the **renal pyramids**, which resemble their namesake, the Egyptian pyramids. The tip of each pyramid points inward toward the hilum. At its tip, called the **renal papilla**, each pyramid opens into a **calyx** (plural is *calyces*), which is continuous with the **renal pelvis**. The calyces and ultimately the renal pelvis collect urine as it is formed. The ureter for each kidney arises from the renal pelvis (see Figure 9.2 ■).

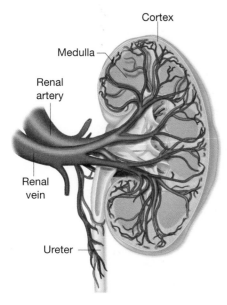

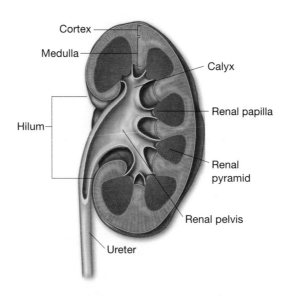

■ **Figure 9.1** Kidney structure. Longitudinal section showing the renal artery entering and the renal vein and ureter exiting at the hilum of the kidney.

■ **Figure 9.2** Longitudinal section of a kidney illustrating the internal structures.

Nephrons

afferent arteriole (AFF-er-ent)
Bowman's capsule
collecting tubule
distal convoluted tubule
      (DISS-tall con-voh-LOOT-ed)
efferent arteriole (EF-er-ent)
glomerular capsule (glom-AIR-yoo-lar)

glomerulus (glom-AIR-yoo-lus)
loop of Henle
proximal convoluted tubule
      (PROK-sim-al con-voh-LOOT-ed)
renal corpuscle (KOR-pus-ehl)
renal tubule

The functional or working unit of the kidney is the nephron. There are more than one million of these microscopic structures in each human kidney.

Each nephron consists of the **renal corpuscle** and the **renal tubule** (see Figure 9.3 ■). The renal corpuscle is the blood-filtering portion of the nephron. It has a double-walled cuplike structure called the **glomerular** or **Bowman's capsule** (also called the *glomerular capsule*) that encases a ball of capillaries called the **glomerulus**. An **afferent arteriole** carries blood to the glomerulus, and an **efferent arteriole** carries blood away from the glomerulus.

Water and substances that were removed from the bloodstream in the renal corpuscle flow into the renal tubules to finish the urine production process. This continuous tubule is divided into four sections: the **proximal convoluted tubule**, followed by the narrow **loop of Henle** (also called the *nephron loop*), then the **distal convoluted tubule**, and finally the **collecting tubule.**

Ureters

As urine drains out of the renal pelvis it enters the ureter, which carries it down to the urinary bladder (see Figure 9.4 ■). Ureters are very narrow tubes measuring less than 1/4 inch wide and 10 to 12 inches long that extend from the renal pelvis to the urinary bladder. Mucous membrane lines the ureters just as it lines most passages that open to the external environment.

Med Term Tip

Afferent, meaning moving toward, and *efferent*, meaning moving away from, are terms used when discussing moving either toward or away from the central point in many systems. For example, there are afferent and efferent nerves in the nervous system.

Med Term Tip

The terms *ureter* and *urethra* are frequently confused. Remember that there are two ureters carrying urine from the kidneys into the bladder. There is only one urethra, and it carries urine from the bladder to the outside of the body.

Figure 9.3 The structure of a nephron, illustrating the nephron structure in relation to the circulatory system.

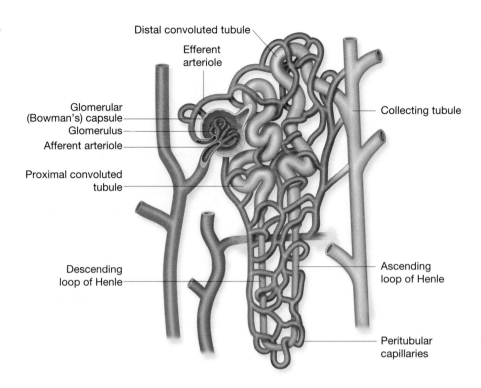

Urinary Bladder

external sphincter (SFINGK-ter)   **rugae** (ROO-gay)
internal sphincter   **urination**

The urinary bladder is an elastic muscular sac that lies in the base of the pelvis just behind the pubic symphysis (see Figure 9.5 ■). It is composed of three layers of smooth muscle tissue lined with mucous membrane containing **rugae** or folds that allow it to stretch. The bladder receives the urine directly from the ureters, stores it, and excretes it by **urination** through the urethra.

Generally, an adult bladder will hold 250 mL of urine. This amount then creates an urge to void or empty the bladder. Involuntary muscle action causes the bladder to contract and the **internal sphincter** to relax. The internal sphincter protects us from having our bladder empty at the wrong time. Voluntary action controls the **external sphincter**, which opens on demand to allow the intentional emptying of the bladder. The act of controlling the emptying of urine is developed sometime after a child is 2 years of age.

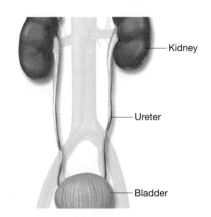

Figure 9.4 The ureters extend from the kidneys to the urinary bladder.

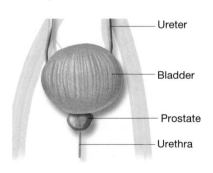

Figure 9.5 The structure of the urinary bladder in a male. (Note the prostate gland.)

Urethra

urinary meatus (mee-AY-tus)

The urethra is a tubular canal that carries the flow of urine from the bladder to the outside of the body (see Figure 9.6 ■ for the male urethra). The external opening through which urine passes out of the body is called the **urinary meatus**. Mucous membrane also lines the urethra as it does other structures of the urinary system. This is one of the reasons that infection spreads up the urinary tract. The urethra is 1½ inches long in the female and 8 inches long in the male. In a woman it functions only as the outlet for urine and is in front of the vagina. In the male, however, it has two functions: an outlet for urine and the passageway for semen to leave the body.

Role of Kidneys in Homeostasis

electrolytes (ee-LEK-troh-lites)   **homeostasis** (hoh-mee-oh-STAY-sis)

The kidneys are responsible for **homeostasis** or balance in your body. They continually adjust the chemical conditions in the body that allow you to survive. Because of its interaction with the bloodstream and its ability to excrete substances from the body, the urinary system maintains the body's proper balance of water and chemicals. If the body is low on water, the kidneys conserve it, or in the opposite case, if there is excess water in the body, the kidneys excrete the excess. In addition to water, the kidneys regulate the level of **electrolytes**—small biologically important molecules such as sodium (Na^+), potassium (K^+), chloride (Cl^-), and bicarbonate (HCO_3^-). Finally, the kidneys play an important role in maintaining the correct pH range within the body, making sure we do not become too acidic or too alkaline. The kidneys accomplish these important tasks through the production of urine.

Stages of Urine Production

filtration   **reabsorption**
glomerular filtrate   **secretion**
peritubular capillaries

As wastes and unnecessary substances are removed from the bloodstream by the nephrons, many desirable molecules are also removed initially. Waste products are eliminated from the body, but other substances such as water, electrolytes, and nutrients must be returned to the bloodstream. Urine, in its final form ready for elimination from the body, is the ultimate product of this entire process.

> **Med Term Tip**
>
> Mucous membranes will carry infections up the urinary tract from the urinary meatus and urethra into the bladder and eventually up the ureters and the kidneys if not stopped. It is never wise to ignore a simple bladder infection or what is called *cystitis*.

> **Med Term Tip**
>
> The amount of water and other fluids processed by the kidneys each day is astonishing. Approximately 190 quarts of fluid are filtered out of the glomerular blood every day. Most of this fluid returns to the body through the reabsorption process. About 99 percent of the water that leaves the blood each day through the filtration process returns to the blood by proximal tubule reabsorption.

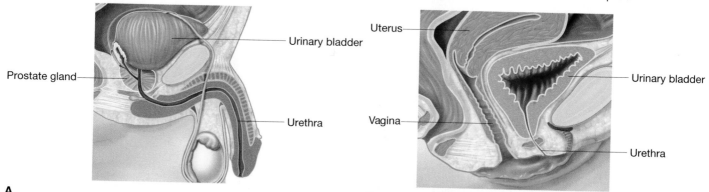

A.   **B.**

■ **Figure 9.6** A) The male urethra extends from the urinary bladder in the floor of the pelvis through the prostate gland and penis to the urinary meatus. B) The much shorter female urethra extends from the urinary bladder to the floor of the pelvis and exits just in front of the vaginal opening.

Urine production occurs in three stages: **filtration**, **reabsorption**, and **secretion**. Each of these steps is performed by a different section of the nephrons (see Figure 9.7 ■).

1. **Filtration.** The first stage is the filtering of particles, which occurs in the renal corpuscle. The pressure of blood flowing through the glomerulus forces material out of the bloodstream, through the wall of Bowman's capsule, and into the renal tubules. This fluid in the tubules is called the **glomerular filtrate** and consists of water, electrolytes, nutrients such as glucose and amino acids, wastes, and toxins.

2. **Reabsorption.** After filtration, the filtrate passes through the four sections of the tubule. As the filtrate moves along its twisted journey, most of the water and much of the electrolytes and nutrients are reabsorbed into the **peritubular capillaries**, a capillary bed that surrounds the renal tubules. They can then reenter the circulating blood.

3. **Secretion.** The final stage of urine production occurs when the special cells of the renal tubules secrete ammonia, uric acid, and other waste substances directly into the renal tubule. Urine formation is now finished; it passes into the collecting tubules, renal papilla, calyx, renal pelvis, and ultimately into the ureter.

Urine

albumin (al-BEW-min)
nitrogenous wastes (nigh-TROJ-eh-nus)

specific gravity
urinalysis (yoo-rih-NAL-ih-sis)

Urine is normally straw colored to clear, and sterile. Although it is 95 percent water, it also contains many dissolved substances, such as electrolytes, toxins, and **nitrogenous wastes**, the byproducts of muscle metabolism. At times the urine also contains substances that should not be there, such as glucose, blood, or **albumin**, a protein that should remain in the blood. This is the reason for performing a **urinalysis**, a physical and chemical analysis of urine, which gives medical personnel important information regarding disease processes occurring in a patient.

■ **Figure 9.7** The three stages of urine production: filtration, reabsorption, and secretion.

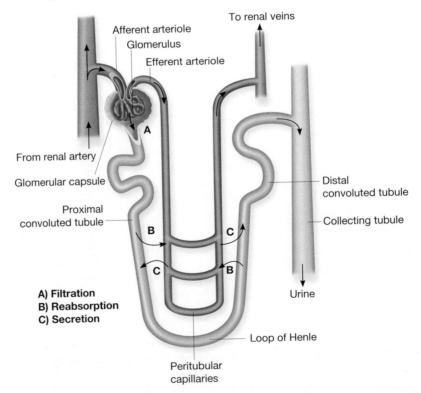

A) Filtration
B) Reabsorption
C) Secretion

Normally, during a 24-hour period the output of urine will be 1,000 to 2,000 mL, depending on the amount of fluid consumed and the general health of the person. Normal urine is acidic because this is one way our bodies dispose of excess acids. **Specific gravity** indicates the amount of dissolved substances in urine. The specific gravity of pure water is 1.000. The specific gravity of urine varies from 1.005 to 1.030. Highly concentrated urine has a higher specific gravity, while the specific gravity of very dilute urine is close to that of water. See Table 9.1 ■ for the normal values for urine testing and Table 9.2 ■ for abnormal findings.

Med Term Tip

The color, odor, volume, and sugar content of urine have been examined for centuries. Color charts for urine were developed by 1140, and "taste testing" was common in the late seventeenth century. By the nineteenth century, urinalysis was a routine part of a physical examination.

Table 9.1 — Values for Urinalysis Testing

ELEMENT	NORMAL FINDINGS
Color	Straw colored, pale yellow to deep gold
Odor	Aromatic
Appearance	Clear
Specific gravity	1.005–1.030
pH	5.0–8.0
Protein	Negative to trace
Glucose	None
Ketones	None
Blood	Negative

Table 9.2 — Abnormal Urinalysis Findings

ELEMENT	IMPLICATIONS
Color	Color varies depending on the patient's fluid intake and output or medication. Brown or black urine color indicates a serious disease process.
Odor	A fetid or foul odor may indicate infection. For instance, a fruity odor may be found in diabetes mellitus, dehydration, or starvation. Other odors may be due to medication or foods.
Appearance	Cloudiness may mean that an infection is present.
Specific gravity	Concentrated urine has a higher specific gravity. Dilute urine, such as can be found with diabetes insipidus, acute tubular necrosis, or salt-restricted diets, has a lower specific gravity.
pH	A pH value below 7.0 (acidic) is common in urinary tract infections, metabolic or respiratory acidosis, diets high in fruits or vegetables, or administration of some drugs. A pH higher than 7.0 (basic or alkaline) is common in metabolic or respiratory alkalosis, fever, high-protein diets, and taking ascorbic acid.
Protein	Protein may indicate glomerulonephritis or preeclampsia in a pregnant woman.
Glucose	Small amounts of glucose may be present as the result of eating a high-carbohydrate meal, stress, pregnancy, and taking some medications, such as aspirin or corticosteroids. Higher levels may indicate poorly controlled diabetes, Cushing's syndrome, or infection.
Ketones	The presence of ketones may indicate poorly controlled diabetes, dehydration, starvation, or ingestion of large amounts of aspirin.
Blood	Blood may indicate some types of anemia, taking of some medications (such as blood thinners), arsenic poisoning, reactions to transfusion, trauma, burns, and convulsions.

Word Building

The following list contains examples of medical terms built directly from word parts. The definition for these terms can be determined by a straightforward translation of the word parts.

COMBINING FORM	COMBINED WITH	MEDICAL TERM	DEFINITION
cyst/o	-algia	**cystalgia** (sis-TAL-jee-ah)	bladder pain

> **Med Term Tip**
>
> Word watch—Be careful using the combining forms *cyst/o* meaning "bladder" and *cyt/o* meaning "cell."

COMBINING FORM	COMBINED WITH	MEDICAL TERM	DEFINITION
	-ectomy	**cystectomy** (sis-TEK-toh-me)	removal of the bladder
	-gram	**cystogram** (SIS-toh-gram)	record of the bladder
	-ic	**cystic** (SIS-tik)	pertaining to the bladder
	-itis	**cystitis** (sis-TYE-tis)	bladder inflammation
	-lith	**cystolith** (SIS-toh-lith)	bladder stone
	-ostomy	**cystostomy** (sis-TOSS-toh-mee)	create a new opening into the bladder
	-otomy	**cystotomy** (sis-TOT-oh-mee)	incision into the bladder
	-pexy	**cystopexy** (SIS-toh-pek-see)	surgical fixation of the bladder
	-plasty	**cystoplasty** (SIS-toh-plas-tee)	surgical repair of the bladder
	-rrhagia	**cystorrhagia** (sis-toh-RAH-jee-ah)	rapid bleeding from the bladder
	-scope	**cystoscope** (SIS-toh-scope)	instrument used to visually examine the bladder
lith/o	-tripsy	**lithotripsy** (LITH-oh-trip-see)	surgical crushing of a stone
	-otomy	**lithotomy** (lith-OT-oh-me)	incision to remove a stone
nephr/o	-ectomy	**nephrectomy** (ne-FREK-toh-mee)	removal of a kidney
	-gram	**nephrogram** (NEH-fro-gram)	x-ray of the kidney
	-itis	**nephritis** (neh-FRYE-tis)	kidney inflammation
	-lith	**nephrolith** (NEF-roh-lith)	kidney stone
	-logist	**nephrologist** (neh-FROL-oh-jist)	specialist in the kidney
	-malacia	**nephromalacia** (nef-roh-mah-LAY-she-ah)	softening of the kidney
	-megaly	**nephromegaly** (nef-roh-MEG-ah-lee)	enlarged kidney
	-oma	**nephroma** (neh-FROH-ma)	kidney tumor
	-osis	**nephrosis** (neh-FROH-sis)	abnormal kidney condition
	-ptosis	**nephroptosis** (nef-rop-TOH-sis)	drooping kidney
	-ostomy	**nephrostomy** (neh-FROS-toh-mee)	create a new opening into the kidney
	-otomy	**nephrotomy** (neh-FROT-oh-mee)	incision into a kidney

Word Building *(continued)*

COMBINING FORM	COMBINED WITH	MEDICAL TERM	DEFINITION
	-pathy	**nephropathy** (neh-FROP-ah-thee)	kidney disease
	-pexy	**nephropexy** (NEF-roh-pek-see)	surgical fixation of kidney
	-lithiasis	**nephrolithiasis** (nef-roh-lith-EE-a-sis)	condition of kidney stones
	-sclerosis	**nephrosclerosis** (nef-roh-skleh-ROH-sis)	hardening of the kidney
pyel/o	-gram	**pyelogram** (PYE-eh-loh-gram)	x-ray record of the renal pelvis
	-itis	**pyelitis** (pye-eh-LYE-tis)	renal pelvis inflammation
	-plasty	**pyeloplasty** (PIE-ah-loh-plas-tee)	surgical repair of the renal pelvis
ren/o	-al	**renal** (REE-nal)	pertaining to the kidney
ur/o	-logist	**urologist** (yoo-RALL-oh-jist)	specialist in urine
	-emia	**uremia** (yoo-REE-mee-ah)	blood condition of urine
ureter/o	-al	**ureteral** (yoo-REE-ter-all)	pertaining to the ureter

Med Term Tip

Word watch—Be particularly careful when using the three very similar combining forms: *uter/o* meaning "uterus," *ureter/o* meaning "ureter," and *urethr/o* meaning "urethra."

	-ectasis	**ureterectasis** (yoo-ree-ter-EK-tah-sis)	ureter dilation
	-lith	**ureterolith** (yoo-REE-teh-roh-lith)	ureter stone
	-stenosis	**ureterostenosis** (yoo-ree-ter-oh-sten-OH-sis)	narrowing of a ureter
urethr/o	-al	**urethral** (yoo-REE-thral)	pertaining to the urethra
	-algia	**urethralgia** (yoo-ree-THRAL-jee-ah)	urethra pain
	-itis	**urethritis** (yoo-ree-THRIGH-tis)	urethra inflammation
	-rrhagia	**urethrorrhagia** (yoo-ree-throh-RAH-jee-ah)	rapid bleeding from the urethra
	-scope	**urethroscope** (yoo-REE-throh-scope)	instrument to visually examine the urethra
	-stenosis	**urethrostenosis** (yoo-ree-throh-steh-NOH-sis)	narrowing of the urethra
urin/o	-meter	**urinometer** (yoo-rin-OH-meter)	instrument to measure urine
	-ary	**urinary** (yoo-rih-NAIR-ee)	pertaining to urine

SUFFIX	COMBINED WITH	MEDICAL TERM	DEFINITION
-uria	an-	**anuria** (an-YOO-ree-ah)	condition of no urine
	bacteri/o	**bacteriuria** (back-teer-ree-YOO-ree-ah)	bacteria in the urine

Word Building (continued)

SUFFIX	COMBINED WITH	MEDICAL TERM	DEFINITION
dys-		**dysuria** (dis-YOO-ree-ah)	condition of difficult or painful urination
	glycos/o	**glycosuria** (glye-kohs-YOO-ree-ah)	condition of sugar in the urine
	hemat/o	**hematuria** (hee-mah-TOO-ree-ah)	condition of blood in the urine
	keton/o	**ketonuria** (key-tone-YOO-ree-ah)	ketones in the urine
	noct/i	**nocturia** (nok-TOO-ree-ah)	condition of frequent nighttime urination
	olig/o	**oliguria** (ol-ig-YOO-ree-ah)	condition of scanty amount of urine
poly-		**polyuria** (pol-ee-YOO-ree-ah)	condition of (too) much urine
	protein	**proteinuria** (pro-ten-YOO-ree-ah)	protein in the urine
	py/o	**pyuria** (pye-YOO-ree-ah)	condition of pus in the urine

Vocabulary

TERM	DEFINITION
anuria (an-YOO-ree-ah)	Complete suppression of urine formed by the kidneys and a complete lack of urine excretion.
azotemia (a-zo-TEE-mee-ah)	Accumulation of nitrogenous waste in the bloodstream. Occurs when the kidney fails to filter these wastes from the blood.
calculus (KAL-kew-lus)	Stone formed within an organ by an accumulation of mineral salts. Found in the kidney, renal pelvis, ureters, bladder, or urethra. Plural is *calculi* (see Figure 9.8 ■).
catheter (KATH-eh-ter)	Flexible tube inserted into the body for the purpose of moving fluids into or out of the body. Most commonly used to refer to a tube threaded through the urethra into the bladder to withdraw urine (see Figure 9.9 ■).

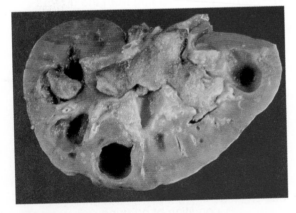

■ **Figure 9.8** Photograph of sectioned kidney specimen illustrating extensive renal calculi.
(Dr. E. Walker/Science Photo Library/Photo Researchers, Inc.)

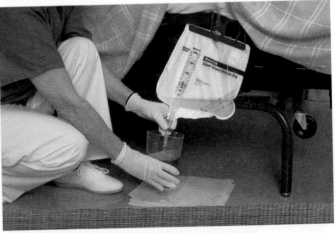

■ **Figure 9.9** Healthcare worker draining urine from a urinary catheter bag.

Vocabulary (continued)

TERM	DEFINITION
diuresis (dye-yoo-REE-sis)	Increased formation and secretion of urine.
enuresis (en-yoo-REE-sis)	Involuntary discharge of urine after the age by which bladder control should have been established. This usually occurs by the age of 5. *Nocturnal enuresis* refers to bed-wetting at night.
frequency	Greater-than-normal occurrence in the urge to urinate, without an increase in the total daily volume of urine. Frequency is an indication of inflammation of the bladder or urethra.
hesitancy	Decrease in the force of the urine stream, often with difficulty initiating the flow. It is often a symptom of a blockage along the urethra, such as an enlarged prostate gland.
micturition (mik-too-RIH-shun)	Another term for urination. **Med Term Tip** Terms such as *micturition*, *voiding*, and *urination* all mean basically the same thing—the process of releasing urine from the body.
nephrology (neh-FROL-oh-jee)	Branch of medicine involved in diagnosis and treatment of diseases and disorders of the kidney. Physician is a *nephrologist*.
renal colic (KOL-ik)	Pain caused by a kidney stone. Can be an excruciating pain and generally requires medical treatment.
stricture (STRIK-chur)	Narrowing of a passageway in the urinary system.
uremia (yoo-REE-me-ah)	Accumulation of waste products (especially nitrogenous wastes) in the bloodstream. Associated with renal failure.
urgency (ER-jen-see)	Feeling the need to urinate immediately.
urinary incontinence (in-CON-tin-ens)	Involuntary release of urine. In some patients an indwelling catheter is inserted into the bladder for continuous urine drainage (see Figure 9.9).
urinary retention	Inability to fully empty the bladder, often indicates a blockage in the urethra.
urology (yoo-RAL-oh-jee)	Branch of medicine involved in diagnosis and treatment of diseases and disorders of the urinary system (and male reproductive system). Physician is a *urologist*.
voiding	Another term for urination.

Pathology

TERM	DEFINITION
■ *Kidney*	
acute tubular necrosis (ATN) (ne-KROH-sis)	Damage to the renal tubules due to presence of toxins in the urine or to ischemia. Results in oliguria.
diabetic nephropathy (ne-FROH-path-ee)	Accumulation of damage to the glomerulus capillaries due to the chronic high blood sugars of diabetes mellitus.

Pathology (continued)

TERM	DEFINITION
glomerulonephritis (gloh-mair-yoo-loh-neh-FRYE-tis)	Inflammation of the kidney (primarily of the glomerulus). Since the glomerular membrane is inflamed, it becomes more permeable and will allow protein and blood cells to enter the filtrate. Results in protein in the urine (proteinuria) and hematuria.
hydronephrosis (high-droh-neh-FROH-sis)	Distention of the renal pelvis due to urine collecting in the kidney; often a result of the obstruction of a ureter.
nephrolithiasis (nef-roh-lith-EE-a-sis)	Presence of calculi in the kidney. Usually begins with the solidification of salts present in the urine.
nephrotic syndrome (NS)	Damage to the glomerulus resulting in protein appearing in the urine, proteinuria, and the corresponding decrease in protein in the bloodstream.
nephroptosis (nef-rop-TOH-sis)	Downward displacement of the kidney out of its normal location; commonly called a *floating kidney*.
polycystic kidneys (POL-ee-sis-tik)	Formation of multiple cysts within the kidney tissue. Results in the destruction of normal kidney tissue and uremia.

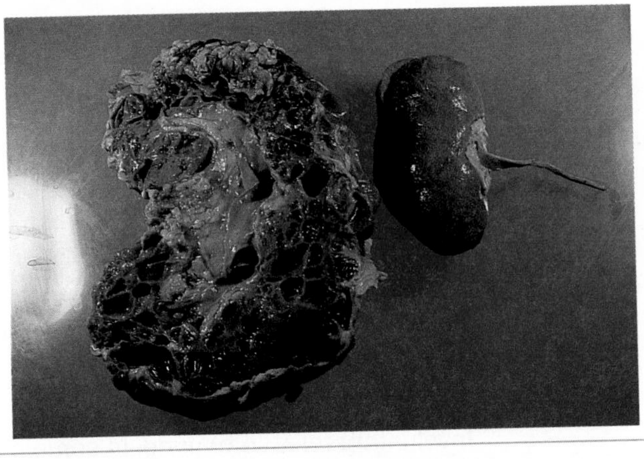

■ **Figure 9.10** Photograph of a polycystic kidney on the left compared to a normal kidney on the right.

(Simon Fraser/Royal Victoria Infirmary, Newcastle/Science Photo Library/Photo Researchers, Inc.)

pyelonephritis (pye-eh-loh-neh-FRYE-tis)	Inflammation of the renal pelvis and the kidney. One of the most common types of kidney disease. It may be the result of a lower urinary tract infection that moved up to the kidney by way of the ureters. There may be large quantities of white blood cells and bacteria in the urine. Blood (hematuria) may even be present in the urine in this condition. Can occur with any untreated or persistent case of cystitis.
renal cell carcinoma	Cancerous tumor that arises from kidney tubule cells.
renal failure	Inability of the kidneys to filter wastes from the blood resulting in uremia. May be acute or chronic. Major reason for a patient being placed on dialysis.
Wilm's tumor (VILMZ TOO-mor)	Malignant kidney tumor found most often in children.
■ *Urinary Bladder*	
bladder cancer	Cancerous tumor that arises from the cells lining the bladder; major sign is hematuria.
bladder neck obstruction (BNO)	Blockage of the bladder outlet. Often caused by an enlarged prostate gland in males.

Pathology *(continued)*

TERM	DEFINITION
cystocele (SIS-toh-seel)	Hernia or protrusion of the urinary bladder into the wall of the vagina.
interstitial cystitis (in-ter-STISH-al sis-TYE-tis)	Disease of unknown cause in which there is inflammation and irritation of the bladder. Most commonly seen in middle-aged women.
neurogenic bladder (noo-roh-JEN-ik)	Loss of nervous control that leads to retention; may be caused by spinal cord injury or multiple sclerosis.
urinary tract infection (UTI)	Infection, usually from bacteria, of any organ of the urinary system. Most often begins with cystitis and may ascend into the ureters and kidneys. Most common in women because of their shorter urethra.

Diagnostic Procedures

TERM	DEFINITION
■ *Clinical Laboratory Tests*	
blood urea nitrogen (BUN) (BLUD yoo-REE-ah NIGH-troh-jen)	Blood test to measure kidney function by the level of nitrogenous waste (urea) that is in the blood.
clean catch specimen (CC)	Urine sample obtained after cleaning off the urinary opening and catching or collecting a urine sample in midstream (halfway through the urination process) to minimize contamination from the genitalia.
creatinine clearance (kree-AT-tih-neen)	Test of kidney function. Creatinine is a waste product cleared from the bloodstream by the kidneys. For this test, urine is collected for 24 hours, and the amount of creatinine in the urine is compared to the amount of creatinine that remains in the bloodstream.
urinalysis (U/A, UA) (yoo-rih-NAL-ih-sis)	Laboratory test that consists of the physical, chemical, and microscopic examination of urine.
urine culture and sensitivity (C&S)	Laboratory test of urine for bacterial infection. Attempt to grow bacteria on a culture medium in order to identify it and determine which antibiotics it is sensitive to.
■ *Diagnostic Imaging*	
cystography (sis-TOG-rah-fee)	Process of instilling a contrast material or dye into the bladder by catheter to visualize the urinary bladder on x-ray.
excretory urography (EU) (EKS-kreh-tor-ee yoo-ROG-rah-fee)	Injecting dye into the bloodstream and then taking an x-ray to trace the action of the kidney as it excretes the dye.
intravenous pyelogram (IVP) (in-trah-VEE-nus PYE-eh-loh-gram)	Injecting a contrast medium into a vein and then taking an x-ray to visualize the renal pelvis.
kidneys, ureters, bladder (KUB)	X-ray taken of the abdomen demonstrating the kidneys, ureters, and bladder without using any contrast dye. Also called a *flat-plate abdomen*.

Diagnostic Prodedures *(continued)*

TERM	DEFINITION
retrograde pyelogram (RP) (RET-roh-grayd PYE-eh-loh-gram)	Diagnostic X-ray in which dye is inserted through the urethra to outline the bladder, ureters, and renal pelvis.

■ **Figure 9.11** Color enhanced retrograde pyelogram X-ray. Radiopaque dye outlines urinary bladder, ureters, and renal pelves. *(Clinique Ste. Catherine/CNRI/Science Photo Library/Photo Researchers, Inc.)*

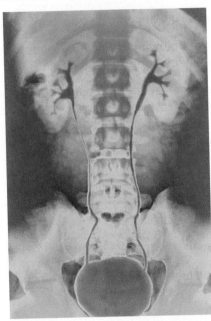

voiding cystourethrography (VCUG) (sis-toh-yoo-ree-THROG-rah-fee)	X-ray taken to visualize the urethra while the patient is voiding after a contrast dye has been placed in the bladder.

■ *Endoscopic Procedure*

cystoscopy (cysto) (sis-TOSS-koh-pee)	Visual examination of the urinary bladder using an instrument called a *cystoscope*.

 ## Therapeutic Procedures

TERM	DEFINITION

■ *Medical Treatments*

catheterization (cath) (kath-eh-ter-ih-ZAY-shun)	Insertion of a tube through the urethra and into the urinary bladder for the purpose of withdrawing urine or inserting dye.
extracorporeal shockwave lithotripsy (ESWL) (eks-trah-cor-POR-ee-al shock-wave LITH-oh-trip-see)	Use of ultrasound waves to break up stones. Process does not require invasive surgery (see Figure 9.12 ■).
hemodialysis (HD) (hee-moh-dye-AL-ih-sis)	Use of an artificial kidney machine that filters the blood of a person to remove waste products. Use of this technique in patients who have defective kidneys is lifesaving (see Figure 9.13 ■).

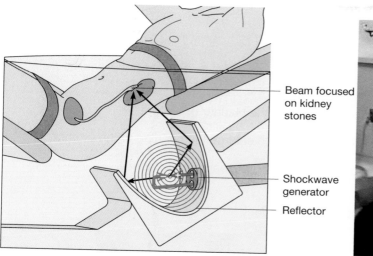

Beam focused
on kidney
stones

Shockwave
generator

Reflector

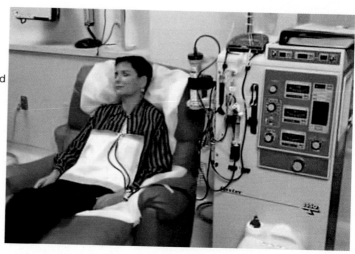

Figure 9.12 Extracorporeal shockwave lithotripsy, a non-invasive procedure using high frequency sound waves to shatter kidney stones.

Figure 9.13 Patient undergoing hemodialysis. Patient's blood passes through hemodialysis machine for cleansing and is then returned to her body.

 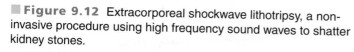

Therapeutic Procedures *(continued)*

TERM	DEFINITION
peritoneal dialysis (pair-ih-TOH-nee-al dye-AL-ih-sis)	Removal of toxic waste substances from the body by placing warm chemically balanced solutions into the peritoneal cavity. Wastes are filtered out of the blood across the peritoneum. Used in treating renal failure and certain poisonings.

Figure 9.14 Peritoneal dialysis. Chemically balanced solution is placed into the abdominal cavity to draw impurities out of the bloodstream. It is removed after several hours.

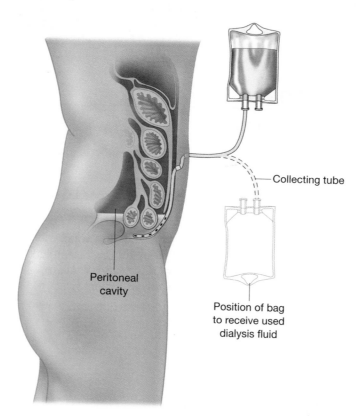

Collecting tube

Peritoneal
cavity

Position of bag
to receive used
dialysis fluid

Therapeutic Procedures *(continued)*

TERM	DEFINITION
■ Surgical Treatments	
lithotripsy (LITH-oh-trip-see)	Destroying or crushing stones in the bladder or urethra.
meatotomy (mee-ah-TOT-oh-me)	Incision into the meatus in order to enlarge the opening of the urethra.
nephrolithotomy (nef-roh-lith-OT-oh-mee)	Surgical incision to directly remove stones from the kidney.
renal transplant	Surgical placement of a donor kidney.

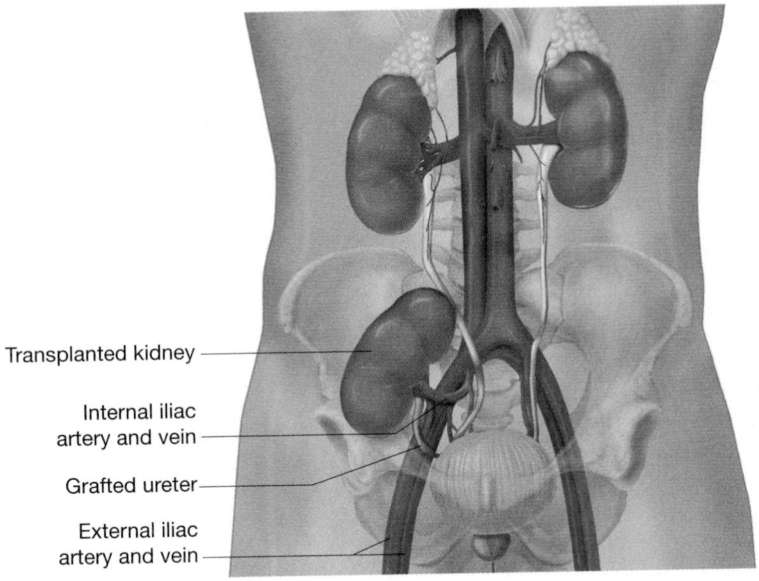

■ Figure 9.15 Figure illustrates location of transplanted donor kidney.

Transplanted kidney

Internal iliac artery and vein

Grafted ureter

External iliac artery and vein

Pharmacology

CLASSIFICATION	ACTION	GENERIC AND BRAND NAMES
antibiotic	Used to treat bacterial infections of the urinary tract.	ciprofloxacin, Cipro; nitrofurantoin, Macrobid
antispasmodic (an-tye-spaz-MAH-dik)	Medication to prevent or reduce bladder muscle spasms.	oxybutynin, Ditropan; neostigmine, Prostigmine
diuretic (dye-yoo-REH-tiks)	Medication that increases the volume of urine produced by the kidneys. Useful in the treatment of edema, kidney failure, heart failure, and hypertension.	furosemide, Lasix; spironolactone, Aldactone

Abbreviations

AGN	acute glomerulonephritis	HD	hemodialysis
ARF	acute renal failure	H_2O	water
ATN	acute tubular necrosis	I&O	intake and output
BNO	bladder neck obstruction	IPD	intermittent peritoneal dialysis
BUN	blood urea nitrogen	IVP	intravenous pyelogram
CAPD	continuous ambulatory peritoneal dialysis	K^+	potassium
cath	catheterization	KUB	kidney, ureter, bladder
CC	clean catch urine specimen	mL	milliliter
Cl^-	chloride	Na^+	sodium
CRF	chronic renal failure	NS	nephrotic syndrome
C&S	culture and sensitivity	pH	acidity or alkalinity of urine
cysto	cystoscopy	RP	retrograde pyelogram
ESRD	end-stage renal disease	SG, sp. gr.	specific gravity
ESWL	extracorporeal shockwave lithotripsy	U/A, UA	urinalysis
EU	excretory urography	UC	urine culture
GU	genitourinary	UTI	urinary tract infection
HCO_3^-	bicarbonate	VCUG	voiding cystourethrography

Chapter Review

Terminology Checklist

Below are all Anatomy and Physiology key terms, Word Building, Vocabulary, Pathology, Diagnostic, Therapeutic, and Pharmacology terms presented in this chapter. Use this list as a study tool by placing a check in the box in front of each term as you master its meaning.

- [ ] acute tubular necrosis
- [ ] afferent arteriole
- [ ] albumin
- [ ] antibiotic
- [ ] antispasmodic
- [ ] anuria
- [ ] azotemia
- [ ] bacteriuria
- [ ] bladder cancer
- [ ] bladder neck obstruction
- [ ] blood urea nitrogen
- [ ] Bowman's capsule
- [ ] calculus
- [ ] calyx
- [ ] catheter
- [ ] catheterization
- [ ] clean catch specimen
- [ ] collecting tubule
- [ ] cortex
- [ ] creatinine clearance
- [ ] cystalgia
- [ ] cystectomy
- [ ] cystic
- [ ] cystitis
- [ ] cystocele
- [ ] cystogram
- [ ] cystography
- [ ] cystolith
- [ ] cystopexy
- [ ] cystoplasty
- [ ] cystorrhagia
- [ ] cystoscope
- [ ] cystoscopy
- [ ] cystostomy
- [ ] cystotomy
- [ ] diabetic nephropathy
- [ ] distal convoluted tubule
- [ ] diuresis

- [ ] diuretic
- [ ] dysuria
- [ ] efferent arteriole
- [ ] electrolyte
- [ ] enuresis
- [ ] excretory urography
- [ ] external sphincter
- [ ] extracorporeal shockwave lithotripsy
- [ ] filtration
- [ ] frequency
- [ ] genitourinary system
- [ ] glomerular capsule
- [ ] glomerular filtrate
- [ ] glomerulonephritis
- [ ] glomerulus
- [ ] glycosuria
- [ ] hematuria
- [ ] hemodialysis
- [ ] hesitancy
- [ ] hilum
- [ ] homeostasis
- [ ] hydronephrosis
- [ ] internal sphincter
- [ ] interstitial cystitis
- [ ] intravenous pyelogram
- [ ] ketonuria
- [ ] kidneys
- [ ] kidneys, ureters, bladder
- [ ] lithotomy
- [ ] lithotripsy
- [ ] loop of Henle
- [ ] meatotomy
- [ ] medulla
- [ ] micturition
- [ ] nephrectomy
- [ ] nephritis
- [ ] nephrogram
- [ ] nephrolith

- [ ] nephrolithiasis
- [ ] nephrolithotomy
- [ ] nephrologist
- [ ] nephrology
- [ ] nephroma
- [ ] nephromalacia
- [ ] nephromegaly
- [ ] nephron
- [ ] nephropathy
- [ ] nephropexy
- [ ] nephroptosis
- [ ] nephrosclerosis
- [ ] nephrosis
- [ ] nephrostomy
- [ ] nephrotic syndrome
- [ ] nephrotomy
- [ ] neurogenic bladder
- [ ] nitrogenous wastes
- [ ] nocturia
- [ ] oliguria
- [ ] peritoneal dialysis
- [ ] peritubular capillaries
- [ ] polycystic kidneys
- [ ] polyuria
- [ ] proteinuria
- [ ] proximal convoluted tubule
- [ ] pyelitis
- [ ] pyelogram
- [ ] pyelonephritis
- [ ] pyeloplasty
- [ ] pyuria
- [ ] reabsorption
- [ ] renal
- [ ] renal artery
- [ ] renal cell carcinoma
- [ ] renal colic
- [ ] renal corpuscle
- [ ] renal failure

- ☐ renal papilla
- ☐ renal pelvis
- ☐ renal pyramid
- ☐ renal transplant
- ☐ renal tubule
- ☐ renal vein
- ☐ retrograde pyelogram
- ☐ retroperitoneal
- ☐ rugae
- ☐ secretion
- ☐ specific gravity
- ☐ stricture
- ☐ uremia
- ☐ ureteral

- ☐ ureterectasis
- ☐ ureterolith
- ☐ ureterostenosis
- ☐ ureters
- ☐ urethra
- ☐ urethral
- ☐ urethralgia
- ☐ urethritis
- ☐ urethrorrhagia
- ☐ urethroscope
- ☐ urethrostenosis
- ☐ urgency
- ☐ urinalysis
- ☐ urinary

- ☐ urinary bladder
- ☐ urinary incontinence
- ☐ urinary meatus
- ☐ urinary retention
- ☐ urinary tract infection
- ☐ urination
- ☐ urine
- ☐ urine culture and sensitivity
- ☐ urinometer
- ☐ urologist
- ☐ urology
- ☐ voiding
- ☐ voiding cystourethrography
- ☐ Wilm's tumor

Practice Exercises

A. Complete the following statements.

1. The functional or working units of the kidneys are the _____.

2. The three stages of urine production are _____, _____, and _____.

3. Na$^+$, K$^+$, and Cl$^-$ are collectively known as _____.

4. The term that describes the location of the kidneys is _____.

5. The center of the concave side of the kidney is the _____.

6. Bowman's capsule surrounds the _____.

7. The tip of each renal pyramid opens into a(n) _____.

8. There are _____ ureters and _____ urethra.

9. Urination can also be referred to as _____ or _____.

10. A(n) _____ is the physical and chemical analysis of urine.

B. State the terms described using the combining forms indicated.

The combining form *nephr/o* refers to the kidney. Use it to write a term that means:

1. surgical fixation of the kidney _____

2. x-ray record of the kidney _____

3. condition of kidney stones _____

4. removal of a kidney _____

5. inflammation of the kidney _____

6. kidney disease _____

7. hardening of the kidney _____

The combining form *cyst/o* refers to the urinary bladder. Use it to write a term that means:

8. inflammation of the bladder _____

9. rapid bleeding from the bladder _____

10. surgical repair of the bladder _____

11. instrument to view inside the bladder _____

12. bladder pain _____

The combining form *pyel/o* refers to the renal pelvis. Use it to write a term that means:

13. surgical repair of the renal pelvis _____

14. inflammation of the renal pelvis _____

15. X-ray record of the renal pelvis _____

The combining form *ureter/o* refers to one or both of the ureters. Use it to write a term that means:

16. a ureteral stone _____

17. ureter dilation _____

18. ureter narrowing _____

The combining form *urethr/o* refers to the urethra. Use it to write a term that means:

19. urethra inflammation _____

20. instrument to view inside the urethra _____

C. Define the following combining forms and use them to form urinary terms.

	Definition	Urinary Term
1. ur/o		
2. meat/o		
3. cyst/o		
4. ren/o		
5. pyel/o		
6. glycos/o		
7. noct/i		
8. olig/o		

9. ureter/o _____ _____

10. glomerul/o _____ _____

D. Define each suffix and use it to form urinary terms.

	Meaning	Urinary Term
1. -ptosis	_____	_____
2. -uria	_____	_____
3. -lith	_____	_____
4. -tripsy	_____	_____
5. -lithiasis	_____	_____

E. Define the following terms.

1. micturition _____

2. diuretic _____

3. renal colic _____

4. catheterization _____

5. pyelitis _____

6. glomerulonephritis _____

7. lithotomy _____

8. enuresis _____

9. meatotomy _____

10. diabetic nephropathy _____

11. urinalysis _____

12. hesitancy _____

F. Write the medical term that means:

1. absence of urine _____

2. blood in the urine _____

3. kidney stone _____

4. crushing a stone _____

5. inflammation of the urethra _____

6. pus in the urine _____

7. bacteria in the urine _____

8. painful urination _____

9. ketones in the urine _____

10. protein in the urine _____

11. (too) much urine _____

G. Write the abbreviation for the following terms.

1. potassium _____

2. sodium _____

3. urinalysis _____

4. blood urea nitrogen _____

5. specific gravity _____

6. intravenous pyelogram _____

7. bladder neck obstruction _____

8. intake and output _____

9. acute tubular necrosis _____

10. end stage renal disease _____

H. Identify the following abbreviations.

1. KUB _____

2. cath _____

3. cysto _____

4. GU _____

5. ESWL _____

6. UTI _____

7. UC _____

8. RP _____

9. ARF _____

10. BUN _____

11. CRF _____

12. H_2O _____

I. Match each term to its definition.

1. _____ Wilm's tumor

2. _____ electrolytes

3. _____ nephrons

a. kidney stones

b. feeling the need to urinate immediately

c. childhood malignant kidney tumor

4. _____ loop of Henle

5. _____ calyx

6. _____ incontinence

7. _____ hydronephrosis

8. _____ urgency

9. _____ nephrolithiasis

10. _____ polycystic kidneys

d. swelling of the kidney due to urine collecting in the renal pelvis

e. involuntary release of urine

f. collects urine as it is produced

g. sodium and potassium

h. functional unit of the kidneys

i. part of the renal tubule

j. multiple cysts in the kidneys

J. Use the following terms in the sentences below.

renal transplant   ureterectomy   intravenous pyelogram (IVP)

cystostomy   pyelolithectomy   nephropexy

renal biopsy   cystoscopy   urinary tract infection

1. Juan suffered from chronic renal failure. His sister, Maria, donated one of her normal kidneys to him, and he had a(n)

   _____.

2. Anesha's floating kidney needed surgical fixation. Her physician performed a surgical procedure known as

   _____.

3. Kenya's physician stated that she had a general infection that he referred to as a UTI. The full name for this infection is

   _____.

4. The surgeons operated on Robert to remove calculi from his renal pelvis. The name of this surgery is

   _____.

5. Charles had to have a small piece of his kidney tissue removed so that the physician could perform a microscopic evaluation. This procedure is called a(n) _____.

6. Naomi had to have one of her ureters removed due to a stricture. This procedure is called _____.

7. The physician had to create a temporary opening between Eric's bladder and his abdominal wall. This procedure is called

   _____.

8. Sally's bladder was visually examined using a special instrument. This procedure is called a(n) _____.

9. The doctors believe that Jacob has a tumor of the right kidney. They are going to do a test called a(n)

   _____ that requires them to inject a radiopaque contrast medium intravenously so that they can see the

   kidney on x-ray.

K. Fill in the classification for each drug description, then match the brand name.

Drug Description	Classification	Brand Name
1. _____ Reduces bladder muscle spasms	_____	a. Lasix
2. _____ Treats bacterial infections	_____	b. Ditropan
3. _____ Increases volume of urine produced	_____	c. Cipro

Medical Record Analysis

Below is an item from a patient's medical record. Read it carefully, make sure you understand all the medical terms used, and then answer the questions that follow.

Discharge Summary

Admitting Diagnosis:	Severe right side pain, visible blood in his urine.
Final Diagnosis:	Pyelonephritis right kidney, complicated by chronic cystitis.
History of Present Illness:	Patient has long history of frequent bladder infections, but denies any recent lower pelvic pain or dysuria. Earlier today he had rapid onset of severe right side pain and is unable to stand fully erect. His temperature was 101°F, and his skin was sweaty and flushed. He was admitted from the ER for further testing and diagnosis.
Summary of Hospital Course:	Clean catch urinalysis revealed gross hematuria and pyuria, but no albuminuria. A culture and sensitivity was ordered to identify the pathogen, and a broad-spectrum IV antibiotic was started. An intravenous pyelogram indicated no calculi or obstructions in the ureters. Cystoscopy showed evidence of chronic cystitis, bladder irritation, and a bladder neck obstruction. The obstruction appears to be congenital and the probable cause of the chronic cystitis. The patient was catheterized to ensure complete emptying of the bladder, and fluids were encouraged. Patient responded well to the antibiotic therapy and fluids, and his symptoms improved.
Discharge Plans:	Patient was discharged home after three days in the hospital. He was switched to an oral antibiotic for the pyelonephritis and chronic cystitis. A repeat urinalysis is scheduled for next week. After all inflammation is corrected, will repeat cystoscopy to reevaluate bladder neck obstruction. Will discuss urethroplasty if it is indicated at that time.

Critical Thinking Questions

1. This patient has a long history of frequent bladder infections. What did the physician discover that explained this? _____
_____

2. Describe, in your own words, the patient's condition when he came to the emergency room. _____
_____
_____

3. This patient has gross hematuria. What do you think the term *gross* means in this context? _____
_____
_____

4. The following terms are not referred to in this chapter. Define each in your own words, using your text as a dictionary.
   a. congenital _____
   b. chronic _____
   c. pathogen _____
   d. oral _____

5. Which of the following substances was not found in the patient's urine?
   a. protein
   b. pus
   c. blood

6. How are pyelonephritis and glomerulonephritis alike? How are they different?

   _____

   _____

   _____

Chart Note Transcription

The chart note below contains eleven phrases that can be reworded with a medical term that you learned in this chapter. Each phrase is identified with an underline. Determine the medical term and write your answers in the space provided.

Current Complaint:	A 36-year-old male was seen by the <u>specialist in the treatment of diseases of the urinary system</u> ❶ because of right flank pain and <u>blood in the urine</u>. ❷
Past History:	Patient has a history of <u>bladder infection</u>; ❸ denies experiencing any symptoms for two years.
Signs and Symptoms:	A <u>technique used to obtain an uncontaminated urine sample</u> ❹ obtained for <u>laboratory analysis of the urine</u> ❺ revealed blood in the urine, but no <u>pus in the urine</u>. ❻ A <u>kidney x-ray made after inserting dye into the bladder</u> ❼ was normal on the left, but dye was seen filling the right <u>tube between the kidney and bladder</u> ❽ only halfway to the kidney.
Diagnosis:	<u>Stone in the tube between the kidney and the bladder</u> ❾ on the right.
Treatment:	Patient underwent <u>the use of ultrasound waves to break up stones</u>.❿ Pieces of dissolved <u>kidney stones</u> ⓫ were flushed out, after which symptoms resolved.

❶ _____

❷ _____

❸ _____

❹ _____

❺ _____

❻ _____

❼ _____

❽ _____

❾ _____

❿ _____

⓫ _____

Labeling Exercise

A. System Review
Write the labels for this figure on the numbered lines provided.

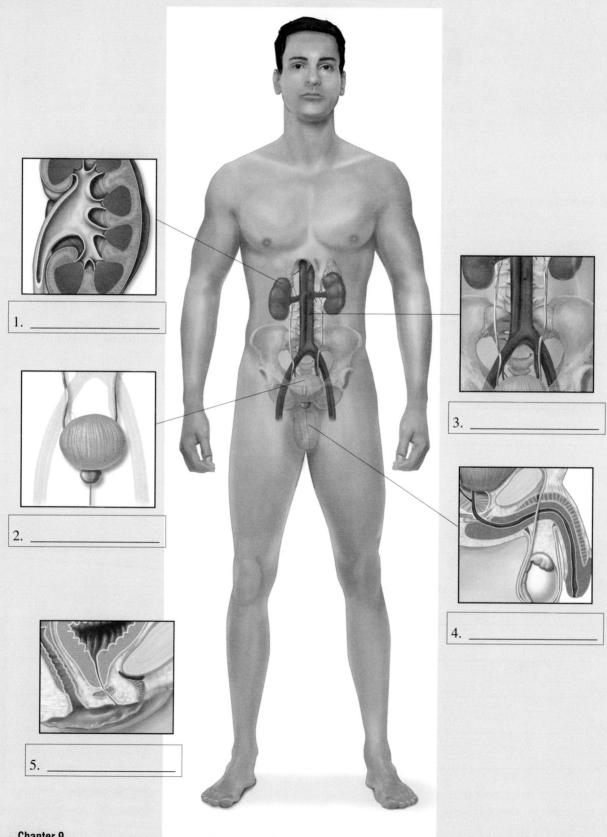

1. _____

2. _____

3. _____

4. _____

5. _____

B. Anatomy Challenge

1. Write the labels for this figure on the numbered lines provided.

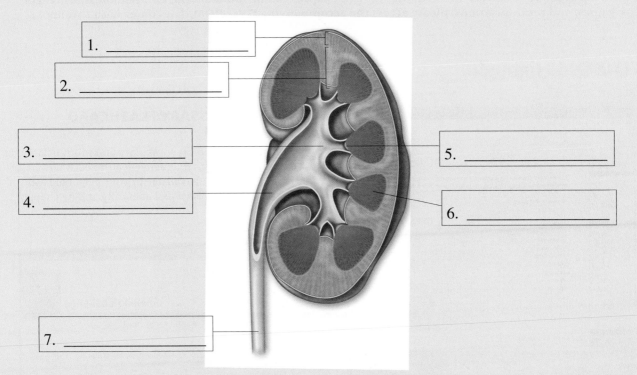

1. _____

2. _____

3. _____

4. _____

5. _____

6. _____

7. _____

2. Write the labels for this figure on the numbered lines provided.

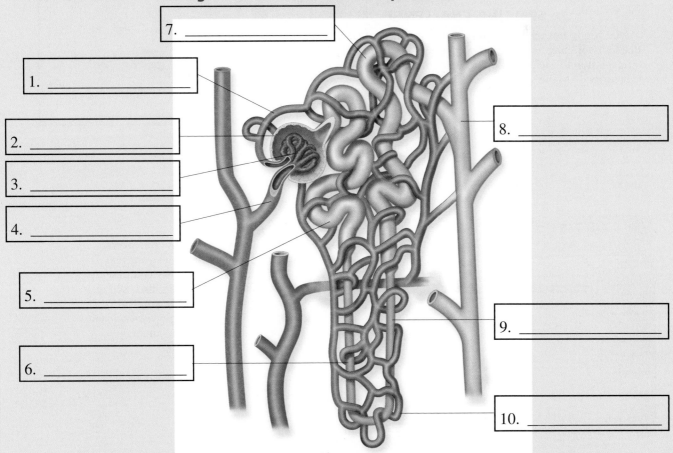

7. _____

1. _____

2. _____

3. _____

4. _____

5. _____

6. _____

8. _____

9. _____

10. _____

Multimedia Preview

Additional interactive resources and activities for this chapter can be found on the Companion Website. For videos, games, and pronunciations, please access the accompanying DVD-ROM that comes with this book.

DVD-ROM Highlights

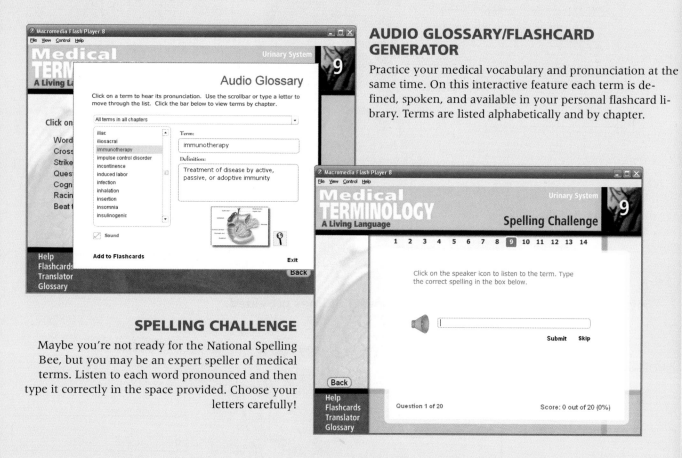

AUDIO GLOSSARY/FLASHCARD GENERATOR

Practice your medical vocabulary and pronunciation at the same time. On this interactive feature each term is defined, spoken, and available in your personal flashcard library. Terms are listed alphabetically and by chapter.

SPELLING CHALLENGE

Maybe you're not ready for the National Spelling Bee, but you may be an expert speller of medical terms. Listen to each word pronounced and then type it correctly in the space provided. Choose your letters carefully!

Website Highlights—www.prenhall.com/fremgen

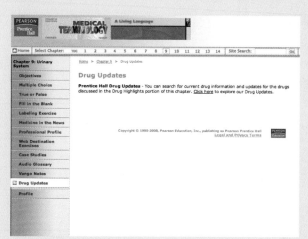

DRUG UPDATES

Click here and take advantage of the free-access on-line study guide that accompanies your textbook. You'll find a feature that allows you to search for current information on the drugs discussed in this chapter. By clicking on this URL you'll also access links to download mp3 audio reviews, current news articles, review questions, and an audio glossary.

10

Reproductive System

Learning Objectives

Upon completion of this chapter, you will be able to:

- Identify and define the combining forms and suffixes introduced in this chapter.
- Correctly spell and pronounce medical terms and major anatomical structures relating to the reproductive systems.
- Locate and describe the major organs of the reproductive systems and their functions.
- Use medical terms to describe circumstances relating to pregnancy.
- Identify the symptoms and origin of sexually transmitted diseases.
- Build and define reproductive system medical terms from word parts.
- Identify and define reproductive system vocabulary terms.
- Identify and define selected reproductive system pathology terms.
- Identify and define selected reproductive system diagnostic procedures.
- Identify and define selected reproductive system therapeutic procedures.
- Identify and define selected medications relating to the reproductive systems.
- Define selected abbreviations associated with the reproductive systems.

Section I: Female Reproductive System at a Glance

Function

The female reproductive system produces ova (the female reproductive cell), provides a location for fertilization and growth of a baby, and secretes female sex hormones. In addition, the breasts produce milk to nourish the newborn.

Organs

breasts
fallopian tubes
ovaries
uterus
vagina
vulva

Combining Forms

amni/o	amnion	**mast/o**	breast
cervic/o	neck, cervix	**men/o**	menses, menstruation
chori/o	chorion	**metr/o**	uterus
colp/o	vagina	**nat/o**	birth
culd/o	cul-de-sac	**oophor/o**	ovary
embry/o	embryo	**ov/o**	egg
episi/o	vulva	**ovari/o**	ovary
fet/o	fetus	**perine/o**	perineum
gynec/o	woman, female	**salping/o**	fallopian tubes, uterine tubes
hymen/o	hymen	**uter/o**	uterus
hyster/o	uterus	**vagin/o**	vagina
lact/o	milk	**vulv/o**	vulva
mamm/o	breast		

Suffixes Relating

-arche	beginning
-cyesis	state of pregnancy
-gravida	pregnancy
-para	to bear (offspring)
-partum	childbirth
-salpinx	fallopian tube
-tocia	labor, childbirth

Female Reproductive System Illustrated

breast, p. 318

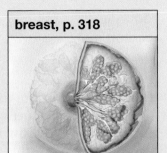

Produces milk

uterus, p. 316

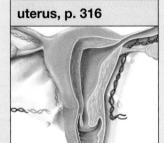

Site of development of fetus

fallopian tube, p. 315

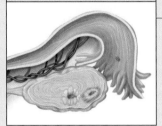

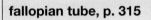

Transports ovum to uterus

ovary, p. 314

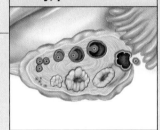

Produces ova and secretes estrogen and progesterone

vagina, p. 317

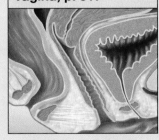

Receives semen during intercourse; birth canal

vulva, p. 317

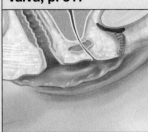

Protects vaginal orifice and urinary meatus

Anatomy and Physiology of the Female Reproductive System

breasts
fallopian tubes (fah-LOH-pee-an TOOBS)
fertilization
genitalia (jen-ih-TAY-lee-ah)
ova (OH-vah)
ovaries (OH-vah-reez)

pregnancy
sex hormones
uterus (YOO-ter-us)
vagina (vah-JIGH-nah)
vulva (VULL-vah)

The female reproductive system plays many vital functions that ensure the continuation of the human race. First, it produces **ova**, the female reproductive cells. It then provides a place for **fertilization** to occur and for a baby to grow during **pregnancy**. The **breasts** provide nourishment for the newborn. Finally, this system secretes the female **sex hormones**.

This system consists of both internal and external **genitalia** or reproductive organs (see Figure 10.1 ■). The internal genitalia are located in the pelvic cavity and consist of the **uterus**, two **ovaries**, two **fallopian tubes**, and the **vagina**, which extends to the external surface of the body. The external genitalia are collectively referred to as the **vulva**.

Internal Genitalia

Ovaries

Med Term Tip

The singular for egg is *ovum*. The plural term for many eggs is *ova*. The term *ova* is not used exclusively when discussing the human reproductive system. For instance, testing the stool for ova and parasites is used to detect the presence of parasites or their ova in the digestive tract, a common cause for severe diarrhea.

estrogen (ESS-troh-jen)
follicle stimulating hormone (FOLL-ih-kl)
luteinizing hormone (loo-teh-NIGH-zing)

ovulation (ov-yoo-LAY-shun)
progesterone (proh-JES-ter-ohn)

There are two ovaries, one located on each side of the uterus within the pelvic cavity (see Figure 10.1). These are small almond-shaped glands that produce ova (singular is *ovum*) and the female sex hormones (see Figure 10.2 ■). In humans, approximately every 28 days, hormones from the anterior pituitary, **follicle stimulating hormone** (FSH) and **luteinizing hormone** (LH), stimulate maturation of ovum and trigger **ovulation**, the process by which one ovary releases an ovum

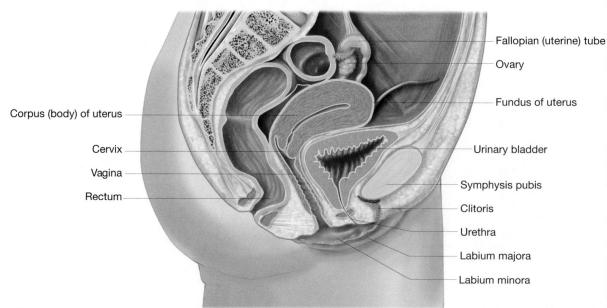

Corpus (body) of uterus
Cervix
Vagina
Rectum

Fallopian (uterine) tube
Ovary
Fundus of uterus
Urinary bladder
Symphysis pubis
Clitoris
Urethra
Labium majora
Labium minora

■ **Figure 10.1** The female reproductive system, sagittal view showing organs of the system in relation to the urinary bladder and rectum.

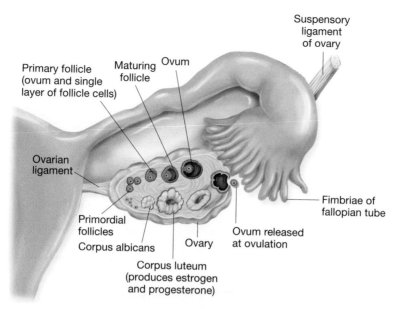

■ **Figure 10.2** Structure of the ovary and fallopian (uterine) tube. Figure illustrates stages of ovum development and the relationship of the ovary to the fallopian tube.

(see Figure 10.3 ■). The principal female sex hormones produced by the ovaries, **estrogen** and **progesterone**, stimulate the lining of the uterus to be prepared to receive a fertilized ovum. These hormones are also responsible for the female secondary sexual characteristics.

Fallopian Tubes

conception (con-SEP-shun)
fimbriae (FIM-bree-ay)

oviducts (OH-vih-ducts)
uterine tubes (YOO-ter-in)

The fallopian tubes, also called the **uterine tubes** or **oviducts**, are approximately 5½ inches long and run from the area around each ovary to either side of the upper portion of the uterus (see Figures 10.4 ■ and 10.5 ■). As they near the ovaries, the unattached ends of these two tubes expand into finger-like projections called

Med Term Tip

When the fertilized egg adheres or implants to the fallopian tube instead of moving into the uterus, a condition called *tubal pregnancy* exists. There is not enough room in the fallopian tube for the fetus to grow normally. Implantation of the fertilized egg in any location other than the uterus is called an *ectopic pregnancy*. *Ectopic* is a general term meaning "in the wrong place."

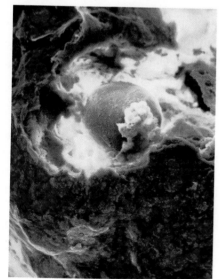

■ **Figure 10.3** Enhanced color scanning electron micrograph showing an ovum (pink) released by the ovary at ovulation surrounded by follicle (white) tissue. The external surface of the ovary is brown in this photo. *(P.M. Motta and J. Van Blekrom/Science Photo Library/Photo Researchers, Inc.)*

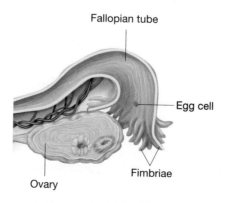

■ **Figure 10.4** Fallopian (uterine) tube, longitudinal view showing released ovum within the fallopian tube.

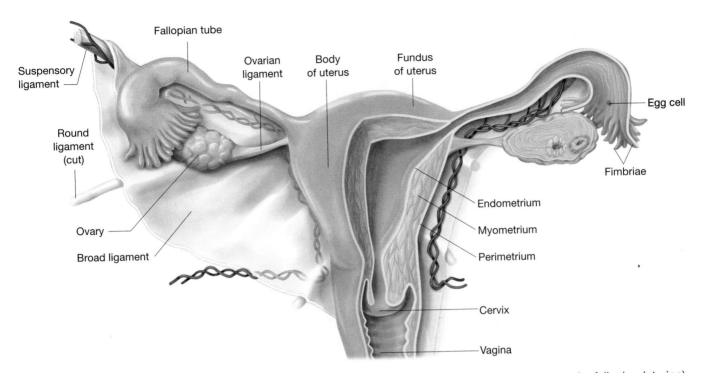

Figure 10.5 The uterus. Cutaway view shows regions of the uterus and cervix and its relationship to the fallopian (uterine) tubes and vagina.

fimbriae. The fimbriae catch an ovum after ovulation and direct it into the fallopian tube. The fallopian tube can then propel the ovum from the ovary to the uterus so that it can implant. The meeting of the egg and sperm, called fertilization or **conception**, normally takes place within the upper one-half of the fallopian tubes.

Uterus

anteflexion (an-tee-FLEK-shun)
cervix (SER-viks)
corpus (KOR-pus)
endometrium (en-doh-MEE-tre-um)
fundus (FUN-dus)
menarche (men-AR-kee)

menopause (MEN-oh-pawz)
menstrual period (MEN-stroo-all)
menstruation (men-stroo-AY-shun)
myometrium (my-oh-MEE-tre-um)
perimetrium (pear-ee-MEE-tre-um)

The uterus is a hollow, pear-shaped organ that contains a thick muscular wall, a mucous membrane lining, and a rich supply of blood (see Figure 10.5). It lies in the center of the pelvic cavity between the bladder and the rectum. It is normally bent slightly forward, which is called **anteflexion**, and is held in position by strong fibrous ligaments anchored in the outer layer of the uterus, called the **perimetrium** (see Figure 10.1). The uterus has three sections: the **fundus** or upper portion, between where the fallopian tubes connect to the uterus; **corpus** or body, which is the central portion; and **cervix** (Cx), or lower portion, also called the neck of the uterus, which opens into the vagina.

The inner layer, or **endometrium**, of the uterine wall contains a rich blood supply. The endometrium reacts to hormonal changes every month that prepare it to receive a fertilized ovum. In a normal pregnancy the fertilized ovum implants in the endometrium, which can then provide nourishment and protection for the developing baby. Contractions of the thick muscular walls of the uterus, called the **myometrium**, assist in propelling the fetus through the birth canal at delivery.

Med Term Tip

During pregnancy, the height of the fundus is an important measurement for estimating the stage of pregnancy and the size of the fetus. Following birth, massaging the fundus with pressure applied in a circular pattern stimulates the uterine muscle to contract to help stop bleeding. Patients may be more familiar with a common term for uterus, *womb*. However, the correct medical term is uterus.

If a pregnancy is not established, the endometrium is sloughed off, resulting in **menstruation** or the **menstrual period**. During a pregnancy, the lining of the uterus does not leave the body but remains to nourish the unborn child. A girl's first menstrual period (usually during her early teenage years) is called **menarche**, while the ending of menstrual activity and childbearing years is called **menopause**. This generally occurs between the ages of 40 and 55.

Med Term Tip

Word watch—Be careful using the combining forms *uter/o* meaning "uterus" and *ureter/o* meaning "ureter."

Vagina

Bartholin's glands (BAR-toh-linz)
hymen (HIGH-men)

vaginal orifice (VAJ-ih-nal OR-ih-fis)

The vagina is a muscular tube, lined with mucous membrane that extends from the cervix of the uterus to the outside of the body (see Figure 10.6 ■). The vagina allows for the passage of the menstrual flow. In addition, during intercourse, it receives the male's penis and semen, which is the fluid containing sperm. The vagina also serves as the birth canal through which the baby passes during a normal vaginal birth.

The **hymen** is a thin membranous tissue that partially covers the external vaginal opening or **vaginal orifice**. This membrane is broken by the use of tampons, during physical activity, or during sexual intercourse. A pair of glands, called **Bartholin's glands**, are located on either side of the vaginal orifice and secrete mucus for lubrication during intercourse.

Med Term Tip

Word watch—Be careful using the combining forms *colp/o* meaning "vagina" and *culd/o* meaning "cul-de-sac (rectouterine pouch)."

Vulva

clitoris (KLIT-oh-ris)
erectile tissue (ee-REK-tile)
labia majora (LAY-bee-ah mah-JOR-ah)

labia minora (LAY-bee-ah min-NOR-ah)
perineum (pair-ih-NEE-um)
urinary meatus (YOO-rih-nair-ee mee-AY-tus)

The vulva is a general term that refers to the group of structures that make up the female external genitalia. The **labia majora** and **labia minora** are folds of skin that serve as protection for the genitalia, the vaginal orifice, and the **urinary meatus** (see Figure 10.7 ■). Since the urinary tract and the reproductive organs are located in proximity to one another and each contains mucous membranes that can transport infection, there is a danger of infection entering the urinary tract. The **clitoris** is a small organ containing sensitive **erectile tissue** that is aroused during sexual stimulation and corresponds to the penis in the male. The region between the vaginal orifice and the anus is referred to as the **perineum**.

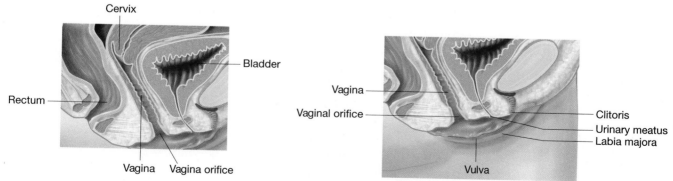

■**Figure 10.6** The vagina, sagittal section showing the location of the vagina and its relationship to the cervix, uterus, rectum, and bladder.

■**Figure 10.7** The vulva, sagittal section illustrating how the labia major and labia minora cover and protect the vaginal orifice, clitoris, and urinary meatus.

Breast

areola (ah-REE-oh-la)   **mammary glands** (MAM-ah-ree)
lactation (lak-TAY-shun)   **nipple**
lactiferous ducts (lak-TIF-er-us)   **nurse**
lactiferous glands (lak-TIF-er-us)

The breasts, or **mammary glands**, play a vital role in the reproductive process because they produce milk, a process called **lactation**, to nourish the newborn. The size of the breasts, which varies greatly from woman to woman, has no bearing on the ability to **nurse** or feed a baby. Milk is produced by the **lactiferous glands** and is carried to the **nipple** by the **lactiferous ducts** (see Figure 10.8 ▓). The **areola** is the pigmented area around the nipple. As long as the breast is stimulated by the nursing infant, the breast will continue to secrete milk.

Pregnancy

amnion (AM-nee-on)   **gestation** (jess-TAY-shun)
amniotic fluid (am-nee-OT-ik)   **placenta** (plah-SEN-tah)
chorion (KOR-ree-on)   **premature**
embryo (EM-bree-oh)   **umbilical cord** (um-BILL-ih-kal KORD)
fetus (FEE-tus)

Pregnancy refers to the period of time during which a baby grows and develops in its mother's uterus (see Figure 10.9 ▓). The normal length of time for a pregnancy, **gestation**, is 40 weeks. If a baby is born before completing at least 37 weeks of gestation, it is considered **premature**.

Mid Term Tip

The term *abortion* (AB) has different meanings for medical professionals and the general population. The general population equates the term *abortion* specifically with the planned termination of a pregnancy. However, to the medical community, abortion is a broader medical term meaning that a pregnancy has ended before a fetus is *viable*, meaning before it can live on its own.

▓ **Figure 10.8** The breast, cutaway view showing both internal and external features.

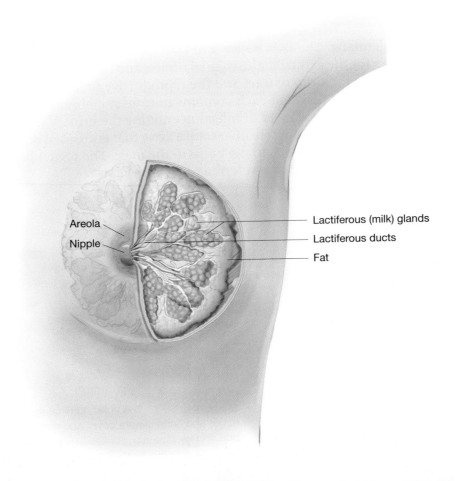

Areola
Nipple

Lactiferous (milk) glands
Lactiferous ducts
Fat

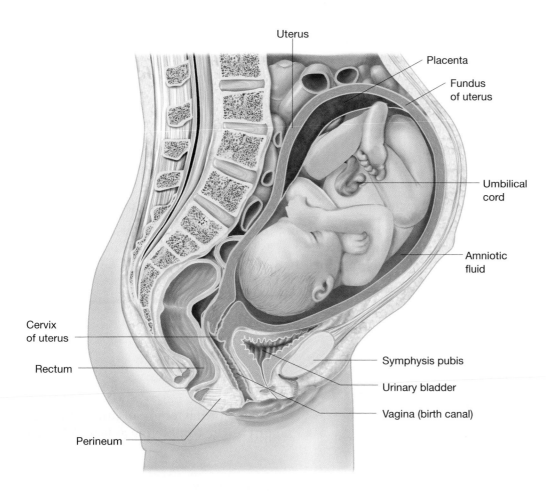

Uterus

Placenta

Fundus
of uterus

Umbilical
cord

Amniotic
fluid

Cervix
of uterus

Rectum

Symphysis pubis

Urinary bladder

Vagina (birth canal)

Perineum

■ **Figure 10.9** A full-term
pregnancy. Images illustrates
position of the fetus and the
structures associated with
pregnancy.

During pregnancy the female body undergoes many changes. In fact, all of the body systems become involved in the development of a healthy infant. From the time the fertilized egg implants in the uterus until approximately the end of the eighth week, the infant is referred to as an **embryo** (see Figure 10.10 ■). During this period all the major organs and body systems are formed. Following the embryo stage and lasting until birth, the infant is called a **fetus** (see Figure 10.11 ■). During this time, the longest period of gestation, the organs mature and begin to function.

The fetus receives nourishment from its mother by way of the **placenta**, which is a spongy, blood-filled organ that forms in the uterus next to the fetus. The

Med Term Tip

During the embryo stage of gestation, the organs and organ systems of the body are formed. Therefore, this is a very common time for *congenital anomalies*, or birth defects, to occur. This may happen before the woman is even aware of being pregnant.

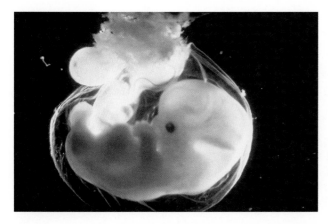

■ **Figure 10.10** Photograph illustrating the development of an embryo. *(Petit Format/Nestle/Photo Researchers, Inc.)*

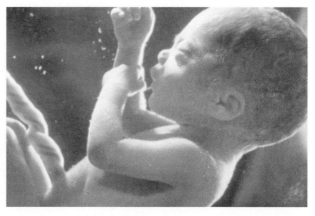

■ **Figure 10.11** Photograph illustrating the development of a fetus. *(Petit Format/Nestle/Photo Researchers, Inc.)*

placenta is commonly referred to as the afterbirth. The fetus is attached to the placenta by way of the **umbilical cord** and is surrounded by two membranous sacs, the **amnion** and the **chorion**. The amnion is the innermost sac, and it holds the **amniotic fluid** in which the fetus floats. The chorion is an outer, protective sac and also forms part of the placenta.

Labor and Delivery

breech presentation	effacement (eh-FACE-ment)
crowning	expulsion stage (ex-PULL-shun)
delivery	labor
dilation stage (dye-LAY-shun)	placental stage (plah-SEN-tal)

Labor is the actual process of expelling the fetus from the uterus and through the vagina. The first stage is referred to as the **dilation stage**, in which the uterine muscle contracts strongly to expel the fetus (see Figure 10.12A ■). During this

A

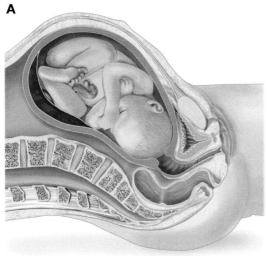

DILATION STAGE:
Uterine contractions dilate cervix

B

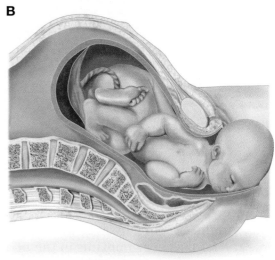

EXPULSION STAGE:
Birth of baby or expulsion

C

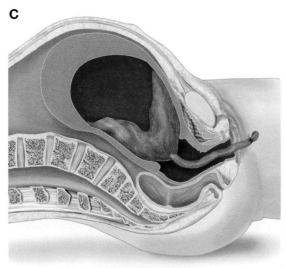

PLACENTAL STAGE:
Delivery of placenta

■ **Figure 10.12** The stages of labor and delivery. A) During the dilation stage the cervix thins and dilates to 10 cm. B) During the expulsion stage the infant is delivered. C) During the placental stage the placenta is delivered.

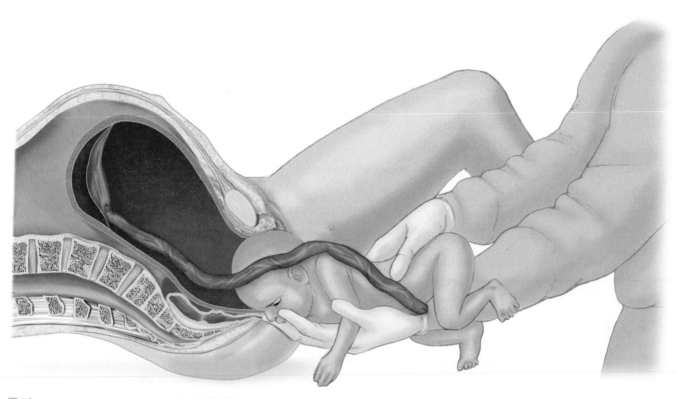

Figure 10.13 A breech birth. This image illustrates a newborn that has been delivered buttocks first.

process the fetus presses on the cervix and causes it to dilate or expand. As the cervix dilates, it also becomes thinner, referred to as **effacement**. When the cervix is completely dilated to 10 centimeters, the second stage of labor begins (see Figure 10.12B ■). This is the **expulsion stage** and ends with **delivery** of the baby. Generally, the head of the baby appears first, which is referred to as **crowning** (see Figure 10.10). In some cases the baby's buttocks will appear first, and this is referred to as a **breech presentation** (see Figure 10.13 ■). The last stage of labor is the **placental stage** (see Figure 10.12C ■). Immediately after childbirth, the uterus continues to contract, causing the placenta to be expelled through the vagina.

 Word Building

The following list contains examples of medical terms built directly from word parts. The definition for these terms can be determined by a straightforward translation of the word parts.

COMBINING FORM	COMBINED WITH	MEDICAL TERM	DEFINITION
amni/o	-otomy	**amniotomy** (am-nee-OT-oh-mee)	incision into amnion
	-tic	**amniotic** (am-nee-OT-ik)	pertaining to the amnion
	-rrhea	**amniorrhea** (am-nee-oh-REE-ah)	flow of fluid from amnion
cervic/o	-ectomy	**cervicectomy** (ser-vih-SEK-toh-mee)	removal of cervix
	-al	**cervical** (SER-vih-kal)	pertaining to the cervix
	endo- -itis	**endocervicitis** (en-doh-ser-vih-SIGH-tis)	inflammation within cervix
chori/o	-nic	**chorionic** (koh-ree-ON-ik)	pertaining to the chorion
colp/o	-scope	**colposcope** (KOL-poh-scope)	instrument to view inside vagina

Word Building *(continued)*

COMBINING FORM	COMBINED WITH	MEDICAL TERM	DEFINITION
embry/o	-nic	**embryonic** (em-bree-ON-ik)	pertaining to the embryo
episi/o	-rrhaphy	**episiorrhaphy** (eh-peez-ee-OR-ah-fee)	suture of vulva
fet/o	-al	**fetal** (FEE-tall)	pertaining to the fetus
gynec/o	-logist	**gynecologist** (gigh-neh-KOL-oh-jist)	specialist in female reproductive system
hymen/o	-ectomy	**hymenectomy** (high-men-EK-toh-mee)	removal of the hymen
hyster/o	-pexy	**hysteropexy** (HISS-ter-oh-pek-see)	surgical fixation of the uterus
	-rrhexis	**hysterorrhexis** (hiss-ter-oh-REK-sis)	ruptured uterus
	-ectomy	**hysterectomy** (hiss-ter-EK-toh-mee)	surgical removal of the uterus
lact/o	-ic	**lactic** (LAK-tik)	pertaining to milk
	-rrhea	**lactorrhea** (lak-toh-REE-ah)	milk discharge
lapar/o	-otomy	**laparotomy** (lap-ah-ROT-oh-mee)	incision into the abdomen
	-scope	**laparoscope** (LAP-ah-row-scope)	instrument to view inside the abdomen
mamm/o	-gram	**mammogram** (MAM-moh-gram)	record of the breast
	-ary	**mammary** (MAM-mah-ree)	pertaining to the breast
	-plasty	**mammoplasty** (MAM-moh-plas-tee)	surgical repair of breast
mast/o	-algia	**mastalgia** (mas-TAL-jee-ah)	breast pain
	-itis	**mastitis** (mas-TYE-tis)	inflammation of the breast
	-ectomy	**mastectomy** (mass-TEK-toh-mee)	removal of the breast
men/o	a- -rrhea	**amenorrhea** (ah-men-oh-REE-ah)	no menstrual flow
	dys- -rrhea	**dysmenorrhea** (dis-men-oh-REE-ah)	painful menstrual flow
	oligo- -rrhea	**oligomenorrhea** (ol-lih-goh-men-oh-REE-ah)	scanty menstrual flow
	-rrhagia	**menorrhagia** (men-oh-RAY-jee-ah)	abnormal, rapid menstrual flow
metr/o	endo- -itis	**endometritis** (en-doh-meh-TRY-tis)	inflammation within the uterus

Med Term Tip

Word watch—Be careful when using the combining form *metr/o* meaning "uterus" and the suffix *–metry* meaning "process of measuring."

	peri- -itis	**perimetritis** (pair-ih-meh-TRY-tis)	inflammation around the uterus
	-rrhea	**metrorrhea** (meh-troh-REE-ah)	flow from uterus
	-rrhagia	**metrorrhagia** (meh-troh-RAY-jee-ah)	rapid (menstrual) blood flow from uterus
nat/o	neo-	**neonate** (NEE-oh-nayt)	newborn
	neo- -logist	**neonatologist** (nee-oh-nay-TALL-oh-jist)	specialist in the study of the newborn
oophor/o	-ectomy	**oophorectomy** (oh-off-oh-REK-toh-mee)	removal of the ovary
	-itis	**oophoritis** (oh-off-oh-RIGH-tis)	inflammation of the ovary

Word Building (continued)

COMBINING FORM	COMBINED WITH	MEDICAL TERM	DEFINITION
ovari/o	-an	**ovarian** (oh-VAIR-ee-an)	pertaining to the ovary
salping/o	-cyesis	**salpingocyesis** (sal-ping-goh-sigh-EE-sis)	tubal pregnancy
	-ectomy	**salpingectomy** (sal-ping-JECK-toh-mee)	removal of the fallopian tube
	-itis	**salpingitis** (sal-ping-JIGH-tis)	inflammation of the fallopian tubes
uter/o	-ine	**uterine** (YOO-ter-in)	pertaining to the uterus
vagin/o	-al	**vaginal** (VAJ-ih-nal)	pertaining to the vagina
	-itis	**vaginitis** (vaj-ih-NIGH-tis)	inflammation of the vagina

PREFIX	SUFFIX	MEDICAL TERM	DEFINITION
pseudo-	-cyesis	**pseudocyesis** (soo-doh-sigh-EE-sis)	false pregnancy
nulli-	-gravida	**nulligravida** (null-ih-GRAV-ih-dah)	no pregnancies
primi-		**primigravida** (prem-ih-GRAV-ih-dah)	first pregnancy
multi-		**multigravida** (mull-tih-GRAV-ih-dah)	multiple pregnancies
nulli-	-para	**nullipara** (null-IP-ah-rah)	no births
primi-		**primipara** (prem-IP-ah-rah)	first birth
multi-		**multipara** (mull-TIP-ah-rah)	multiple births
ante-	-partum	**antepartum** (an-tee-PAR-tum)	before birth
post-		**postpartum** (post-PAR-tum)	after birth
hemato-	-salpinx	**hematosalpinx** (hee-mah-toh-SAL-pinks)	blood in fallopian tube
pyo-		**pyosalpinx** (pie-oh-SAL-pinks)	pus in fallopian tube
dys-	-tocia	**dystocia** (dis-TOH-she-ah)	difficult labor and childbirth

Vocabulary

TERM	DEFINITION
atresia (ah-TREE-she-ah)	Congenital lack of a normal body opening.
barrier contraception (kon-trah-SEP-shun)	Prevention of a pregnancy using a device to prevent sperm from meeting an ovum. Examples include condoms, diaphragms, and cervical caps.
colostrum (kuh-LOS-trum)	Thin fluid first secreted by the breast after delivery. It does not contain much protein, but is rich in antibodies.
fraternal twins	Twins that develop from two different ova fertilized by two different sperm. Although twins, these siblings do not have identical DNA.
gynecology (GYN) (gigh-neh-KOL-oh-jee)	Branch of medicine specializing in the diagnosis and treatment of conditions of the female reproductive system. Physician is called a *gynecologist*.
hormonal conception	Use of hormones to block ovulation and prevent contraception. May be in the form of a pill, a patch, an implant under the skin, or injection.
identical twins	Twins that develop from the splitting of one fertilized ovum. These siblings have identical DNA.

Vocabulary (continued)

TERM	DEFINITION
infertility	Inability to produce children. Generally defined as no pregnancy after properly timed intercourse for 1 year.
intrauterine device (IUD) (in-trah-YOO-ter-in)	Device that is inserted into the uterus by a physician for the purpose of contraception.

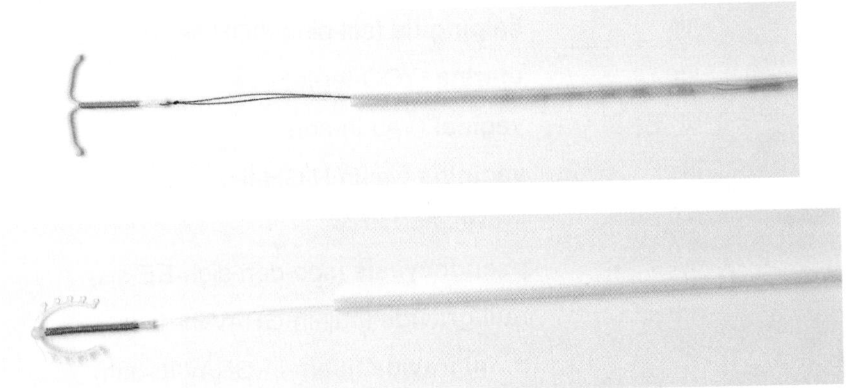

Figure 10.14 Photographs illustrating the shape of two different intrauterine devices (IUDs). *(Jules Selmes and Debi Treloar/Dorling Kindersley Media Library)*

TERM	DEFINITION
meconium (meh-KOH-nee-um)	First bowel movement of a newborn. It is greenish-black in color and consists of mucus and bile.
neonatology (nee-oh-nay-TALL-oh-jee)	Branch of medicine specializing in the diagnosis and treatment of conditions involving newborns. Physician is called a *neonatologist*.
obstetrics (OB) (ob-STET-riks)	Branch of medicine specializing in the diagnosis and treatment of women during pregnancy and childbirth, and immediately after childbirth. Physician is called an *obstetrician*.
premenstrual syndrome (PMS) (pre-MEN-stroo-al SIN-drohm)	Symptoms that develop just prior to the onset of a menstrual period, which can include irritability, headache, tender breasts, and anxiety.
puberty (PEW-ber-tee)	Beginning of menstruation and the ability to reproduce.

Pathology

TERM	DEFINITION
■ *Ovary*	
ovarian carcinoma (oh-VAY-ree-an kar-sih-NOH-mah)	Cancer of the ovary.
ovarian cyst (oh-VAY-ree-an SIST)	Cyst that develops within the ovary. These may be multiple cysts and may rupture, causing pain and bleeding.
■ *Uterus*	
cervical cancer (SER-vih-kal CAN-ser)	Malignant growth in the cervix. Some cases are caused by the *human papilloma virus* (HPV), a sexually transmitted virus for which there is now a vaccine. An especially difficult type of cancer to treat that causes 5 percent of the cancer deaths in women. Pap smear tests have helped to detect early cervical cancer.
endometrial cancer (en-doh-MEE-tree-al CAN-ser)	Cancer of the endometrial lining of the uterus.

Pathology *(continued)*

TERM	DEFINITION
fibroid tumor (FIGH-broyd TOO-mor) ■ **Figure 10.15** Common sites for the development of fibroid tumors.	Benign tumor or growth that contains fiber-like tissue. Uterine fibroid tumors are the most common tumors in women.

Under the perimetrium

Within the myometrium

Under the endometrium

TERM	DEFINITION
menometrorrhagia (men-oh-met-thro-RAY-jee-ah)	Excessive bleeding during the menstrual period and at intervals between menstrual periods.
prolapsed uterus (pro-LAPS'D YOO-ter-us)	Fallen uterus that can cause the cervix to protrude through the vaginal opening. Generally caused by weakened muscles from vaginal delivery or as the result of pelvic tumors pressing down.
■ *Vagina*	
candidiasis (kan-dih-DYE-ah-sis)	Yeast infection of the skin and mucous membranes that can result in white plaques on the tongue and vagina.

> **Med Term Tip**
>
> The term *candida* comes from a Latin term meaning "dazzling white." Candida is the scientific name for yeast and refers to the very white discharge that is the hallmark of a yeast infection.

TERM	DEFINITION
cystocele (SIS-toh-seel)	Hernia or outpouching of the bladder that protrudes into the vagina. This may cause urinary frequency and urgency.
rectocele (REK-toh-seel)	Protrusion or herniation of the rectum into the vagina.
toxic shock syndrome (TSS)	Rare and sometimes fatal staphylococcus infection that generally occurs in menstruating women. Initial infection of the vagina is associated with prolonged wearing of a super-absorbent tampon.
■ *Pelvic Cavity*	
endometriosis (en-doh-mee-tree-OH-sis)	Abnormal condition of endometrium tissue appearing throughout the pelvis or on the abdominal wall. This tissue is normally found within the uterus.
pelvic inflammatory disease (PID) (PELL-vik in-FLAM-mah-toh-ree dih-ZEEZ)	Chronic or acute infection, usually bacterial, that has ascended through the female reproductive organs and out into the pelvic cavity. May result in scarring that interferes with fertility.
■ *Breast*	
breast cancer	Malignant tumor of the breast. Usually forms in the milk-producing gland tissue or the lining of the milk ducts (see Figure 10.16A ■).

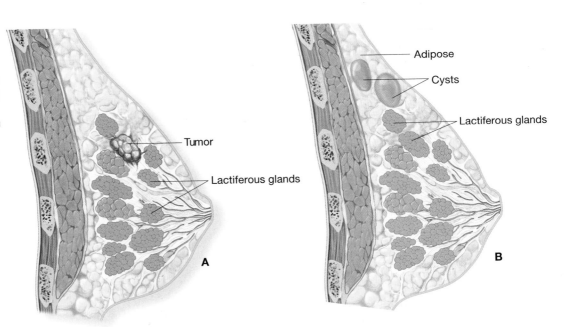

Figure 10.16
Comparison of breast cancer and fibrocystic disease. A) Breast with a malignant tumor growing in the lactiferous gland and duct. B) The location of a fibrocystic lump in the adipose tissue covering the breast.

 Pathology *(continued)*

TERM	DEFINITION
fibrocystic breast disease (figh-bro-SIS-tik)	Benign cysts forming in the breast (see Figure 10.16B ■).
■ *Pregnancy*	
abruptio placentae (ah-BRUP-tee-oh plah-SEN-tee)	Emergency condition in which the placenta tears away from the uterine wall prior to delivery of the infant. Requires immediate delivery of the baby.
eclampsia (eh-KLAMP-see-ah)	Convulsive seizures and coma occurring in the woman between the twentieth week of pregnancy and the first week of postpartum. Preceded by preeclampsia.
hemolytic disease of the newborn (HDN) (hee-moh-LIT-ik)	Condition developing in the baby when the mother's blood type is Rh-negative and the baby's blood is Rh-positive. Antibodies in the mother's blood enter the fetus's bloodstream through the placenta and destroy fetus's red blood cells causing anemia, jaundice, and enlargement of the spleen. Treatment is early diagnosis and blood transfusion. Also called *erythroblastosis fetalis*.
placenta previa (plah-SEN-tah PREE-vee-ah)	A placenta that is implanted in the lower portion of the uterus and, in turn, blocks the birth canal.

■ **Figure 10.17** Placenta previa, longitudinal section showing the placenta growing over the opening into the cervix.

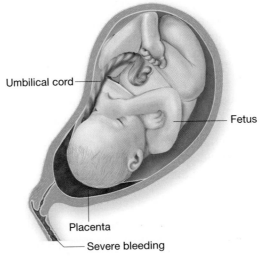

Pathology *(continued)*

TERM	DEFINITION
preeclampsia (pre-eh-KLAMP-see-ah)	Metabolic disease of pregnancy. If untreated, it may result in true eclampsia. Symptoms include hypertension, headaches, albumin in the urine, and edema. Also called *toxemia*.
prolapsed umbilical cord (pro-LAPS'D um-BILL-ih-kal)	When the umbilical cord of the baby is expelled first during delivery and is squeezed between the baby's head and the vaginal wall. This presents an emergency situation since the baby's circulation is compromised.
spontaneous abortion	Unplanned loss of a pregnancy due to the death of the embryo or fetus before the time it is viable, commonly referred to as a *miscarriage*.
stillbirth	Birth in which a viable-aged fetus dies shortly before or at the time of delivery.

 # Diagnostic Procedures

TERM	DEFINITION
■ Clinical Laboratory Tests	
Pap (Papanicolaou) **smear** (pap-ah-NIK-oh-low)	Test for the early detection of cancer of the cervix named after the developer of the test, George Papanicolaou, a Greek physician. A scraping of cells is removed from the cervix for examination under a microscope.
pregnancy test (PREG-nan-see)	Chemical test that can determine a pregnancy during the first few weeks. Can be performed in a physician's office or with a home-testing kit.
■ Diagnostic Imaging	
hysterosalpingography (HSG) (hiss-ter-oh-sal-pin-GOG-rah-fee)	Taking of an X-ray after injecting radiopaque material into the uterus and fallopian tubes.
mammography (mam-OG-rah-fee)	Using X-ray to diagnose breast disease, especially breast cancer.
pelvic ultrasonography (PELL-vik-ull-trah-son-OG-rah-fee)	Use of ultrasound waves to produce an image or photograph of an organ, such as the uterus, ovaries, or fetus.
■ Endoscopic Procedures	
colposcopy	Examination of vagina using an instrument called a *colposcope*.
culdoscopy (kul-DOS-koh-pee)	Examination of the female pelvic cavity, particularly behind the uterus, by introducing an endoscope through the wall of the vagina.
laparoscopy (lap-ar-OS-koh-pee)	Examination of the peritoneal cavity using an instrument called a *laparoscope*. The instrument is passed through a small incision made by the surgeon into the abdominopelvic cavity.

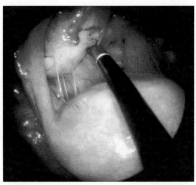

■ **Figure 10.18** Photograph taken during a laparoscopic procedure. The fundus of the uterus is visible below the probe, the ovary is at the tip of the probe, and the fallopian tube extends along the left side of the photo. *(Southern Illinois University/Photo Researchers, Inc.)*

Diagnostic Procedures *(continued)*

TERM	DEFINITION
■ *Obstetrical Diagnostic Procedures*	
amniocentesis (am-nee-oh-sen-TEE-sis)	Puncturing of the amniotic sac using a needle and syringe for the purpose of withdrawing amniotic fluid for testing. Can assist in determining fetal maturity, development, and genetic disorders.
Apgar score (AP-gar)	Evaluation of a neonate's adjustment to the outside world. Observes color, heart rate, muscle tone, respiratory rate, and response to stimulus at one minute and five minutes after birth.
chorionic villus sampling (CVS) (kor-ree-ON-ik vill-us)	Removal of a small piece of the chorion for genetic analysis. May be done at an earlier stage of pregnancy than amniocentesis.
fetal monitoring (FEE-tal)	Using electronic equipment placed on the mother's abdomen or the fetus' scalp to check the fetal heart rate (FHR) and fetal heart tone (FHT) during labor. The normal heart rate of the fetus is rapid, ranging from 120 to 160 beats per minute. A drop in the fetal heart rate indicates the fetus is in distress.
■ *Additional Diagnostic Procedures*	
cervical biopsy (SER-vih-kal BYE-op-see)	Taking a sample of tissue from the cervix to test for the presence of cancer cells.
endometrial biopsy (EMB) (en-doh-MEE-tre-al BYE-op-see)	Taking a sample of tissue from the lining of the uterus to test for abnormalities.
pelvic examination (PELL-vik)	Physical examination of the vagina and adjacent organs performed by a physician placing the fingers of one hand into the vagina. An instrument called a *speculum* is used to open the vagina.

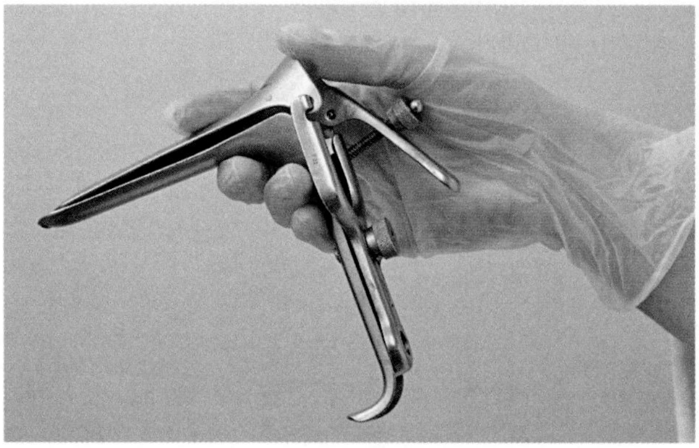

■ **Figure 10.19** A speculum used to hold the vagina open in order to visualize the cervix.

Therapeutic Procedures

TERM	DEFINITION
■ *Surgical Procedures*	
cesarean section (CS, C-section) (see-SAYR-ee-an)	Surgical delivery of a baby through an incision into the abdominal and uterine walls. Legend has it that the Roman emperor, Julius Caesar, was the first person born by this method.
conization (kon-ih-ZAY-shun)	Surgical removal of a core of cervical tissue. Also refers to partial removal of the cervix.

Therapeutic Procedures *(continued)*

TERM	DEFINITION
dilation and curettage (D & C) (dye-LAY-shun and koo-reh-TAHZ)	Surgical procedure in which the opening of the cervix is dilated and the uterus is scraped or suctioned of its lining or tissue. Often performed after a spontaneous abortion and to stop excessive bleeding from other causes.
elective abortion	Legal termination of a pregnancy for nonmedical reasons.
episiotomy (eh-peez-ee-OT-oh-mee)	Surgical incision of the perineum to facilitate the delivery process. Can prevent an irregular tearing of tissue during birth. Note: the combining form *episi/o* actually means vulva, however, in this term it is referring to the perineum instead.
lumpectomy (lump-EK-toh-mee)	Removal of only a breast tumor and the tissue immediately surrounding it.
radical mastectomy (mast-EK-toh-mee)	Surgical removal of the breast tissue plus chest muscles and axillary lymph nodes.
simple mastectomy (mast-EK-toh-mee)	Surgical removal of the breast tissue.
therapeutic abortion	Termination of a pregnancy for the health of the mother or another medical reason.
total abdominal hysterectomy— bilateral salpingo-oophorectomy (TAH-BSO) (hiss-ter-EK-toh-me sal-ping-goh oh-oh-foe-REK-toh-mee)	Removal of the entire uterus, cervix, both ovaries, and both fallopian tubes.
tubal ligation (TOO-bal lye-GAY-shun)	Surgical tying off of the fallopian tubes to prevent conception from taking place. Results in sterilization of the female.
vaginal hysterectomy (VAJ-ih-nal hiss-ter-EK-toh-me)	Removal of the uterus through the vagina rather than through an abdominal incision.

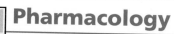

Pharmacology

CLASSIFICATION	ACTION	GENERIC AND BRAND NAMES
abortifacient (ah-bore-tih-FAY-shee-ent)	Medication that terminates a pregnancy.	mifepristone, Mifeprex; dinoprostone, Prostin E2
fertility drug	Medication that triggers ovulation. Also called *ovulation stimulant*.	clomiphene, Clomid; follitropin alfa, Gonal-F
hormone replacement therapy (HRT)	Menopause or the surgical loss of the ovaries results in the lack of estrogen production. Replacing this hormone may prevent some of the consequences of menopause, especially in younger women who have surgically lost their ovaries.	conjugated estrogens, Cenestin, Premarin
oral contraceptive pills (OCPs) (kon-trah-SEP-tive)	Birth control medication that uses low doses of female hormones to prevent conception by blocking ovulation.	desogestrel/ethinyl estradiol, Ortho-Cept; ethinyl estradiol/norgestrel, Lo/Ovral
oxytocin (ox-ee-TOH-sin)	Oxytocin is a natural hormone that begins or improves uterine contractions during labor and delivery.	oxytocin, Pitocin, Syntocinon

■ Abbreviations

AB	abortion	**HPV**	human papilloma virus
AI	artificial insemination	**HRT**	hormone replacement therapy
BSE	breast self-examination	**HSG**	hysterosalpingography
CS, C-section	cesarean section	**IUD**	intrauterine device
CVS	chorionic villus sampling	**IVF**	*in vitro* fertilization
Cx	cervix	**LBW**	low birth weight
D & C	dilation and curettage	**LH**	luteinizing hormone
EDC	estimated date of confinement	**LMP**	last menstrual period
EMB	endometrial biopsy	**NB**	newborn
ERT	estrogen replacement therapy	**OB**	obstetrics
FEKG	fetal electrocardiogram	**OCPs**	oral contraceptive pills
FHR	fetal heart rate	**PAP**	Papanicolaou test
FHT	fetal heart tone	**PI, para I**	first delivery
FSH	follicle-stimulating hormone	**PID**	pelvic inflammatory disease
FTND	full-term normal delivery	**PMS**	premenstrual syndrome
GI, grav I	first pregnancy	**TAH-BSO**	total abdominal hysterectomy–bilateral salpingo-oophorectomy
GYN, gyn	gynecology		
HCG, hCG	human chorionic gonadotropin	**TSS**	toxic shock syndrome
HDN	hemolytic disease of the newborn	**UC**	uterine contractions

Section II: Male Reproductive System at a Glance

Function

Similar to the female reproductive system, the male reproductive system is responsible for producing sperm, the male reproductive cell, secreting the male sex hormones, and delivering sperm to the female reproductive tract.

Organs

bulbourethral glands
epididymis
penis
prostate gland
seminal vesicles
testes
vas deferens

Combining Forms

andr/o	male	**prostat/o**	prostate
balan/o	glans penis	**spermat/o**	sperm
crypt/o	hidden	**testicul/o**	testes
epididym/o	epididymis	**varic/o**	varicose veins
orch/o	testes	**vas/o**	vas deferens
orchi/o	testes	**vesicul/o**	seminal vesicle
orchid/o	testes		

Suffixes Relating

-spermia	condition of sperm

Male Reproductive System Illustrated

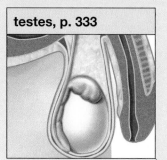

testes, p. 333

Produces sperm and secretes testosterone

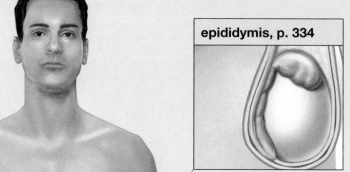

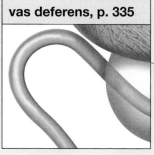

vas deferens, p. 335

Transports sperm to urethra

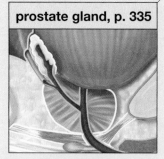

prostate gland, p. 335

Secretes fluid for semen

epididymis, p. 334

Stores sperm

seminal vesicles, p. 335

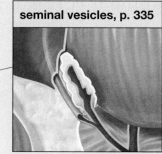

Secretes fluid for semen

bulbourethral gland, p. 335

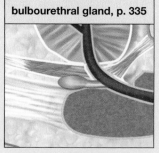

Secretes fluid for semen

penis, p. 334

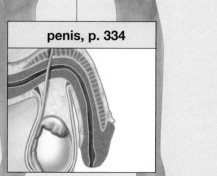

Delivers semen during intercourse

Anatomy and Physiology of the Male Reproductive System

bulbourethral glands
  (buhl-boh-yoo-REE-thral)
epididymis (ep-ih-DID-ih-mis)
genitourinary system
  (jen-ih-toh-YOO-rih-nair-ee)
penis (PEE-nis)
prostate gland (PROSS-tayt)

semen (SEE-men)
seminal vesicles (SEM-ih-nal VESS-ih-kls)
sex hormones
sperm
testes (TESS-teez)
vas deferens (VAS DEF-er-enz)

The male reproductive system has two main functions. The first is to produce **sperm**, the male reproductive cell. The second is to secrete the male **sex hormones**. In the male, the major organs of reproduction are located outside the body: the **penis**, and the two **testes**, each with an **epididymis** (see Figure 10.20 ■). The penis contains the urethra, which carries both urine and **semen** to the outside of the body. For this reason, this system is sometimes referred to as the **genitourinary system** (GU).

The internal organs of reproduction include two **seminal vesicles**, two **vas deferens**, the **prostate gland**, and two **bulbourethral glands**.

External Organs of Reproduction

Testes

perineum
scrotum (SKROH-tum)
seminiferous tubules
  (sem-ih-NIF-er-us TOO-byools)

spermatogenesis (sper-mat-oh-JEN-eh-sis)
testicles (test-IH-kles)
testosterone (tess-TOSS-ter-ohn)

The testes (singular is *testis*) or **testicles** are oval in shape and are responsible for the production of sperm (see Figure 10.20). This process, called **spermatogenesis**,

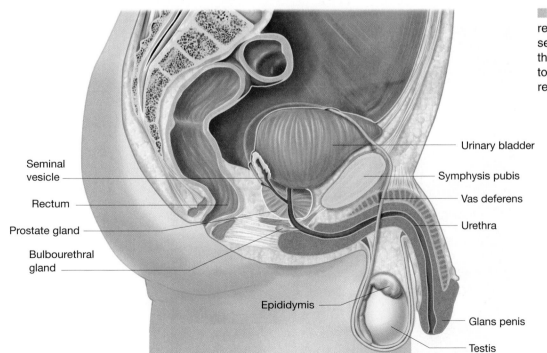

■ **Figure 10.20** The male reproductive system, sagittal section showing the organs of the system and their relation to the urinary bladder and rectum.

Seminal vesicle

Rectum

Prostate gland

Bulbourethral gland

Epididymis

Urinary bladder

Symphysis pubis

Vas deferens

Urethra

Glans penis

Testis

takes place within the **seminiferous tubules** that make up the insides of the testes (see Figure 10.21 ■). The testes must be maintained at the proper temperature for the sperm to survive. This lower temperature level is achieved by the placement of the testes suspended in the **scrotum,** a sac outside the body. The **perineum** of the male is similar to that in the female. It is the area between the scrotum and the anus. The male sex hormone **testosterone**, which is responsible for the development of the male reproductive organs, sperm, and secondary sex characteristics, is also produced by the testes.

Epididymis

Each epididymis is a coiled tubule that lies on top of the testes within the scrotum (see Figure 10.20). This elongated structure serves as the location for sperm maturation and storage until they are ready to be released into the vas deferens.

Penis

circumcision (ser-kum-SIH-zhun)   **prepuce** (PREE-pyoos)
ejaculation (ee-jak-yoo-LAY-shun)   **sphincter** (SFINGK-ter)
erectile tissue (ee-REK-tile)   **urinary meatus** (YOO-rih-nair-ee me-AY-tus)
glans penis (GLANS PEE-nis)

The penis is the male sex organ containing **erectile tissue** that is encased in skin (see Figure 10.20). This organ delivers semen into the female vagina. The soft tip of the penis is referred to as the **glans penis**. It is protected by a covering called the **prepuce** or foreskin. It is this covering of skin that is removed during the procedure known as **circumcision**. The penis becomes erect during sexual stimulation, which allows it to be placed within the female for the **ejaculation** of semen. The male urethra extends from the urinary bladder to the external opening in the penis, the **urinary meatus**, and serves a dual function: the elimination of urine and the ejaculation of semen. During the ejaculation process, a **sphincter** closes to keep urine from escaping.

■ **Figure 10.21**
Electronmicrograph of human sperm. *(Juergen Berger, Max-Planck Institute/Science Photo Library/Photo Researchers, Inc.)*

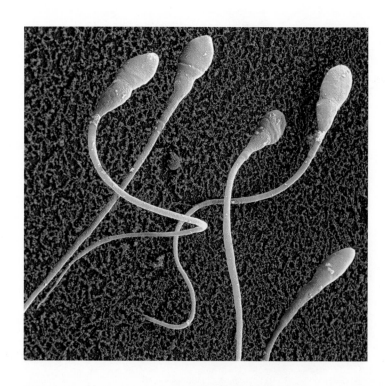

Internal Organs of Reproduction

Vas Deferens

spermatic cord (sper-MAT-ik)

Each vas deferens carries sperm from the epididymis up into the pelvic cavity. They travel up in front of the urinary bladder, over the top, and then back down the posterior side of the bladder to empty into the urethra (see Figure 10.20). They, along with nerves, arteries, veins, and lymphatic vessels running between the pelvic cavity and the testes, form the **spermatic cord**.

Seminal Vesicles

The two seminal vesicles are small glands located at the base of the urinary bladder (see Figure 10.20). These vesicles are connected to the vas deferens just before it empties into the urethra. The seminal vesicles secrete a glucose-rich fluid that nourishes the sperm. This liquid, along with the sperm, constitutes semen, the fluid that is eventually ejaculated during sexual intercourse.

Prostate Gland

The single prostate gland is located just below the urinary bladder (see Figure 10.20). It surrounds the urethra and when enlarged can cause difficulty in urination. The prostate is important for the reproductive process since it secretes an alkaline fluid that assists in keeping the sperm alive by neutralizing the pH of the urethra and vagina.

Bulbourethral Glands

Cowper's glands (KOW-perz)

The bulbourethral glands, also known as **Cowper's glands**, are two small glands located on either side of the urethra just below the prostate (see Figure 10.20). They produce a mucuslike lubricating fluid that joins with semen to become a part of the ejaculate.

Word Building

The following list contains examples of medical terms built directly from word parts. The definition for these terms can be determined by a straightforward translation of the word parts.

COMBINING FORM	COMBINED WITH	MEDICAL TERM	DEFINITION
andr/o	-gen	**androgen** (AN-droh-jen)	male producing
	-pathy	**andropathy** (an-DROP-ah-thee)	male disease
balan/o	-itis	**balanitis** (bal-ah-NYE-tis)	inflammation of glans penis
	-plasty	**balanoplasty** (BAL-ah-noh-plas-tee)	surgical repair of glans penis
	-rrhea	**balanorrhea** (bah-lah-noh-REE-ah)	discharge from glans penis
epididym/o	-ectomy	**epididymectomy** (ep-ih-did-ih-MEK-toh-mee)	removal of epididymis
	-al	**epididymal** (ep-ih-DID-ih-mal)	pertaining to the epididymis
	-itis	**epididymitis** (ep-ih-did-ih-MYE-tis)	inflammation of the epididymis

Word Building *(continued)*

COMBINING FORMS	COMBINED WITH	MEDICAL TERM	DEFINITION
orch/o	an- -ism	**anorchism** (an-OR-kizm)	condition of no testes
orchi/o	-ectomy	**orchiectomy** (or-kee-EK-toh-mee)	removal of testes
	-otomy	**orchiotomy** (or-kee-OT-oh-mee)	incision into testes
	-plasty	**orchioplasty** (OR-kee-oh-plas-tee)	surgical repair of testes
orchid/o	-ectomy	**orchidectomy** (or-kid-EK-toh-mee)	removal of the testes
	-pexy	**orchidopexy** (OR-kid-oh-peck-see)	surgical fixation of testes
prostat/o	-itis	**prostatitis** (pross-tah-TYE-tis)	prostate inflammation
	-ectomy	**prostatectomy** (pross-tah-TEK-toh-mee)	removal of prostate
	-ic	**prostatic** (pross-TAT-ik)	pertaining to the prostate
spermat/o	-ic	**spermatic** (sper-MAT-ik)	pertaining to sperm
	-lysis	**spermatolysis** (sper-mah-TOL-ih-sis)	sperm destruction
testicul/o	-ar	**testicular** (tes-TIK-yoo-lar)	pertaining to the testes
vesicul/o	-ar	**vesicular** (veh-SIC-yoo-lar)	pertaining to the seminal vesicle

Med Term Tip

Word watch—Be careful using the combining forms *vesic/o* meaning "bladder" and *vesicul/o* meaning "seminal vesicle."

PREFIX	SUFFIX	MEDICAL TERM	DEFINITION
a-	-spermia	**aspermia** (ah-SPER-mee-ah)	condition of no sperm
oligo-		**oligospermia** (ol-ih-goh-SPER-mee-ah)	condition of scanty (few) sperm

Vocabulary

TERM	DEFINITION
erectile dysfunction (ED) (ee-REK-tile)	Inability to engage in sexual intercourse due to inability to maintain an erection. Also called *impotence*.
sterility	Inability to father children due to a problem with spermatogenesis.

Pathology

TERM	DEFINITION
■ *Testes*	
cryptorchidism (kript-OR-kid-izm)	Failure of the testes to descend into the scrotal sac before birth. Usually, the testes will descend before birth. A surgical procedure called orchidopexy may be required to bring the testes down into the scrotum permanently. Failure of the testes to descend could result in sterility in the male or an increased risk of testicular cancer.
hydrocele (HIGH-droh-seel)	Accumulation of fluid around the testes or along the spermatic cord. Common in infants.

Pathology *(continued)*

TERM	DEFINITION
testicular carcinoma (kar-sih-NOH-mah)	Cancer of one or both testicles; most common cancer in men under age 40.
testicular torsion	A twisting of the spermatic cord.
varicocele (VAIR-ih-koh-seel)	Enlargement of the veins of the spermatic cord that commonly occurs on the left side of adolescent males.

■ *Prostate Gland*

benign prostatic hypertrophy (BPH) (bee-NINE pross-TAT-ik high-PER-troh-fee)	Noncancerous enlargement of the prostate gland commonly seen in males over age 50.
prostate cancer (PROSS-tayt CAN-ser)	Slow-growing cancer that affects a large number of males after age 50. The prostate-specific antigen (PSA) test is used to assist in early detection of this disease.

■ *Penis*

epispadias (ep-ih-SPAY-dee-as)	Congenital opening of the urethra on the dorsal surface of the penis.
hypospadias (high-poh-SPAY-dee-as)	Congenital opening of the male urethra on the underside of the penis.
phimosis (fih-MOH-sis)	Narrowing of the foreskin over the glans penis resulting in difficulty with hygiene. This condition can lead to infection or difficulty with urination. The condition is treated with circumcision, the surgical removal of the foreskin.
priapism (pri-ah-pizm)	A persistent and painful erection due to pathological causes, not sexual arousal.

■ *Sexually Transmitted Diseases*

chancroid (SHANG-kroyd) ■ **Figure 10.22** Photograph showing a chancroid on the glans penis. *(Joe Miller/Centers for Disease Control and Prevention [CDC])*	Highly infectious nonsyphilitic venereal ulcer. 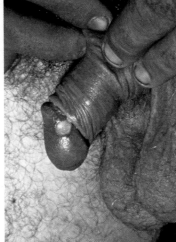
chlamydia (klah-MID-ee-ah)	Bacterial infection causing genital inflammation in males and females. Can lead to pelvic inflammatory disease in females and eventual infertility.
genital herpes (JEN-ih-tal HER-peez)	Creeping skin disease that can appear like a blister or vesicle, caused by a sexually transmitted virus.

Pathology *(continued)*

TERM	DEFINITION
genital warts (JEN-ih-tal)	Growth of warts on the genitalia of both males and females that can lead to cancer of the cervix in females. Caused by the sexual transmission of the human papilloma virus (HPV).
gonorrhea (GC) (gon-oh-REE-ah)	Sexually transmitted bacterial infection of the mucous membranes of either sex. Can be passed on to an infant during the birth process.
human immunodeficiency virus (HIV)	Sexually transmitted virus that attacks the immune system.
sexually transmitted disease (STD)	Disease usually acquired as the result of sexual intercourse. Formerly referred to as *venereal disease* (VD).
syphilis (SIF-ih-lis)	Infectious, chronic, bacterial venereal disease that can involve any organ. May exist for years without symptoms, but is fatal if untreated. Treated with the antibiotic penicillin.
trichomoniasis (trik-oh-moh-NYE-ah-sis)	Genitourinary infection caused by a single-cell protist that is usually without symptoms (asymptomatic) in both males and females. In women the disease can produce itching and/or burning, a foul-smelling discharge, and result in vaginitis.

Diagnostic Procedures

TERM	DEFINITION
■ Clinical Laboratory Tests	
prostate-specific antigen (PSA) (PROSS-tayt-specific AN-tih-jen)	A blood test to screen for prostate cancer. Elevated blood levels of PSA are associated with prostate cancer.
semen analysis (SEE-men ah-NAL-ih-sis)	Procedure used when performing a fertility workup to determine if the male is able to produce sperm. Semen is collected by the patient after abstaining from sexual intercourse for a period of three to five days. The sperm in the semen are analyzed for number, swimming strength, and shape. Also used to determine if a vasectomy has been successful. After a period of six weeks, no further sperm should be present in a sample from the patient.
■ Additional Diagnostic Procedures	
digital rectal exam (DRE) (DIJ-ih-tal REK-tal)	Manual examination for an enlarged prostate gland performed by palpating (feeling) the prostate gland through the wall of the rectum.

Therapeutic Procedures

TERM	DEFINITION
■ Surgical Procedures	
castration (kass-TRAY-shun)	Removal of the testicles in the male or the ovaries in the female.
circumcision (ser-kum-SIH-zhun)	Surgical removal of the end of the prepuce or foreskin of the penis. Generally performed on the newborn male at the request of the parents. The primary reason is for ease of hygiene. Circumcision is also a ritual practice in some religions.

Therapeutic Procedures *(continued)*

TERM	DEFINITION
orchidopexy (OR-kid-oh-peck-see)	Surgical fixation to move undescended testes into the scrotum and to attach them to prevent retraction. Used to treat cryptorchidism.
sterilization (ster-ih-lih-ZAY-shun)	Process of rendering a male or female sterile or unable to conceive children.
transurethral resection of the prostate (TUR, TURP) (trans-yoo-REE-thrall REE-sek-shun of the PROSS-tayt)	Surgical removal of the prostate gland by inserting a device through the urethra and removing prostate tissue.
vasectomy (vas-EK-toh-mee)	Removal of a segment or all of the vas deferens to prevent sperm from leaving the male body. Used for contraception purposes.

Med Term Tip

The vas deferens is the tubing that is severed during a procedure called a *vasectomy*. A vasectomy results in the sterilization of the male since the sperm are no longer able to travel into the urethra and out of the penis during sexual intercourse. The surgical procedure to reverse a vasectomy is a *vasovasostomy*. A new opening is created in order to reconnect one section of the vas deferens to another section of the vas deferens, thereby reestablishing an open tube for sperm to travel through.

■**Figure 10.23** A vasectomy, showing how each vas deferens is tied off in two places and then a section is removed from the middle. This prevents sperm from traveling through the vas deferens during ejaculation.

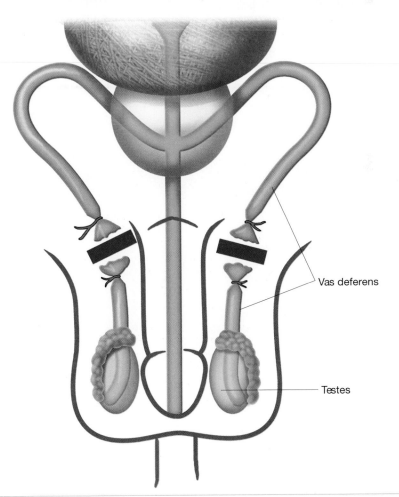

Vas deferens

Testes

vasovasostomy (vas-oh-vay-ZOS-toh-mee)	Surgical procedure to reconnect the vas deferens to reverse a vasectomy.

Pharmacology

CLASSIFICATION	ACTION	GENERIC AND BRAND NAME
androgen therapy (AN-droh-jen)	Replacement of male hormones to treat patients who produce insufficient hormone naturally.	testosterone cypionate, Andronate, depAndro
antiprostatic agents (an-tye-pross-TAT-ik)	Medication to treat early cases of benign prostatic hypertrophy. May prevent surgery for mild cases.	finasteride, Proscar; dutasteride, Avodart
erectile dysfunction agents (ee-REK-tile)	Medication that temporarily produces an erection in patients with erectile dysfunction.	sildenafil citrate, Viagra; tadalafil, Cialis
spermatocide (sper-mah-toh-LIT-ik)	Destruction of sperm. One form of birth control is the use of spermatolytic creams.	nonoxynol 9, Semicid, Ortho-Gynol

Abbreviations

BPH	benign prostatic hypertrophy	**RPR**	rapid plasma reagin (test for syphilis)
DRE	digital rectal exam	**SPP**	suprapubic prostatectomy
ED	erectile dysfunction	**STD**	sexually transmitted disease
GC	gonorrhea	**TUR**	transurethral resection
GU	genitourinary	**TURP**	transurethral resection of the prostate
PSA	prostate-specific antigen	**VD**	venereal disease

Chapter Review

Terminology Checklist

 Below are all Anatomy and Physiology key terms, Word Building, Vocabulary, Pathology, Diagnostic, Therapeutic, and Pharmacology terms presented in this chapter. Use this list as a study tool by placing a check in the box in front of each term as you master its meaning.

- ☐ abortifacient
- ☐ abruptio placentae
- ☐ amenorrhea
- ☐ amniocentesis
- ☐ amnion
- ☐ amniorrhea
- ☐ amniotic
- ☐ amniotic fluid
- ☐ amniotomy
- ☐ androgen
- ☐ androgen therapy
- ☐ andropathy
- ☐ anorchism
- ☐ anteflexion
- ☐ antepartum
- ☐ antiprostatic agents
- ☐ Apgar score
- ☐ areola
- ☐ aspermia
- ☐ atresia
- ☐ balanitis
- ☐ balanoplasty
- ☐ balanorrhea
- ☐ barrier contraception
- ☐ Bartholin's glands
- ☐ benign prostatic hypertrophy
- ☐ breast cancer
- ☐ breasts
- ☐ breech presentation
- ☐ bulbourethral gland
- ☐ candidiasis
- ☐ castration
- ☐ cervical
- ☐ cervical biopsy
- ☐ cervical cancer
- ☐ cervicectomy
- ☐ cervix
- ☐ cesarean section

- ☐ chancroid
- ☐ chlamydia
- ☐ chorion
- ☐ chorionic
- ☐ chorionic villus sampling
- ☐ circumcision
- ☐ clitoris
- ☐ colostrum
- ☐ colposcope
- ☐ colposcopy
- ☐ conception
- ☐ conization
- ☐ corpus
- ☐ Cowper's glands
- ☐ crowning
- ☐ cryptorchidism
- ☐ culdoscopy
- ☐ cystocele
- ☐ delivery
- ☐ digital rectal exam
- ☐ dilation and curettage
- ☐ dilation stage
- ☐ dysmenorrhea
- ☐ dystocia
- ☐ eclampsia
- ☐ effacement
- ☐ ejaculation
- ☐ elective abortion
- ☐ embryo
- ☐ embryonic
- ☐ endocervicitis
- ☐ endometrial biopsy
- ☐ endometrial cancer
- ☐ endometriosis
- ☐ endometritis
- ☐ endometrium
- ☐ epididymal
- ☐ epididymectomy

- ☐ epididymis
- ☐ epididymitis
- ☐ episiorrhaphy
- ☐ episiotomy
- ☐ epispadias
- ☐ erectile dysfunction
- ☐ erectile dysfunction agents
- ☐ erectile tissue
- ☐ estrogen
- ☐ expulsion stage
- ☐ fallopian tubes
- ☐ fertility drug
- ☐ fertilization
- ☐ fetal
- ☐ fetal monitoring
- ☐ fetus
- ☐ fibrocystic breast disease
- ☐ fibroid tumor
- ☐ fimbriae
- ☐ follicle stimulating hormone
- ☐ fraternal twins
- ☐ fundus
- ☐ genital herpes
- ☐ genitalia
- ☐ genital warts
- ☐ genitourinary system
- ☐ gestation
- ☐ glans penis
- ☐ gonorrhea
- ☐ gynecologist
- ☐ gynecology
- ☐ hematosalpinx
- ☐ hemolytic disease of the newborn
- ☐ hormonal contraception
- ☐ hormone replacement therapy
- ☐ human immunodeficiency virus
- ☐ hydrocele

- hymen
- hymenectomy
- hypospadias
- hysterectomy
- hysteropexy
- hysterorrhexis
- hysterosalpingography
- identical twins
- infertility
- intrauterine device
- labia majora
- labia minora
- labor
- lactation
- lactic
- lactiferous ducts
- lactiferous glands
- lactorrhea
- laparoscope
- laparoscopy
- laparotomy
- lumpectomy
- luteinizing hormone
- mammary
- mammary glands
- mammogram
- mammography
- mammoplasty
- mastalgia
- mastectomy
- mastitis
- meconium
- menarche
- menometrorrhagia
- menopause
- menorrhagia
- menstrual period
- menstruation
- metrorrhagia
- metrorrhea
- multigravida
- multipara
- myometrium
- neonate
- neonatologist

- neonatology
- nipple
- nulligravida
- nullipara
- nurse
- obstetrics
- oligomenorrhea
- oligospermia
- oophorectomy
- oophoritis
- oral contraceptive pills
- orchidectomy
- orchidopexy
- orchiectomy
- orchioplasty
- orchiotomy
- ova
- ovarian
- ovarian carcinoma
- ovarian cyst
- ovaries
- oviducts
- ovulation
- oxytocin
- Pap (Papanicolaou) smear
- pelvic examination
- pelvic inflammatory disease
- pelvic ultrasonography
- penis
- perimetritis
- perimetrium
- perineum
- phimosis
- placenta
- placenta previa
- placental stage
- postpartum
- preeclampsia
- pregnancy
- pregnancy test
- premature
- premenstrual syndrome
- prepuce
- priapism
- primigravida

- primipara
- progesterone
- prolapsed umbilical cord
- prolapsed uterus
- prostate cancer
- prostate gland
- prostatectomy
- prostate-specific antigen
- prostatic
- prostatitis
- pseudocyesis
- puberty
- pyosalpinx
- radical mastectomy
- rectocele
- salpingectomy
- salpingitis
- salpingocyesis
- scrotum
- semen
- semen analysis
- seminal vesicles
- seminiferous tubules
- sex hormones
- sexually transmitted disease
- simple mastectomy
- sperm
- spermatic
- spermatic cord
- spermatocide
- spermatogenesis
- spermatolysis
- sphincter
- spontaneous abortion
- sterility
- sterilization
- stillbirth
- syphilis
- testes
- testicles
- testicular
- testicular carcinoma
- testicular torsion
- testosterone
- therapeutic abortion

- ☐ total abdominal hysterectomy–bilateral salpingo-oophorectomy
- ☐ toxic shock syndrome
- ☐ transurethral resection of the prostate
- ☐ trichomoniasis
- ☐ tubal ligation
- ☐ umbilical cord
- ☐ urinary meatus
- ☐ uterine
- ☐ uterine tubes
- ☐ uterus
- ☐ vagina
- ☐ vaginal
- ☐ vaginal hysterectomy
- ☐ vaginal orifice
- ☐ vaginitis
- ☐ varicocele
- ☐ vas deferens
- ☐ vasectomy
- ☐ vasovasostomy
- ☐ vesicular
- ☐ vulva

Practice Exercises

A. Complete the following statements.

1. The study of the female reproductive system is the medical specialty of _____.

2. A physician who specializes in the treatment of women is called a(n) _____.

3. The three stages of labor and delivery are the _____ stage, the _____ stage, and the

   _____ stage.

4. The time required for the development of a fetus is called _____.

5. The cessation of menstruation is called _____.

6. The female sex cell is a(n) _____.

7. The inner lining of the uterus is called the _____.

8. The organ in which the developing fetus resides is called the _____.

9. The tubes that extend from the outer edges of the uterus and assist in transporting the ova and sperm are called

   _____.

10. One of the longest terms used in medical terminology refers to the removal of the uterus, cervix, ovaries, and fallopian

    tubes. This term is _____.

B. State the terms described using the combining forms provided.

The combining form *colp/o* refers to the vagina. Use it to write a term that means:

1. visual examination of the vagina _____

2. instrument used to examine the vagina _____

The combining form *cervic/o* refers to the cervix. Use it to write a term that means:

3. removal of the cervix _____

4. inflammation of the cervix _____

5. pertaining to the cervix _____

The combining form *hyster/o* also refers to the uterus. Use it to write a term that means:

6. surgical fixation of the uterus _____

7. removal of the uterus _____

8. rupture of the uterus _____

The combining form *oophor/o* refers to the ovaries. Use it to write a term that means:

9. inflammation of an ovary _____

10. removal of an ovary _____

The combining form *mamm/o* refers to the breasts. Use it to write a term that means:

11. pertaining to the breasts _____

12. record of breast _____

13. surgical repair of breast _____

The combining form *amni/o* refers to the amnion. Use it to write a term that means:

14. pertaining to the amnion _____

15. incision into amnion _____

16. flow from amnion _____

C. Identify the following abbreviations.

1. Cx _____

2. LMP _____

3. FHR _____

4. PID _____

5. GYN _____

6. CS _____

7. NB _____

8. PMS _____

9. TSS _____

10. LBW _____

D. Write the abbreviations for the following terms.

1. first pregnancy _____

2. artificial insemination _____

3. uterine contractions _____

4. full-term normal delivery _____

5. intrauterine device _____

6. dilation and curettage _____

7. hormone replacement therapy _____   9. abortion _____

8. gynecology _____   10. oral contraception pills _____

E. Define the following combining forms and use them to form female reproductive terms.

	Definition	Female Reproductive Term
1. metr/o	_____	_____
2. hyster/o	_____	_____
3. gynec/o	_____	_____
4. episi/o	_____	_____
5. oophor/o	_____	_____
6. ovari/o	_____	_____
7. salping/o	_____	_____
8. men/o	_____	_____
9. vagin/o	_____	_____
10. mast/o	_____	_____

F. Match each term to its definition.

1. _____ hemolytic disease of the newborn   a. lack of a normal body opening

2. _____ ovary   b. erythroblastosis fetalis

3. _____ vagina   c. detached placenta

4. _____ abruption placentae   d. female erectile tissue

5. _____ placenta   e. produces eggs

6. _____ endometrium   f. normal place for fertilization

7. _____ clitoris   g. buttocks first to appear in birth canal

8. _____ candidiasis   h. birth canal

9. _____ Pap smear   i. nourishes fetus

10. _____ fallopian tube   j. uterine lining

11. _____ dysmenorrhea   k. measures newborn's adjustment to outside world

12. _____ breech presentation   l. test for cervical cancer

13. _____ Apgar   m. newborn

14. _____ neonate   n. yeast infection

15. _____ atresia   o. painful menstruation

G. Use the following terms in the sentences below.

premenstrual syndrome   stillbirth   conization   laparoscopy

D & C   puberty   endometriosis   eclampsia

fibroid tumor   cesarean section

1. Kesha had a core of tissue from her cervix removed for testing. This is called _____.

2. Joan delivered a baby that had died while still in the uterus. She had a(n) _____.

3. Ashley has just started her first menstrual cycle. She is said to have entered _____.

4. Kimberly is experiencing tender breasts, headaches, and some irritability just prior to her monthly menstrual cycle. This may be _____.

5. Ana has been scheduled for an examination in which her physician will use an instrument to observe her abdominal cavity to rule out the diagnosis of severe endometriosis. The physician will insert the instrument through a small incision. This procedure is called a(n) _____.

6. Lenora is scheduled to have a hysterectomy as a result of a long history of large benign growths in her uterus that have caused pain and bleeding. Lenora has a(n) _____.

7. Tiffany's physician has recommended that she have a uterine scraping to stop excessive bleeding after a miscarriage. She will be scheduled for a _____.

8. Stacey is having frequent prenatal checkups to prevent the serious condition of pregnancy called _____.

9. Marion has experienced painful menstrual periods as a result of the lining of her uterus being displaced into her pelvic cavity. This is called _____.

10. Because her cervix was not dilating, Shataundra was informed that she will probably require a(n) _____ for her baby's delivery.

H. Define the following suffixes and use them to form reproductive system terms.

Definition	Reproductive Term
1. -tocia _____	_____
2. -gravida _____	_____
3. -arche _____	_____
4. -cyesis _____	_____
5. -partum _____	_____
6. -para _____	_____
7. -salpinx _____	_____
8. -spermia _____	_____

I. Match each term to its definition.

1. _____ gonorrhea

2. _____ genital herpes

3. _____ human immunodeficiency virus

4. _____ syphilis

5. _____ venereal disease

6. _____ genital warts

7. _____ chancroid

8. _____ chlamydia

9. _____ trichomoniasis

a. also called STD

b. caused by parasitic microorganism

c. treated with penicillin

d. caused by human papilloma virus

e. can pass to infant during birth

f. genitourinary infection

g. venereal ulcer

h. attacks the immune system

i. skin disease with vesicles

J. Complete the following statements.

1. The male reproductive system is a combination of the _____ and _____ systems.

2. The male's external organs of reproduction consist of the _____, _____, and the

   _____.

3. Another term for the prepuce is the _____.

4. The organs responsible for developing the sperm cells are the _____.

5. The glands of lubrication and fluid production at each side of the male urethra are the _____.

6. The male sex hormone is _____.

7. The area between the scrotum and the anus is called the _____.

K. State the terms described using the combining forms provided.

The combining form *prostat/o* refers to the prostate. Use this to write a term that means:

1. removal of prostate _____

2. pertaining to the prostate _____

3. inflammation of the prostate _____

The combining form *orchi/o* refers to the testes. Use this to write a term that means:

4. removal of the testes _____

5. surgical repair of the testes _____

6. incision into the testes _____

The combining form *andr/o* refers to male. Use this to write a term that means:

7. disease of the male _____

8. male producing _____

The combining form *spermat/o* refers to sperm. Use this to write a term that means:

9. sperm forming _____

10. sperm destruction _____

L. Identify the following abbreviations.

1. SPP _____

2. TUR _____

3. GU _____

4. BPH _____

5. DRE _____

6. PSA _____

M. Define the following terms.

1. spermatogenesis _____

2. hydrocele _____

3. transurethral resection of the prostate (TURP) _____

4. aspermia _____

5. orchiectomy _____

6. vasectomy _____

7. castration _____

N. Fill in the classification for each drug description, then match the brand name.

Drug Description	Classification	Brand Name
1. _____ replacement male hormone	_____	a. Pitocin
2. _____ improves uterine contractions	_____	b. Avodart
3. _____ treats early BPH	_____	c. Clomid
4. _____ blocks ovulation	_____	d. nonoxynol 9
5. _____ kills sperm	_____	e. Mifeprex
6. _____ produces an erection	_____	f. Andronate
7. _____ replaces estrogen	_____	g. Ortho-Cept
8. _____ terminates a pregnancy	_____	h. Viagra
9. _____ triggers ovulation	_____	i. Premarin

Medical Record Analysis

Below is an item from a patient's medical record. Read it carefully, make sure you understand all the medical terms used, and then answer the questions that follow.

High-Risk Obstetrics Consultation Report

Reason for Consultation:	High-risk pregnancy with late-term bleeding
History of Present Illness:	Patient is 23 years old. She is currently estimated to be at 175 days of gestation. She has had a 23-lb weight gain with this pregnancy. Amniocentesis at 20 weeks indicated male fetus with no evidence of genetic or developmental disorders. She noticed a moderate degree of vaginal bleeding this morning but denies any cramping or pelvic pain. She immediately saw her obstetrician who referred her for high-risk evaluation.
Past Medical History:	This patient is multigravida but nullipara with three early miscarriages without obvious cause. She was diagnosed with cancer of the left ovary four years ago. It was treated with a left oophorectomy and chemotherapy. She continues to undergo full-body CT scan every six months, and there has been no evidence of metastasis since that time. Menarche was at age 13, and her menstrual history is significant for menorrhagia resulting in chronic anemia.
Results of Physical Examination:	Patient appears well nourished and abdominal girth appears consistent with length of gestation. She is understandably quite anxious regarding the sudden spotting. Pelvic ultrasound indicates placenta previa with placenta almost completely overlying cervix. However, there is no evidence of abruptio placentae at this time. Fetal size estimate is consistent with 25 weeks of gestation. The fetus is turned head down, and the umbilical cord is not around the neck. The fetal heart tones are strong with a rate of 130 beats/minute. There is no evidence of cervical effacement or dilation at this time.
Recommendations:	Fetus appears to be developing well and in no distress at this time. The placenta appears to be well attached on ultrasound, but the bleeding is cause for concern. With the extremely low position of the placenta, this patient is at very high risk for abruptio placentae when cervix begins effacement and dilation. She may require early delivery by cesarean section at that time. She will definitely require C-section at onset of labor. At this time, recommend bed rest with bathroom privileges. She is to return every other day for two weeks and every day after that for evaluation of cervix and fetal condition. She is to call immediately if she notes any further bleeding or change in activity level of the fetus.

Critical Thinking Questions

1. Describe in your own words the treatment this patient received for her ovarian cancer. What procedure does she continue to have every six months?

_____

_____

2. Describe in your own words this patient's menstrual history. _____

_____

3. Which of the following choices describes this patient (choose all that apply)?

    a. She has never been pregnant.
    b. She has several live children.
    c. She has no live children.
    d. She has been pregnant several times.

4. This patient has placenta previa. What procedure discovered this condition? The physician, however, is much more concerned about abruptio placentae. Explain why.

    _____

    _____

5. Describe the condition of the fetus. _____

    _____

6. The following two phrases are not specifically defined by your text. Explain what you believe them to mean based on the context of this consultation report.

    a. high-risk pregnancy _____

    _____

    b. abdominal girth appears consistent with length of gestation _____

    _____

Chart Note Transcription

The chart note below contains ten phrases that can be reworded with a medical term that you learned in this chapter. Each phrase is identified with an underline. Determine the medical term and write your answers in the space provided.

Current Complaint: Patient is a 77-year-old male seen by the urologist with complaints of nocturia and difficulty with <u>the release of semen from the urethra</u>. ❶

Past History: Medical history revealed that the patient had <u>failure of the testes to descend into the scrotum</u> ❷ at birth, which was repaired by <u>surgical fixation of the testes</u>. ❸ He had also undergone elective sterilization <u>by removal of a segment of the vas deferens</u> ❹ at the age of 41.

Signs and Symptoms: Patient states he first noted these symptoms about five years ago. They have become increasingly severe and now he is not able to sleep without waking to urinate up to 20 times a night. He has difficulty with <u>release of semen</u>. ❺ <u>Palpation of the prostate gland through the rectum</u> ❻ revealed multiple round firm nodules in prostate gland. A needle biopsy was negative for <u>slow-growing cancer that frequently affects males over 50</u> ❼ and a <u>blood test for prostate cancer</u> ❽ was normal.

Diagnosis: <u>Noncancerous enlargement of the prostate gland</u>. ❾

Treatment: Patient was scheduled for a <u>surgical removal of prostate tissue through the urethra</u>. ❿

❶ _____

❷ _____

❸ _____

❹ _____

❺ _____

❻ _____

❼ _____

❽ _____

❾ _____

❿ _____

Labeling Exercise

A. System Review

1. Write the labels for this figure on the numbered lines provided.

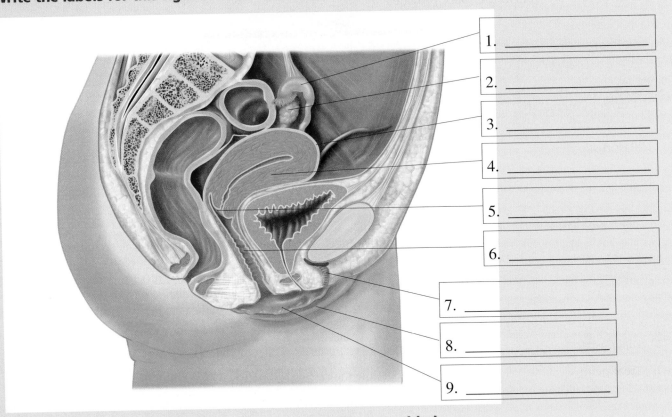

1. _____

2. _____

3. _____

4. _____

5. _____

6. _____

7. _____

8. _____

9. _____

2. Write the labels for this figure on the numbered lines provided.

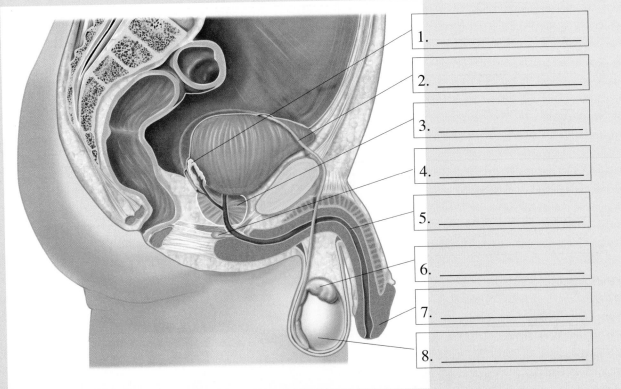

1. _____

2. _____

3. _____

4. _____

5. _____

6. _____

7. _____

8. _____

B. Anatomy Challenge

Write the labels for this figure on the numbered lines provided.

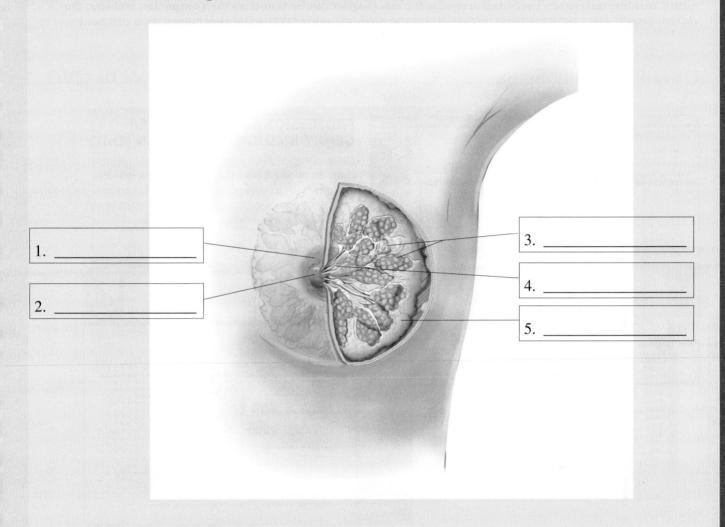

1. _____

2. _____

3. _____

4. _____

5. _____

Multimedia Preview

Additional interactive resources and activities for this chapter can be found on the Companion Website. For videos, games, and pronunciations, please access the accompanying DVD-ROM that comes with this book.

DVD-ROM Highlights

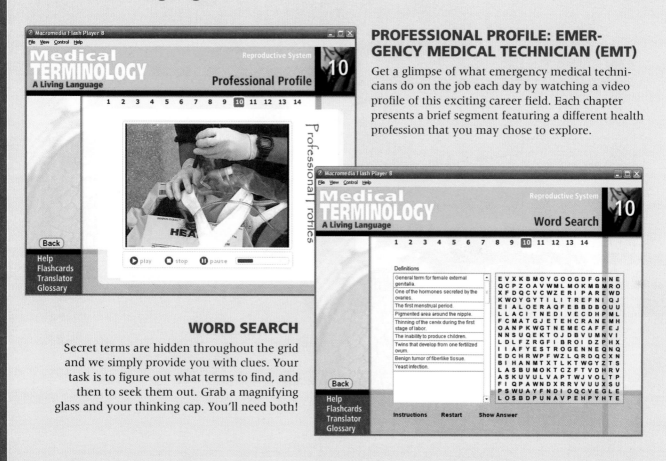

PROFESSIONAL PROFILE: EMERGENCY MEDICAL TECHNICIAN (EMT)

Get a glimpse of what emergency medical technicians do on the job each day by watching a video profile of this exciting career field. Each chapter presents a brief segment featuring a different health profession that you may chose to explore.

WORD SEARCH

Secret terms are hidden throughout the grid and we simply provide you with clues. Your task is to figure out what terms to find, and then to seek them out. Grab a magnifying glass and your thinking cap. You'll need both!

Website Highlights—www.prenhall.com/fremgen

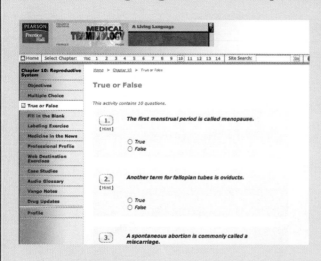

TRUE/FALSE QUIZ

Take advantage of the free-access on-line study guide that accompanies your textbook. You'll find a true/false quiz that provides instant feedback that allows you to check your score and see what you got right or wrong. By clicking on this URL you'll also access links to download mp3 audio reviews, current news articles, and an audio glossary.

11

Endocrine System

Learning Objectives

Upon completion of this chapter, you will be able to:

- Identify and define the combining forms and suffixes introduced in this chapter.
- Correctly spell and pronounce medical terms and major anatomical structures relating to the endocrine system.
- Locate and describe the major organs of the endocrine system and their functions.
- List the major hormones secreted by each endocrine gland and describe their functions.
- Build and define endocrine system medical terms from word parts.
- Identify and define endocrine system vocabulary terms.
- Identify and define selected endocrine system pathology terms.
- Identify and define selected endocrine system diagnostic procedures.
- Identify and define selected endocrine system therapeutic procedures.
- Identify and define selected medications relating to the endocrine system.
- Define selected abbreviations associated with the endocrine system.

Endocrine System at a Glance

Function

Endocrine glands secrete hormones that regulate many body activities such as metabolic rate, water and mineral balance, immune system reactions, and sexual functioning.

Organs

adrenal glands
ovaries
pancreas (islets of Langerhans)
parathyroid glands
pineal gland
pituitary gland
testes
thymus gland
thyroid gland

Combining Forms

acr/o	extremities	kal/i	potassium
adren/o	adrenal glands	natr/o	sodium
adrenal/o	adrenal glands	ophthalm/o	eye
andr/o	male	pancreat/o	pancreas
calc/o	calcium	parathyroid/o	parathyroid gland
crin/o	secrete	pineal/o	pineal gland
estr/o	female	pituitar/o	pituitary gland
glyc/o	sugar	thym/o	thymus gland
glycos/o	sugar	thyr/o	thyroid gland
gonad/o	sex glands	thyroid/o	thyroid gland
home/o	sameness	toxic/o	poison

Suffixes

-crine	to secrete
-dipsia	thirst
-prandial	relating to a meal
-tropin	stimulate

Endocrine System Illustrated

pineal gland, p. 362

Regulates circadian rhythm

pituitary gland, p. 363

Regulates many other
endocrine glands

thyroid gland, p. 366
parathyroid glands, p. 362

Thyroid

Parathyroid

Regulates metabolic rate
Regulate blood calcium level

thymus gland, p. 364

Development of
immune system

adrenal glands, p. 360

Cortex
Medulla

Regulate water and
electrolyte levels

ovaries, p. 360

Regulate female
reproductive system

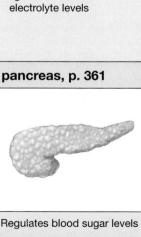
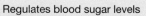

pancreas, p. 361

Regulates blood sugar levels

testes, p. 364

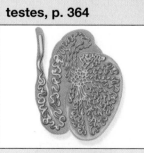

Regulate male
reproductive system

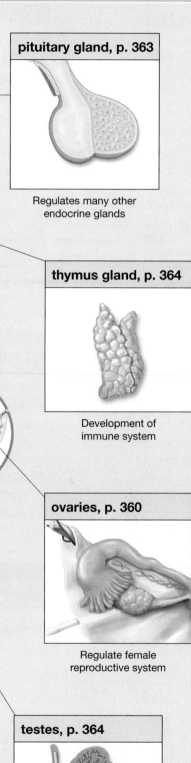
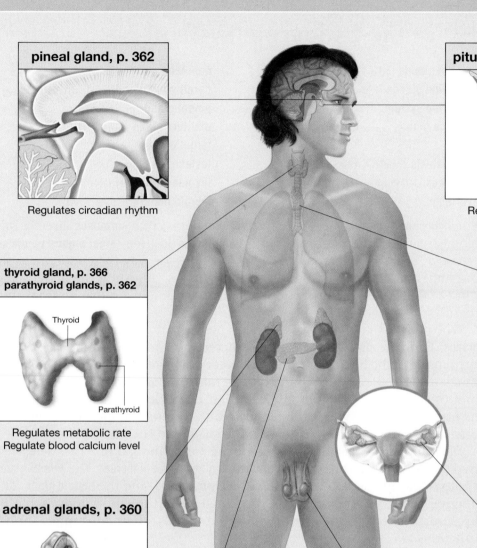

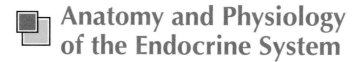

Anatomy and Physiology of the Endocrine System

adrenal glands (ad-REE-nal)
endocrine glands (EN-doh-krin)
endocrine system
exocrine glands (EKS-oh-krin)
glands
homeostasis (hoe-me-oh-STAY-sis)
hormones (HOR-mohnz)
ovaries (OH-vah-reez)

pancreas (PAN-kree-ass)
parathyroid glands (pair-ah-THIGH-royd)
pineal gland (pih-NEAL)
pituitary gland (pih-TOO-ih-tair-ee)
target organs
testes (TESS-teez)
thymus gland (THIGH-mus)
thyroid gland (THIGH-royd)

Med Term Tip

The terms *endocrine* and *exocrine* were constructed to reflect the function of each type of gland. As glands, they both secrete, indicated by the combining form *crin/o*. The prefix *exo-*, meaning "external" or "outward," tells us that exocrine gland secretions are carried to the outside of the body. However, the prefix *endo-*, meaning "within" or "internal," indicates that endocrine gland secretions are carried to other internal body structures by the bloodstream.

The **endocrine system** is a collection of **glands** that secrete **hormones** directly into the bloodstream. Hormones are chemicals that act on their **target organs** to either increase or decrease the target's activity level. In this way the endocrine system is instrumental in maintaining **homeostasis**—that is, adjusting the activity level of most of the tissues and organs of the body to maintain a stable internal environment.

The body actually has two distinct types of glands: **exocrine glands** and **endocrine glands**. Exocrine glands release their secretions into a duct that carries them to the outside of the body. For example, sweat glands release sweat into a sweat duct that travels to the surface of the body. Endocrine glands, however, release hormones directly into the bloodstream. For example, the thyroid gland secretes its hormones directly into the bloodstream. Because endocrine glands have no ducts, they are also referred to as *ductless glands*.

The endocrine system consists of the following glands: two **adrenal glands**, two **ovaries** in the female, four **parathyroid glands**, the **pancreas**, the **pineal gland**, the **pituitary gland**, two **testes** in the male, the **thymus gland**, and the **thyroid gland**. The endocrine glands as a whole affect the functions of the entire body. Table 11.1 ■ presents a description of the endocrine glands, their hormones, and their functions.

Table 11.1 Endocrine Glands and Their Hormones

GLAND AND HORMONE	FUNCTION
Adrenal cortex	
Glucocorticoids	
Cortisol	Regulates carbohydrate levels in the body
Mineralocorticoids	
Aldosterone	Regulates electrolytes and fluid volume in body
Steroid sex hormones	
Androgen, estrogen, progesterone	Responsible for reproduction and secondary sexual characteristics
Adrenal medulla	
Epinephrine (adrenaline)	Intensifies response during stress; "fight or flight" response
Norepinephrine	Chiefly a vasoconstrictor

Table 11.1 — Endocrine Glands and Their Hormones *(continued)*

GLAND AND HORMONE	FUNCTION
Ovaries	
Estrogen	Stimulates development of secondary sex characteristics in females; regulates menstrual cycle
Progesterone	Prepares for conditions of pregnancy
Pancreas	
Glucagon	Stimulates liver to release glucose into the blood
Insulin	Regulates and promotes entry of glucose into cells
Parathyroid glands	
Parathyroid hormone (PTH)	Stimulates bone breakdown; regulates calcium level in the blood
Pituitary anterior lobe	
Adrenocorticotropin hormone (ACTH)	Regulates function of adrenal cortex
Follicle-stimulating hormone (FSH)	Stimulates growth of eggs in female and sperm in males
Growth hormone (GH)	Stimulates growth of the body
Luteinizing hormone (LH)	Regulates function of male and female gonads and plays a role in releasing ova in females
Melanocyte-stimulating hormone (MSH)	Stimulates pigment in skin
Prolactin	Stimulates milk production
Thyroid-stimulating hormone (TSH)	Regulates function of thyroid gland
Pituitary posterior lobe	
Antidiuretic hormone (ADH)	Stimulates reabsorption of water by the kidneys
Oxytocin	Stimulates uterine contractions and releases milk into ducts
Testes	
Testosterone	Promotes sperm production and development of secondary sex characteristics in males
Thymus	
Thymosin	Promotes development of cells in immune system
Thyroid gland	
Calcitonin	Stimulates deposition of calcium into bone
Thyroxine (T_4)	Stimulates metabolism in cells
Triiodothyronine (T_3)	Stimulates metabolism in cells

Adrenal Glands

adrenal cortex (KOR-tex)
adrenal medulla (meh-DOOL-lah)
adrenaline (ah-DREN-ah-lin)
aldosterone (al-DOSS-ter-ohn)
androgens (AN-druh-jenz)
corticosteroids (kor-tih-koh-STAIR-oydz)
cortisol (KOR-tih-sal)
epinephrine (ep-ih-NEF-rin)

estrogen (ESS-troh-jen)
glucocorticoids (gloo-koh-KOR-tih-koydz)
mineralocorticoids
    (min-er-al-oh-KOR-tih-koydz)
norepinephrine (nor-ep-ih-NEF-rin)
progesterone (proh-JESS-ter-ohn)
steroid sex hormones (STAIR-oyd)

Med Term Tip

The term *cortex* is frequently used in anatomy to indicate the outer portion of an organ such as the adrenal gland or the kidney. The term *cortex* means "bark," as in the bark of a tree. The term *medulla* means "marrow." Because marrow is found in the inner cavity of bones, the term came to stand for the middle of an organ.

The two adrenal glands are located above each of the kidneys (see Figure 11.1 ▦). Each gland is composed of two sections: **adrenal cortex** and **adrenal medulla**.

The outer adrenal cortex manufactures several different families of hormones: **mineralocorticoids**, **glucocorticoids**, and **steroid sex hormones**. However, because they are all produced by the cortex, they are collectively referred to as **corticosteroids**. The mineralocorticoid hormone, **aldosterone**, regulates sodium (Na^+) and potassium (K^+) levels in the body. The glucocorticoid hormone, **cortisol**, regulates carbohydrates in the body. The adrenal cortex of both men and women secretes steroid sex hormones: **androgens**, **estrogen**, and **progesterone**. These hormones regulate secondary sexual characteristics. All hormones secreted by the adrenal cortex are steroid hormones.

The inner adrenal medulla is responsible for secreting the hormones **epinephrine**, also called **adrenaline**, and **norepinephrine**. These hormones are critical during emergency situations because they increase blood pressure, heart rate, and respiration levels. This helps the body perform better during emergencies or otherwise stressful times.

Ovaries

estrogen
gametes (gam-EATS)
gonads (GOH-nadz)

menstrual cycle (men-STROO-all)
ova
progesterone

The two ovaries are located in the lower abdominopelvic cavity of the female (see Figure 11.2 ▦). They are the female **gonads**. Gonads are organs that produce **gametes** or the reproductive sex cells. In the case of females, the gametes are the **ova**. Of importance to the endocrine system, the ovaries produce the female sex hormones, **estrogen** and **progesterone**. Estrogen is responsible for the appearance of the female sexual characteristics and regulation of the **menstrual cycle**. Progesterone helps to maintain a suitable uterine environment for pregnancy.

▦ **Figure 11.1** The adrenal glands. These glands sit on top of each kidney. Each adrenal is subdivided into an outer cortex and an inner medulla. Each region secretes different hormones.

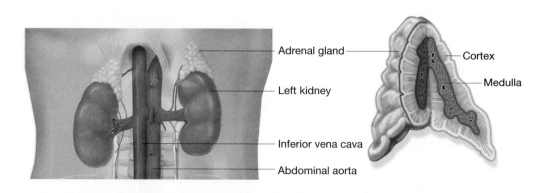

Adrenal gland
Left kidney
Inferior vena cava
Abdominal aorta
Cortex
Medulla

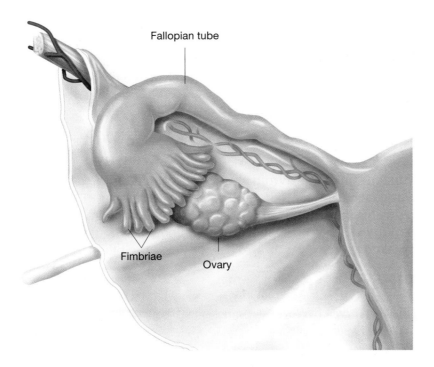

■ **Figure 11.2** The ovaries. In addition to producing ova, the ovaries secrete the female sex hormones, estrogen and progesterone.

Fallopian tube

Fimbriae

Ovary

Pancreas

glucagon (GLOO-koh-gon)

insulin (IN-suh-lin)

islets of Langerhans
(EYE-lets of LAHNG-er-hahnz)

The pancreas is located along the lower curvature of the stomach (see Figure 11.3A ■). It is the only organ in the body that has both endocrine and exocrine functions. The exocrine portion of the pancreas releases digestive enzymes through a duct into the duodenum of the small intestine. The endocrine sections of the pancreas, **islets of Langerhans**, are named after Dr. Paul Langerhans, a German anatomist. The islets cells produce two different hormones: **insulin** and **glucagon** (see Figure 11.3B ■). Insulin, produced by beta (β) islet cells, stimulates the cells of the body to take in glucose from the bloodstream, lowering your blood sugar level. This occurs after you have eaten a meal and absorbed the carbohydrates into your bloodstream. In this way the cells obtain the glucose they need for cellular respiration.

Another set of islet cells, the alpha (α) cells, secrete a different hormone, glucagon, which stimulates the liver to release glucose, thereby raising the blood

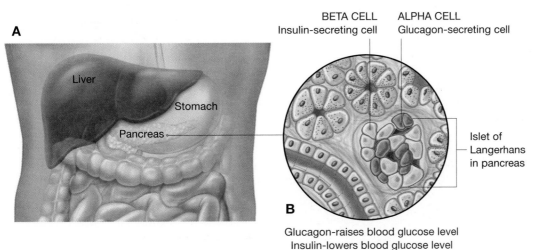

A

Liver

Stomach

Pancreas

BETA CELL
Insulin-secreting cell

ALPHA CELL
Glucagon-secreting cell

Islet of
Langerhans
in pancreas

B

Glucagon-raises blood glucose level
Insulin-lowers blood glucose level

■ **Figure 11.3** The pancreas. This organ sits just below the stomach and is both an exocrine and an endocrine gland. The endocrine regions of the pancreas are called the islets of Langerhans and they secrete insulin and glucagon.

glucose level. Glucagon is released when the body needs more sugar, such as at the beginning of strenuous activity or several hours after the last meal has been digested. Insulin and glucagon have opposite effects on blood sugar level. Insulin will reduce the blood sugar level, while glucagon will increase it.

Parathyroid Glands

calcium   **parathyroid hormone**
                                                 (pair-ah-THIGH-royd HOR-mohn)

The four tiny parathyroid glands are located on the dorsal surface of the thyroid gland (see Figure 11.4 ■). The **parathyroid hormone** (PTH) secreted by these glands regulates the amount of **calcium** in the blood. If blood calcium levels fall too low, parathyroid hormone levels in the blood are increased and will stimulate bone breakdown to release more calcium into the blood.

Pineal Gland

circadian rhythm (seer-KAY-dee-an)   **thalamus** (THALL-mus)
melatonin (mel-ah-TOH-nin)

The pineal gland is a small pine-cone-shaped gland that is part of the **thalamus** region of the brain (see Figure 11.5 ■). The pineal gland secretes **melatonin**, a hormone not well understood, but that plays a role in regulating the body's **circadian rhythm**. This is the 24-hour clock that governs our periods of wakefulness and sleepiness.

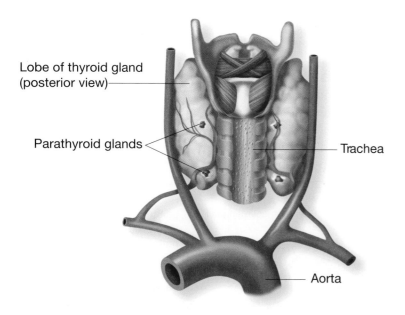

Lobe of thyroid gland (posterior view)

Parathyroid glands

Trachea

Aorta

■ **Figure 11.4** The parathyroid glands. These four glands are located on the posterior side of the thyroid gland. They secrete parathyroid hormone.

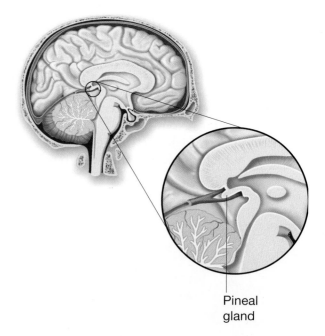

Pineal gland

■ **Figure 11.5** The pineal gland is a part of the thalamus region of the brain. It secretes melatonin.

Pituitary Gland

adrenocorticotropin hormone
  (ah-dree-noh-kor-tih-koh-TROH-pin)
anterior lobe
antidiuretic hormone (an-tye-dye-yoo-RET-ik)
follicle-stimulating hormone
  (FOLL-ih-kl STIM-yoo-lay-ting)
gonadotropins (go-nad-oh-TROH-pins)
growth hormone
hypothalamus (high-poh-THAL-ah-mus)

luteinizing hormone (LOO-tee-in-eye-zing)
melanocyte-stimulating hormone
oxytocin (ok-see-TOH-sin)
posterior lobe
prolactin (proh-LAK-tin)
somatotropin (so-mat-oh-TROH-pin)
thyroid-stimulating hormone

The pituitary gland is located underneath the brain (see Figure 11.6 ■). The small marble-shaped gland is divided into an **anterior lobe** and a **posterior lobe**. Both lobes are controlled by the **hypothalamus**, a region of the brain active in regulating automatic body responses.

The anterior pituitary secretes several different hormones (see Figure 11.7 ■). **Growth hormone** (GH), also called **somatotropin**, promotes growth of the body by stimulating cells to rapidly increase in size and divide. **Thyroid-stimulating hormone** (TSH) regulates the function of the thyroid gland. **Adrenocorticotropin hormone** (ACTH) regulates the function of the adrenal cortex. **Prolactin** (PRL) stimulates milk production in the breast following pregnancy and birth. **Follicle-stimulating hormone** (FSH) and **luteinizing hormone** (LH) both exert their influence on the male and female gonads. Therefore, these two hormones together are referred to as the **gonadotropins**. Follicle-stimulating hormone is responsible for the develop-

Med Term Tip

The pituitary gland is sometimes referred to as the "master gland" because several of its secretions regulate other endocrine glands.

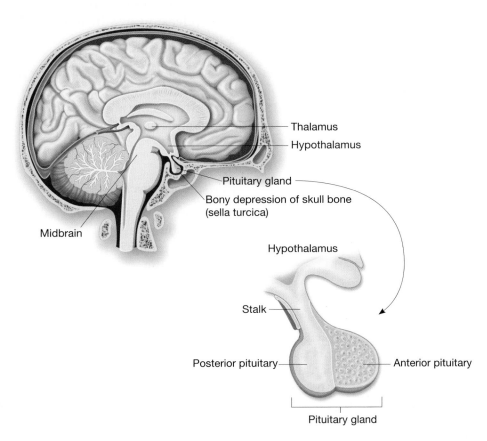

■ **Figure 11.6** The pituitary gland lies just underneath the brain. It is subdivided into anterior and posterior lobes. Each lobe secretes different hormones.

Thalamus
Hypothalamus
Pituitary gland
Bony depression of skull bone (sella turcica)
Midbrain
Hypothalamus
Stalk
Posterior pituitary
Anterior pituitary
Pituitary gland

■ **Figure 11.7** The anterior pituitary is sometimes called the master gland because it secretes many hormones that regulate other glands. This figure illustrates the different hormones and target tissues for the anterior pituitary.

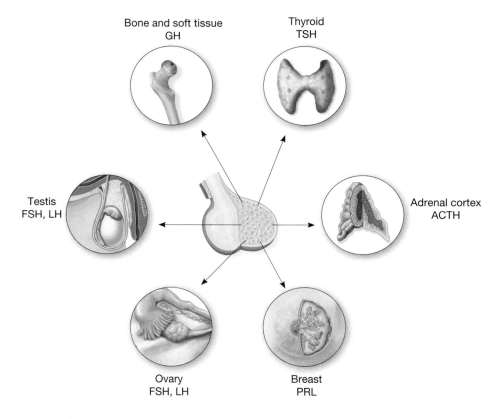

Bone and soft tissue
GH

Thyroid
TSH

Testis
FSH, LH

Adrenal cortex
ACTH

Ovary
FSH, LH

Breast
PRL

Med Term Tip

Many people use the term *diabetes* to refer to diabetes mellitus (DM). But there is another type of diabetes, called *diabetes insipidus* (DI) that is a result of the inadequate secretion of the antidiuretic hormone (ADH) from the pituitary gland.

ment of ova in ovaries and sperm in testes. It also stimulates the ovary to secrete estrogen. Luteinizing hormone stimulates secretion of sex hormones in both males and females and plays a role in releasing ova in females. **Melanocyte-stimulating hormone** (MSH) stimulates melanocytes to produce more melanin, thereby darkening the skin.

The posterior pituitary secretes two hormones, **antidiuretic hormone** (ADH) and **oxytocin**. Antidiuretic hormone promotes water reabsorption by the kidney tubules. Oxytocin stimulates uterine contractions during labor and delivery, and after birth the release of milk from the mammary glands.

Testes

sperm   **testosterone** (tess-TOSS-ter-own)

The testes are two oval glands located in the scrotal sac of the male (see Figure 11.8 ■). They are the male gonads, which produce the male gametes, **sperm**, and the male sex hormone, **testosterone**. Testosterone produces the male secondary sexual characteristics and regulates sperm production.

Thymus Gland

T cells   **thymosin** (thigh-MOH-sin)

In addition to its role as part of the immune system, the thymus is also one of the endocrine glands because it secretes the hormone **thymosin**. Thymosin, like the rest of the thymus gland, is important for proper development of the immune system. The thymus gland is located in the mediastinal cavity anterior and superior to the heart (see Figure 11.9 ■). The thymus is present at birth and grows to its largest size during puberty. At puberty it begins to shrink and eventually is replaced with connective and adipose tissue.

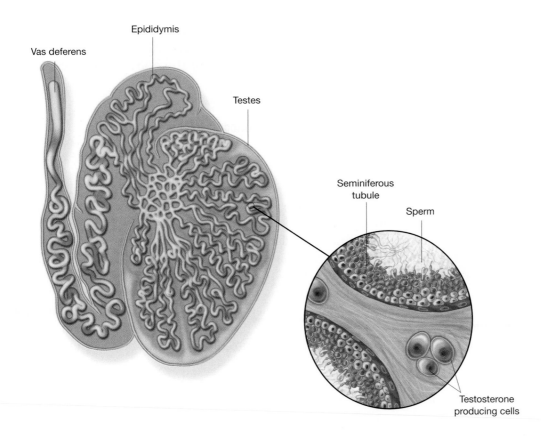

Figure 11.8 The testes. In addition to producing sperm, the testes secrete the male sex hormones, primarily testosterone.

Vas deferens

Epididymis

Testes

Seminiferous tubule

Sperm

Testosterone producing cells

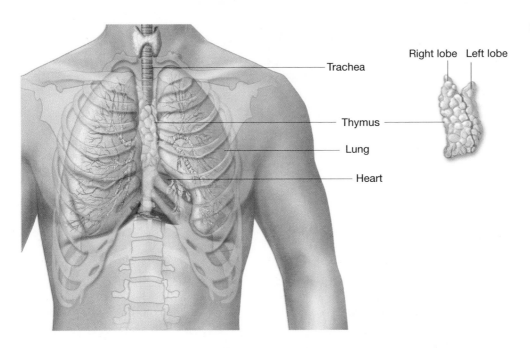

Figure 11.9 The thymus gland. This gland lies in the mediastinum of the thoracic cavity, just above the heart. It secretes thymosin.

Trachea

Thymus

Lung

Heart

Right lobe   Left lobe

The most important function of the thymus is the development of the immune system in the newborn. It is essential to the growth and development of thymic lymphocytes or **T cells**, which are critical for the body's immune system.

Thyroid Gland

calcitonin (kal-sih-TOH-nin)

iodine

thyroxine (thigh-ROKS-in)

triiodothyronine
    (try-eye-oh-doh-THIGH-roh-neen)

The thyroid gland, which resembles a butterfly in shape, has right and left lobes (see Figure 11.10 ■). It is located on either side of the trachea and larynx. The thyroid cartilage, or Adam's apple, is located just above the thyroid gland. This gland produces the hormones **thyroxine** (T_4) and **triiodothyronine** (T_3). These hormones are produced in the thyroid gland from the mineral **iodine** (**EYE** oh dine). Thyroxine and triiodothyronine help to regulate the production of energy and heat in the body to adjust the body's metabolic rate.

The thyroid gland also secretes **calcitonin** in response to hypercalcemia (too high blood calcium level). Its action is the opposite of parathyroid hormone and stimulates the increased deposition of calcium into bone, thereby lowering blood levels of calcium.

■ **Figure 11.10** The thyroid gland is subdivided into two lobes, one on each side of the trachea.

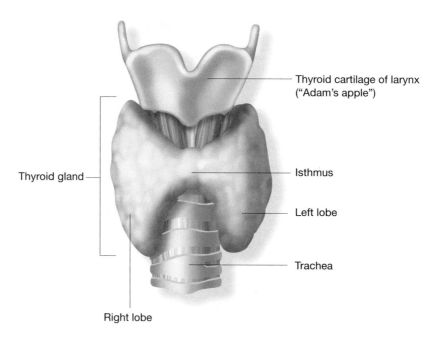

Thyroid cartilage of larynx ("Adam's apple")

Thyroid gland

Isthmus

Left lobe

Trachea

Right lobe

Word Building

The following list contains examples of medical terms built directly from word parts. The definitions of these terms can be determined by a straightforward translation of the word parts.

COMBINING FORM	COMBINED WITH	MEDICAL TERM	DEFINITION
adren/o	-al	**adrenal** (ah-DREE-nall)	pertaining to the adrenal glands
	-megaly	**adrenomegaly** (ad-ree-noh-MEG-ah-lee)	enlarged adrenal gland
	-pathy	**adrenopathy** (ad-ren-OP-ah-thee)	adrenal gland disease

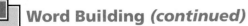
Word Building *(continued)*

COMBINING FORM	COMBINED WITH	MEDICAL TERM	DEFINITION
adrenal/o	-ectomy	**adrenalectomy** (ad-ree-nal-EK-toh-mee)	removal of adrenal glands
	-itis	**adrenalitis** (ad-ree-nal-EYE-tis)	inflammation of an adrenal gland
calc/o	hyper- -emia	**hypercalcemia** (high-per-kal-SEE-mee-ah)	excessive calcium in the blood
	hypo- -emia	**hypocalcemia** (high-poh-kal-SEE-mee-ah)	low calcium in the blood
crin/o	endo- -logist	**endocrinologist** (en-doh-krin-ALL-oh-jist)	specialist in the endocrine system
	endo- -pathy	**endocrinopathy** (en-doh-krin-OP-ah-thee)	endocrine system disease
glyc/o	hyper- -emia	**hyperglycemia** (high-per-glye-SEE-mee-ah)	excessive sugar in the blood
	hypo- -emia	**hypoglycemia** (high-poh-glye-SEE-mee-ah)	low sugar in the blood
kal/i	hyper- -emia	**hyperkalemia** (high-per-kal-EE-mee-ah)	excessive potassium in the blood
natr/o	hypo- -emia	**hyponatremia** (high-poh-nah-TREE-mee-ah)	low sodium in the blood
pancreat/o	-ic	**pancreatic** (pan-kree-AT-ik)	pertaining to the pancreas
parathyroid/o	-al	**parathyroidal** (pair-ah-THIGH-roy-dall)	pertaining to the parathyroid gland
	-ectomy	**parathyroidectomy** (pair-ah-thigh-royd-EK-toh-mee)	removal of the parathyroid gland
	hyper- -ism	**hyperparathyroidism** (HIGH-per-pair-ah-THIGH-royd-izm)	state of excessive parathyroid
	hypo- -ism	**hypoparathyroidism** (HIGH-poh-pair-ah-THIGH-royd-izm)	state of insufficient parathyroid
pituitar/o	-ary	**pituitary** (pih-TOO-ih-tair-ee)	pertaining to the pituitary gland
	hypo- -ism	**hypopituitarism** (HIGH-poh-pih-TOO-ih-tuh-rizm)	state of insufficient pituitary
	hyper- -ism	**hyperpituitarism** (HIGH-per-pih-TOO-ih-tuh-rizm)	state of excessive pituitary
thym/o	-ic	**thymic** (THIGH-mik)	pertaining to the thymus gland
	-ectomy	**thymectomy** (thigh-MEK-toh-mee)	removal of the thymus
	-itis	**thymitis** (thigh-MY-tis)	thymus inflammation
	-oma	**thymoma** (thigh-MOH-mah)	thymus tumor
thyr/o	-megaly	**thyromegaly** (thigh-roh-MEG-ah-lee)	enlarged thyroid
thyroid/o	-al	**thyroidal** (thigh-ROYD-all)	pertaining to the thyroid gland

Word Building *(continued)*

COMBINING FORM	COMBINED WITH	MEDICAL TERM	DEFINITION
	-ectomy	**thyroidectomy** (thigh-royd-EK-toh-mee)	removal of the thyroid
	hyper- -ism	**hyperthyroidism** (hi-per-THIGH-royd-izm)	state of excessive thyroid
	hypo- -ism	**hypothyroidism** (high-poh-THIGH-royd-izm)	state of insufficient thyroid

SUFFIX	COMBINED WITH	MEDICAL TERM	DEFINITION
-dipsia	poly-	**polydipsia** (pall-ee-DIP-see-ah)	many (excessive) thirst
-uria	poly-	**polyuria** (pall-ee-YOO-ree-ah)	condition of (too) much urine
	glycos/o	**glycosuria** (glye-kohs-YOO-ree-ah)	sugar in the urine

Vocabulary

TERM	DEFINITION
acidosis (as-ih-DOH-sis)	Excessive acidity of body fluids due to the accumulation of acids, as in diabetic acidosis.
edema (eh-DEE-mah)	Condition in which the body tissues contain excessive amounts of fluid.
endocrinology (en-doh-krin-ALL-oh-jee)	Branch of medicine involving diagnosis and treatment of conditions and diseases of endocrine glands. Physician is an *endocrinologist*.
exophthalmos (eks-off-THAL-mohs)	Condition in which the eyeballs protrude, such as in Graves' disease. This is generally caused by an overproduction of thyroid hormone.

Figure 11.11 A photograph of a woman with exophthalmos. This condition is associated with hypersecretion of the thyroid gland. *(Custom Medical Stock Photo, Inc.)*

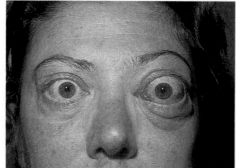

TERM	DEFINITION
gynecomastia (gigh-neh-koh-MAST-ee-ah)	Development of breast tissue in males. May be a symptom of adrenal feminization (see Pathology table).
hirsutism (HER-soot-izm)	Condition of having an excessive amount of hair. Term generally used to describe females who have the adult male pattern of hair growth. Can be the result of a hormonal imbalance.
hypersecretion	Excessive hormone production by an endocrine gland.
hyposecretion	Deficient hormone production by an endocrine gland.
obesity (oh-BEE-sih-tee)	Having an abnormal amount of fat in the body.
syndrome (SIN-drohm)	Group of symptoms and signs that, when combined, present a clinical picture of a disease or condition.

Pathology

TERM	DEFINITION
■ Adrenal Glands	
Addison's disease (AD-ih-sons dih-ZEEZ)	Disease named for British physician Thomas Addison that results from a deficiency in adrenocortical hormones. There may be an increased pigmentation of the skin, generalized weakness, and weight loss.
adrenal feminization (ad-REE-nal fem-ih-nigh-ZAY-shun)	Development of female secondary sexual characteristics (such as breasts) in a male. Often as a result of increased estrogen secretion by the adrenal cortex.
adrenal virilism (ad-REE-nal VIR-ill-izm)	Development of male secondary sexual characteristics (such as deeper voice and facial hair) in a female. Often as a result of increased androgen secretion by the adrenal cortex.
Cushing's syndrome (CUSH-ings SIN-drohm)	Set of symptoms, named after U.S. neurosurgeon Harvey Cushing, that result from hypersecretion of the adrenal cortex. This may be the result of a tumor of the adrenal glands. The syndrome may present symptoms of weakness, edema, excess hair growth, skin discoloration, and osteoporosis.

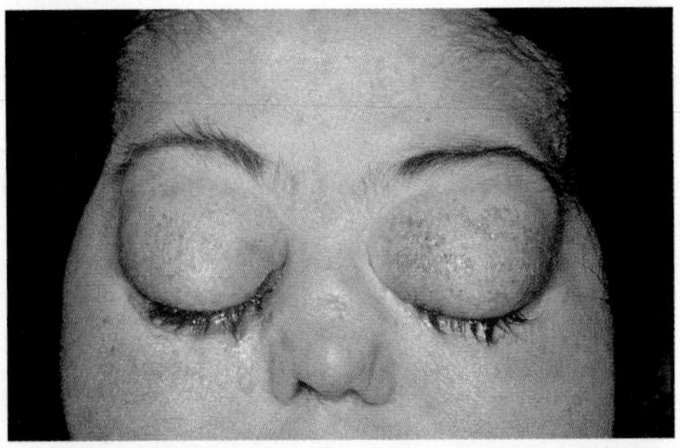

■ Figure 11.12 Cushing's syndrome. A photograph of a woman with the characteristic facial features of Cushing's syndrome. *(Biophoto Associates/ Science Source/Photo Researchers, Inc.)*

TERM	DEFINITION
pheochromocytoma (fee-oh-kroh-moh-sigh-TOH-ma)	Usually benign tumor of the adrenal medulla that secretes epinephrine. Symptoms include anxiety, heart palpitations, dyspnea, profuse sweating, headache, and nausea.
■ Pancreas	
diabetes mellitus (DM) (dye-ah-BEE-teez MELL-ih-tus)	Chronic disorder of carbohydrate metabolism that results in hyperglycemia and glycosuria. There are two distinct forms of diabetes mellitus: *insulin-dependent diabetes mellitus* (IDDM) or *type 1*, and *non–insulin-dependent diabetes mellitus* (NIDDM) or *type 2*.
diabetic retinopathy (dye-ah-BET-ik ret-in-OP-ah-thee)	Secondary complication of diabetes that affects the blood vessels of the retina, resulting in visual changes and even blindness.
insulin-dependent diabetes mellitus (IDDM) (dye-ah-BEE-teez MELL-ih-tus)	Also called *type 1 diabetes mellitus.* It develops early in life when the pancreas stops insulin production. Patient must take daily insulin injections.
insulinoma (in-sue-lin-OH-mah)	Tumor of the islets of Langerhans cells of the pancreas that secretes an excessive amount of insulin.
ketoacidosis (kee-toh-ass-ih-DOH-sis)	Acidosis due to an excess of acidic ketone bodies (waste products). A serious condition requiring immediate treatment that can result in death for the diabetic patient if not reversed. Also called *diabetic acidosis.*

Pathology (continued)

TERM	DEFINITION
non–insulin-dependent diabetes mellitus (dye-ah-BEE-teez MELL-ih-tus)	Also called *type 2 diabetes mellitus.* It typically develops later in life. The pancreas produces normal to high levels of insulin, but the cells fail to respond to it. Patients may take oral hypoglycemics to improve insulin function, or may eventually have to take insulin.
peripheral neuropathy (per-IF-eh-rall new-ROP-ah-thee)	Damage to the nerves in the lower legs and hands as a result of diabetes mellitus. Symptoms include either extreme sensitivity or numbness and tingling.

■ Parathyroid Glands

tetany (TET-ah-nee)	Nerve irritability and painful muscle cramps resulting from hypocalcemia. Hypoparathyroidism is one cause of tetany.
Recklinghausen disease (REK-ling-how-zenz)	Excessive production of parathyroid hormone, which results in degeneration of the bones. Named for German histologist Friedrich von Recklinghausen.

■ Pituitary Gland

acromegaly (ak-roh-MEG-ah-lee)	Chronic disease of adults that results in an elongation and enlargement of the bones of the head and extremities. There can also be mood changes. Due to an excessive amount of growth hormone in an adult.

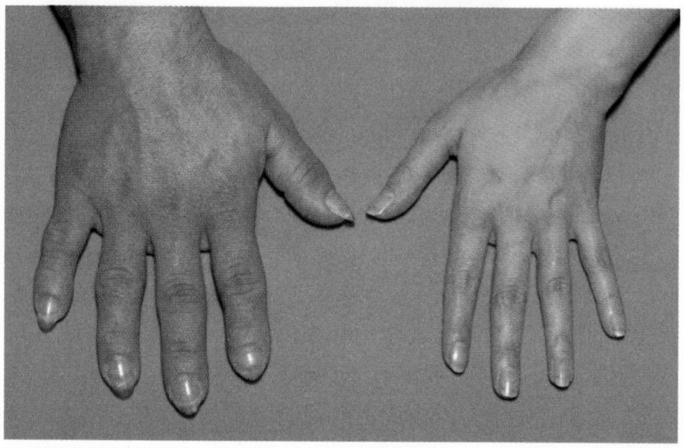

■ **Figure 11.13** Acromegaly. The hand on the right is from an adult with normal levels of growth hormone. The hand on the left is from an adult with excessive levels of growth hormone. This results in an increase in the size of the hands, feet, and jaw. *(Bart's Medical Library/Phototake NYC)*

diabetes insipidus (DI) (dye-ah-BEE-teez in-SIP-ih-dus)	Disorder caused by the inadequate secretion of antidiuretic hormone by the posterior lobe of the pituitary gland. There may be polyuria and polydipsia.
dwarfism (DWARF-izm)	Condition of being abnormally short in height. It may be the result of a hereditary condition or a lack of growth hormone.
gigantism (JYE-gan-tizm)	Excessive development of the body due to the overproduction of the growth hormone by the pituitary gland in a child or teenager. The opposite of *dwarfism.*
panhypopituitarism (pan-high-poh-pih-TOO-ih-tair-izm)	Deficiency in all the hormones secreted by the pituitary gland. Often recognized because of problems with the glands regulated by the pituitary–adrenal cortex, thyroid, ovaries, and testes.

■ Thyroid Gland

cretinism (KREE-tin-izm)	Congenital condition in which a lack of thyroid hormones may result in arrested physical and mental development.

Pathology *(continued)*

TERM	DEFINITION
goiter (GOY-ter)	Enlargement of the thyroid gland.

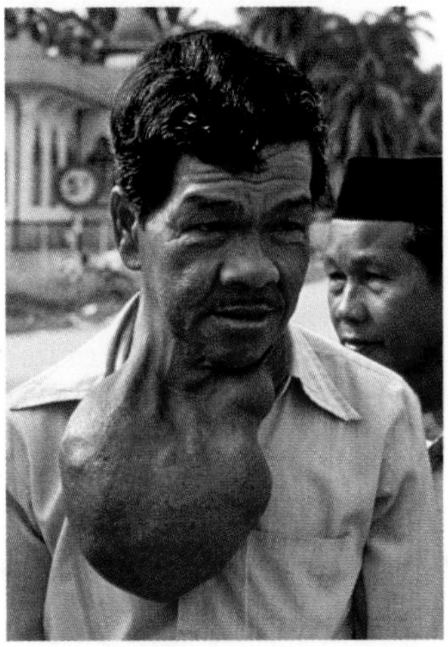

■ **Figure 11.14** Goiter. A photograph of a male with an extreme goiter or enlarged thyroid gland.

TERM	DEFINITION
Graves' disease	Condition named for Irish physician Robert Graves that results in overactivity of the thyroid gland and can cause a crisis situation. Symptoms include exophthalmos and goiter. A type of *hyperthyroidism.*
Hashimoto's disease (hash-ee-MOH-tohz dih-ZEEZ)	Chronic autoimmune form of thyroiditis, results in hyposecretion of thyroid hormones.
myxedema (miks-eh-DEE-mah)	Condition resulting from a hyposecretion of the thyroid gland in an adult. Symptoms can include anemia, slow speech, swollen facial features, edematous skin, drowsiness, and mental lethargy.
thyrotoxicosis (thigh-roh-toks-ih-KOH-sis)	Condition resulting from marked overproduction of the thyroid gland. Symptoms include rapid heart action, tremors, enlarged thyroid gland, exophthalmos, and weight loss.

■ *All Glands*

TERM	DEFINITION
adenocarcinoma (ad-eh-no-car-sih-NO-mah)	Cancerous tumor in a gland that is capable of producing the hormones secreted by that gland. One cause of hypersecretion pathologies.

Diagnostic Procedures

TERM	DEFINITION
■ *Clinical Laboratory Tests*	
blood serum test	Blood test to measure the level of substances such as calcium, electrolytes, testosterone, insulin, and glucose. Used to assist in determining the function of various endocrine glands.
fasting blood sugar (FBS)	Blood test to measure the amount of sugar circulating throughout the body after a 12-hour fast.

Diagnostic Procedures *(continued)*

TERM	DEFINITION
glucose tolerance test (GTT) (GLOO-kohs)	Test to determine the blood sugar level. A measured dose of glucose is given to a patient either orally or intravenously. Blood samples are then drawn at certain intervals to determine the ability of the patient to use glucose. Used for diabetic patients to determine their insulin response to glucose.
protein-bound iodine test (PBI)	Blood test to measure the concentration of thyroxine (T_4) circulating in the bloodstream. The iodine becomes bound to the protein in the blood and can be measured. Useful in establishing thyroid function.
radioimmunoassay (RIA) (ray-dee-oh-im-yoo-noh-ASS-ay)	Test used to measure the levels of hormones in the plasma of the blood.
thyroid function test (TFT) (THIGH-royd)	Blood test used to measure the levels of thyroxine, triiodothyronine, and thyroid-stimulating hormone in the bloodstream to assist in determining thyroid function.
total calcium	Blood test to measure the total amount of calcium to assist in detecting parathyroid and bone disorders.
two-hour postprandial glucose tolerance test (post-PRAN-dee-al)	Blood test to assist in evaluating glucose metabolism. The patient eats a high carbohydrate diet and then fasts overnight before the test. Then the blood sample is taken two hours after a meal.
■ *Diagnostic Imaging*	
thyroid echogram (THIGH-royd EK-oh-gram)	Ultrasound examination of the thyroid that can assist in distinguishing a thyroid nodule from a cyst.
thyroid scan (THIGH-royd)	Test in which radioactive iodine is administered that localizes in the thyroid gland. The gland can then be visualized with a scanning device to detect pathology such as tumors.

Therapeutic Procedures

TERM	DEFINITION
■ *Medical Procedures*	
chemical thyroidectomy (thigh-royd-EK-toh-mee)	Large dose of radioactive iodine is given in order to kill thyroid gland cells without having to actually do surgery.
hormone replacement therapy	Artificial replacement of hormones in patients with hyposecretion disorders. May be oral pills, injections, or adhesive skin patches.
■ *Surgical Procedures*	
laparoscopic adrenalectomy (lap-row-SKOP-ik ad-ree-nal-EK-toh-mee)	Removal of the adrenal gland through a small incision in the abdomen and using endoscopic instruments.
lobectomy (lobe-EK-toh-mee)	Removal of a lobe from an organ. In this case, one lobe of the thyroid gland.

Pharmacology

CLASSIFICATION	ACTION	GENERIC AND BRAND NAMES
antithyroid agents	Medication given to block production of thyroid hormones in patients with hypersecretion disorders.	methimazole, Tapazole; propylthiouracil
corticosteroids (kor-tih-koh-STAIR-oydz)	Although the function of these hormones in the body is to regulate carbohydrate metabolism, they also have a strong anti-inflammatory action. Therefore they are used to treat severe chronic inflammatory diseases such as rheumatoid arthritis. Long-term use of corticosteroids has adverse side effects such as osteoporosis and the symptoms of Cushing's disease. Also used to treat adrenal cortex hyposecretion disorders such as Addison's disease.	prednisone, Deltasone
human growth hormone therapy	Hormone replacement therapy with human growth hormone in order to stimulate skeletal growth. Used to treat children with abnormally short stature.	somatropin, Genotropin; somatrem, Protropin
insulin (IN-suh-lin)	Administered to replace insulin for type 1 diabetics or to treat severe type 2 diabetics.	human insulin, Humulin L
oral hypoglycemic agents (high-poh-glye-SEE-mik)	Medications taken by mouth that cause a decrease in blood sugar; not used for insulin-dependent patients.	metformin, Glucophage; glipizide, Glucotrol
thyroid replacement hormone	Hormone replacement therapy for patients with hypothyroidism or who have had a thyroidectomy.	levothyroxine, Levo-T; liothyronine, Cytomel
vasopressin (vaz-oh-PRESS-in)	Given to control diabetes insipidus and promote reabsorption of water in the kidney tubules.	desmopressin acetate, Desmopressin; conivaptan, Vaprisol

Abbreviations

α	alpha	MSH	melanocyte-stimulating hormone
ACTH	adrenocorticotropin hormone	Na⁺	sodium
ADH	antidiuretic hormone	NIDDM	non–insulin-dependent diabetes mellitus
β	beta	NPH	neutral protamine Hagedorn (insulin)
BMR	basal metabolic rate	PBI	protein-bound iodine
DI	diabetes insipidus	PRL	prolactin
DM	diabetes mellitus	PTH	parathyroid hormone
FBS	fasting blood sugar	RAI	radioactive iodine
FSH	follicle-stimulating hormone	RIA	radioimmunoassay
GH	growth hormone	T$_3$	triiodothyronine
GTT	glucose tolerance test	T$_4$	thyroxine
IDDM	insulin-dependent diabetes mellitus	TFT	thyroid function test
K⁺	potassium	TSH	thyroid-stimulating hormone
LH	luteinizing hormone		

Chapter Review

Terminology Checklist

Below are all Anatomy and Physiology key terms, Word Building, Vocabulary, Pathology, Diagnostic, Therapeutic, and Pharmacology terms presented in this chapter. Use this list as a study tool by placing a check in the box in front of each term as you master its meaning.

- ☐ acidosis
- ☐ acromegaly
- ☐ Addison's disease
- ☐ adenocarcinoma
- ☐ adrenal
- ☐ adrenal cortex
- ☐ adrenalectomy
- ☐ adrenal feminization
- ☐ adrenal glands
- ☐ adrenaline
- ☐ adrenalitis
- ☐ adrenal medulla
- ☐ adrenal virilism
- ☐ adrenocorticotropin hormone
- ☐ adrenomegaly
- ☐ adrenopathy
- ☐ aldosterone
- ☐ androgen
- ☐ anterior lobe
- ☐ antidiuretic hormone
- ☐ antithyroid agents
- ☐ blood serum test
- ☐ calcitonin
- ☐ calcium
- ☐ chemical thyroidectomy
- ☐ circadian rhythm
- ☐ corticosteroids
- ☐ cortisol
- ☐ cretinism
- ☐ Cushing's syndrome
- ☐ diabetes insipidus
- ☐ diabetes mellitus
- ☐ diabetic retinopathy
- ☐ dwarfism
- ☐ edema
- ☐ endocrine glands
- ☐ endocrine system
- ☐ endocrinologist
- ☐ endocrinology

- ☐ endocrinopathy
- ☐ epinephrine
- ☐ estrogen
- ☐ exocrine glands
- ☐ exophthalmos
- ☐ fasting blood sugar
- ☐ follicle-stimulating hormone
- ☐ gametes
- ☐ gigantism
- ☐ glands
- ☐ glucagon
- ☐ glucocorticoids
- ☐ glucose tolerance test
- ☐ glycosuria
- ☐ goiter
- ☐ gonadotropins
- ☐ gonads
- ☐ Graves' disease
- ☐ growth hormone
- ☐ gynecomastia
- ☐ Hashimoto's disease
- ☐ hirsutism
- ☐ homeostasis
- ☐ hormone
- ☐ hormone replacement therapy
- ☐ human growth hormone therapy
- ☐ hypercalcemia
- ☐ hyperglycemia
- ☐ hyperkalemia
- ☐ hyperparathyroidism
- ☐ hyperpituitarism
- ☐ hypersecretion
- ☐ hyperthyroidism
- ☐ hypocalcemia
- ☐ hypoglycemia
- ☐ hyponatremia
- ☐ hypoparathyroidism
- ☐ hypopituitarism

- ☐ hyposecretion
- ☐ hypothalamus
- ☐ hypothyroidism
- ☐ insulin
- ☐ insulin-dependent diabetes mellitus
- ☐ insulinoma
- ☐ iodine
- ☐ islets of Langerhans
- ☐ ketoacidosis
- ☐ laparoscopic adrenalectomy
- ☐ lobectomy
- ☐ luteinizing hormone
- ☐ melanocyte-stimulating hormone
- ☐ melatonin
- ☐ menstrual cycle
- ☐ mineralocorticoids
- ☐ myxedema
- ☐ non–insulin-dependent diabetes mellitus
- ☐ norepinephrine
- ☐ obesity
- ☐ oral hypoglycemic agent
- ☐ ova
- ☐ ovaries
- ☐ oxytocin
- ☐ pancreas
- ☐ pancreatic
- ☐ panhypopituitarism
- ☐ parathyroid glands
- ☐ parathyroidal
- ☐ parathyroidectomy
- ☐ parathyroid hormone
- ☐ peripheral neuropathy
- ☐ pheochromocytoma
- ☐ pineal gland
- ☐ pituitary
- ☐ pituitary gland
- ☐ polydipsia

□ polyuria	□ testes	□ thyroid function tests
□ posterior lobe	□ testosterone	□ thyroid gland
□ progesterone	□ tetany	□ thyroid replacement hormone
□ prolactin	□ thalamus	□ thyroid scan
□ protein-bound iodine test	□ thymectomy	□ thyroid-stimulating hormone
□ radioimmunoassay	□ thymic	□ thyromegaly
□ Recklinghausen disease	□ thymitis	□ thyrotoxicosis
□ somatotropin	□ thymoma	□ thyroxine
□ sperm	□ thymosin	□ total calcium
□ steroid sex hormones	□ thymus gland	□ triiodothyronine
□ syndrome	□ thyroidal	□ two-hour postprandial glucose tolerance test
□ target organs	□ thyroid echogram	□ vasopressin
□ T cells	□ thyroidectomy	

Practice Exercises

A. Complete the following statements.

1. The study of the endocrine system is called _____.

2. The master endocrine gland is the _____.

3. _____ is a general term for the sexual organs that produce gametes.

4. The term for the hormones produced by the outer portion of the adrenal cortex is _____.

5. The hormone produced by the testes is _____.

6. The two hormones produced by the ovaries are _____ and _____.

7. An inadequate supply of the hormone _____ causes diabetes insipidus.

8. The endocrine gland associated with the immune system is the _____.

9. The term for a protrusion of the eyeballs in Graves' disease is _____.

10. A general medical term for a hormone-secreting cancerous tumor is _____.

B. State the terms described using the combining forms provided.

The combining form *thyroid/o* refers to the thyroid. Use it to write a term that means:

1. removal of the thyroid _____

2. pertaining to the thyroid _____

3. state of excessive thyroid _____

The combining form *pancreat/o* refers to the pancreas. Use it to write a term that means:

4. pertaining to the pancreas _____

5. inflammation of the pancreas _____

6. removal of the pancreas _____

7. incision into the pancreas _____

The combining form *adren/o* refers to the adrenal glands. Use it to write a term that means:

8. pertaining to the adrenal gland _____

9. enlargement of the adrenal glands _____

10. adrenal gland disease _____

The combining form *thym/o* refers to the thymus glands. Use it to write a term that means:

11. tumor of the thymus gland _____

12. removal of the thymus gland _____

13. pertaining to the thymus gland _____

14. inflammation of the thymus gland _____

C. Match each term to its definition.

1. _____ Cushing's disease   a. enlarged thyroid

2. _____ goiter   b. overactive adrenal cortex

3. _____ acidosis   c. hyperthyroidism

4. _____ gigantism   d. underactive adrenal cortex

5. _____ cretinism   e. associated with diabetes

6. _____ myxedema   f. causes polyuria and polydipsia

7. _____ diabetes mellitus   g. thyroiditis

8. _____ diabetes insipidus   h. arrested growth

9. _____ Hashimoto's disease   i. poor carbohydrate metabolism

10. _____ Graves' disease   j. enlarged facial features and edematous skin

11. _____ Addison's disease   k. excessive growth hormone

D. Identify the following abbreviations.

1. PBI _____

2. K^+ _____

3. T_4 _____

4. GTT _____

5. DM _____

6. BMR _____

7. Na⁺ _____

8. ADH _____

E. Write the abbreviations for the following terms.

1. non–insulin-dependent diabetes mellitus _____

2. insulin-dependent diabetes mellitus _____

3. adrenocorticotropin hormone _____

4. parathyroid hormone _____

5. triiodothyronine _____

6. thyroid stimulating hormone _____

7. fasting blood sugar _____

8. prolactin _____

F. Build an endocrine system term using one of the following suffixes.

| -crine | -uria | -tropin |
| -dipsia | -emia | -prandial |

1. the presence of sugar or glucose in the urine _____

2. the glandular system that secretes directly into the bloodstream _____

3. excessive urination _____

4. condition of excessive calcium in the blood _____

5. excessive thirst _____

6. stimulate adrenal cortex _____

7. after a meal _____

G. Define the following terms.

1. corticosteroid _____

2. hirsutism _____

3. tetany _____

4. diabetic retinopathy _____

5. hyperglycemia _____

6. hypoglycemia _____

7. adrenaline _____

8. insulin _____

9. thyrotoxicosis _____

10. hypersecretion _____

H. Define the following combining forms and use them to form endocrine terms.

	Definition	Endocrine System Term
1. natr/o	_____	_____
2. estr/o	_____	_____
3. pineal/o	_____	_____
4. pituitar/o	_____	_____
5. kal/i	_____	_____
6. calc/o	_____	_____
7. parathyroid/o	_____	_____
8. acr/o	_____	_____
9. glyc/o	_____	_____
10. gonad/o	_____	_____

I. Match each term to its definition.

1. _____ protein bound iodine test

2. _____ fasting blood sugar

3. _____ radioimmunoassay

4. _____ thyroid scan

5. _____ 2-hour postprandial glucose tolerance test

6. _____ gluose tolerance test

a. measures levels of hormones in the blood

b. determines glucose metabolism after patient receives a measure dose of glucose

c. test of glucose metabolism two hours after eating a meal

d. measures blood sugar level after 12-hour fast

e. measures T4 concentration in the blood

f. uses radioactive iodine

J. Use the following terms in the sentences below.

insulinoma   ketoacidosis   pheochromocytoma

gynecomastia   panhypopituitarinism   Hashimoto's disease

1. The doctor found that Marsha's high level of insulin and hypoglycemia was caused by a(n) _____.

2. Kevin developed _____ as a result of his diabetes mellitus and required emergency treatment.

3. It was determined that Karen had _____ when doctors realized she had problems with her thyroid gland, adrenal cortex, and ovaries.

4. Luke's high epinephrine level was caused by a(n) _____.

5. When it was determined that Carl's thyroiditis was an autoimmune condition, it became obvious that he had

   _____.

6. Excessive sex hormones caused Jack to develop _____.

K. Fill in the classification for each drug description, then match the brand name.

Drug Description	Classification	Brand Name
1. _____ strong anti-inflammatory	_____	a. genotropin
2. _____ stimulates skeletal growth	_____	b. Desmopressin
3. _____ treats type II diabetes mellitus	_____	c. Tapazole
4. _____ blocks production of thyroid hormone	_____	d. glucophage
5. _____ treats type I diabetes mellitus	_____	e. Deltasone
6. _____ controls diabetes insipidus	_____	f. Humulin L

Medical Record Analysis

Below is an item from a patient's medical record. Read it carefully, make sure you understand all the medical terms used, and then answer the questions that follow.

Discharge Summary

Admitting Diagnosis:	Hyperglycemia, ketoacidosis, glycosuria
Final Diagnosis:	New-onset type 1 diabetes mellitus
History of Present Illness:	Patient presented to pediatrician's office with a two-month history of weight loss, fatigue, polyuria, and polydipsia. Her family history is significant for a grandfather, mother, and older brother with type 1 diabetes mellitus. The pediatrician found hyperglycemia with a fasting blood sugar and glycosuria with a urine dipstick. Patient was also noted to be dehydrated and extremely lethargic. She is being admitted at this time for management of new-onset diabetes mellitus.
Summary of Hospital Course:	At the time of admission, the FBS was 300 mg/100 mL and she was in ketoacidosis. She rapidly improved after receiving insulin; her serum glucose level normalized, and her lethargy disappeared. The next day a two-hour postprandial glucose tolerance test confirmed the diagnosis of diabetes mellitus while an abdominal x-ray and a pancreas CT scan were normal. There was no evidence of diabetic retinopathy. The patient was started on insulin injections. She was discharged three days later on a protocol of b.i.d. (twice a day) insulin injections. The patient and her family were instructed in diet, exercise, symptoms of hypoglycemic coma, insulin shock, and long-term complications of diabetes mellitus.
Discharge Plans:	Patient was discharged to home with her parents. She is on a 2,000-calorie ADA diet with three meals and two snacks. She may engage in any activity and may return to school next Monday. Her parents are to check her serum glucose levels b.i.d. and call the office for insulin dosage. She is to return to the office in two weeks.

Critical Thinking Questions

1. The patient's admitting diagnosis is three symptoms related to her final diagnosis. List the three symptoms and describe each in your own words.

   a._____

   b._____

   c._____

2. This patient has type 1 diabetes mellitus. Use your text or other resource, such as the Internet, to explain the difference between type 1 and type 2.

   _____

   _____

3. This discharge summary contains four medical terms that have not been introduced yet. Describe each of these terms in your own words. Use your text as a dictionary.

a. retinopathy _____

b. protocol _____

c. coma _____

d. b.i.d. _____

4. This patient had three different types of blood tests during her hospital stay. List the three blood tests and describe the differences among them in your own words.

a. _____

b. _____

c. _____

5. This patient had two imaging procedures conducted by the radiology department while she was in the hospital. List them and describe the differences between the two.

a. _____

b. _____

6. Describe the patient's discharge instructions in your own words. _____

_____

Chart Note Transcription

The chart note below contains eleven phrases that can be reworded with a medical term that you learned in this chapter. Each phrase is identified with an underline. Determine the medical term and write your answers in the space provided.

Current Complaint:	A 56-year-old female was referred to the <u>specialist in the treatment of diseases of the endocrine glands</u> ❶ for evaluation of weakness, edema, <u>an abnormal amount of fat in the body</u>, ❷ and <u>an excessive amount of hair for a female</u>. ❸
Past History:	Patient reports she has been overweight most of her life in spite of a healthy diet and regular exercise. She was diagnosed with osteoporosis after incurring a pathological rib fracture following a coughing attack.
Signs and Symptoms:	Patient has moderate edema in bilateral feet and lower legs as well as a puffy face and an upper lip moustache. She is 100 lbs. over normal body weight for her age and height. She moves slowly and appears generally lethargic. A test to <u>measure the hormone levels in the blood plasma</u> ❹ reports increased <u>steroid hormone that regulates carbohydrates in the body</u> ❺ levels in the blood. A CT scan demonstrates a <u>gland tumor</u> ❻ in the right <u>outer layer of the adrenal gland</u>. ❼
Diagnosis:	<u>A group of symptoms associated with hypersecretion of the adrenal cortex</u> ❽ secondary to a <u>gland tumor</u> ❾ in the right <u>outer layer of the adrenal gland</u> ❿
Treatment:	<u>Surgical removal of the right adrenal gland</u>. ⓫

❶ _____

❷ _____

❸ _____

❹ _____

❺ _____

❻ _____

❼ _____

❽ _____

❾ _____

❿ _____

⓫ _____

Labeling Exercise

A. System Review

Write the labels for this figure on the numbered lines provided.

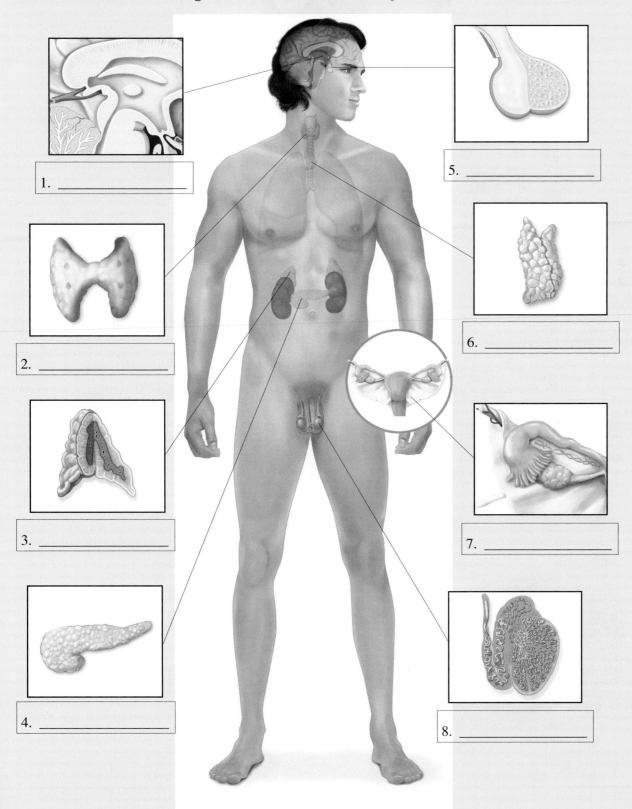

1. _____

2. _____

3. _____

4. _____

5. _____

6. _____

7. _____

8. _____

B. Anatomy Challenge

1. Write the labels for this figure on the numbered lines provided.

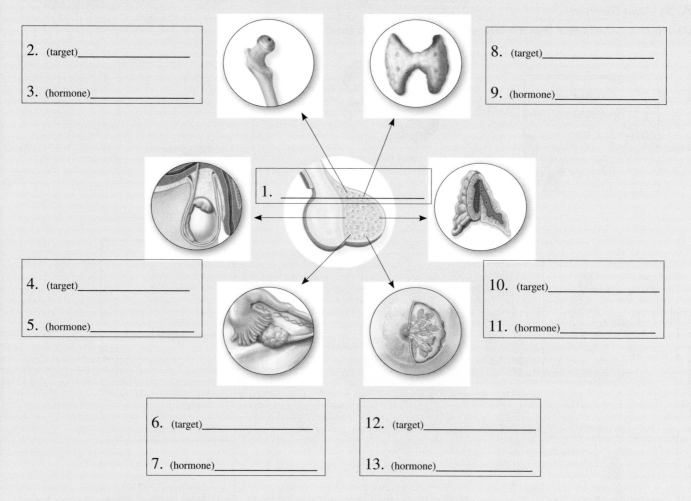

2. (target)_____

3. (hormone)_____

8. (target)_____

9. (hormone)_____

1. _____

4. (target)_____

5. (hormone)_____

10. (target)_____

11. (hormone)_____

6. (target)_____

7. (hormone)_____

12. (target)_____

13. (hormone)_____

2. Write the labels for this figure on the numbered lines provided.

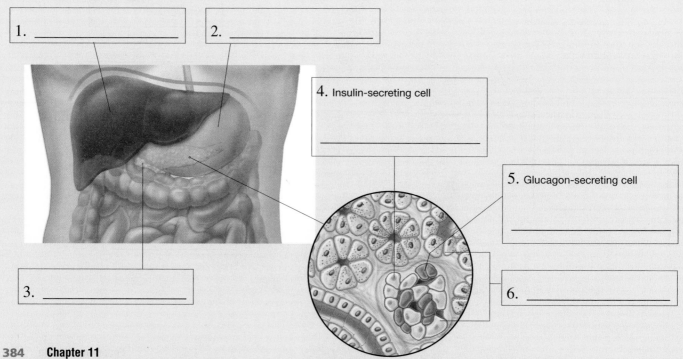

1. _____

2. _____

4. Insulin-secreting cell

_____

5. Glucagon-secreting cell

_____

3. _____

6. _____

Multimedia Preview

Additional interactive resources and activities for this chapter can be found on the Companion Website. For videos, games, and pronunciations, please access the accompanying DVD-ROM that comes with this book.

DVD-ROM Highlights

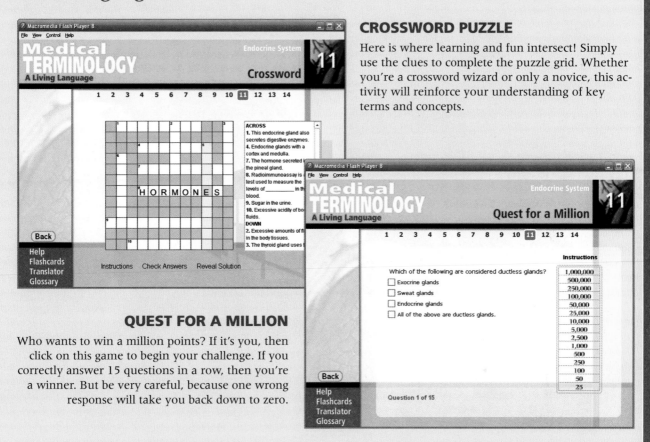

CROSSWORD PUZZLE

Here is where learning and fun intersect! Simply use the clues to complete the puzzle grid. Whether you're a crossword wizard or only a novice, this activity will reinforce your understanding of key terms and concepts.

QUEST FOR A MILLION

Who wants to win a million points? If it's you, then click on this game to begin your challenge. If you correctly answer 15 questions in a row, then you're a winner. But be very careful, because one wrong response will take you back down to zero.

Website Highlights—www.prenhall.com/fremgen

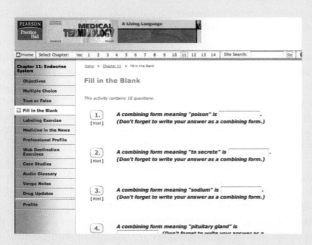

FILL-IN-THE-BLANKS EXERCISE

Take advantage of the free-access on-line study guide that accompanies your textbook. You'll find a fill-in-the-blank quiz that provides instant feedback that allows you to check your score and see what you got right or wrong. By clicking on this URL you'll also access links to download mp3 audio reviews, current news articles, and an audio glossary.

12

Nervous System

Learning Objectives

Upon completion of this chapter, you will be able to:

- Identify and define the combining forms and suffixes introduced in this chapter.
- Correctly spell and pronounce medical terms and major anatomical structures relating to the nervous system.
- Locate and describe the major organs of the nervous system and their functions.
- Describe the components of a neuron.
- Distinguish between the central nervous system, peripheral nervous system, and autonomic nervous system.
- Build and define nervous system medical terms from word parts.
- Identify and define nervous system vocabulary terms.
- Identify and define selected nervous system pathology terms.
- Identify and define selected nervous system diagnostic procedures.
- Identify and define selected nervous system therapeutic procedures.
- Identify and define selected medications relating to the nervous system.
- Define selected abbreviations associated with the nervous system.

Nervous System at a Glance

Function

The nervous system coordinates and controls body function. It receives sensory input, makes decisions, and then orders body responses.

Organs

brain
nerves
spinal cord

Combining Forms

cephal/o	head
cerebell/o	cerebellum
cerebr/o	cerebrum
encephal/o	brain
gli/o	glue
medull/o	medulla oblongata
mening/o	meninges
meningi/o	meninges
myel/o	spinal cord
neur/o	nerve
phas/o	speech
poli/o	gray matter
pont/o	pons
radicul/o	nerve root
thalam/o	thalamus
thec/o	sheath (meninges)
ventricul/o	brain ventricle

Suffixes

-algesia	pain, sensitivity
-esthesia	feeling, sensation
-paresis	weakness
-phasia	speech
-plegia	paralysis
-taxia	muscle coordination

Nervous System Illustrated

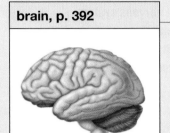

Coordinates body functions

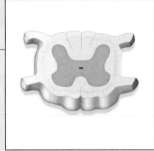

Transmits messages to and from the brain

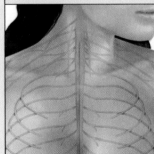

Transmit messages to and from the central nervous system

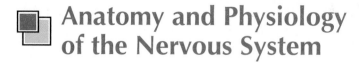

Anatomy and Physiology of the Nervous System

brain	nerves
central nervous system	peripheral nervous system (per-IF-er-al)
cranial nerves (KRAY-nee-al)	sensory receptors
glands	spinal cord
muscles	spinal nerves

The nervous system is responsible for coordinating all the activity of the body. To do this, it first receives information from both external and internal **sensory receptors** and then uses that information to adjust the activity of **muscles** and **glands** to match the needs of the body.

The nervous system can be subdivided into the **central nervous system** (CNS) and the **peripheral nervous system** (PNS). The central nervous system consists of the **brain** and **spinal cord**. Sensory information comes into the central nervous system, where it is processed. Motor messages then exit the central nervous system carrying commands to muscles and glands. The **nerves** of the peripheral nervous system are **cranial nerves** and **spinal nerves**. Sensory nerves carry information to the central nervous system, and motor nerves carry commands away from the central nervous system. All portions of the nervous system are composed of nervous tissue.

Nervous Tissue

axon (AK-son)	neuron (NOO-ron)
dendrites (DEN-drights)	neurotransmitter (noo-roh-TRANS-mit-ter)
myelin (MY-eh-lin)	synapse (sih-NAPSE)
nerve cell body	synaptic cleft (sih-NAP-tik)
neuroglial cells (noo-ROH-glee-all)	

Nervous tissue consists of two basic types of cells: **neurons** and **neuroglial cells**. Neurons are individual nerve cells. These are the cells that are capable of conducting electrical impulses in response to a stimulus. Neurons have three basic parts: **dendrites**, a **nerve cell body**, and an **axon** (see Figure 12.1A ■). Dendrites are highly branched projections that receive impulses. The nerve cell body contains the nucleus and many of the other organelles of the cell (see Figure 12.1B ■). A neuron has only a single axon, a projection from the nerve cell body that conducts the electrical impulse toward its destination. The point at which the axon of one neuron meets the dendrite of the next neuron is called a **synapse**. Electrical impulses cannot pass directly across the gap between two neurons, called the **synaptic cleft**. They instead require the help of a chemical messenger, called a **neurotransmitter**.

A variety of neuroglial cells are found in nervous tissue. Each has a different support function for the neurons. For example, some neuroglial cells produce **myelin**, a fatty substance that acts as insulation for many axons so that they conduct electrical impulses faster. Neuroglial cells *do not* conduct electrical impulses.

Central Nervous System

gray matter	tract
meninges (men-IN-jeez)	white matter
myelinated (MY-eh-lih-nayt-ed)	

Because the central nervous system is a combination of the brain and spinal cord, it is able to receive impulses from all over the body, process this informa-

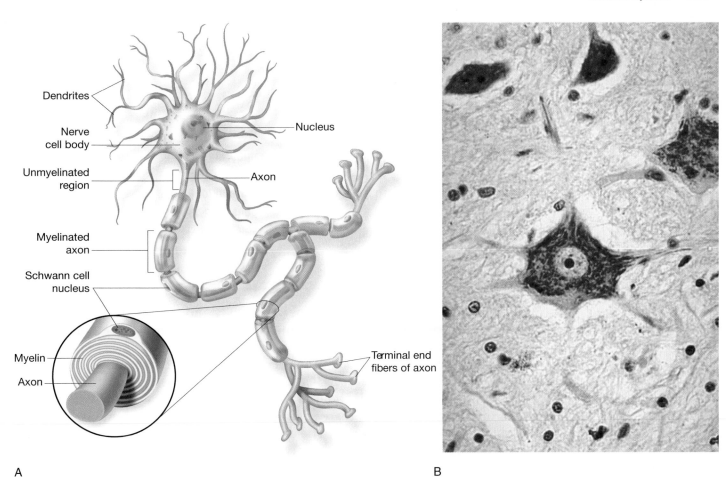

A   B

Figure 12.1 A) The structure of a neuron, showing the dendrites, nerve cell body, and axon. B) Photomicrograph of typical neuron showing the nerve cell body, nucleus, and dendrites.

tion, and then respond with an action. This system consists of both **gray** and **white matter.** Gray matter is comprised of unsheathed or uncovered cell bodies and dendrites. White matter is **myelinated** nerve fibers (see Figure 12.2 ■). The myelin sheath makes the nervous tissue appear white. Bundles of nerve fibers inter-

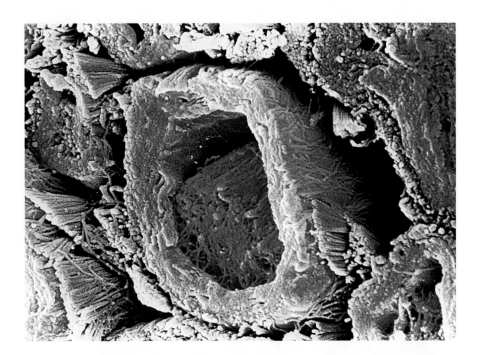

Figure 12.2
Electronmicrograph illustrating an axon (red) wrapped in its myelin sheath (blue). *(Quest/Science Photo Library/Photo Researchers, Inc.)*

Med Term Tip

Myelin is a lipid and a very white molecule. This is why myelinated neurons are called *white matter*.

connecting different parts of the central nervous system are called **tracts**. The central nervous system is encased and protected by three membranes known as the **meninges**.

The Brain

brain stem	**medulla oblongata**
cerebellum (ser-eh-BELL-um)	(meh-DULL-ah ob-long-GAH-tah)
cerebral cortex (seh-REE-bral KOR-teks)	**midbrain**
cerebral hemisphere	**occipital lobe** (ock-SIP-ih-tal)
cerebrospinal fluid (ser-eh-broh-SPY-nal)	**parietal lobe** (pah-RYE-eh-tal)
cerebrum (SER-eh-brum)	**pons** (PONZ)
diencephalon (dye-en-SEFF-ah-lon)	**sulci** (SULL-kye)
frontal lobe	**temporal lobe** (TEM-por-al)
gyri (JYE-rye)	**thalamus** (THAL-ah-mus)
hypothalamus (high-poh-THAL-ah-mus)	**ventricles** (VEN-trik-lz)

The brain is one of the largest organs in the body and coordinates most body activities. It is the center for all thought, memory, judgment, and emotion. Each part of the brain is responsible for controlling different body functions, such as temperature regulation, blood pressure, and breathing. There are four sections to the brain: **cerebrum**, **cerebellum**, **diencephalon**, and **brain stem** (see Figure 12.3 ▇).

The largest section of the brain is the cerebrum. It is located in the upper portion of the brain and is the area that processes thoughts, judgment, memory, problem solving, and language. The outer layer of the cerebrum is the **cerebral cortex**, which is composed of folds of gray matter. The elevated portions of the cerebrum, or convolutions, are called **gyri** and are separated by fissures, or valleys, called **sulci**. The cerebrum is subdivided into left and right halves called **cerebral hemispheres**. Each hemisphere has four lobes. The lobes and their locations and functions are as follows (see Figure 12.4 ▇):

▇ **Figure 12.3** The regions of the brain.

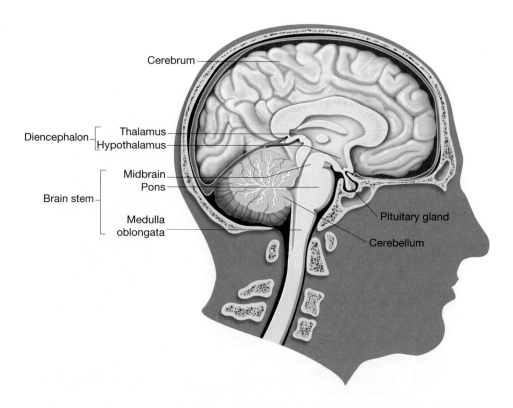

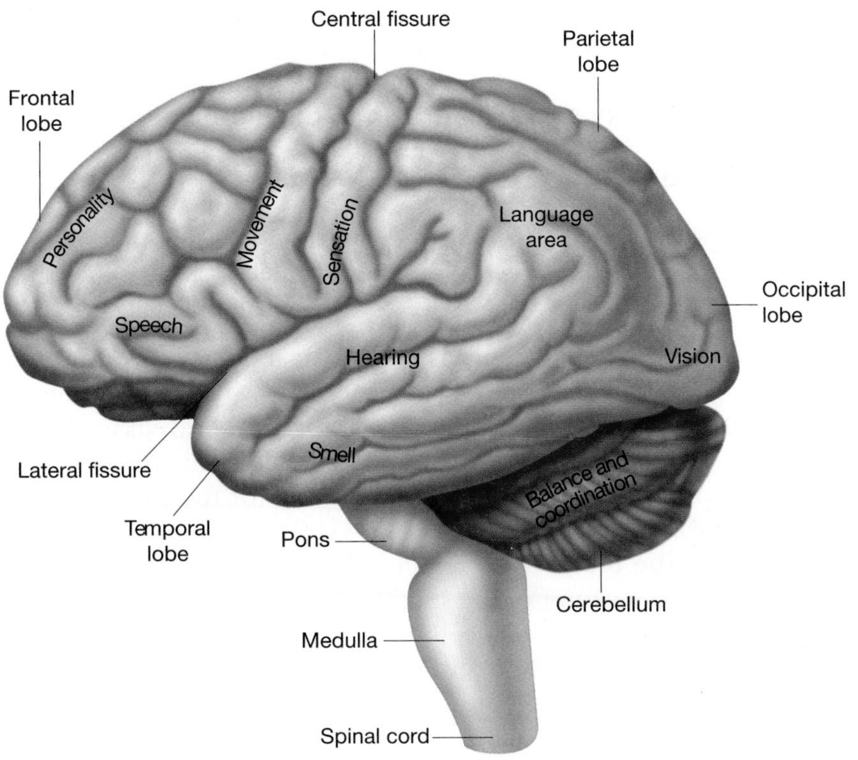

■ **Figure 12.4** The functional regions of the cerebrum.

1. **Frontal lobe:** Most anterior portion of the cerebrum; controls motor function, personality, and speech
2. **Parietal lobe:** Most superior portion of the cerebrum; receives and interprets nerve impulses from sensory receptors and interprets language
3. **Occipital lobe:** Most posterior portion of the cerebrum; controls vision
4. **Temporal lobe:** Left and right lateral portion of the cerebrum; controls hearing and smell

The diencephalon, located below the cerebrum, contains two of the most critical areas of the brain, the **thalamus** and the **hypothalamus**. The thalamus is composed of gray matter and acts as a center for relaying impulses from the eyes, ears, and skin to the cerebrum. Our pain perception is controlled by the thalamus. The hypothalamus located just below the thalamus controls body temperature, appetite, sleep, sexual desire, and emotions. The hypothalamus is actually responsible for controlling the autonomic nervous system, cardiovascular system, digestive system, and the release of hormones from the pituitary gland.

The cerebellum, the second largest portion of the brain, is located beneath the posterior part of the cerebrum. This part of the brain aids in coordinating voluntary body movements and maintaining balance and equilibrium. The cerebellum refines the muscular movement that is initiated in the cerebrum.

The final portion of the brain is the brain stem. This area has three components: **midbrain, pons,** and **medulla oblongata**. The midbrain acts as a pathway for impulses to be conducted between the brain and the spinal cord. The pons—a term meaning bridge—connects the cerebellum to the rest of the brain. The medulla oblongata is the most inferior positioned portion of the brain; it connects the brain to the spinal cord. However, this vital area contains the centers that control respiration, heart rate, temperature, and blood pressure. Additionally, this is the site where nerve tracts cross from one side of the brain to control functions and movement on the other side of the body. In other words, with few exceptions, the left side of the brain controls the right side of the body and vice versa.

The brain has four interconnected cavities called **ventricles**: one in each cerebral hemisphere, one in the thalamus, and one in front of the cerebellum. These contain **cerebrospinal fluid** (CSF), which is the watery, clear fluid that provides protection from shock or sudden motion to the brain and spinal cord.

Spinal Cord

ascending tracts	spinal cavity
central canal	vertebral canal
descending tracts	vertebral column

The function of the spinal cord is to provide a pathway for impulses traveling to and from the brain. The spinal cord is actually a column of nervous tissue that extends from the medulla oblongata of the brain down to the level of the second lumbar vertebra within the **vertebral column**. The thirty-three vertebrae of the backbone line up to form a continuous canal for the spinal cord called the **spinal cavity** or **vertebral canal** (see Figure 12.5 ■).

Similar to the brain, the spinal cord is also protected by cerebrospinal fluid. It flows down the center of the spinal cord within the **central canal**. The inner core of the spinal cord consists of cell bodies and dendrites of peripheral nerves and therefore is gray matter. The outer portion of the spinal cord is myelinated white matter. The white matter is either **ascending tracts** carrying sensory information up to the brain or **descending tracts** carrying motor commands down from the brain to a peripheral nerve.

Med Term Tip

Certain disease processes attack the gray matter and the white matter of the central nervous system. For instance, *poliomyelitis* is a viral infection of the gray matter of the spinal cord. The combining term *poli/o* means "gray matter." This disease has almost been eradicated, due to the polio vaccine.

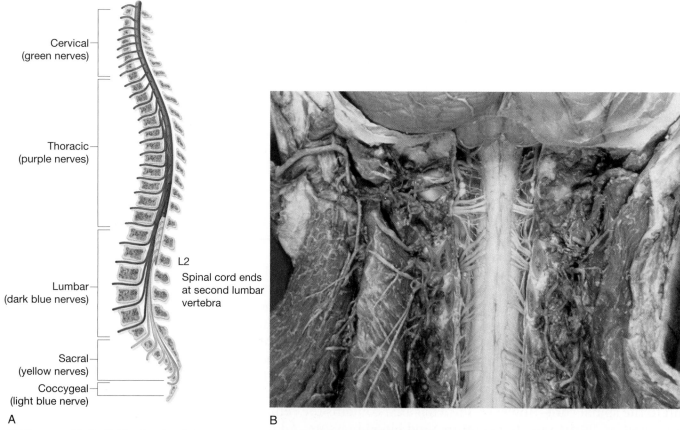

Cervical (green nerves)

Thoracic (purple nerves)

Lumbar (dark blue nerves)

Sacral (yellow nerves)

Coccygeal (light blue nerve)

L2
Spinal cord ends at second lumbar vertebra

A   B

■ **Figure 12.5** A) The levels of the spinal cord and spinal nerves. B) Photograph of the spinal cord as it descends from the brain. The spinal nerve roots are clearly visible branching off from the spinal cord. *(Video Surgery/Photo Researchers, Inc.)*

Meninges

arachnoid layer (ah-RAK-noyd)
dura mater (DOO-rah MATE-er)
pia mater (PEE-ah MATE-er)

subarachnoid space (sub-ah-RAK-noyd)
subdural space (sub-DOO-ral)

The meninges are three layers of connective tissue membranes that surround the brain and spinal cord (see Figure 12.6 ■). Moving from external to internal, the meninges are:

1. **Dura mater**: Meaning *tough mother*; it forms a tough, fibrous sac around the central nervous system
2. **Subdural space**: Actual space between the dura mater and arachnoid layers
3. **Arachnoid layer**: Meaning *spiderlike*; it is a thin, delicate layer attached to the pia mater by weblike filaments
4. **Subarachnoid space**: Space between the arachnoid layer and the pia mater; it contains cerebrospinal fluid that cushions the brain from the outside
5. **Pia mater**: Meaning *soft mother*; it is the innermost membrane layer and is applied directly to the surface of the brain and spinal cord

Peripheral Nervous System

afferent neurons (AFF-er-ent)
autonomic nervous system (aw-toh-NOM-ik)
efferent neurons (EFF-er-ent)
ganglion (GANG-lee-on)

motor neurons
nerve root
sensory neurons
somatic nerves

The peripheral nervous system (PNS) includes both the twelve pairs of cranial nerves and the thirty-one pairs of spinal nerves. A nerve is a group or bundle of axon fibers located outside the central nervous system that carries messages between the central nervous system and the various parts of the body. Whether a nerve is cranial or spinal is determined by where the nerve originates. Cranial nerves arise from the brain, mainly at the medulla oblongata. Spinal nerves split off from the spinal cord, and one pair (a left and a right) exits between each pair of vertebrae. The point where either type of nerve is attached to the central nervous system is called the **nerve root**. The names of most nerves reflect either

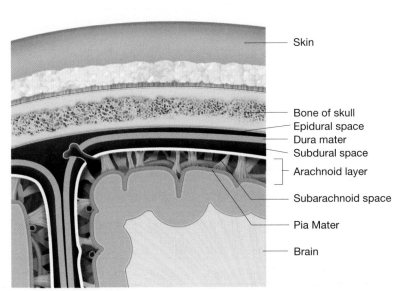

Skin

Bone of skull
Epidural space
Dura mater
Subdural space
Arachnoid layer

Subarachnoid space

Pia Mater

Brain

■ **Figure 12.6** The meninges. This figure illustrates the location and structure of each layer of the meninges and their relationship to the skull and brain.

Med Term Tip

Because nerve tracts cross from one side of the body to the other side of the brain, damage to one side of the brain results in symptoms appearing on the opposite side of the body. Since nerve cells that control the movement of the right side of the body are located in the left side of the medulla oblongata, a stroke that paralyzed the right side of the body would actually have occurred in the left side of the brain.

the organ the nerve serves or the portion of the body the nerve is traveling through. The entire list of cranial nerves is found in Table 12.1 ■. Figure 12.7 ■ illustrates some of the major spinal nerves in the human body.

Although most nerves carry information to and from the central nervous system, individual neurons carry information in only one direction. **Afferent neurons**, also called **sensory neurons**, carry sensory information from a sensory receptor to the central nervous system. **Efferent neurons**, also called **motor neurons**, carry activity instructions from the central nervous system to muscles or glands out in the body (see Figure 12.8 ■). The nerve cell bodies of the neurons forming the nerve are grouped together in a knot-like mass, called a **ganglion**, located outside the central nervous system.

The nerves of the peripheral nervous system are subdivided into two divisions, the **autonomic nervous system** (ANS) and **somatic nerves**, each serving a different area of the body.

Autonomic Nervous System

parasympathetic branch
(pair-ah-sim-pah-THET-ik)

sympathetic branch (sim-pah-THET-ik)

The autonomic nervous system is involved with the control of involuntary or unconscious bodily functions. It may increase or decrease the activity of the smooth muscle found in viscera and blood vessels, cardiac muscle, and glands. The autonomic nervous system is divided into two branches: **sympathetic branch** and **parasympathetic branch**. The sympathetic nerves control the "fight or flight" reaction during times of stress and crisis. These nerves increase heart rate, dilate airways, increase blood pressure, inhibit digestion, and stimulate the production of adrenaline during a crisis. The parasympathetic nerves serve as a counterbalance for the sympathetic nerves, the "rest and digest" reaction. Therefore, they cause heart rate to slow down, lower blood pressure, and stimulate digestion.

Table 12.1	Cranial Nerves	
NUMBER	**NAME**	**FUNCTION**
I	Olfactory	Transports impulses for sense of smell
II	Optic	Carries impulses for sense of sight
III	Oculomotor	Motor impulses for eye muscle movement and the pupil of eye
IV	Trochlear	Controls oblique muscle of eye on each side
V	Trigeminal	Carries sensory facial impulses and controls muscles for chewing; branches into eyes, forehead, upper and lower jaw
VI	Abducens	Controls an eyeball muscle to turn eye to side
VII	Facial	Controls facial muscles for expression, salivation, and taste on two-thirds of tongue (anterior)
VIII	Vestibulocochlear	Responsible for impulses of equilibrium and hearing; also called auditory nerve
IX	Glossopharyngeal	Carries sensory impulses from pharynx (swallowing) and taste on one-third of tongue
X	Vagus	Supplies most organs in abdominal and thoracic cavities
XI	Accessory	Controls the neck and shoulder muscles
XII	Hypoglossal	Controls tongue muscles

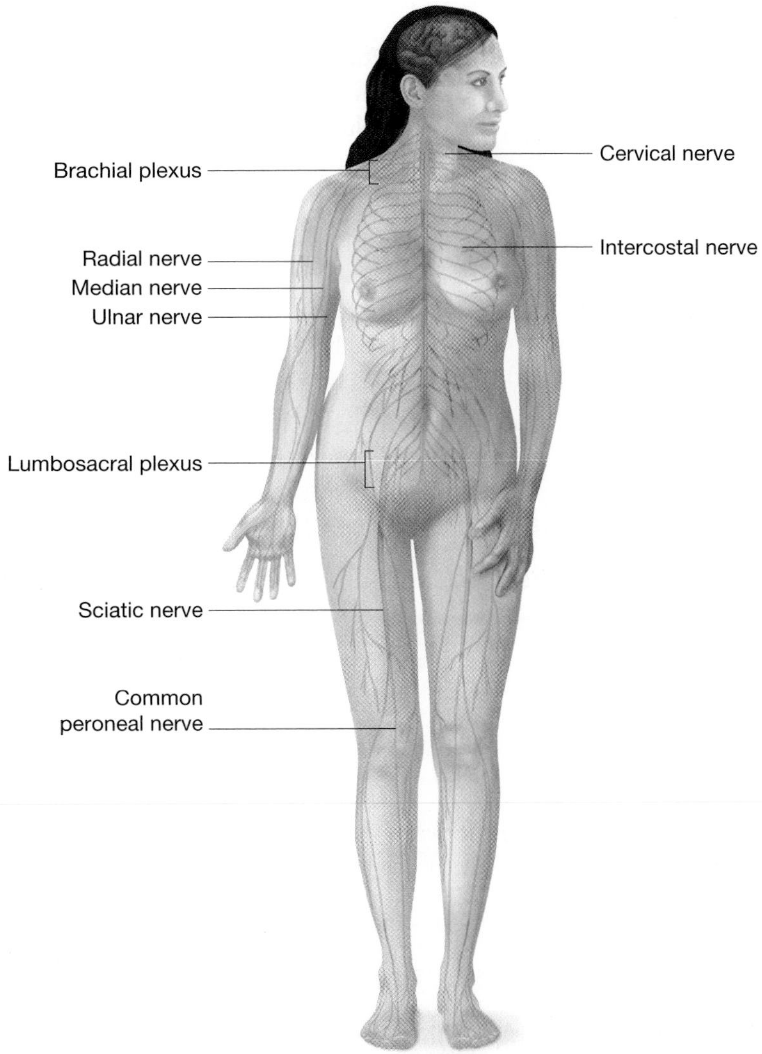

■ **Figure 12.7** The major spinal nerves.

Brachial plexus —

— Cervical nerve

Radial nerve —
Median nerve —
Ulnar nerve —

— Intercostal nerve

Lumbosacral plexus —

Sciatic nerve —

Common peroneal nerve —

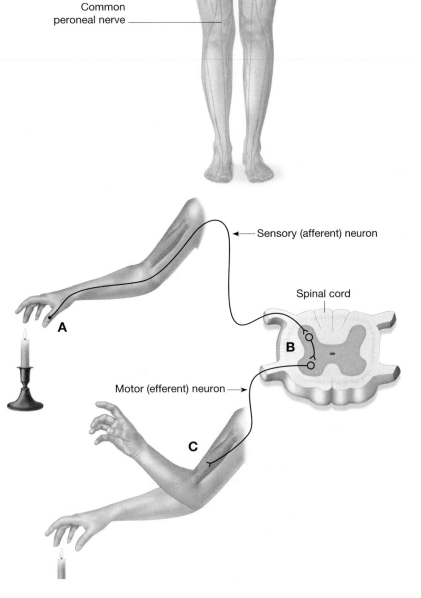

Sensory (afferent) neuron

Spinal cord

A

B

Motor (efferent) neuron

C

■ **Figure 12.8** The functional structure of the peripheral nervous system. A) Afferent or sensory neurons carry sensory information to the spinal cord. B) The spinal cord receives incoming sensory information and delivers motor messages. C) Efferent or motor neurons deliver motor commands to muscles and glands.

Somatic Nerves

Somatic nerves serve the skin and skeletal muscles and are mainly involved with the conscious and voluntary activities of the body. The large variety of sensory receptors found in the dermis layer of the skin use somatic nerves to send their information, such as touch, temperature, pressure, and pain, to the brain. These are also the nerves that carry motor commands to skeletal muscles.

Word Building

The following list contains examples of medical terms built directly from word parts. The definition for these terms can be determined by a straightforward translation of the word parts.

COMBINING FORM	COMBINED WITH	MEDICAL TERM	DEFINITION
cephal/o	-algia	**cephalalgia** (seff-al-AL-jee-ah)	head pain (headache)
cerebell/o	-ar	**cerebellar** (ser-eh-BELL-ar)	pertaining to the cerebellum
	-itis	**cerebellitis** (ser-eh-bell-EYE-tis)	cerebellum inflammation
cerebr/o	-al	**cerebral** (seh-REE-bral)	pertaining to the cerebrum
	spin/o -al	**cerebrospinal** (ser-eh-broh-SPY-nal)	pertaining to the cerebrum and spine
encephal/o	electr/o -gram	**electroencephalogram** (EEG) (ee-lek-troh-en-SEFF-ah-loh-gram)	record of brain's electricity
	-itis	**encephalitis** (en-seff-ah-LYE-tis)	brain inflammation
meningi/o	-oma	**meningioma** (meh-nin-jee-OH-mah)	meninges tumor
mening/o	-eal	**meningeal** (meh-NIN-jee-all)	pertaining to the meninges
	-itis	**meningitis** (men-in-JYE-tis)	meninges inflammation
myel/o	-gram	**myelogram** (MY-eh-loh-gram)	record of spinal cord

Med Term Tip

The combining form *myel/o* means "marrow" and is used for both the spinal cord and bone marrow. To the ancient Greek philosophers and physicians, the spinal cord appeared to be much like the marrow found in the medullary cavity of a long bone.

	-itis	**myelitis** (my-eh-LYE-tis)	spinal cord inflammation
neur/o	-al	**neural** (NOO-rall)	pertaining to nerves
	-algia	**neuralgia** (noo-RAL-jee-ah)	nerve pain
	-ectomy	**neurectomy** (noo-REK-toh-mee)	removal of nerve
	-ologist	**neurologist** (noo-RAL-oh-jist)	specialist in nerves
	-oma	**neuroma** (noo-ROH-mah)	nerve tumor
	-pathy	**neuropathy** (noo-ROP-ah-thee)	nerve disease
	-plasty	**neuroplasty** (NOOR-oh-plas-tee)s	surgical repair of nerves
	poly- -itis	**polyneuritis** (pol-ee-noo-RYE-tis)	inflammation of many nerves

Word Building *(continued)*

COMBINING FORM	COMBINED WITH	MEDICAL TERM	DEFINITION
	-rrhaphy	**neurorrhaphy** (noo-ROR-ah-fee)	suture of nerve
pont/o	-ine	**pontine** (pon-TEEN)	pertaining to the pons
radicul/o	-itis	**radiculitis** (rah-dick-yoo-LYE-tis)	nerve root inflammation
	-pathy	**radiculopathy** (rah-dick-yoo-LOP-ah-thee)	nerve root disease
thalam/o	-ic	**thalamic** (tha-LAM-ik)	pertaining to the thalamus
thec/o	intra- -al	**intrathecal** (in-tra-THEE-kal)	pertaining to within the meninges

SUFFIX	COMBINED WITH	MEDICAL TERM	DEFINITION
-algesia	an-	**analgesia** (an-al-JEE-zee-ah)	absence of pain or sensation
-esthesia	an-	**anesthesia** (an-ess-THEE-zee-ah)	lack of sensations
	hyper-	**hyperesthesia** (high-per-ess-THEE-zee-ah)	excessive sensations
-paresis	mono-	**monoparesis** (mon-oh-pah-REE-sis)	weakness of one
-phasia	a-	**aphasia** (ah-FAY-zee-ah)	lack of speech
	dys-	**dysphasia** (dis-FAY-zee-ah)	difficult speech
-plegia	mono-	**monoplegia** (mon-oh-PLEE-jee-ah)	paralysis of one
	quadri-	**quadriplegia** (kwod-rih-PLEE-jee-ah)	paralysis of four
-taxia	a-	**ataxia** (ah-TAK-see-ah)	lack of muscle coordination

Vocabulary

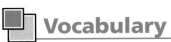

TERM	DEFINITION
anesthesiology (an-es-thee-zee-ol-oh-jee)	Branch of medicine specializing in all aspects of anesthesia, including for surgical procedures, resuscitation measures, and the management of acute and chronic pain. Physician is an *anesthesiologist*.
aura (AW-ruh)	Sensations, such as seeing colors or smelling an unusual odor, that occur just prior to an epileptic seizure or migraine headache.
coma (COH-mah)	Profound unconsciousness or stupor resulting from an illness or injury.
conscious (KON-shus)	Condition of being awake and aware of surroundings.
convulsion (kon-VULL-shun)	Severe involuntary muscle contractions and relaxations. These have a variety of causes, such as epilepsy, fever, and toxic conditions.
delirium (dee-LEER-ee-um)	Abnormal mental state characterized by confusion, disorientation, and agitation.

Vocabulary *(continued)*

TERM	DEFINITION
dementia (dee-MEN-she-ah)	Progressive impairment of intellectual function that interferes with performing activities of daily living. Patients have little awareness of their condition. Found in disorders such as Alzheimer's.
focal seizure (FOE-kal)	Localized seizure often affecting one limb.
hemiparesis (hem-ee-par-EE-sis)	Weakness or loss of motion on one side of the body.
hemiplegia (hem-ee-PLEE-jee-ah)	Paralysis on only one side of the body.
neurology (noo-rol-oh-jee)	Branch of medicine concerned with diagnosis and treatment of diseases and conditions of the nervous system. Physician is a *neurologist*.
neurosurgery (noo-roh-SIR-jury)	Branch of medicine concerned with treating conditions and diseases of the nervous systems by surgical means. Physician is a *neurosurgeon*.
palsy (PAWL-zee)	Temporary or permanent loss of the ability to control movement.
paralysis (pah-RAL-ih-sis)	Temporary or permanent loss of function or voluntary movement.
paraplegia (pair-ah-PLEE-jee-ah)	Paralysis of the lower portion of the body and both legs.
paresthesia (par-es-THEE-zee-ah)	Abnormal sensation such as burning or tingling.
seizure (SEE-zyoor)	Sudden, uncontrollable onset of symptoms; such as in an epileptic seizure.
syncope (SIN-koh-pee)	Fainting.
tremor (TREM-or)	Involuntary repetitive alternating movement of a part of the body.
unconscious (un-KON-shus)	Condition or state of being unaware of surroundings, with the inability to respond to stimuli.

Pathology

TERM	DEFINITION
■ *Brain*	
absence seizure	Type of epileptic seizure that lasts only a few seconds to half a minute, characterized by a loss of awareness and an absence of activity. It is also called a *petit mal seizure*.
Alzheimer's disease (ALTS-high-merz)	Chronic, organic mental disorder consisting of dementia, which is more prevalent in adults between ages 40 and 60. Involves progressive disorientation, apathy, speech and gait disturbances, and loss of memory. Named for German neurologist Alois Alzheimer.
astrocytoma (ass-troh-sigh-TOH-mah)	Tumor of the brain or spinal cord that is composed of astrocytes, one of the types of neuroglial cells.

Pathology *(continued)*

TERM	DEFINITION
brain tumor	Intracranial mass, either benign or malignant. A benign tumor of the brain can still be fatal since it will grow and cause pressure on normal brain tissue.

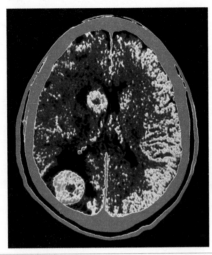

Figure 12.9 Color enhanced CT-scan showing two malignant tumors in the brain. *(Scott Camazine/Photo Researchers, Inc.)*

TERM	DEFINITION
cerebral aneurysm (AN-yoo-rizm)	Localized abnormal dilation of a blood vessel, usually an artery; the result of a congenital defect or weakness in the wall of the vessel. A ruptured aneurysm is a common cause of a hemorrhagic cerebrovascular accident.

Figure 12.10 Common locations for cerebral artery aneurysms in the Circle of Willis.

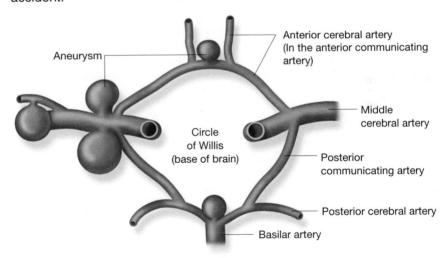

TERM	DEFINITION
cerebral contusion (kon-TOO-shun)	Bruising of the brain from a blow or impact. Symptoms last longer than 24 hours and include unconsciousness, dizziness, vomiting, unequal pupil size, and shock.
cerebral palsy (CP) (ser-REE-bral PAWL-zee)	Nonprogressive brain damage resulting from a defect, trauma, or oxygen deprivation at the time of birth.
cerebrovascular accident (CVA) (ser-eh-broh-VASS-kyoo-lar AK-sih-dent)	The development of an infarct due to loss in the blood supply to an area of the brain. Blood flow can be interrupted by a ruptured blood vessel (hemorrhage), a floating clot (embolus), a stationary clot (thrombosis), or compression (see Figure 12.11 ■). The extent of damage depends on the size and location of the infarct and often includes dysphasia and hemiplegia. Commonly called a *stroke*.

■ **Figure 12.11** The four common causes for cerebrovascular accidents.

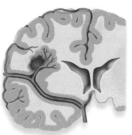
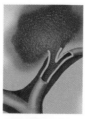
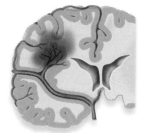
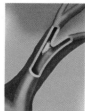

Cerebral hemorrhage: Cerebral artery ruptures and bleeds into brain tissue.

Cerebral embolism: Embolus from another area lodges in cerebral artery and blocks blood flow.

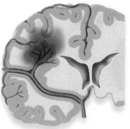
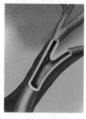
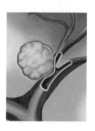

Cerebral thrombosis: Blood clot forms in cerebral artery and blocks blood flow.

Compression: Pressure from tumor squeezes adjacent blood vessel and blocks blood flow.

Pathology *(continued)*

TERM	DEFINITION
concussion (kon-KUSH-un)	Injury to the brain resulting from the brain being shaken inside the skull from a blow or impact. Can result in unconsciousness, dizziness, vomiting, unequal pupil size, and shock. Symptoms last 24 hours or less.
epilepsy (EP-ih-lep-see)	Recurrent disorder of the brain in which seizures and loss of consciousness occur as a result of uncontrolled electrical activity of the neurons in the brain.
hydrocephalus (high-droh-SEFF-ah-lus)	Accumulation of cerebrospinal fluid within the ventricles of the brain, causing the head to be enlarged. It is treated by creating an artificial shunt for the fluid to leave the brain. If left untreated, it may lead to seizures and mental retardation.

■ **Figure 12.12** Hydrocephalus. The figure on the left is a child with the enlarged ventricles of hydrocephalus. The figure on the right is the same child with a shunt to send the excess cerebrospinal fluid to the abdominal cavity.

Bulging fontanel

Enlarged ventricles

Catheter tip in ventricle

Valve

Blocked aqueduct

Shunt

Pathology (continued)

TERM	DEFINITION
migraine (MY-grain)	Specific type of headache characterized by severe head pain, sensitivity to light, dizziness, and nausea.
Parkinson's disease (PARK-in-sons dih-ZEEZ)	Chronic disorder of the nervous system with fine tremors, muscular weakness, rigidity, and a shuffling gait. Named for British physician Sir James Parkinson.
Reye syndrome (RISE SIN-drohm)	Combination of symptoms first recognized by Australian pathologist R. D. K. Reye that includes acute encephalopathy and damage to various organs, especially the liver. This occurs in children under age 15 who have had a viral infection. It is also associated with taking aspirin. For this reason, it's not recommended for children to use aspirin.
tonic-clonic seizure	Type of severe epileptic seizure characterized by a loss of consciousness and convulsions. The seizure alternates between strong continuous muscle spasms (tonic) and rhythmic muscle contraction and relaxation (clonic). It is also called a *grand mal seizure*.
transient ischemic attack (TIA) (TRAN-shent iss-KEM-ik)	Temporary interference with blood supply to the brain, causing neurological symptoms such as dizziness, numbness, and hemiparesis. May eventually lead to a full-blown stroke (cerebrovascular accident).

■ Spinal Cord

amyotrophic lateral sclerosis (ALS) (ah-my-oh-TROFF-ik LAT-er-al skleh-ROH-sis)	Disease with muscular weakness and atrophy due to degeneration of motor neurons of the spinal cord. Also called *Lou Gehrig's disease,* after the New York Yankees baseball player who died from the disease.
meningocele (men-IN-goh-seel)	Congenital condition in which the meninges protrude through an opening in the vertebral column (see Figure 12.13B ■). See *spina bifida.*

■ **Figure 12.13** Spina bifida. A) Spina bifica occulta, the vertebra is not complete, but there is not protrusion of nervous system structures. B) Meningocele, the meninges sac protrudes through the opening in the vertebra. C) Myelomeningocele, the meninges sac and spinal cord protrude through the opening in the vertebra.

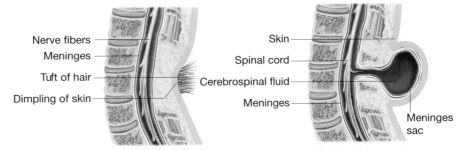

A. Spina bifida

B. Meningocele

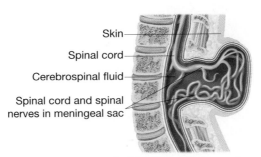

C. Myelomeningocele

Pathology *(continued)*

TERM	DEFINITION
myelomeningocele (my-eh-loh-meh-NIN-goh-seel)	Congenital condition in which the meninges and spinal cord protrude through an opening in the vertebral column (see Figure 12.13C ■). See *spina bifida*.
poliomyelitis (poh-lee-oh-my-eh-lye-tis)	Viral inflammation of the gray matter of the spinal cord. Results in varying degrees of paralysis, may be mild and reversible or may be severe and permanent. This disease has been almost eliminated due to the discovery of a vaccine in the 1950s.
spina bifida (SPY-nah BIFF-ih-dah)	Congenital defect in the walls of the spinal canal in which the laminae of the vertebra do not meet or close (see Figure 12.13A ■). May result in a meningocele or a myelomeningocele—meninges or the spinal cord being pushed through the opening.
spinal cord injury (SCI)	Damage to the spinal cord as a result of trauma. Spinal cord may be bruised or completely severed.

■ *Nerves*

TERM	DEFINITION
Bell's palsy (BELLZ PAWL-zee)	One-sided facial paralysis due to inflammation of the facial nerve, probably viral in nature. The patient cannot control salivation, tearing of the eyes, or expression, but most will eventually recover.
Guillain-Barré syndrome (GHEE-yan bah-RAY)	Disease of the nervous system in which nerves lose their myelin covering. May be caused by an autoimmune reaction. Characterized by loss of sensation and/or muscle control starting in the legs. Symptoms then move toward the trunk and may even result in paralysis of the diaphragm.
multiple sclerosis (MS) (MULL-tih-pl skleh-ROH-sis)	Inflammatory disease of the central nervous system in which there is extreme weakness and numbness due to loss of myelin insulation from nerves.
myasthenia gravis (my-ass-THEE-nee-ah GRAV-iss)	Disease with severe muscular weakness and fatigue due to insufficient neurotransmitter at a synapse.
shingles (SHING-lz)	Eruption of painful blisters on the body along a nerve path. Thought to be caused by a *Herpes zoster* virus infection of the nerve root. 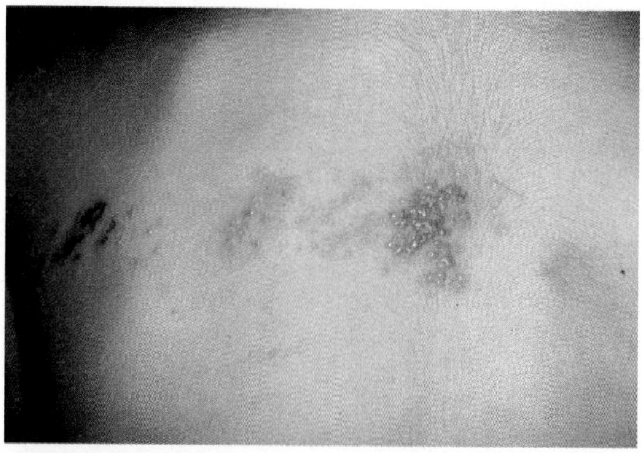

■ **Figure 12.14** Photograph of the skin eruptions associated with shingles.

■ *Meninges*

TERM	DEFINITION
epidural hematoma (ep-ih-DOO-ral hee-mah-TOH-mah)	Mass of blood in the space outside the dura mater of the brain and spinal cord.

Pathology *(continued)*

TERM	DEFINITION
subdural hematoma (sub-DOO-ral hee-mah-TOH-mah) **Figure 12.15** A subdural hematoma. A meningeal vein is ruptured and blood has accumulated in the subdural space producing pressure on the brain.	Mass of blood forming beneath the dura mater if the meninges are torn by trauma. May exert fatal pressure on the brain if the hematoma is not drained by surgery. 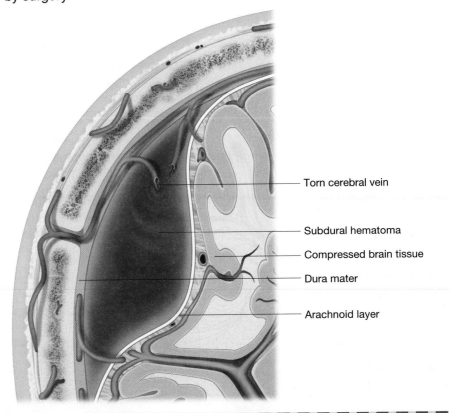

Torn cerebral vein

Subdural hematoma

Compressed brain tissue

Dura mater

Arachnoid layer

Diagnostic Procedures

TERM	DEFINITION
■ *Clinical Laboratory Tests*	
cerebrospinal fluid analysis (ser-eh-broh-SPY-nal FLOO-id an-NAL-ih-sis)	Laboratory examination of the clear, watery, colorless fluid from within the brain and spinal cord. Infections and the abnormal presence of blood can be detected in this test.
■ *Diagnostic Imaging*	
brain scan	Image of the brain taken after injection of radioactive isotopes into the circulation.
cerebral angiography (seh-REE-bral-an-jee-OG-rah-fee)	X-ray of the blood vessels of the brain after the injection of radiopaque dye.
echoencephalography (ek-oh-en-SEFF-ah-log-rah-fee)	Recording of the ultrasonic echoes of the brain. Useful in determining abnormal patterns of shifting in the brain.
myelography (my-eh-LOG-rah-fee)	Injection of radiopaque dye into the spinal canal. An X-ray is then taken to examine the normal and abnormal outlines made by the dye.

Diagnostic Procedures *(continued)*

TERM	DEFINITION
positron emission tomography (PET) (PAHZ-ih-tron ee-MISH-un toh-MOG-rah-fee)	Use of positive radionuclides to reconstruct brain sections. Measurement can be taken of oxygen and glucose uptake, cerebral blood flow, and blood volume. The amount of glucose the brain uses indicates how metabolically active the tissue is.

■ *Additional Diagnostic Tests*

Babinski reflex (bah-BIN-skeez)	Reflex test developed by French neurologist Joseph Babinski to determine lesions and abnormalities in the nervous system. The Babinski reflex is present if the great toe extends instead of flexes when the lateral sole of the foot is stroked. The normal response to this stimulation is flexion of the toe.
electroencephalography (EEG) (ee-lek-troh-en-SEFF-ah-LOG-rah-fee)	Recording the electrical activity of the brain by placing electrodes at various positions on the scalp. Also used in sleep studies to determine if there is a normal pattern of activity during sleep.
lumbar puncture (LP) (LUM-bar PUNK-chur)	Puncture with a needle into the lumbar area (usually the fourth intervertebral space) to withdraw fluid for examination and for the injection of anesthesia. Also called *spinal puncture* or *spinal tap*.

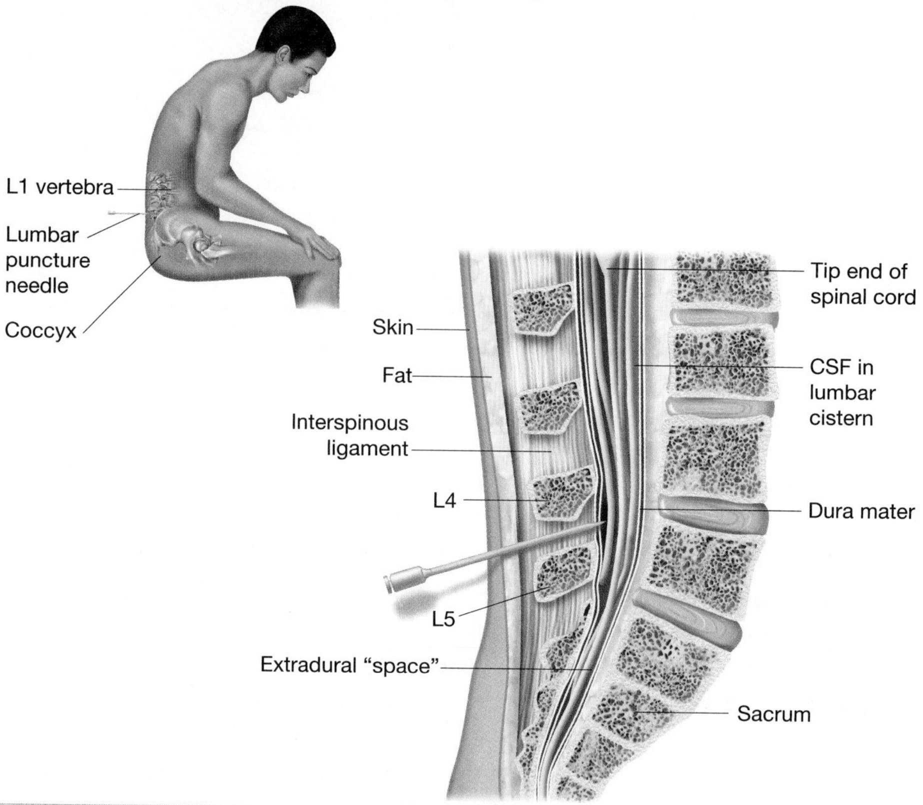

■ **Figure 12.16** A lumbar puncture. The needle is inserted between the lumbar vertebrae and into the spinal canal.

L1 vertebra

Lumbar puncture needle

Coccyx

Skin

Fat

Interspinous ligament

L4

L5

Extradural "space"

Tip end of spinal cord

CSF in lumbar cistern

Dura mater

Sacrum

| **nerve conduction velocity** | Test that measures how fast an impulse travels along a nerve. Can pinpoint an area of nerve damage. |

Therapeutic Procedures

TERM	DEFINITION
■ Medical Procedures	
nerve block	Injection of regional anesthetic to stop the passage of sensory or pain impulses along a nerve path.
■ Surgical Procedures	
carotid endarterectomy (kah-ROT-id end-ar-ter-EK-toh-mee)	Surgical procedure for removing an obstruction within the carotid artery, a major artery in the neck that carries oxygenated blood to the brain. Developed to prevent strokes, but is found to be useful only in severe stenosis with transient ischemic attack.
cerebrospinal fluid shunts (ser-eh-broh SPY-nal FLOO-id)	Surgical procedure in which a bypass is created to drain cerebrospinal fluid. It is used to treat hydrocephalus by draining the excess cerebrospinal fluid from the brain and diverting it to the abdominal cavity.
laminectomy (lam-ih-NEK-toh-mee)	Removal of a portion of a vertebra in order to relieve pressure on the spinal nerve.
tractotomy (track-OT-oh-mee)	Surgical interruption of a nerve tract in the spinal cord. Used to treat intractable pain or muscle spasms.

Pharmacology

CLASSIFICATION	ACTION	GENERIC AND BRAND NAMES
analgesic (an-al-JEE-zik)	Non-narcotic medication to treat minor to moderate pain. Includes aspirin, acetaminophen, and ibuprofen.	aspirin, Bayer, Ecotrin; acetaminophen, Tylenol; ibuprofen, Aleve
anesthetic (an-ess-THET-ik)	Drug that produces a loss of sensation or a loss of consciousness.	lidocaine, Xylocaine; pentobarbital, Nembutal; propofol, Diprivan; procaine, Novocain
anticonvulsant (an-tye-kon-VULL-sant)	Substance that reduces the excitability of neurons and therefore prevents the uncontrolled neuron activity associated with seizures.	carbamazepine, Tegretol; phenobarbital, Nembutal
dopaminergic drugs (dope-ah-men-ER-gik)	Group of medications to treat Parkinson's disease by either replacing the dopamine that is lacking or increasing the strength of the dopamine that is present.	levodopa; L-dopa, Larodopa; levodopa/carbidopa, Sinemet
hypnotic (hip-NOT-tik)	Drug that promotes sleep.	secobarbital, Seconal; temazepam, Restoril
narcotic analgesic (nar-KOT-tik)	Drug used to treat severe pain; has the potential to be habit forming if taken for a prolonged time. Also called *opiates*.	morphine, MS Contin; oxycodone, OxyContin; meperidine, Demerol
sedative (SED-ah-tiv)	Drug that has a relaxing or calming effect.	amobarbital, Amytal; butabarbital, Butisol

Abbreviations

ALS	amyotrophic lateral sclerosis	**HA**	headache
ANS	autonomic nervous system	**ICP**	intracranial pressure
CNS	central nervous system	**LP**	lumbar puncture
CP	cerebral palsy	**MS**	multiple sclerosis
CSF	cerebrospinal fluid	**PET**	positron emission tomography
CVA	cerebrovascular accident	**PNS**	peripheral nervous system
CVD	cerebrovascular disease	**SCI**	spinal cord injury
EEG	electroencephalogram, electroencephalography	**TIA**	transient ischemic attack

Chapter Review

Terminology Checklist

Below are all Anatomy and Physiology key terms, Word Building, Vocabulary, Pathology, Diagnostic, Therapeutic, and Pharmacology terms presented in this chapter. Use this list as a study tool by placing a check in the box in front of each term as you master its meaning.

☐ absence seizure
☐ afferent neurons
☐ Alzheimer's disease
☐ amyotrophic lateral sclerosis
☐ analgesia
☐ analgesic
☐ anesthesia
☐ anesthesiology
☐ anesthetic
☐ anticonvulsant
☐ aphasia
☐ arachnoid layer
☐ ascending tracts
☐ astrocytoma
☐ ataxia
☐ aura
☐ autonomic nervous system
☐ axon
☐ Babinski reflex
☐ Bell's palsy
☐ brain
☐ brain scan
☐ brain stem
☐ brain tumor
☐ carotid endarterectomy
☐ central canal
☐ central nervous system
☐ cephalalgia
☐ cerebellar
☐ cerebellitis
☐ cerebellum
☐ cerebral
☐ cerebral aneurysm
☐ cerebral angiography
☐ cerebral contusion
☐ cerebral cortex
☐ cerebral hemispheres
☐ cerebral palsy
☐ cerebrospinal

☐ cerebrospinal fluid
☐ cerebrospinal fluid analysis
☐ cerebrospinal fluid shunts
☐ cerebrovascular accident
☐ cerebrum
☐ coma
☐ concussion
☐ conscious
☐ convulsion
☐ cranial nerves
☐ delirium
☐ dementia
☐ dendrite
☐ descending tracts
☐ diencephalon
☐ dopaminergic drugs
☐ dura mater
☐ dysphasia
☐ echoencephalography
☐ efferent neurons
☐ electroencephalogram
☐ electroencephalography
☐ encephalitis
☐ epidural hematoma
☐ epilepsy
☐ focal seizure
☐ frontal lobe
☐ ganglion
☐ glands
☐ gray matter
☐ Guillain-Barré syndrome
☐ gyri
☐ hemiparesis
☐ hemiplegia
☐ hydrocephalus
☐ hyperesthesia
☐ hypnotic
☐ hypothalamus
☐ intrathecal

☐ laminectomy
☐ lumbar puncture
☐ medulla oblongata
☐ meningeal
☐ meninges
☐ meningioma
☐ meningitis
☐ meningocele
☐ midbrain
☐ migraine
☐ monoparesis
☐ monoplegia
☐ motor neurons
☐ multiple sclerosis
☐ muscles
☐ myasthenia gravis
☐ myelin
☐ myelinated
☐ myelitis
☐ myelogram
☐ myelography
☐ myelomeningocele
☐ narcotic analgesic
☐ nerve block
☐ nerve cell body
☐ nerve conduction velocity
☐ nerve root
☐ nerves
☐ neural
☐ neuralgia
☐ neurectomy
☐ neuroglial cells
☐ neurologist
☐ neurology
☐ neuroma
☐ neuron
☐ neuropathy
☐ neuroplasty
☐ neurorrhaphy

☐ neurosurgery	☐ radiculitis	☐ sympathetic branch
☐ neurotransmitter	☐ radiculopathy	☐ synapse
☐ occipital lobe	☐ Reye syndrome	☐ synaptic cleft
☐ palsy	☐ sedative	☐ syncope
☐ paralysis	☐ seizure	☐ temporal lobe
☐ paraplegia	☐ sensory neurons	☐ thalamic
☐ parasympathetic branch	☐ sensory receptors	☐ thalamus
☐ paresthesia	☐ shingles	☐ tonic-clonic seizure
☐ parietal lobe	☐ somatic nerves	☐ tract
☐ Parkinson's disease	☐ spina bifida	☐ tractotomy
☐ peripheral nervous system	☐ spinal cavity	☐ transient ischemic attack
☐ pia mater	☐ spinal cord	☐ tremor
☐ poliomyelitis	☐ spinal cord injury	☐ unconscious
☐ polyneuritis	☐ spinal nerves	☐ ventricles
☐ pons	☐ subarachnoid space	☐ vertebral canal
☐ pontine	☐ subdural hematoma	☐ vertebral column
☐ positron emission tomography	☐ subdural space	☐ white matter
☐ quadriplegia	☐ sulci	

Practice Exercises

A. Complete the following statements.

1. The study of the nervous system is called _____.

2. The organs of the nervous system are the _____, _____, and _____.

3. The two divisions of the nervous system are the _____ and _____.

4. The neurons that carry impulses away from the brain and spinal cord are called _____ neurons.

5. The neurons that carry impulses to the brain and spinal cord are called _____ neurons.

6. The largest portion of the brain is the _____.

7. The second largest portion of the brain is the _____.

8. The occipital lobe controls _____.

9. The temporal lobe controls _____ and _____.

10. The two divisions of the autonomic nervous system are the _____ and _____.

B. State the described terms using the combining forms provided.

The combining form *neur/o* refers to the nerve. Use it to write a term that means:

1. inflammation of the nerve _____

2. specialist in nerves _____

3. pain in the nerve _____

4. inflammation of many nerves _____

5. removal of a nerve _____

6. surgical repair of a nerve _____

7. nerve tumor _____

8. suture of a nerve _____

The combining form *mening/o* refers to the meninges or membranes. Use it to write a term that means:

9. inflammation of the meninges _____

10. protrusion of the meninges _____

11. protrusion of the spinal cord and the meninges _____

The combining form *encephal/o* refers to the brain. Use it to write a term that means:

12. X-ray record of the brain _____

13. disease of the brain _____

14. inflammation of the brain _____

15. protrusion of the brain _____

The combining form *cerebr/o* refers to the cerebrum. Use it to write a term that means:

16. pertaining to the cerebrum and spinal cord _____

17. pertaining to the cerebrum _____

C. Match each term to its definition.

1. _____ aura

2. _____ meningitis

3. _____ coma

4. _____ shingles

5. _____ syncope

6. _____ palsy

7. _____ absence seizure

8. _____ tonic-clonic seizure

9. _____ meningocele

a. loss of ability to control movement

b. sensations before a seizure

c. seizure with convulsions

d. congenital hernia of meninges

e. form of epilepsy without convulsion

f. inflammation of meninges

g. profound stupor

h. painful virus on nerves

i. fainting

D. Identify the following abbreviations.

1. TIA _____

2. MS _____

3. SCI _____

4. CNS _____

5. PNS _____

6. HA _____

7. CP _____

8. LP _____

9. ALS _____

E. Write the abbreviation for the following terms.

1. cerebrospinal fluid _____

2. cerebrovascular disease _____

3. electroencephalogram _____

4. intracranial pressure _____

5. positron emission tomography _____

6. cerebrovascular accident _____

7. subarachnoid hemorrhage _____

8. autonomic nervous system _____

F. Match each cranial nerves to its function.

1. _____ olfactory

2. _____ optic

3. _____ oculomotor

4. _____ trochlear

5. _____ trigeminal

6. _____ abducens

7. _____ facial

8. _____ vestibulocochlear

a. carries facial sensory impulses

b. turn eye to side

c. controls tongue muscles

d. eye muscles and controls pupils

e. swallowing

f. controls facial muscles

g. controls oblique eye muscles

h. smell

9. _____ glossopharyngeal   i.   controls neck and shoulder muscles

10. _____ vagus   j.   hearing and equilibrium

11. _____ accessory   k.   vision

12. _____ hypoglossal   l.   organs in lower body cavities

G. Define the following procedures and tests.

1. myelography _____

2. cerebral angiography _____

3. Babinski's reflex _____

4. nerve conduction velocity _____

5. cerebrospinal fluid analysis _____

6. PET scan _____

7. echoencephalography _____

8. lumbar puncture _____

H. Define each suffix and provide an example of its use in the nervous system.

	Meaning	Example
1. -plegia	_____	_____
2. -taxia	_____	_____
3. -algesia	_____	_____
4. -paresis	_____	_____
5. -phasia	_____	_____
6. -esthesia	_____	_____

I. Define the following combining forms and use them to form nervous system terms.

	Definition	Nervous System Term
1. mening/o	_____	_____
2. encephal/o	_____	_____
3. cerebell/o	_____	_____
4. myel/o	_____	_____
5. cephal/o	_____	_____
6. thalam/o	_____	_____

7. neur/o _____   _____

8. radicul/o _____   _____

9. cerebr/o _____   _____

10. pont/o _____   _____

J. Define the following terms.

1. astrocytoma _____

2. epilepsy _____

3. anesthesia _____

4. hemiparesis _____

5. neurosurgeon _____

6. analgesia _____

7. focal seizure _____

8. quadriplegia _____

9. subdural hematoma _____

10. intrathecal _____

K. Match each term to its definition.

1. _____ neurologist

2. _____ cerebrovascular accident

3. _____ concussion

4. _____ aphasia

5. _____ migraine

6. _____ seizure

7. _____ dementia

8. _____ ataxia

9. _____ spina bifida

10. _____ unconscious

a. sudden attack

b. a type of severe headache

c. loss of intellectual ability

d. physician who treats nervous problem

e. stroke

f. brain injury from a blow to the head

g. loss of ability to speak

h. congenital anomaly

i. state of being unaware

j. lack of muscle coordination

L. Use the following terms in the sentences below.

Parkinson's disease	transient ischemic attack	cerebral palsy	cerebrospinal fluid shunt
Bell's palsy	subdural hematoma	amyotrophic lateral sclerosis	nerve conduction velocity
delirium	cerebral aneurysm		

1. Dr. Martin noted that the 96-year-old patient suffered from _____ when she determined that he was confused, disoriented, and agitated.

2. Lucinda's _____ resulted in increasing muscle weakness as the motor neurons in her spinal cord degenerated.

3. The diagnosis of _____ was correct because the weakness affected only one side of Charles' face.

4. A cerebral angiogram was ordered because Dr. Larson suspected Mrs. Constantine had a(n) _____.

5. Roberta's symptoms included fine tremors, muscular weakness, rigidity, and a shuffling gait, leading to a diagnosis of _____.

6. Matthew's hydrocephalus required the placement of a(n) _____.

7. Because Mae's hemiparesis was temporary, the final diagnosis was _____.

8. Following the car accident, a CT scan showed a(n) _____ was putting pressure on the brain, necessitating immediate neurosurgery.

9. Birth trauma resulted in the newborn developing _____.

10. A(n) _____ test was performed in order to pinpoint the exact position of the nerve damage.

M. Fill in the classification for each drug description, then match the brand name.

Drug Description	Classification	Brand Name
1. _____ produces loss of sensation	_____	a. L-Dopa
2. _____ treats Parkinson's disease	_____	b. Amytal
3. _____ promotes sleep	_____	c. OxyContin
4. _____ non-narcotic pain medication	_____	d. Seconal
5. _____ produces a calming effect	_____	e. Xylocaine
6. _____ treats severe pain	_____	f. Tegretol
7. _____ treats seizures	_____	g. Aleve

Medical Record Analysis

Below is an item from a patient's medical record. Read it carefully, make sure you understand all the medical terms used, and then answer the questions that follow.

Discharge Summary

Admitting Diagnosis:	Paraplegia following motorcycle accident.
Final Diagnosis:	Comminuted L2 fracture with epidural hematoma and spinal cord damage resulting in complete paraplegia at the L2 level.
History of Present Illness:	Patient is a 23-year-old male who was involved in a motorcycle accident. He was unconscious for 35 minutes but was fully aware of his surroundings upon regaining consciousness. He was immediately aware of total anesthesia and paralysis below the waist.
Summary of Hospital Course:	CT scan revealed extensive bone destruction at the fracture site and that the spinal cord was severed. Lumbar puncture revealed sanguinous cerebrospinal fluid. Patient was unable to voluntarily contract any lower extremity muscles and was not able to feel touch or pinpricks. Lumbar laminectomy with spinal fusion was performed to stabilize the fracture and remove the epidural hematoma. The immediate postoperative recovery period proceeded normally with one incidence of pneumonia due to extended bed rest. It responded to antibiotics and respiratory therapy treatments. Patient began intensive rehabilitation with physical therapy and occupational therapy to strengthen upper extremities, as well as transfer and ADL training. After two months, X-rays indicated full healing of the spinal fusion and patient was transferred to a rehabilitation institute.
Discharge Plans:	Patient was transferred to a rehabilitation institute to continue intensive PT and OT. He will require skilled nursing care to assess his skin for the development of decubitus ulcers and intermittent urinary catheterization for incontinence. Since spinal cord was severed, it is not expected that this patient will regain muscle function and sensation. However, long-term goals include independent transfers, independent mobility with a wheelchair, and independent ADLs.

Critical Thinking Questions

1. The final diagnosis of "paraplegia at the L2 level" is not specifically defined by your text. Explain what you believe it to mean in the context of this discharge summary.

_____

_____

2. Is this patient expected to regain use of his muscles? Explain why or why not. _____

_____

3. The following medical terms are not specifically referred to in this chapter. Using your text as a dictionary, define each term in your own words.

a. comminuted _____

b. sanguinous _____

c. decubitus ulcer _____

d. catheterization _____

4. Which of the following is NOT part of this patient's rehabilitation therapy?
   a. arm strengthening
   b. transfer training
   c. instruction in activities of daily living
   d. leg strengthening

5. Describe, in your own words, the patient's long-term goals. _____

_____

6. Name and describe the complete surgical procedure this patient underwent. Then describe the purpose for this surgery. _____

_____

Chart Note Transcription

The chart note below contains eleven phrases that can be reworded with a medical term that you learned in this chapter. Each phrase is identified with an underline. Determine the medical term and write your answers in the space provided.

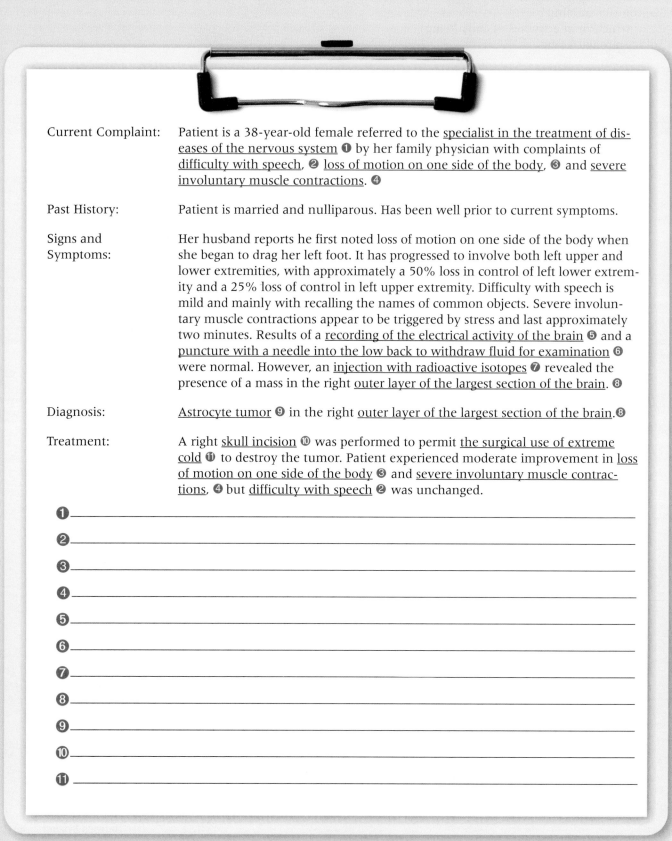

Current Complaint: Patient is a 38-year-old female referred to the <u>specialist in the treatment of diseases of the nervous system</u> ❶ by her family physician with complaints of <u>difficulty with speech,</u> ❷ <u>loss of motion on one side of the body,</u> ❸ and <u>severe involuntary muscle contractions.</u> ❹

Past History: Patient is married and nulliparous. Has been well prior to current symptoms.

Signs and Symptoms: Her husband reports he first noted loss of motion on one side of the body when she began to drag her left foot. It has progressed to involve both left upper and lower extremities, with approximately a 50% loss in control of left lower extremity and a 25% loss of control in left upper extremity. Difficulty with speech is mild and mainly with recalling the names of common objects. Severe involuntary muscle contractions appear to be triggered by stress and last approximately two minutes. Results of a <u>recording of the electrical activity of the brain</u> ❺ and a <u>puncture with a needle into the low back to withdraw fluid for examination</u> ❻ were normal. However, an <u>injection with radioactive isotopes</u> ❼ revealed the presence of a mass in the right <u>outer layer of the largest section of the brain.</u> ❽

Diagnosis: <u>Astrocyte tumor</u> ❾ in the right <u>outer layer of the largest section of the brain.</u>❽

Treatment: A right <u>skull incision</u> ❿ was performed to permit <u>the surgical use of extreme cold</u> ⓫ to destroy the tumor. Patient experienced moderate improvement in <u>loss of motion on one side of the body</u> ❸ and <u>severe involuntary muscle contractions,</u> ❹ but <u>difficulty with speech</u> ❷ was unchanged.

❶ _____

❷ _____

❸ _____

❹ _____

❺ _____

❻ _____

❼ _____

❽ _____

❾ _____

❿ _____

⓫ _____

Labeling Exercise

A. System Review

Write the labels for this figure on the numbered lines provided.

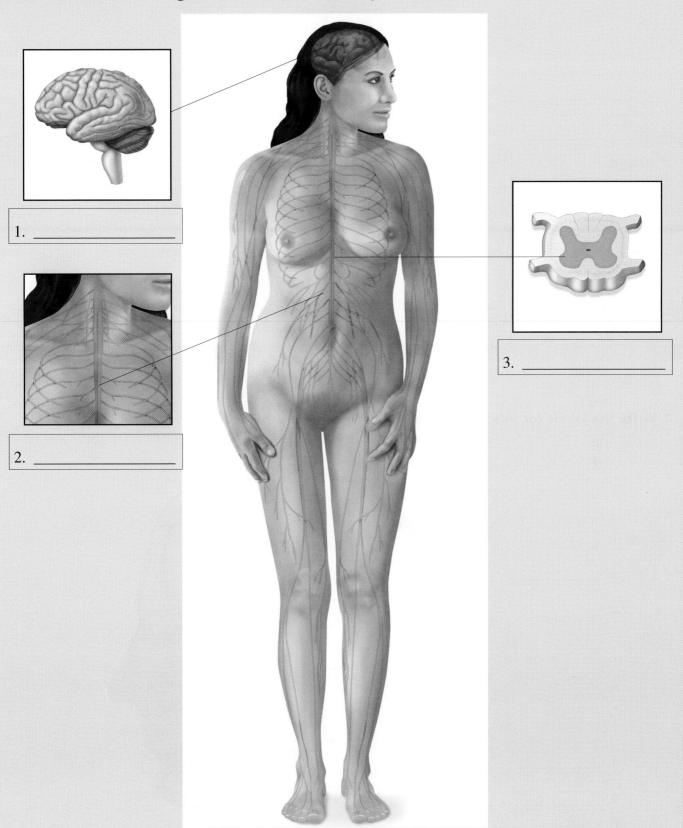

1. _____

2. _____

3. _____

B. Anatomy Challenge

1. Write the labels for this figure on the numbered lines provided.

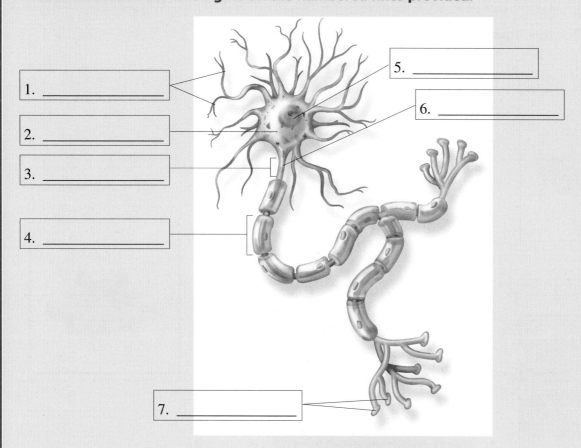

1. _____

2. _____

3. _____

4. _____

5. _____

6. _____

7. _____

2. Write the labels for this figure on the numbered lines provided.

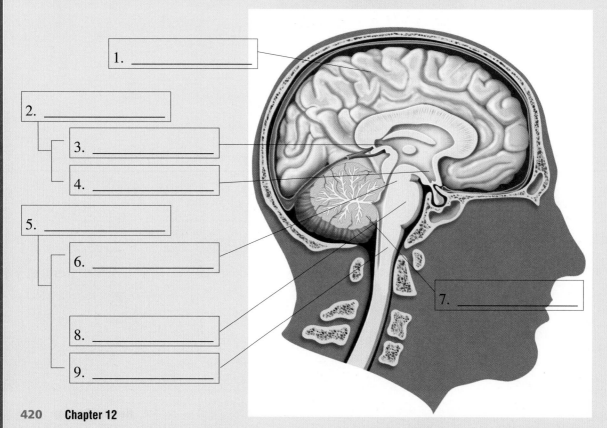

1. _____

2. _____

3. _____

4. _____

5. _____

6. _____

7. _____

8. _____

9. _____

Multimedia Preview

Additional interactive resources and activities for this chapter can be found on the Companion Website. For videos, games, and pronunciations, please access the accompanying **DVD-ROM** that comes with this book.

DVD-ROM Highlights

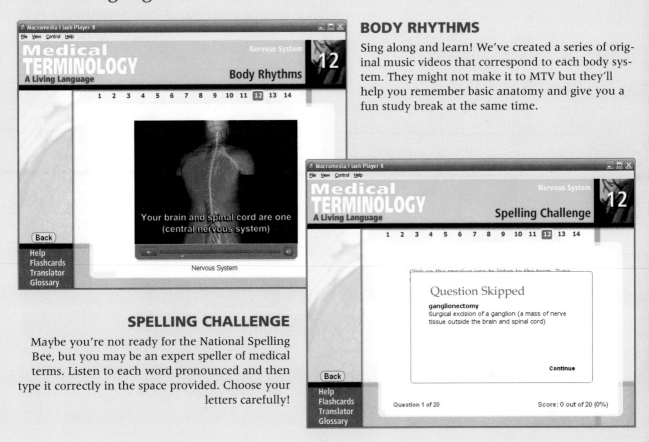

BODY RHYTHMS

Sing along and learn! We've created a series of original music videos that correspond to each body system. They might not make it to MTV but they'll help you remember basic anatomy and give you a fun study break at the same time.

SPELLING CHALLENGE

Maybe you're not ready for the National Spelling Bee, but you may be an expert speller of medical terms. Listen to each word pronounced and then type it correctly in the space provided. Choose your letters carefully!

Website Highlights—www.prenhall.com/fremgen

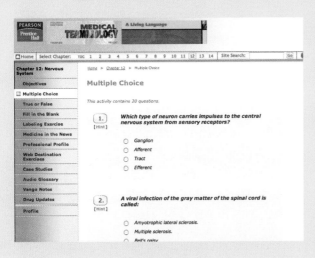

MULTIPLE CHOICE QUIZ

Take advantage of the free-access on-line study guide that accompanies your textbook. You'll find a multiple-choice quiz that provides instant feedback that allows you to check your score and see what you got right or wrong. By clicking on this URL you'll also access links to download mp3 audio reviews, current news articles, and an audio glossary.

13

Special Senses: The Eye and Ear

Learning Objectives

Upon completion of this chapter, you will be able to:

- Identify and define the combining forms and suffixes introduced in this chapter.

- Correctly spell and pronounce medical terms and major anatomical structures relating to the eye and ear.

- Locate and describe the major structures of the eye and ear and their functions.

- Describe how we see.

- Describe the path of sound vibration.

- Build and define eye and ear medical terms from word parts.

- Identify and define eye and ear vocabulary terms.

- Identify and define selected eye and ear pathology terms.

- Identify and define selected eye and ear diagnostic procedures.

- Identify and define selected eye and ear therapeutic procedures.

- Identify and define selected medications relating to the eye and ear.

- Define selected abbreviations associated with the eye and ear.

Section I: The Eye at a Glance

Function

The eye contains the sensory receptor cells for vision.

Structures

choroid
conjunctiva
eye muscles
eyeball
eyelids
lacrimal apparatus
retina
sclera

Combining Forms

ambly/o	dull, dim	**ocul/o**	eye
aque/o	water	**ophthalm/o**	eye
blephar/o	eyelid	**opt/o**	eye, vision
chrom/o	color	**optic/o**	eye
conjunctiv/o	conjunctiva	**nyctal/o**	night
core/o	pupil	**papill/o**	optic disk
corne/o	cornea	**phac/o**	lens
cycl/o	ciliary muscle	**phot/o**	light
dacry/o	tear, tear duct	**presby/o**	old age
dipl/o	double	**pupill/o**	pupil
glauc/o	gray	**retin/o**	retina
ir/o	iris	**scler/o**	sclera
irid/o	iris	**uve/o**	choroid
kerat/o	cornea	**vitre/o**	glassy
lacrim/o	tears		

Suffixes

-metrist	one who measures
-opia	vision
-tropia	to turn

The Eye Illustrated

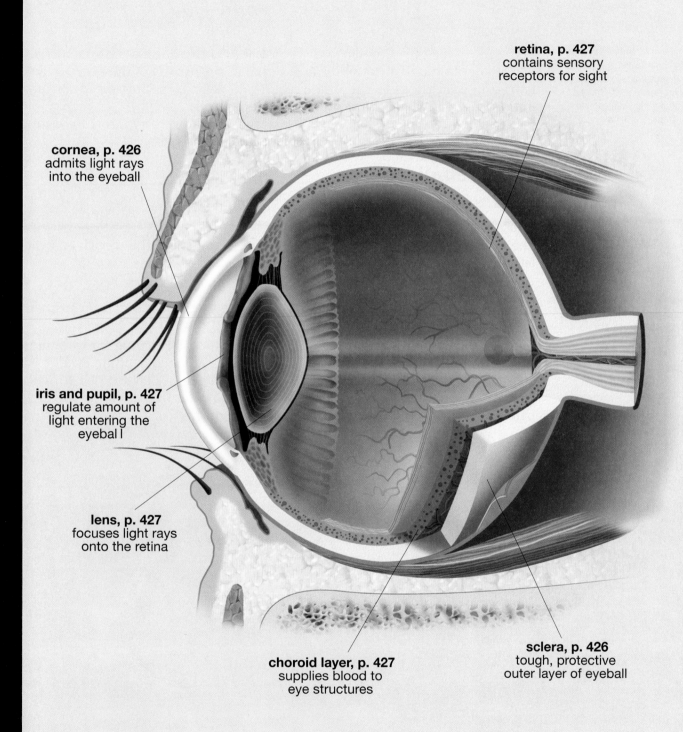

retina, p. 427
contains sensory
receptors for sight

cornea, p. 426
admits light rays
into the eyeball

iris and pupil, p. 427
regulate amount of
light entering the
eyebal l

lens, p. 427
focuses light rays
onto the retina

choroid layer, p. 427
supplies blood to
eye structures

sclera, p. 426
tough, protective
outer layer of eyeball

Anatomy and Physiology of the Eye

conjunctiva (kon-JUNK-tih-vah)   **lacrimal apparatus** (LAK-rim-al)
eyeball   **ophthalmology** (off-thal-MALL-oh-gee)
eyelids   **optic nerve** (OP-tik)
eye muscles

The study of the eye is known as **ophthalmology** (Ophth). The **eyeball** is the incredible organ of sight that transmits an external image by way of the nervous system—the **optic nerve**—to the brain. The brain then translates these sensory impulses into an image with computerlike accuracy.

In addition to the eyeball, several external structures play a role in vision. These are the **eye muscles**, **eyelids**, **conjunctiva**, and **lacrimal apparatus**.

The Eyeball

choroid (KOR-oyd)   **sclera** (SKLAIR-ah)
retina (RET-in-ah)

The actual eyeball is composed of three layers: the **sclera**, the **choroid**, and the **retina**.

Sclera

cornea (COR-nee-ah)   **refracts**

The outer layer, the sclera, provides a tough protective coating for the inner structures of the eye. Another term for the sclera is the white of the eye.

The anterior portion of the sclera is called the **cornea** (see Figure 13.1 ■). This clear, transparent area of the sclera allows light to enter the interior of the eyeball. The cornea actually bends, or **refracts**, the light rays.

■ **Figure 13.1** The internal structures of the eye.

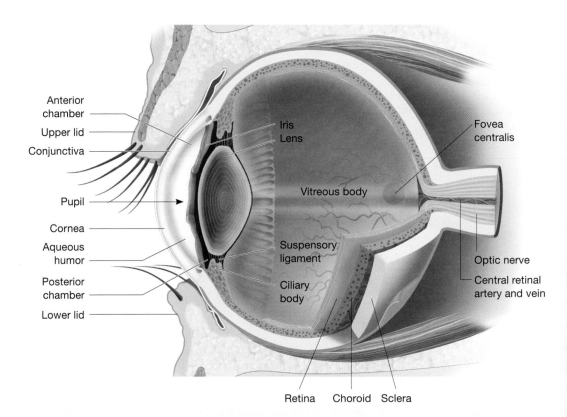

Choroid

ciliary body (SIL-ee-ar-ee)   **lens**
iris   **pupil**

The second or middle layer of the eyeball is called the choroid. This opaque layer provides the blood supply for the eye.

The anterior portion of the choroid layer consists of the **iris**, **pupil**, and **ciliary body** (see Figure 13.1). The iris is the colored portion of the eye and contains smooth muscle. The pupil is the opening in the center of the iris that allows light rays to enter the eyeball. The iris muscle contracts or relaxes to change the size of the pupil, thereby controlling how much light enters the interior of the eyeball. Behind the iris is the **lens**. The lens is not actually part of the choroid layer, but it is attached to the muscular ciliary body. By pulling on the edge of the lens, these muscles change the shape of the lens so it can focus incoming light onto the retina.

Retina

aqueous humor (AY-kwee-us)   **optic disk**
cones   **retinal blood vessels** (RET-in-al)
fovea centralis (FOH-vee-ah sen-TRAH-lis)   **rods**
macula lutea (MAK-yoo-lah loo-TEE-ah)   **vitreous humor** (VIT-ree-us)

The third and innermost layer of the eyeball is the retina. It contains the sensory receptor cells, **rods** and **cones**, that respond to light rays. Rods are active in dim light and help us to see in gray tones. Cones are active only in bright light and are responsible for color vision. When the lens projects an image onto the retina, it strikes an area called the **macula lutea**, or yellow spot (see Figure 13.1). In the center of the macula lutea is a depression called the **fovea centralis**, meaning central pit. This pit contains a high concentration of sensory receptor cells and, therefore, is the point of clearest vision. Also visible on the retina is the **optic disk**. This is the point where the **retinal blood vessels** enter and exit the eyeball and where the optic nerve leaves the eyeball (see Figure 13.2 ■). There are no sensory receptor cells in the optic disk and therefore it causes a blind spot in each eye's field of vision. The interior spaces of the eyeball are not empty. The spaces between the cornea and lens are filled with **aqueous humor**, a watery fluid, and the large open area between the lens and retina contains **vitreous humor**, a semisolid gel.

Med Term Tip

The function of the choroid, to provide the rest of the eyeball with blood, is responsible for an alternate name for this layer—*uvea*. The combining form *uve/o* means "vascular."

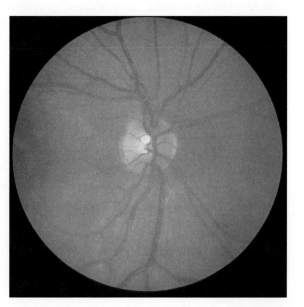

■ **Figure 13.2** Photograph of the retina of the eye. The optic disk appears yellow and the retinal arteries are clearly visible radiating out from it.

(Rory McClenaghan/Science Photo Library/ Photo Researchers, Inc.)

Figure 13.3 The arrangement of the external eye muscles, A) lateral and B) anterior views.

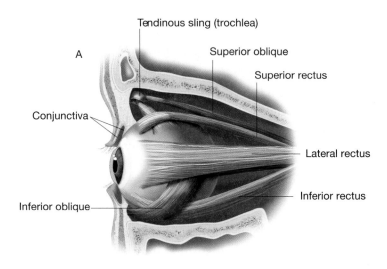
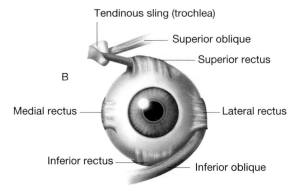

Muscles of the Eye

oblique muscles (oh-BLEEK)   **rectus muscles** (REK-tus)

Med Term Tip

Like many other muscles, the names *rectus* and *oblique* provide clues regarding the direction of their fibers, or their *line of pull*. Rectus means straight and oblique means slanted. Rectus muscles have a straight line of pull. Since the fibers of an oblique muscle are slanted on an angle, they produce rotation.

Six muscles connect the actual eyeball to the skull (see Figure 13.3 ■). These muscles allow for change in the direction of each eye's sightline. In addition, they provide support for the eyeball in the eye socket. Children may be born with a weakness in some of these muscles and may require treatments such as eye exercises or even surgery to correct this problem commonly referred to as crossed eyes or *strabismus* (see Figure 13.4 ■). The muscles involved are the four **rectus** and two **oblique muscles**. Rectus muscles (meaning straight) pull the eye up, down, left, or right in a straight line. Oblique muscles are on an angle and produce diagonal eye movement.

Figure 13.4 Photograph of an infant with strabismus. The left eye is turned inward, called esotropia. *(Bart's Medical Library/Phototake NYC)*

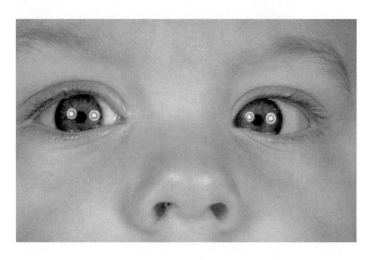

The Eyelids

cilia (SIL-ee-ah)   **sebaceous glands** (see-BAY-shus)
eyelashes

A pair of eyelids over each eyeball provides protection from foreign particles, injury from the sun and intense light, and trauma (see Figure 13.1). Both the upper and lower edges of the eyelids have **eyelashes** or **cilia** that protect the eye from foreign particles. In addition, **sebaceous glands** located in the eyelids secrete lubricating oil onto the eyeball.

Conjunctiva

mucous membrane

The conjunctiva of the eye is a **mucous membrane** lining. It forms a continuous covering on the underside of each eyelid and across the anterior surface of each eyeball (see Figure 13.1). This serves as protection for the eye by sealing off the eyeball in the socket.

Lacrimal Apparatus

lacrimal ducts   **nasolacrimal duct** (naz-oh-LAK-rim-al)
lacrimal gland   **tears**
nasal cavity

The **lacrimal gland** is located under the outer upper corner of each eyelid. These glands produce **tears**. Tears serve the important function of washing and lubricating the anterior surface of the eyeball. **Lacrimal ducts** located in the inner corner of the eye socket then collect the tears and drain them into the **nasolacrimal duct**. This duct ultimately drains the tears into the **nasal cavity** (see Figure 13.5 ■).

How We See

When light rays strike the eye, they first pass through the cornea, pupil, aqueous humor, lens, and vitreous humor (see Figure 13.6 ■). They then strike the retina and stimulate the rods and cones. When the light rays hit the retina, an upside-down image is sent along nerve impulses to the optic nerve (see

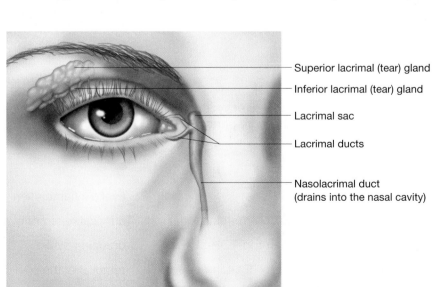

■ **Figure 13.5** The structure of the lacrimal apparatus.

Superior lacrimal (tear) gland

Inferior lacrimal (tear) gland

Lacrimal sac

Lacrimal ducts

Nasolacrimal duct
(drains into the nasal cavity)

Figure 13.6 The path of light through the cornea, pupil, lens, and striking the retina.

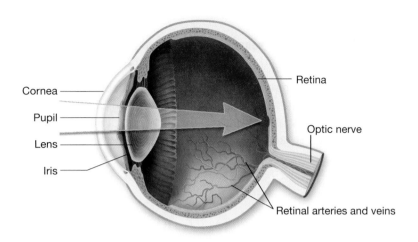

Figure 13.7 ■). The optic nerve transmits these impulses to the brain, where the upside-down image is translated into the right-side-up image we are looking at.

Vision requires proper functioning of four mechanisms:

1. Coordination of the external eye muscles so that both eyes move together.
2. The correct amount of light admitted by the pupil.
3. The correct focus of light on the retina by the lens.
4. The optic nerve transmitting sensory images to the brain.

Figure 13.7 The image formed on the retina is inverted. The brain rights the image as part of the interpretation process.

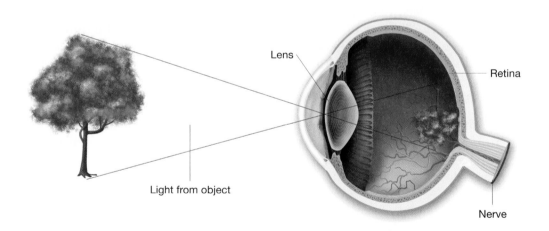

Word Building

The following list contains examples of medical terms built directly from word parts. The definitions of these terms can be determined by a straightforward translation of the word parts.

COMBINING FORM	COMBINED WITH	MEDICAL TERM	DEFINITION
blephar/o	-itis	**blepharitis** (blef-ah-RYE-tis)	eyelid inflammation
	-plasty	**blepharoplasty** (BLEF-ah-roh-plass-tee)	surgical repair of eyelid
	-ptosis	**blepharoptosis** (blef-ah-rop-TOH-sis)	drooping eyelid
	-ectomy	**blepharectomy** (blef-ah-REK-toh-mee)	removal of the eyelid
conjuctiv/o	-al	**conjunctival** (kon-JUNK-tih-vall)	pertaining to the conjunctiva

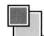

Word Building *(continued)*

COMBINING FORM	COMBINED WITH	MEDICAL TERM	DEFINITION
	-itis	**conjunctivitis** (kon-junk-tih-VYE-tis)	conjunctiva inflammation (pink eye)
	-plasty	**conjunctivoplasty** (kon-junk-tih-VOH-plas-tee)	surgical repair of the conjunctiva
corne/o	-al	**corneal** (KOR-nee-all)	pertaining to the cornea

Med Term Tip

Word watch — Be careful using the combining forms *core/o* meaning "pupil" and *corne/o* meaning "cornea."

cycl/o	-plegia	**cycloplegia** (sigh-kloh-PLEE-jee-ah)	paralysis of the ciliary body
dacry/o	cyst/o -itis	**dacryocystitis** (dak-ree-oh-sis-TYE-tis)	tear bladder inflammation
dipl/o	-opia	**diplopia** (dip-LOH-pee-ah)	double vision
ir/o	-itis	**iritis** (eye-RYE-tis)	iris inflammation
irid/o	-al	**iridal** (ir-id-all)	pertaining to the iris
	-ectomy	**iridectomy** (ir-id-EK-toh-mee)	removal of iris
	-plegia	**iridoplegia** (ir-id-oh-PLEE-jee-ah)	paralysis of iris
	scler/o -otomy	**iridosclerotomy** (ir-ih-doh-skleh-ROT-oh-mee)	incision into iris and sclera
kerat/o	-itis	**keratitis** (kair-ah-TYE-tis)	cornea inflammation

Med Term Tip

Word watch — Be careful using the combining form *kerat/o*, which means both "cornea" and "hard protein keratin."

	-meter	**keratometer** (KAIR-ah-toh-mee-ter)	instrument to measure (curve of) cornea
	-otomy	**keratotomy** (kair-ah-TOT-oh-mee)	incision into the cornea
lacrim/o	-al	**lacrimal** (LAK-rim-al)	pertaining to tears
ocul/o	-ar	**ocular** (OCK-yoo-lar)	pertaining to the eye
	intra- -ar	**intraocular** (in-trah-OCK-yoo-lar)	pertaining to within the eye
	myc/o -osis	**oculomycosis** (ok-yoo-loh-my-KOH-sis)	abnormal condition of eye fungus
ophthalm/o	-algia	**ophthalmalgia** (off-thal-MAL-jee-ah)	eye pain
	-ic	**ophthalmic** (off-THAL-mik)	pertaining to the eye
	-ologist	**ophthalmologist** (off-thal-MALL-oh-jist)	specialist in the eye
	-plegia	**ophthalmoplegia** (off-thal-moh-PLEE-jee-ah)	eye paralysis
	-rrhagia	**ophthalmorrhagia** (off-thal-moh-RAH-jee-ah)	rapid bleeding from the eye
	-scope	**ophthalmoscope** (off-THAL-moh-scope)	instrument to view inside the eye
opt/o	-ic	**optic** (OP-tik)	pertaining to the eye or vision
	-meter	**optometer** (op-TOM-eh-ter)	instrument to measure vision
	-metrist	**optometrist** (op-TOM-eh-trist)	one who measures vision

Word Building *(continued)*

COMBINING FORM	COMBINED WITH	MEDICAL TERM	DEFINITION
pupill/o	-ary	**pupillary** (PYOO-pih-lair-ee)	pertaining to the pupil
retin/o	-al	**retinal** (RET-in-al)	pertaining to the retina
	-pathy	**retinopathy** (ret-in-OP-ah-thee)	retina disease
	-pexy	**retinopexy** (ret-ih-noh-PEX-ee)	surgical fixation of the retina
scler/o	-al	**scleral** (SKLAIR-all)	pertaining to the sclera
	-malacia	**scleromalacia** (sklair-oh-mah-LAY-she-ah)	softening of the sclera
	-otomy	**sclerotomy** (skleh-ROT-oh-mee)	incision into the sclera
	-itis	**scleritis** (skler-EYE-tis)	inflammation of the sclera
uve/o	-itis	**uveitis** (yoo-vee-EYE-tis)	inflammation of the choroid

Vocabulary

TERM	DEFINITION
emmetropia (EM) (em-eh-TROH-pee-ah)	State of normal vision.
legally blind	Describes a person who has severely impaired vision. Usually defined as having visual acuity of 20/200 that cannot be improved with corrective lenses or having a visual field of less than 20 degrees.
nyctalopia (nik-tah-LOH-pee-ah)	Difficulty seeing in dim light; also called *night-blindness.* Usually due to damaged rods. **Med Term Tip** The simple translation of *nyctalopia* is "night vision." However, it is used to mean "night blindness."
ophthalmology (opf-thal-MOLL-oh-jee)	Branch of medicine involving the diagnosis and treatment of conditions and diseases of the eye and surrounding structures. The physician is an *ophthalmologist.*
optician (op-TISH-an)	Specialist in grinding corrective lenses.
optometry (op-TOM-eh-tree)	Medical profession specializing in examining the eyes, testing visual acuity, and prescribing corrective lenses. A doctor of optometry is an *optometrist.*
papilledema (pah-pill-eh-DEEM-ah)	Swelling of the optic disk. Often as a result of increased intraocular pressure. Also called *choked disk.*
photophobia (foh-toh-FOH-bee-ah)	Although the term translates into *fear of light,* it actually means a strong sensitivity to bright light.
presbyopia (prez-bee-OH-pee-ah)	Visual loss due to old age, resulting in difficulty in focusing for near vision (such as reading).
xerophthalmia (zee-ROP-thal-mee-ah)	Dry eyes.

Pathology

TERM	DEFINITION
■ Eyeball	
achromatopsia (ah-kroh-mah-TOP-see-ah)	Condition of color blindness—unable to perceive one or more colors; more common in males.
amblyopia (am-blee-OH-pee-ah)	Loss of vision not as a result of eye pathology. Usually occurs in patients who see two images. In order to see only one image, the brain will no longer recognize the image being sent to it by one of the eyes. May occur if strabismus is not corrected. This condition is not treatable with a prescription lens. Commonly referred to as *lazy eye*.
astigmatism (Astigm) (ah-STIG-mah-tizm)	Condition in which light rays are focused unevenly on the retina, causing a distorted image, due to an abnormal curvature of the cornea.
cataract (KAT-ah-rakt)	Damage to the lens causing it to become opaque or cloudy, resulting in diminished vision. Treatment is usually surgical removal of the cataract or replacement of the lens.

Med Term Tip

The term *cataract* comes from the Latin word meaning "waterfall." This refers to how a person with a cataract sees the world—as if looking through a waterfall.

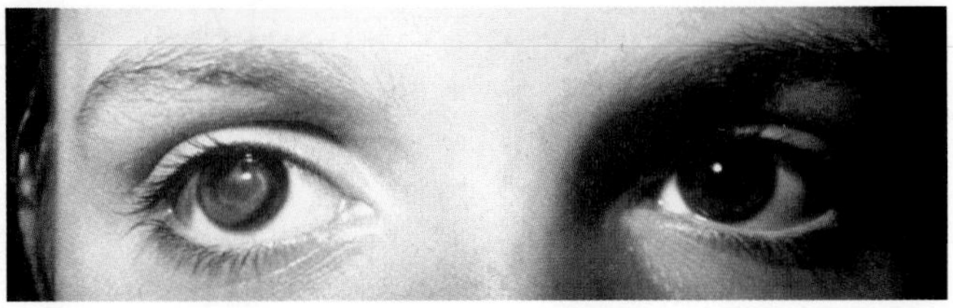

Figure 13.8 Photograph of a person with a cataract in the right eye.

TERM	DEFINITION
corneal abrasion	Scraping injury to the cornea. If it does not heal, it may develop into an ulcer.
glaucoma (glau-KOH-mah)	Increase in intraocular pressure, which, if untreated, may result in atrophy (wasting away) of the optic nerve and blindness. Glaucoma is treated with medication and surgery. There is an increased risk of developing glaucoma in persons over age 60, of African ancestry, who have sustained a serious eye injury, and in anyone with a family history of diabetes or glaucoma.
hyperopia (high-per-OH-pee-ah)	With this condition a person can see things in the distance but has trouble reading material at close range. Also known as *farsightedness*. This condition is corrected with converging or biconvex lenses.

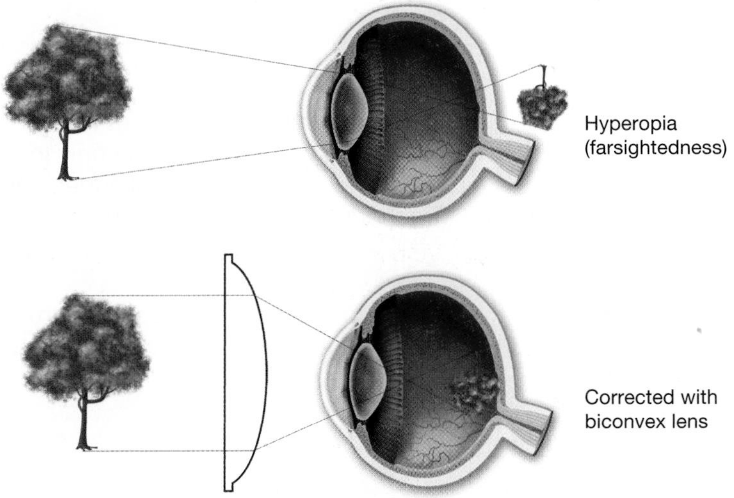

Figure 13.9 Hyperopia (farsightedness). In the uncorrected top figure, the image would come into focus behind the retina, making the image on the retina blurry. The bottom image shows how a biconvex lens corrects this condition.

Hyperopia (farsightedness)

Corrected with biconvex lens

Pathology *(continued)*

TERM	DEFINITION
macular degeneration (MAK-yoo-lar)	Deterioration of the macular area of the retina of the eye. May be treated with laser surgery to destroy the blood vessels beneath the macula.
monochromatism (mon-oh-KROH-mah-tizm)	Unable to perceive one color.
myopia (MY) (my-OH-pee-ah)	With this condition a person can see things close up but distance vision is blurred. Also known as *nearsightedness.* This condition is corrected with diverging or biconcave lenses.

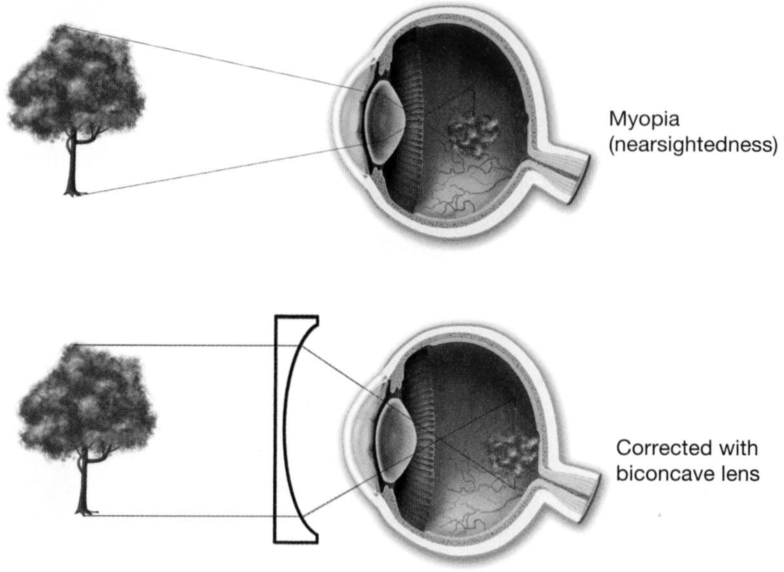

Figure 13.10 Myopia (nearsightedness). In the uncorrected top figure, the image comes into focus in front of the lens, making the image on the retina blurry. The bottom image shows how a biconcave lens corrects this condition.

Myopia (nearsightedness)

Corrected with biconcave lens

TERM	DEFINITION
retinal detachment (RET-in-al)	Occurs when the retina becomes separated from the choroid layer. This separation seriously damages blood vessels and nerves, resulting in blindness. May be treated with surgical or medical procedures to stabilize the retina and prevent separation.
retinitis pigmentosa (ret-in-EYE-tis pig-men-TOH-sah)	Progressive disease of the eye resulting in the retina becoming hard (sclerosed), pigmented (colored), and atrophying (wasting away). There is no known cure for this condition.
retinoblastoma (RET-in-noh-blast-OH-mah)	Malignant eye tumor occurring in children, usually under the age of 3. Requires enucleation.

■ *Conjunctiva*

TERM	DEFINITION
pterygium (the-RIJ-ee-um)	Hypertrophied conjunctival tissue in the inner corner of the eye.
trachoma (tray-KOH-mah)	Chronic infectious disease of the conjunctiva and cornea caused by bacteria. Occurs more commonly in those living in hot, dry climates. Untreated, it may lead to blindness when the scarring invades the cornea. Trachoma can be treated with antibiotics.

■ *Eyelids*

TERM	DEFINITION
hordeolum (hor-DEE-oh-lum)	Refers to a *stye* (or *sty*), a small purulent inflammatory infection of a sebaceous gland of the eyelid; treated with hot compresses and/or surgical incision.

Pathology *(continued)*

TERM	DEFINITION
■ *Eye Muscles*	
esotropia (ST) (ess-oh-TROH-pee-ah)	Inward turning of the eye; also called *cross-eyed*. An example of a form of strabismus (muscle weakness of the eye).
exotropia (XT) (eks-oh-TROH-pee-ah)	Outward turning of the eye; also called *wall-eyed*. Also an example of strabismus (muscle weakness of the eye).
strabismus (strah-BIZ-mus)	Eye muscle weakness commonly seen in children resulting in the eyes looking in different directions at the same time. May be corrected with glasses, eye exercises, and/or surgery.
■ *Brain-Related Vision Pathologies*	
hemianopia (hem-ee-ah-NOP-ee-ah)	Loss of vision in half of the visual field. A stroke patient may suffer from this disorder.
nystagmus (niss-TAG-mus)	Jerky-appearing involuntary eye movements, usually left and right. Often an indication of brain injury.

Diagnostic Procedures

TERM	DEFINITION
■ *Eye Examination Tests*	
color vision tests	Use of polychromic (multicolored) charts to determine the ability of the patient to recognize color.

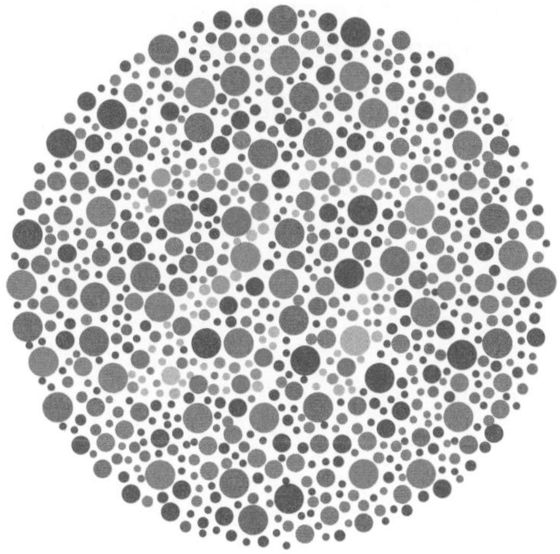

Figure 13.11 An example of color blindness test. A person with red-green color blindness would not be able to distinguish the green 27 from the surrounding red circles.

TERM	DEFINITION
fluorescein angiography (floo-oh-RESS-ee-in an-jee-OG-rah-fee)	Process of injecting a dye (fluorescein) to observe the movement of blood and detect lesions in the macular area of the retina. Used to determine if there is a detachment of the retina.
fluorescein staining (floo-oh-RESS-ee-in)	Applying dye eye drops that are a bright green fluorescent color. Used to look for corneal abrasions or ulcers.
keratometry (kair-ah-TOM-eh-tree)	Measurement of the curvature of the cornea using an instrument called a *keratometer*.
ophthalmoscopy (off-thal-MOSS-koh-pee)	Examination of the interior of the eyes using an instrument called an *ophthalmoscope* (see Figure 13.12 ■). The physician dilates the pupil in order to see the cornea, lens, and retina. Used to identify abnormalities in the blood vessels of the eye and some systemic diseases.

Figure 13.12 Examination of the interior of the eye using an ophthalmoscope.

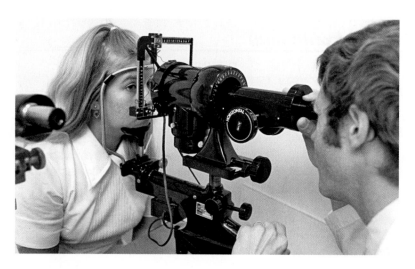

Diagnostic Procedures *(continued)*

TERM	DEFINITION
refractive error test (ree-FRAK-tiv)	Vision test for a defect in the ability of the eye to accurately focus the image that is hitting it. Refractive errors result in myopia and hyperopia.
slit lamp microscopy	Examining the posterior surface of the cornea.
Snellen chart (SNEL-enz)	Chart used for testing distance vision named for Dutch ophthalmologist Hermann Snellen. It contains letters of varying size and is administered from a distance of 20 feet. A person who can read at 20 feet what the average person can read at this distance is said to have 20/20 vision.
tonometry (tohn-OM-eh-tree)	Measurement of the intraocular pressure of the eye using a *tonometer* to check for the condition of glaucoma. The physician places the tonometer lightly on the eyeball and a pressure measurement is taken. Generally part of a normal eye exam for adults.
visual acuity (VA) **test** (VIZH-oo-al ah-KYOO-ih-tee)	Measurement of the sharpness of a patient's vision. Usually, a Snellen chart is used for this test in which the patient identifies letters from a distance of 20 feet.

Therapeutic Procedures

TERMS	DEFINITION
■ Surgical Procedures	
cryoextraction (cry-oh-eks-TRAK-shun)	Procedure in which cataract is lifted from the lens with an extremely cold probe.
cryoretinopexy (cry-oh-RET-ih-noh-pek-see)	Surgical fixation of the retina by using extreme cold.
enucleation (ee-new-klee-AH-shun)	Surgical removal of an eyeball.
keratoplasty (KAIR-ah-toh-plass-tee)	Surgical repair of the cornea is the simple translation of this term that is utilized to mean corneal transplant.
laser-assisted in-situ keratomileusis (LASIK) (in-SIH-tyoo kair-ah-toh-mih-LOO-sis)	Correction of myopia using laser surgery to remove corneal tissue (see Figure 13.13 ■).

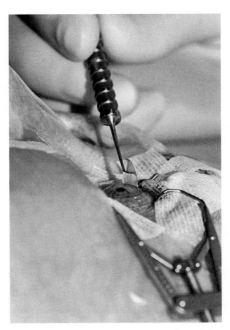

Figure 13.13 LASIK surgery. The cornea has been lifted in order to reshape it. *(Chris Barry/Phototake NYC)*

Therapeutic Procedures *(continued)*

TERM	DEFINITION
laser photocoagulation (LAY-zer foh-toh-koh-ag-yoo-LAY-shun)	Use of a laser beam to destroy very small precise areas of the retina. May be used to treat retinal detachment or macular degeneration.
phacoemulsification (fak-oh-ee-mull-sih-fih-KAY-shun)	Use of high-frequency sound waves to emulsify (liquefy) a lens with a cataract, which is then aspirated (removed by suction) with a needle.
photorefractive keratectomy (PRK) (foh-toh-ree-FRAK-tiv kair-ah-TEK-toh-mee)	Use of a laser to reshape the cornea and correct errors of refraction.
radial keratotomy (RK) (RAY-dee-all kair-ah-TOT-oh-mee)	Spokelike incisions around the cornea that result in it becoming flatter. A surgical treatment for myopia.
scleral buckling (SKLAIR-al)	Placing a band of silicone around the outside of the sclera that stabilizes a detaching retina.
strabotomy (strah-BOT-oh-mee)	Incision into the eye muscles in order to correct strabismus.

Pharmacology

CLASSIFICATION	ACTION	GENERIC AND BRAND NAMES
anesthetic ophthalmic solution (off-THAL-mik)	Eye drops for pain relief associated with eye infections, corneal abrasions, or surgery.	proparacain, Ak-Taine, Ocu-Caine; tetracaine, Opticaine, Pontocaine
antibiotic ophthalmic solution (off-THAL-mik)	Eye drops for the treatment of bacterial eye infections.	erythromycin, Del-Mycin, Ilotycin Ophthalmic
antiglaucoma medications (an-tye-glau-KOH-mah)	Group of drugs that reduce intraocular pressure by lowering the amount of aqueous humor in the eyeball. May achieve this by either reducing the production of aqueous humor or increasing its outflow.	timolol, Betimol, Timoptic; acetazolamide, Ak-Zol, Dazamide; prostaglandin analogs, Lumigan, Xalatan

Pharmacology *(continued)*

CLASSIFICATION	ACTION	GENERIC AND BRAND NAMES
artificial tears	Medications, many of them over the counter, to treat dry eyes.	buffered isotonic solutions, Akwa Tears, Refresh Plus, Moisture Eyes
miotic (my-OT-ik)	Any substance that causes the pupil to constrict. These medications may also be used to treat glaucoma.	physostigmine, Eserine Sulfate, Isopto Eserine; carbachol, Carbastat, Miostat
mydriatic (mid-ree-AT-ik)	Any substance that causes the pupil to dilate by paralyzing the iris and/or ciliary body muscles. Particularly useful during eye examinations and eye surgery.	atropine sulfate, Atropine-Care Ophthalmic, Atropisol Ophthalmic
ophthalmic decongestants	Over-the-counter medications that constrict the arterioles of the eye, reduce redness and itching of the conjunctiva.	tetrahydrozoline, Visine, Murine

Abbreviations

ARMD	age-related macular degeneration	**Ophth.**	ophthalmology
Astigm	astigmatism	**OS**	left eye
c.gl.	correction with glasses	**OU**	each eye/both eyes
D	diopter (lens strength)	**PERRLA**	pupils equal, round, react to light and accommodation
DVA	distance visual acuity		
ECCE	extracapsular cataract extraction	**PRK**	photorefractive keratectomy
EENT	eye, ear, nose, and throat	**REM**	rapid eye movement
EM	emmetropia	**s.gl.**	without correction or glasses
EOM	extraocular movement	**SMD**	senile macular degeneration
ICCE	intracapsular cataract extraction	**ST**	esotropia
IOP	intraocular pressure	**VA**	visual acuity
LASIK	laser-assisted in-situ keratomileusis	**VF**	visual field
OD	right eye	**XT**	exotropia

Med Term Tip

The abbreviations for right eye (OD) and left eye (OS) are easy to remember when we know their origins. OD stands for *oculus* (eye) *dexter* (right). OS has its origin in *oculus* (eye) *sinister* (left). At one time in history it was considered to be sinister if a person looked at another from only the left side. Hence the term *oculus sinister* (OS) means left eye.

Section II: The Ear at a Glance

Function

The ear contains the sensory receptors for hearing and equilibrium (balance).

Structures

auricle
external ear
inner ear
middle ear

Combining Forms

acous/o	hearing
audi/o	hearing
audit/o	hearing
aur/o	ear
auricul/o	ear
cerumin/o	cerumen
cochle/o	cochlea
labyrinth/o	labyrinth (inner ear)
myring/o	eardrum
ot/o	ear
salping/o	eustachian tube
staped/o	stapes
tympan/o	eardrum, middle ear

Suffixes

-cusis	hearing
-otia	ear condition

The Ear Illustrated

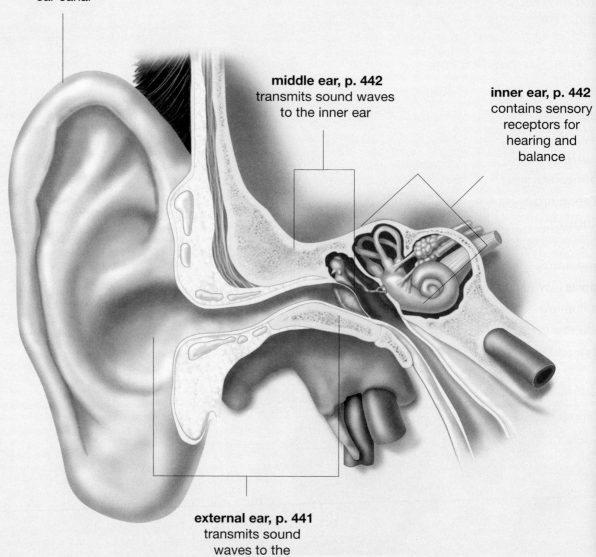

auricle, p. 441
directs sound
waves into the
ear canal

middle ear, p. 442
transmits sound waves
to the inner ear

inner ear, p. 442
contains sensory
receptors for
hearing and
balance

external ear, p. 441
transmits sound
waves to the
middle ear

Anatomy and Physiology of the Ear

audiology (aw-dee-OL-oh-jee)
cochlear nerve (KOK-lee-ar)
equilibrium (ee-kwih-LIB-ree-um)
external ear
hearing
inner ear

middle ear
otology (oh-TOL-oh-jee)
vestibular nerve (ves-TIB-yoo-lar)
vestibulocochlear nerve
(ves-tib-yoo-loh-KOK-lee-ar)

The study of the ear is referred to as **otology** (Oto), and the study of hearing disorders is called **audiology**. While there is a large amount of overlap between these two areas, there are also examples of ear problems that do not affect hearing. The ear is responsible for two senses: **hearing** and **equilibrium**, or our sense of balance. Hearing and equilibrium sensory information is carried to the brain by cranial nerve VIII, the **vestibulocochlear nerve**. This nerve is divided into two major branches. The **cochlear nerve** carries hearing information, and the **vestibular nerve** carries equilibrium information.

The ear is subdivided into three areas:

1. **external ear**
2. **middle ear**
3. **inner ear**

External Ear

auditory canal (AW-dih-tor-ee)
auricle (AW-rih-k'l)
cerumen (seh-ROO-men)
external auditory meatus
(AW-dih-tor-ee me-A-tus)

pinna (PIN-ah)
tympanic membrane (tim-PAN-ik)

The external ear consists of three parts: the **auricle**, the **auditory canal**, and the **tympanic membrane** (see Figure 13.14 ■). The auricle or **pinna** is what is commonly referred to as *the ear* because this is the only visible portion. The auricle with its

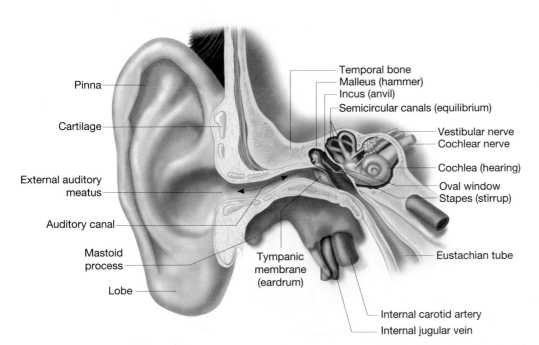

■ **Figure 13.14** The internal structures of the outer, middle, and inner ear.

Pinna
Cartilage
External auditory meatus
Auditory canal
Mastoid process
Lobe

Temporal bone
Malleus (hammer)
Incus (anvil)
Semicircular canals (equilibrium)
Vestibular nerve
Cochlear nerve
Cochlea (hearing)
Oval window
Stapes (stirrup)
Eustachian tube
Internal carotid artery
Internal jugular vein

Tympanic membrane (eardrum)

earlobe has a unique shape in each person and functions like a funnel to capture sound waves as they go past the outer ear and channel them through the **external auditory meatus**. The sound then moves along the auditory canal and causes the tympanic membrane (eardrum) to vibrate. The tympanic membrane actually separates the external ear from the middle ear. Ear wax or **cerumen** is produced in oil glands in the auditory canal. This wax helps to protect and lubricate the ear. It is also just barely liquid at body temperature. This causes cerumen to slowly flow out of the auditory canal, carrying dirt and dust with it. Therefore, the auditory canal is self-cleaning.

Middle Ear

auditory tube (AW-dih-tor-ee)   **ossicles** (OSS-ih-kls)
eustachian tube (yoo-STAY-she-en)   **oval window**
incus (ING-kus)   **stapes** (STAY-peez)
malleus (MAL-ee-us)

The middle ear is located in a small cavity in the temporal bone of the skull. This air-filled cavity contains three tiny bones called **ossicles** (see Figure 13.15 ■). These three bones, the **malleus**, **incus**, and **stapes**, are vital to the hearing process. They amplify the vibrations in the middle ear and transmit them to the inner ear from the malleus to the incus and finally to the stapes. The stapes, the last of the three ossicles, is attached to a very thin membrane that covers the opening to the inner ear called the **oval window**.

The **eustachian tube** or **auditory tube** connects the nasopharynx with the middle ear (see Figure 13.14). Each time you swallow the eustachian tube opens. This connection allows pressure to equalize between the middle ear cavity and the atmospheric pressure.

Inner Ear

cochlea (KOK-lee-ah)   **saccule** (SAK-yool)
labyrinth (LAB-ih-rinth)   **semicircular canals**
organs of Corti (KOR-tee)   **utricle** (YOO-trih-k'l)

The inner ear is also located in a cavity within the temporal bone (see Figure 13.14). This fluid-filled cavity is referred to as the **labyrinth** because of its shape. The labyrinth contains the hearing and equilibrium sensory organs: the **cochlea** for hearing and the **semicircular canals**, **utricle**, and **saccule** for equilibrium. Each of these organs contains hair cells, which are the actual sensory receptor cells. In the cochlea, the hair cells are referred to as **organs of Corti**.

■ **Figure 13.15** Close-up view of the ossicles within the middle ear. These three bones extend from the tympanic membrane to the oval window.

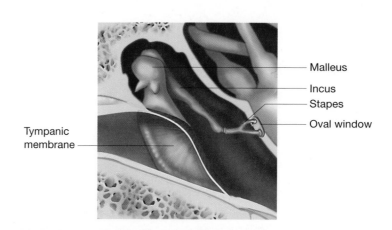

Tympanic membrane

Malleus
Incus
Stapes
Oval window

How We Hear

conductive hearing loss (kon-DUK-tiv)   **sensorineural hearing loss**
(sen-soh-ree-NOO-ral)

Figure 13.16 ▪ outlines the path of sound through the outer ear and middle ear and into the cochlea of the inner ear. Sound waves traveling down the external auditory canal strike the eardrum, causing it to vibrate. The ossicles conduct these vibrations across the middle ear from the eardrum to the oval window. Oval window movements initiate vibrations in the fluid that fills the cochlea. As the fluid vibrations strike a hair cell, they bend the small hairs and stimulate the nerve ending. The nerve ending then sends an electrical impulse to the brain on the cochlear portion of the vestibulocochlear nerve.

Hearing loss can be divided into two main categories: **conductive hearing loss** and **sensorineural hearing loss.** Conductive refers to disease or malformation of the outer or middle ear. All sound is weaker and muffled in conductive hearing loss since it is not conducted correctly to the inner ear. Sensorineural hearing loss is the result of damage or malformation of the inner ear (cochlea) or the cochlear nerve. In this hearing loss, some sounds are distorted and heard incorrectly. There can also be a combination of both conductive and sensorineural hearing loss.

Med Term Tip

Hearing impairment is becoming a greater problem for the general population for several reasons. First, people are living longer. Hearing loss can accompany old age, and there are a greater number of people over 50 years of age requiring hearing assistance. In addition, sound technology has produced music quality that was never available before. However, listening to loud music either naturally or through earphones can cause gradual damage to the hearing mechanism.

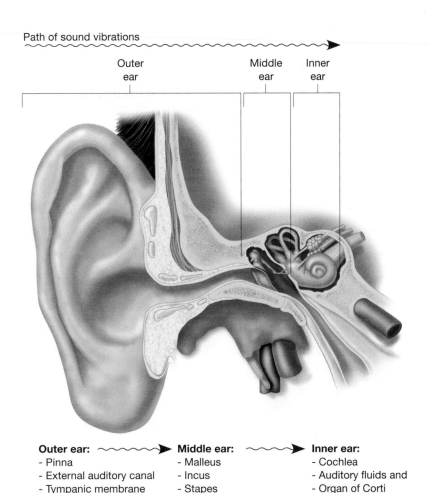

Path of sound vibrations

Outer ear   Middle ear   Inner ear

Outer ear:
- Pinna
- External auditory canal
- Tympanic membrane

Middle ear:
- Malleus
- Incus
- Stapes
- Oval window

Inner ear:
- Cochlea
- Auditory fluids and
- Organ of Corti
- Auditory nerve fibers
- Cerebral cortex

▪ **Figure 13.16** The path of sound waves through the outer, middle, and inner ear.

Word Building

The following list contains examples of medical terms built directly from word parts. The definitions of these terms can be determined by a straightforward translation of the word parts.

COMBINING FORM	COMBINED WITH	MEDICAL TERM	DEFINITION
acous/o	-tic	**acoustic** (ah-KOOS-tik)	pertaining to hearing
audi/o	-gram	**audiogram** (AW-dee-oh-gram)	record of hearing
	-meter	**audiometer** (aw-dee-OM-eh-ter)	instrument to measure hearing
	-ologist	**audiologist** (aw-dee-OL-oh-jist)	hearing specialist
audit/o	-ory	**auditory** (AW-dih-tor-ee)	pertaining to hearing
aur/o	-al	**aural** (AW-ral)	pertaining to the ear

> **Med Term Tip**
> Word watch—Be careful when using two terms that sound the same — *aural* meaning "pertaining to the ear" and *oral* meaning "pertaining to the mouth."

auricul/o	-ar	**auricular** (aw-RIK-cu-lar)	pertaining to the ear
cochle/o	-ar	**cochlear** (KOK-lee-ar)	pertaining to the cochlea
labyrinth/o	-ectomy	**labyrinthectomy** (lab-ih-rin-THEK-toh-mee)	removal of the labyrinth
	-otomy	**labyrinthotomy** (lab-ih-rinth-OT-oh-mee)	incision into the labyrinth
myring/o	-itis	**myringitis** (mir-ing-JYE-tis)	eardrum inflammation
	-ectomy	**myringectomy** (mir-in-GEK-toh-mee)	removal of the eardrum
	-plasty	**myringoplasty** (mir-IN-goh-plass-tee)	surgical repair of eardrum
ot/o	-algia	**otalgia** (oh-TAL-jee-ah)	ear pain
	-ic	**otic** (OH-tik)	pertaining to the ear
	-itis	**otitis** (oh-TYE-tis)	ear inflammation
	myc/o -osis	**otomycosis** (oh-toh-my-KOH-sis)	abnormal condition of ear fungus
	-ologist	**otologist** (oh-TOL-oh-jist)	ear specialist
	py/o -rrhea	**otopyorrhea** (oh-toh-pye-oh-REE-ah)	pus discharge from ear
	-rrhagia	**otorrhagia** (oh-toh-RAH-jee-ah)	bleeding from the ear
	-scope	**otoscope** (OH-toh-scope)	instrument to view inside the ear
	-plasty	**otoplasty** (OH-toh-plas-tee)	surgical repair of the (external) ear
salping/o	-itis	**salpingitis** (sal-pin-JIH-tis)	eustachian tube inflammation

> **Med Term Tip**
> Word watch—Be careful using the combining form *salping/o*, which can mean either "Eustachian tube" or "fallopian tube."

	-otomy	**salpingotomy** (sal-pin-GOT-oh-mee)	incision into eustachian tube
tympan/o	-ic	**tympanic** (tim-PAN-ik)	pertaining to the eardrum
	-itis	**tympanitis** (tim-pan-EYE-tis)	eardrum inflammation
	-meter	**tympanometer** (tim-pah-NOM-eh-ter)	instrument to measure eardrum
	-plasty	**tympanoplasty** (tim-pan-oh-PLASS-tee)	surgical repair of eardrum

Word Building *(continued)*

COMBINING FORM	COMBINED WITH	MEDICAL TERM	DEFINITION
	-rrhexis	**tympanorrhexis** (tim-pan-oh-REK-sis)	eardrum rupture
	-otomy	**tympanotomy** (tim-pan-OT-oh-mee)	incision into the eardrum
	-ectomy	**tympanectomy** (tim-pan-EK-toh-mee)	removal of the eardrum

SUFFIX	COMBINED WITH	MEDICAL TERM	DEFINITION
-otia	micro-	**microtia** (my-KROH-she-ah)	(abnormally) small ears
	macro-	**macrotia** (mah-KROH-she-ah)	(abnormally) large ears

Vocabulary

TERM	DEFINITION
American Sign Language (ASL)	Nonverbal method of communicating in which the hands and fingers are used to indicate words and concepts. Used by both persons who are deaf and persons with speech impairments.

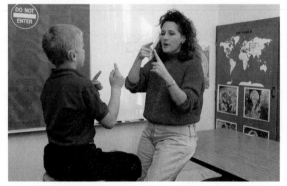

■ **Figure 13.17** Photograph of a teacher and student communicating using American Sign Language. *(Trevon Baker/Baker Consulting and Design)*

TERM	DEFINITION
binaural (bin-AW-rall)	Referring to both ears.
decibel (dB) (DES-ih-bel)	Measures the intensity or loudness of a sound. Zero decibels is the quietest sound measured and 120 dB is the loudest sound commonly measured.
hertz (Hz)	Measurement of the frequency or pitch of sound. The lowest pitch on an audiogram is 250 Hz. The measurement can go as high as 8000 Hz, which is the highest pitch measured.
monaural (mon-AW-rall)	Referring to one ear.
otorhinolaryngology (ENT) (oh-toh-rye-rye-noh-lair-in-GOL-oh-jee)	Branch of medicine involving the diagnosis and treatment of conditions and diseases of the ear, nose, and throat. Also referred to as *ENT*. Physician is an *otorhinolaryngologist*.
presbycusis (pres-bih-KOO-sis)	Normal loss of hearing that can accompany the aging process.
residual hearing (rih-ZID-yoo-al)	Amount of hearing that is still present after damage has occurred to the auditory mechanism.
tinnitus (tin-EYE-tus)	Ringing in the ears.
vertigo (VER-tih-goh)	Dizziness.

Pathology

TERM	DEFINITION
■ *Hearing Loss*	
anacusis (an-ah-KOO-sis)	Total absence of hearing; inability to perceive sound. Also called *deafness.*
deafness	Inability to hear or having some degree of hearing impairment.
■ *External Ear*	
ceruminoma (seh-roo-men-oh-ma)	Excessive accumulation of ear wax resulting in a hard wax plug. Sound becomes muffled.
otitis externa (OE) (oh-TYE-tis ex-TERN-ah)	External ear infection. Most commonly caused by fungus. Also called *otomycosis* and commonly referred to as *swimmer's ear.*
■ *Middle Ear*	
otitis media (OM) (oh-TYE-tis MEE-dee-ah)	Seen frequently in children; commonly referred to as a *middle ear infection.* Often preceded by an upper respiratory infection during which pathogens move from the pharynx to the middle ear via the eustachian tube. Fluid accumulates in the middle ear cavity. The fluid may be watery, *serous otitis media,* or full of pus, *purulent otitis media.*
otosclerosis (oh-toh-sklair-OH-sis)	Loss of mobility of the stapes bone, leading to progressive hearing loss.
■ *Inner Ear*	
acoustic neuroma (ah-KOOS-tik noor-OH-mah)	Benign tumor of the eighth cranial nerve sheath. The pressure causes symptoms such as tinnitus, headache, dizziness, and progressive hearing loss.
labyrinthitis (lab-ih-rin-THIGH-tis)	May affect both the hearing and equilibrium portions of the inner ear. Also referred to as an *inner ear infection.*
Ménière's disease (may-nee-ARZ dih-ZEEZ)	Abnormal condition within the labyrinth of the inner ear that can lead to a progressive loss of hearing. The symptoms are dizziness or vertigo, hearing loss, and tinnitus (ringing in the ears). Named for French physician Prosper Ménière.

Diagnostic Procedures

TERM	DEFINITION
■ *Audiology Tests*	
audiometry (aw-dee-OM-eh-tree)	Test of hearing ability by determining the lowest and highest intensity (decibels) and frequencies (hertz) that a person can distinguish. The patient may sit in a soundproof booth and receive sounds through earphones as the technician decreases the sound or lowers the tones.

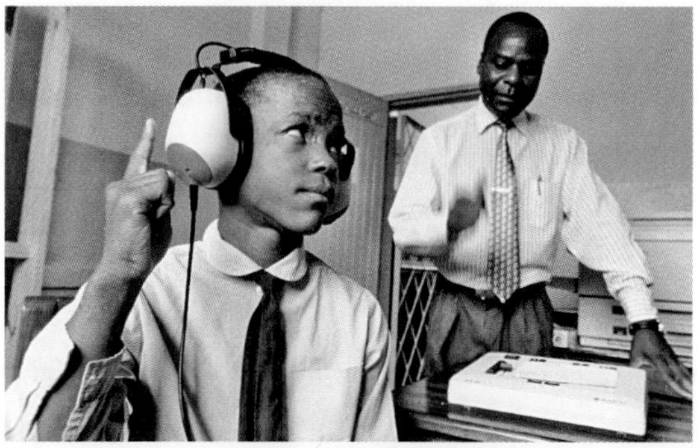

■ Figure 13.18 Audiometry exam. Photograph of a young person holding up his hand to indicate in which ear he is able to hear the sound. *(Jorgen Shytte/Peter Arnold, Inc.)*

Diagnostic Procedures (*continued*)

TERM	DEFINITION
Rinne and Weber tuning-fork tests (RIN-eh)	These tests assess both nerve and bone conduction of sound. The physician holds a tuning fork, an instrument that produces a constant pitch when it is struck, against or near the bones on the side of the head. Friedrich Rinne was a German otologist, and Ernst Weber was a German physiologist.

■ Otology Tests

otoscopy (oh-TOSS-koh-pee)	Examination of the ear canal, eardrum, and outer ear using an *otoscope*.

> **Med Term Tip**
>
> Small children are prone to placing objects in their ears. In some cases, as with peas and beans, these become moist in the ear canal and swell, which makes removal difficult. *Otoscopy*, or the examination of the ear using an *otoscope*, can aid in identifying and removing the cause of hearing loss if it is due to foreign bodies (see Figure 13.14).

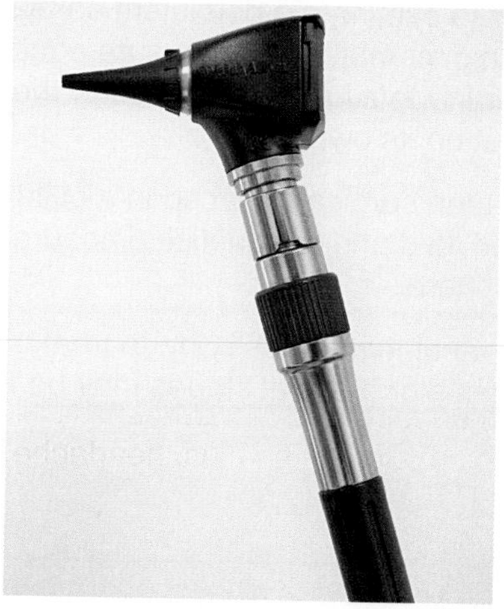

■ **Figure 13.19** An otoscope, used to visually examine the external auditory ear canal and tympanic membrane.

tympanometry (tim-pah-NOM-eh-tree)	Measurement of the movement of the tympanic membrane. Can indicate the presence of pressure in the middle ear.

■ Balance Tests

falling test	Test used to observe balance and equilibrium. The patient is observed balancing on one foot, then with one foot in front of the other, and then walking forward with eyes open. The same test is conducted with the patient's eyes closed. Swaying and falling with the eyes closed can indicate an ear and equilibrium malfunction.

Therapeutic Procedures

TERM	DEFINITION

■ Audiology Procedures

hearing aid	Apparatus or mechanical device used by persons with impaired hearing to amplify sound. Also called an *amplification device*.

■ Surgical Procedures

cochlear implant (KOK-lee-ar)	Mechanical device surgically placed under the skin behind the outer ear (pinna) that converts sound signals into magnetic impulses to stimulate the auditory nerve (see Figure 13.20 ■). Can be beneficial for those with profound sensorineural hearing loss.

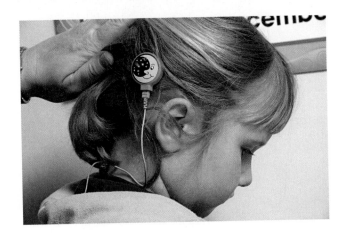

Figure 13.20 Photograph of a child with a cochlear implant. This device sends electrical impulses directly to the brain.

Therapeutic Procedures *(continued)*

TERM	DEFINITION
myringotomy (mir-in-GOT-oh-mee)	Surgical puncture of the eardrum with removal of fluid and pus from the middle ear to eliminate a persistent ear infection and excessive pressure on the tympanic membrane. A pressure equalizing tube is placed in the tympanic membrane to allow for drainage of the middle ear cavity; this tube typically falls out on its own.
pressure equalizing tube (pressure equalizing tube)	Small tube surgically placed in a child's eardrum to assist in drainage of trapped fluid and to equalize pressure between the middle ear cavity and the atmosphere.
stapedectomy (stay-pee-DEK-toh-mee)	Removal of the stapes bone to treat otosclerosis (hardening of the bone). A prosthesis or artificial stapes may be implanted.

Pharmacology

CLASSIFICATION	ACTION	GENERIC AND BRAND NAMES
antibiotic otic solution (OH-tik)	Eardrops to treat otitis externa.	Neomycin, polymyxin B, and hydrocortisone solution, Otocort, Cortisporin, Otic Care
antiemetics (an-tye-ee-mit-tiks)	Medications that are effective in treating the nausea associated with vertigo.	meclizine, Antivert, Meni-D; phenothiazine, Compazine
anti-inflammatory otic solution (OH-tik)	Reduces inflammation, itching, and edema associated with otitis externa.	antipyrine & benzoaine, Allergan Ear Drops, A/B Otic
wax emulsifiers	Substances used to soften ear wax to prevent buildup within the external ear canal.	carbamide peroxide, Debrox Drops, Murine Ear Drops

Abbreviations

AD	right ear	**HEENT**	head, ears, eyes, nose, throat
AS	left ear	**Hz**	hertz
ASL	American Sign Language	**OM**	otitis media
AU	both ears	**Oto**	otology
BC	bone conduction	**PE tube**	pressure tube equalizing
dB	decibel	**PORP**	partial ossicular replacement prosthesis
EENT	eyes, ears, nose, throat	**SOM**	serous otitis media
ENT	ear, nose, and throat	**TORP**	total ossicular replacement prosthesis

Chapter Review

Terminology Checklist

 Below are all Anatomy and Physiology key terms, Word Building. Vocabulary, Pathology, Diagnostic, Therapeutic, and Pharmacology terms presented in this chapter. Use this list as a study tool by placing a check in the box in front of each term as you master its meaning.

- ☐ achromatopsia
- ☐ acoustic
- ☐ acoustic neuroma
- ☐ amblyopia
- ☐ American Sign Language
- ☐ anacusis
- ☐ anesthetic ophthalmic solution
- ☐ antibiotic ophthalmic solution
- ☐ antibiotic otic solution
- ☐ antiemetic
- ☐ antiglaucoma medications
- ☐ anti-inflammatory otic solution
- ☐ aqueous humor
- ☐ artificial tears
- ☐ astigmatism
- ☐ audiogram
- ☐ audiologist
- ☐ audiology
- ☐ audiometer
- ☐ audiometry
- ☐ auditory
- ☐ auditory canal
- ☐ auditory tube
- ☐ aural
- ☐ auricle
- ☐ auricular
- ☐ binaural
- ☐ blepharectomy
- ☐ blepharitis
- ☐ blepharoplasty
- ☐ blepharoptosis
- ☐ cataract
- ☐ cerumen
- ☐ ceruminoma
- ☐ choroid
- ☐ cilia
- ☐ ciliary body
- ☐ cochlea
- ☐ cochlear
- ☐ cochlear implant

- ☐ cochlear nerve
- ☐ color vision tests
- ☐ conductive hearing loss
- ☐ cones
- ☐ conjunctiva
- ☐ conjunctival
- ☐ conjunctivitis
- ☐ conjunctivoplasty
- ☐ cornea
- ☐ corneal
- ☐ corneal abrasion
- ☐ cryoextraction
- ☐ cryoretinopexy
- ☐ cycloplegia
- ☐ dacryocystitis
- ☐ deafness
- ☐ decibel
- ☐ diplopia
- ☐ emmetropia
- ☐ enucleation
- ☐ equilibrium
- ☐ esotropia
- ☐ eustachian tube
- ☐ exotropia
- ☐ external auditory meatus
- ☐ external ear
- ☐ eyeball
- ☐ eyelashes
- ☐ eyelids
- ☐ eye muscles
- ☐ falling test
- ☐ fluorescein angiography
- ☐ fluorescein staining
- ☐ fovea centralis
- ☐ glaucoma
- ☐ hearing
- ☐ hearing aid
- ☐ hemianopia
- ☐ hertz
- ☐ hordeolum

- ☐ hyperopia
- ☐ incus
- ☐ inner ear
- ☐ intraocular
- ☐ iridal
- ☐ iridectomy
- ☐ iridoplegia
- ☐ iridosclerotomy
- ☐ iris
- ☐ iritis
- ☐ keratitis
- ☐ keratometer
- ☐ keratometry
- ☐ keratoplasty
- ☐ keratotomy
- ☐ labyrinth
- ☐ labyrinthectomy
- ☐ labyrinthitis
- ☐ labyrinthotomy
- ☐ lacrimal
- ☐ lacrimal apparatus
- ☐ lacrimal ducts
- ☐ lacrimal gland
- ☐ laser-assisted in-situ keratomileusis
- ☐ laser photocoagulation
- ☐ legally blind
- ☐ lens
- ☐ macrotia
- ☐ macula lutea
- ☐ macular degeneration
- ☐ malleus
- ☐ Ménière's disease
- ☐ microtia
- ☐ middle ear
- ☐ miotic
- ☐ monaural
- ☐ monochromatism
- ☐ mucous membrane

- mydriatic
- myopia
- myringectomy
- myringitis
- myringoplasty
- myringotomy
- nasal cavity
- nasolacrimal duct
- nyctalopia
- nystagmus
- oblique muscles
- ocular
- oculomycosis
- ophthalmalgia
- ophthalmic
- ophthalmic decongestants
- ophthalmologist
- ophthalmology
- ophthalmoplegia
- ophthalmorrhagia
- ophthalmoscope
- ophthalmoscopy
- optic
- optic disk
- optician
- optic nerve
- optometer
- optometrist
- optometry
- organs of Corti
- ossicles
- otalgia
- otic
- otitis
- otitis externa
- otitis media
- otologist
- otology

- otomycosis
- otoplasty
- otopyorrhea
- otorhinolaryngology
- otorrhagia
- otosclerosis
- otoscope
- otoscopy
- oval window
- papilledema
- phacoemulsification
- photophobia
- photorefractive keratectomy
- pinna
- pressure equalizing tube
- presbycusis
- presbyopia
- pterygium
- pupil
- pupillary
- radial keratotomy
- rectus muscles
- refractive error test
- refracts
- residual hearing
- retina
- retinal
- retinal blood vessels
- retinal detachment
- retinitis pigmentosa
- retinoblastoma
- retinopathy
- retinopexy
- Rinne and Weber tuning-fork tests
- rods
- saccule
- salpingitis

- salpingotomy
- sclera
- scleral
- scleral buckling
- scleritis
- scleromalacia
- sclerotomy
- sebaceous glands
- semicircular canals
- sensorineural hearing loss
- slit lamp microscopy
- Snellen chart
- stapedectomy
- stapes
- strabismus
- strabotomy
- tears
- tinnitus
- tonometry
- trachoma
- tympanectomy
- tympanic
- tympanic membrane
- tympanitis
- tympanometer
- tympanometry
- tympanoplasty
- tympanorrhexis
- tympanotomy
- utricle
- uveitis
- vertigo
- vestibular nerve
- vestibulocochlear nerve
- visual acuity test
- vitreous humor
- wax emulsifiers
- xerophthalmia

Practice Exercises

A. Complete the following statements.

1. The study of the eye is _____.

2. Another term for eyelashes is _____.

3. The glands responsible for tears are called _____ glands.

4. The clear, transparent portion of the sclera is called the _____.

5. The innermost layer of the eye, which is composed of sensory receptors, is the _____.

6. The pupil of the eye is actually a hole in the _____.

7. The three bones in the middle ear are the _____, _____, and _____.

8. The study of the ear is called _____.

9. Another term for the eardrum is _____.

10. _____ is produced in the oil glands in the auditory canal.

11. The _____ tube connects the nasopharynx with the middle ear.

12. The _____ is responsible for conducting impulses from the ear to the brain.

B. State the terms described using the combining forms provided.

The combining form *blephar/o* refers to the eyelid. Use it to write a term that means:

1. inflammation of the eyelid _____

2. surgical repair of the eyelid _____

3. drooping of the upper eyelid _____

The combining form *retin/o* refers to the retina. Use it to write a term that means:

4. a disease of the retina _____

5. surgical fixation of the retina _____

The combining form *ophthalm/o* refers to the eye. Use it to write a term that means:

6. the study of the eye _____

7. pertaining to the eye _____

8. an eye examination using a scope _____

The combining form *irid/o* refers to the iris. Use it to write a term that means:

9. iris paralysis _____

10. removal of the iris _____

The combining form *ot/o* refers to the ear. Write a word that means:

11. ear surgical repair _____

12. pus flow from the ear _____

13. pain in the ear _____

14. inflammation of the ear _____

The combining form *tympan/o* refers to eardrum. Write a word that means:

15. eardrum rupture _____

16. eardrum incision _____

17. eardrum inflammation _____

The combining form *audi/o* refers to hearing. Write a word that means:

18. record of hearing _____

19. instrument to measure hearing _____

20. study of hearing _____

C. Answer the following questions.

1. Describe the difference between conductive hearing loss and sensorineural hearing loss. _____

_____

_____

2. List in order the eyeball structures light rays pass through: _____, _____,

_____, _____

3. Describe the role of the conjunctiva. _____

_____

_____

4. List the ossicles and what they do. _____

_____

_____

D. Write the suffix for each expression and provide an example of its use from this chapter.

	Suffix	Example
1. to turn	_____	_____
2. vision	_____	_____
3. inflammation of	_____	_____
4. the study of	_____	_____
5. incision into	_____	_____

6. surgical repair   _____   _____

7. surgical fixation   _____   _____

8. pain   _____   _____

9. ear condition   _____   _____

10. hearing   _____   _____

E. Define the following combining forms and use them in words from this chapter.

	Meaning	Example
1. dacry/o		
2. uve/o		
3. aque/o		
4. phot/o		
5. kerat/o		
6. vitre/o		
7. dipl/o		
8. glauc/o		
9. presby/o		
10. ambly/o		
11. aur/o		
12. staped/o		
13. acous/o		
14. salping/o		
15. myring/o		

F. Define the following terms.

1. amblyopia _____

2. diplopia _____

3. mydriatic _____

4. miotic _____

5. presbyopia _____

6. tinnitus _____

7. stapes _____

8. tympanometry _____

9. eustachian tube _____

10. labyrinth _____

11. audiogram _____

12. otitis media _____

G. Match each term to its definition.

1.	_____ emmetropia	a.	opacity of the lens
2.	_____ sclera	b.	muscle regulating size of pupil
3.	_____ cataract	c.	nearsightedness
4.	_____ conjunctiva	d.	protective membrane of eye
5.	_____ iris	e.	blind spot
6.	_____ xerophthalmia	f.	involuntary movements of eye
7.	_____ myopia	g.	white of eye
8.	_____ nystagmus	h.	normal vision
9.	_____ optic disk	i.	dry eyes
10.	_____ vitreous humor	j.	material filling eyeball

H. Match each term to its definition.

1.	_____ myringotomy	a.	removal of stapes bone
2.	_____ tympanoplasty	b.	reconstruction of eardrum
3.	_____ otoplasty	c.	surgical puncture of eardrum
4.	_____ stapedectomy	d.	change size of pinna
5.	_____ anacusis	e.	absence of hearing
6.	_____ falling test	f.	treats sensorineural hearing loss
7.	_____ PE tube	g.	tuning fork tests
8.	_____ cochlear implant	h.	swimmer's ear
9.	_____ otitis externa	i.	drains off fluid
10.	_____ Rinne & Weber	j.	balance test

I. Identify the following abbreviations.

1. Oto _____

2. OU _____

3. REM _____

4. Hz _____

5. SMD _____

6. PERRLA _____

7. IOP _____

8. dB _____

9. OD _____

10. VF _____

J. Write the abbreviation for the following terms.

1. pressure equalizing tube _____

2. eye, ear, nose, and throat _____

3. bone conduction _____

4. both ears _____

5. otitis media _____

6. emmetropia _____

7. exotropia _____

8. left eye _____

9. extraocular movement _____

10. visual acuity _____

K. Use the following terms in the sentences below.

emmetropia   hyperopia   acoustic neuroma   otorhinolaryngologist

conjunctivitis   tonometry   cataract   strabismus

presbycusis   inner ear   Ménière's disease   hordeolum

myopia

1. Cheri is having a regular eye checkup. The pressure reading test that the physician will do to detect glaucoma is _____.

2. Carlos's ophthalmologist tells him that he has normal vision. This is called _____.

3. Ana has been given an antibiotic eye ointment for pink eye. The medical term for this condition is _____.

4. Adrian is nearsighted and cannot read signs in the distance. This is called _____.

5. Ivan is scheduled to have surgery to have the opaque lens of his right eye removed. This condition is a(n) _____.

6. Roberto has developed a stye on the corner of his left eye. He has been told to treat it with hot compresses. This condition is called a(n) _____.

7. Judith has twin boys with crossed eyes that will require surgical correction. The medical term for this condition is _____.

8. Beth is farsighted and has difficulty reading textbooks. Her eyeglass correction will be for _____.

9. Grace was told by her physician that her hearing loss was a part of the aging process. The term for this is _____.

10. Stacey is having frequent middle ear infections and wishes to be treated by a specialist. She would go to a(n) _____.

11. Warren was told that his dizziness may be caused by a problem in the _____ area.

12. Shantel is suffering from an abnormal condition of the inner ear, vertigo, and tinnitus. She may have _____.

13. Keisha was told that her tumor of the eighth cranial nerve was benign, but she still experienced a hearing loss as a result of the tumor. This tumor is called a(n) _____.

L. Fill in the classification for each drug description, then match the brand name.

Drug Description	Classification	Brand Name
1. _____ treats dry eyes	_____	a. Atropine-Care
2. _____ reduces intraocular pressure	_____	b. Allergan Ear Drops
3. _____ ear drops for ear infection	_____	c. Timoptic
4. _____ dilates pupil	_____	d. Opticaine
5. _____ treats nausea from vertigo	_____	e. Debrox Drops
6. _____ eye drops for bacterial infection	_____	f. Eserine Sulfate
7. _____ treats ear itching	_____	g. Antivert
8. _____ constricts pupil	_____	h. Refresh Plus
9. _____ softens cerumen	_____	i. Otocort
10. _____ eye drops for pain	_____	j. Del-Mycin

Medical Record Analysis

Below is an item from a patient's medical record. Read it carefully, make sure you understand all the medical terms used, and then answer the questions that follow.

Ophthalmology Consultation Report

Reason for Consultation:	Evaluation of progressive loss of vision in right eye.
History of Present Illness:	Patient is a 79-year-old female who has noted gradual deterioration of vision and increasing photophobia during the past year, particularly in the right eye. She states that it feels like there is a film over her right eye. She denies any change in vision in her left eye.
Past Medical History:	Patient has used corrective lenses her entire adult life to correct hyperopia. She is not married and is nulligravida. Past medical history includes left breast cancer successfully treated with left breast mastectomy ten years ago and cholelithiasis necessitating a cholecystectomy two years ago. She has no history of cardiac problems or hypertension.
Results of Physical Examination:	Visual acuity test showed no change in this patient's long-standing hyperopia. The eye muscles function properly, and there is no evidence of conjunctivitis or nystagmus. The pupils react properly to light. Intraocular pressure is normal. Ophthalmoscopy after application of mydriatic drops revealed presence of large opaque cataract in lens of right eye. There is a very small cataract forming in the left eye. There is no evidence of retinopathy, macular degeneration, or keratitis.
Assessment:	Diminished vision in OD secondary to cataract.
Recommendations:	Phacoemulsification of cataract followed by aspiration of lens and prosthetic lens implant.

Critical Thinking Questions

1. The results of the physical exam state that the patient's pupils react properly to light. What does this mean? How do pupils react in bright and dim light? Why is this important? _____
_____
_____

2. Carefully read the results of the physical examination and list the eye structures that do not have any problems. _____
_____

3. Briefly describe the pathologies that form the patient's past medical history that required surgery, and the surgeries. _____
_____

4. The ophthalmologist placed mydriatic drops in her eyes. For what purpose? What is the general name for drops with the opposite effect? _____
_____

5. This patient wears corrective lenses for which condition?
   a. farsightedness
   b. nearsightedness
   c. abnormal curvature of the cornea

6. Her cataract was removed by phacoemulsification. Using your text as a reference, what other procedure could have been used to remove a cataract? _____
_____

Chart Note Transcription

The chart note below contains ten phrases that can be reworded with a medical term that you learned in this chapter. Each phrase is identified with an underline. Determine the medical term and write your answers in the space provided.

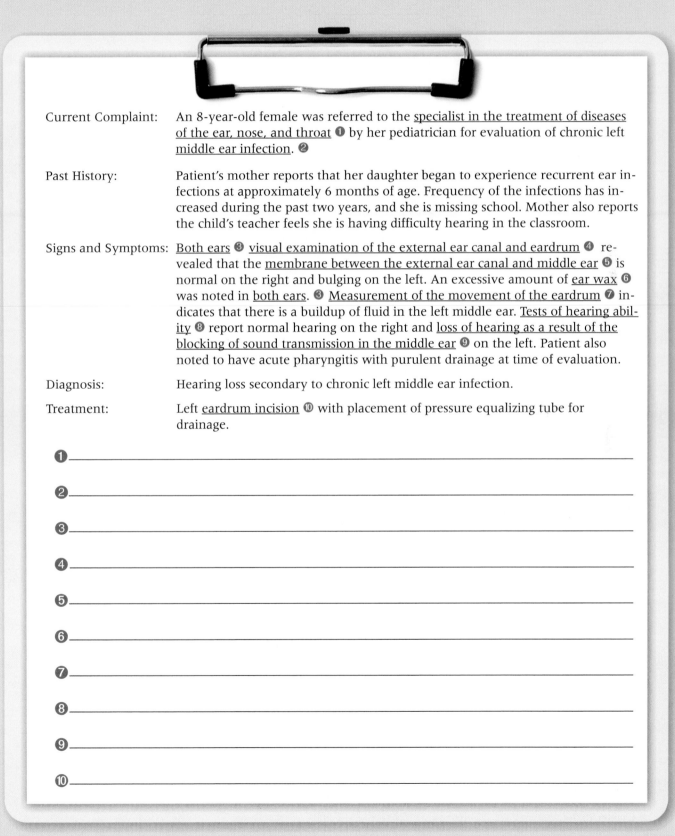

Current Complaint:	An 8-year-old female was referred to the <u>specialist in the treatment of diseases of the ear, nose, and throat</u> ❶ by her pediatrician for evaluation of chronic left <u>middle ear infection</u>. ❷
Past History:	Patient's mother reports that her daughter began to experience recurrent ear infections at approximately 6 months of age. Frequency of the infections has increased during the past two years, and she is missing school. Mother also reports the child's teacher feels she is having difficulty hearing in the classroom.
Signs and Symptoms:	<u>Both ears</u> ❸ <u>visual examination of the external ear canal and eardrum</u> ❹ revealed that the <u>membrane between the external ear canal and middle ear</u> ❺ is normal on the right and bulging on the left. An excessive amount of <u>ear wax</u> ❻ was noted in <u>both ears</u>. ❸ <u>Measurement of the movement of the eardrum</u> ❼ indicates that there is a buildup of fluid in the left middle ear. <u>Tests of hearing ability</u> ❽ report normal hearing on the right and <u>loss of hearing as a result of the blocking of sound transmission in the middle ear</u> ❾ on the left. Patient also noted to have acute pharyngitis with purulent drainage at time of evaluation.
Diagnosis:	Hearing loss secondary to chronic left middle ear infection.
Treatment:	Left <u>eardrum incision</u> ❿ with placement of pressure equalizing tube for drainage.

❶ _____

❷ _____

❸ _____

❹ _____

❺ _____

❻ _____

❼ _____

❽ _____

❾ _____

❿ _____

Labeling Exercise

A. System Review

1. Write the labels for this figure on the numbered lines provided.

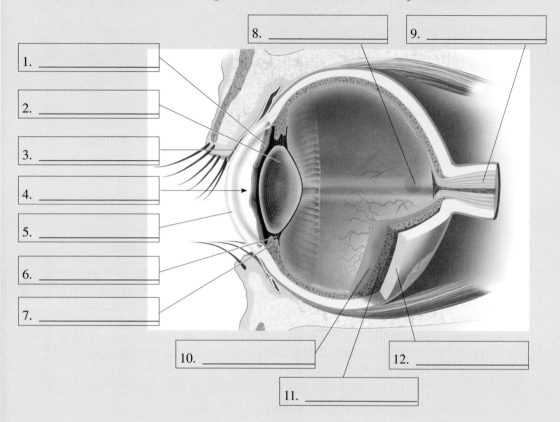

8. _____

9. _____

1. _____

2. _____

3. _____

4. _____

5. _____

6. _____

7. _____

10. _____

12. _____

11. _____

2. Write the labels for this figure on the numbered lines provided.

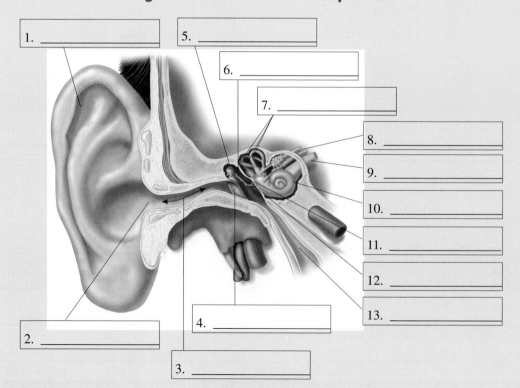

1. _____

5. _____

6. _____

7. _____

8. _____

9. _____

10. _____

11. _____

12. _____

13. _____

2. _____

4. _____

3. _____

B. Anatomy Challenge
Write the labels for this figure on the numbered lines provided.

1. _____

2. _____

3. _____

4. _____

5. _____

Multimedia Preview

Additional interactive resources and activities for this chapter can be found on the Companion Website. For videos, games, and pronunciations, please access the accompanying DVD-ROM that comes with this book.

DVD-ROM Highlights

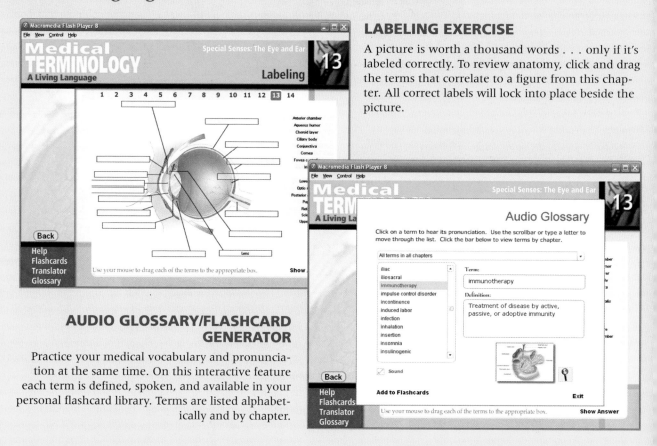

LABELING EXERCISE

A picture is worth a thousand words . . . only if it's labeled correctly. To review anatomy, click and drag the terms that correlate to a figure from this chapter. All correct labels will lock into place beside the picture.

AUDIO GLOSSARY/FLASHCARD GENERATOR

Practice your medical vocabulary and pronunciation at the same time. On this interactive feature each term is defined, spoken, and available in your personal flashcard library. Terms are listed alphabetically and by chapter.

Website Highlights—www.prenhall.com/fremgen

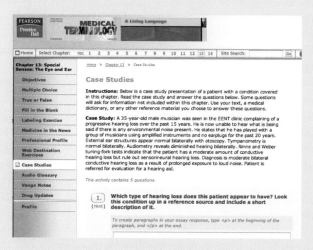

CASE STUDY

Put your understanding of medical terms to the test within a real-world scenario. Here you'll be presented with a clinical case followed by a series of questions that quiz your grasp of the situation.

14

Special Topics

Learning Objectives

Upon completion of this chapter, you will be able to:

- Identify and define the combining forms and suffixes introduced in this chapter.
- Correctly spell and pronounce medical terms relating to the medical fields introduced in this chapter.
- Describe pertinent information relating to Pharmacology.
- Describe pertinent information relating to Mental Health.
- Describe pertinent information relating to Diagnostic Imaging.
- Describe pertinent information relating to Rehabilitation Services.
- Describe pertinent information relating to Surgery.
- Describe pertinent information relating to Oncology.
- Identify and define vocabulary terms relating to the topics.
- Identify and define selected pathology terms relating to the topics.
- Identify and define selected diagnostic procedures relating to the topics.
- Identify and define selected therapeutic procedures relating to the topics.
- Define selected abbreviations associated with the topics.

Introduction

There are many specialized areas within medicine, and each has medical terms relating to that field. This chapter presents medical terminology from six of these fields:

1. Pharmacology, p. 465
2. Mental Health, p. 473
3. Diagnostic Imaging, p. 478
4. Rehabilitation Services, p. 484
5. Surgery, p. 490
6. Oncology, p. 495

Section I: Pharmacology at a Glance

Combining Forms

aer/o	air
bucc/o	cheek
chem/o	drug
cutane/o	skin
derm/o	skin
lingu/o	tongue
muscul/o	muscle
or/o	mouth
pharmac/o	drug
rect/o	rectum
toxic/o	poison
vagin/o	vagina
ven/o	vein

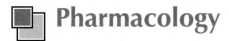 Pharmacology

pharmacology (far-ma-KALL-oh-jee)

Pharmacology is the study of the origin, characteristics, and effects of drugs. Drugs are obtained from many different sources. Some drugs, such as vitamins, are found naturally in the foods we eat. Others, such as hormones, are obtained from animals. Penicillin and some of the other antibiotics are developed from mold, which is a fungus. Plants have been the source of many of today's drugs. Many drugs, such as those used in chemotherapy, are synthetic, meaning they are developed by artificial means in a laboratory.

Drug Names

brand name
chemical name
generic name
nonproprietary name
(non-prah-PRYE-ah-tair-ee)

pharmaceutical (far-mih-SOO-tih-kal)
pharmacist (FAR-mah-sist)
proprietary name (proh-PRYE-ah-tair-ee)
trademark

All drugs are chemicals. The **chemical name** describes the chemical formula or molecular structure of a particular drug. For example, the chemical name for ibuprofen, an over-the-counter pain medication, is 2-*p*-isobutylphenyl propionic acid. Just as in this case, chemical names are usually very long, so a shorter name is given to the drug. This name is the **generic** or **nonproprietary name**, and it is recognized and accepted as the official name for a drug.

Each drug has only one generic name, such as ibuprofen, and this name is not subject to copyright protection, so any **pharmaceutical** manufacturer may use it. However, the pharmaceutical company that originally developed the drug has exclusive rights to produce it for seventeen years. After that time, any manufacturer may produce and sell the drug. When a company manufactures a drug for sale, it must choose a **brand**, or **proprietary**, **name** for its product. This is the company's **trademark** for the drug. For example, ibuprofen is known by several brand names, including Motrin™, Advil™, and Nuprin™. All three contain the same ibuprofen; they are just marketed by different pharmaceutical companies. (See Table 14.1 ■ for examples of different drug names.)

Generic drugs are usually priced lower than brand name drugs. A physician can indicate on the prescription if the **pharmacist** may substitute a generic drug for a brand name. The physician may prefer that a particular brand name drug be used if he or she believes it to be more effective than the generic drug.

Legal Classification of Drugs

controlled substances
Drug Enforcement Agency
over-the-counter drug

prescription (prih-SKRIP-shun)
prescription drug (prih-SKRIP-shun)

A **prescription drug** can only be ordered by licensed healthcare practitioners such as physicians, dentists, or physician assistants. These drugs must include the words "Caution: Federal law prohibits dispensing without prescription" on their labels. Antibiotics, such as penicillin, and heart medications, such as digoxin, are available only by prescription. A **prescription** is the written explanation to the pharmacist regarding the name of the medication, the dosage, and the times of administration. A licensed practitioner can also give a prescription order orally to the pharmacist.

A drug that does not require a prescription is referred to as an **over-the-counter drug** (OTC) Many medications or drugs can be purchased without a prescription,

Table 14.1	Examples of Different Drug Names	
CHEMICAL NAME	**GENERIC NAME**	**BRAND NAMES**
2-*p*-isobutylphenyl propionic acid	Ibuprofen	Motrin™
		Advil™
		Nuprin™
Acetylsalicylic acid	Aspirin	Anacin™
		Bufferin™
		Excedrin™
S-2-[1-(methylamino) ethyl] benzenemethanol hydrochloride	Pseudoephedrine hydrochloride	Sudafed™
		Actifed™
		Nucofed™

for example, aspirin, antacids, and antidiarrheal medications. However, taking aspirin along with an anticoagulant, such as coumadin, can cause internal bleeding in some people, and OTC antacids interfere with the absorption of the prescription drug tetracycline into the body. It is better for the physician or pharmacist to advise the patient on the proper OTC drugs to use with prescription drugs.

Certain drugs are **controlled substances** if they have a potential for being addictive (habit forming) or can be abused. The **Drug Enforcement Agency** (DEA) enforces the control of these drugs. Some of the more commonly prescribed controlled substances are:

- butabarbital
- chloral hydrate
- codeine
- diazepam
- oxycontin
- morphine
- phenobarbital
- secobarbital

Controlled drugs are classified as Schedule I through Schedule V, indicating their potential for abuse. The differences between each schedule are listed in Table 14.2 ■.

Table 14.2	Schedule for Controlled Substances
CLASSIFICATION	**MEANING**
Schedule I	Drugs with the highest potential for addiction and abuse. They are not accepted for medical use. Examples are heroin and LSD.
Schedule II	Drugs with a high potential for addiction and abuse accepted for medical use in the United States. Examples are codeine, cocaine, morphine, opium, and secobarbital.
Schedule III	Drugs with a moderate to low potential for addiction and abuse. Examples are butabarbital, anabolic steroids, and acetaminophen with codeine.
Schedule IV	Drugs with a lower potential for addiction and abuse than Schedule III drugs. Examples are chloral hydrate, phenobarbital, and diazepam.
Schedule V	Drugs with a low potential for addiction and abuse. An example is low-strength codeine combined with other drugs to suppress coughing.

How to Read a Prescription

A prescription is not difficult to read once you understand the symbols that are used. Symbols and abbreviations based on Latin and Greek words are used to save time for the physician. For example, the abbreviation po, meaning to be taken by mouth, comes from the Latin term *per os,* which means by mouth.

See Figure 14.1 ■ for an example of a prescription. In this example, the prescribed medication (Rx) is Tagamet (a medication to reduce stomach acid) in the 800 milligram (mg) size. The instructions on the label are to say (Sig) to take 1 (ī) by mouth (po) every (q) bedtime (hs). The pharmacist is to dispense (disp) 30 tablets (#30). The prescription concludes by informing the pharmacist to refill the prescription two times, and he or she may substitute with another medication. Each prescription must contain the date, physician's name, address, and Drug Enforcement Agency number as well as the patient's name and date of birth. The physician must also sign his or her name at the bottom of the prescription. A blank prescription cannot be handed to a patient.

The physician's instruction to the patient will be placed on the label. The pharmacist will also include instructions about the medication and alert the patient to side effects that may need to be reported to the physician. In addition, any special instructions regarding the medication (i.e., take with meals, do not take along with dairy products) will also be supplied by the pharmacist.

Routes and Methods of Drug Administration

aerosol (AIR-oh-sol)

buccal (BUCK-al)

eardrops

eyedrops

inhalation (in-hah-LAY-shun)

oral (OR-al)

parenteral (par-EN-ter-al)

rectal (REK-tal)

sublingual (sub-LING-gwal)

suppositories (suh-POZ-ih-tor-ees)

topical (TOP-ih-kal)

transdermal (tranz-DER-mal)

vaginal (VAJ-in-al)

The method by which a drug is introduced into the body is referred to as the *route of administration.* To be effective, drugs must be administered by a particular route. In some cases, there may be a variety of routes by which a drug can be

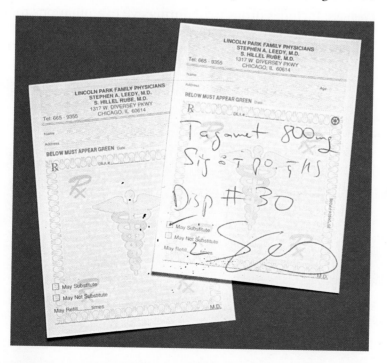

■ **Figure 14.1** A sample prescription written by a physician.

administered. For instance, the female hormone estrogen can be administered orally in pill form or by a patch applied to the skin. In general, the routes of administration are as follows:

Oral: Includes all drugs that are given by mouth. The advantages are ease of administration and a slow rate of absorption via the stomach and intestinal wall. The disadvantages include slowness of absorption and destruction of some chemical compounds by gastric juices. In addition, some medications, such as aspirin, can have a corrosive action on the stomach lining.

Sublingual: Includes drugs that are held under the tongue and not swallowed. The medication is absorbed by the blood vessels on the underside of the tongue as the saliva dissolves it. The rate of absorption is quicker than the oral route. Nitroglycerin to treat angina pectoris (chest pain) is administered by this route (see Figure 14.2 ■).

Inhalation: Includes drugs that are inhaled directly into the nose and mouth. **Aerosol** sprays are administered by this route (see Figure 14.3 ■).

Parenteral: Is an invasive method of administering drugs since it requires the skin to be punctured by a needle. The needle with syringe attached is introduced either under the skin or into a muscle, vein, or body cavity. See Table 14.3 ■ for a description of the methods for parenteral administration.

Transdermal: Includes medications that coat the underside of a patch, which is applied to the skin where it is then absorbed. Examples include birth control patches, nicotine patches, and sea sickness patches.

Rectal: Includes medications introduced directly into the rectal cavity in the form of **suppositories** or solution. Drugs may have to be administered by this route if the patient is unable to take them by mouth due to nausea, vomiting, or surgery.

Topical: Includes medications applied directly to the skin or mucous membranes. They are distributed in ointment, cream, or lotion form, and are used to treat skin infections and eruptions.

Vaginal: Includes tablets and suppositories that may be inserted vaginally to treat vaginal yeast infections and other irritations.

Eyedrops: Includes drops used during eye examinations to dilate the pupil of the eye for better examination of the interior of the eye. They are also placed into the eye to control eye pressure in glaucoma and treat infections.

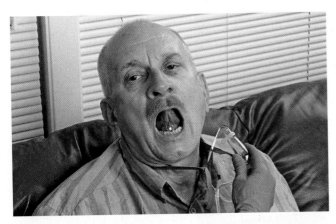

■ **Figure 14.2** Sublingual medication administration. Photograph of a male patient placing a nitroglycerine tablet under his tongue.

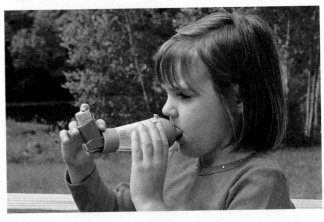

■ **Figure 14.3** Inhalation medication administration. Photograph of a young girl using a metered dose inhaler.

Table 14.3 Methods for Parenteral Administration of Drugs

METHOD	DESCRIPTION
intracavitary (in-trah-KAV-ih-tair-ee)	Injection into a body cavity such as the peritoneal and chest cavity.
intradermal (ID) (in-trah-DER-mal)	Very shallow injection just under the top layer of skin. Commonly used in skin testing for allergies and tuberculosis testing (see Figure 14.4 ■).
intramuscular (IM) (in-trah-MUSS-kyoo-lar)	Injection directly into the muscle of the buttocks, thigh, or upper arm. Used when there is a large amount of medication or it is irritating (see Figure 14.4).
intrathecal (in-trah-THEE-kal)	Injection into the meningeal space surrounding the brain and spinal cord.
intravenous (IV) (in-trah-VEE-nus)	Injection into the veins. This route may be set up to deliver medication very quickly or to deliver a continuous drip of medication (see Figure 14.4).
subcutaneous (SC) (sub-kyoo-TAY-nee-us)	Injection into the subcutaneous layer of the skin, usually the upper, outer arm or abdomen (see Figure 14.4); for example, insulin injection.

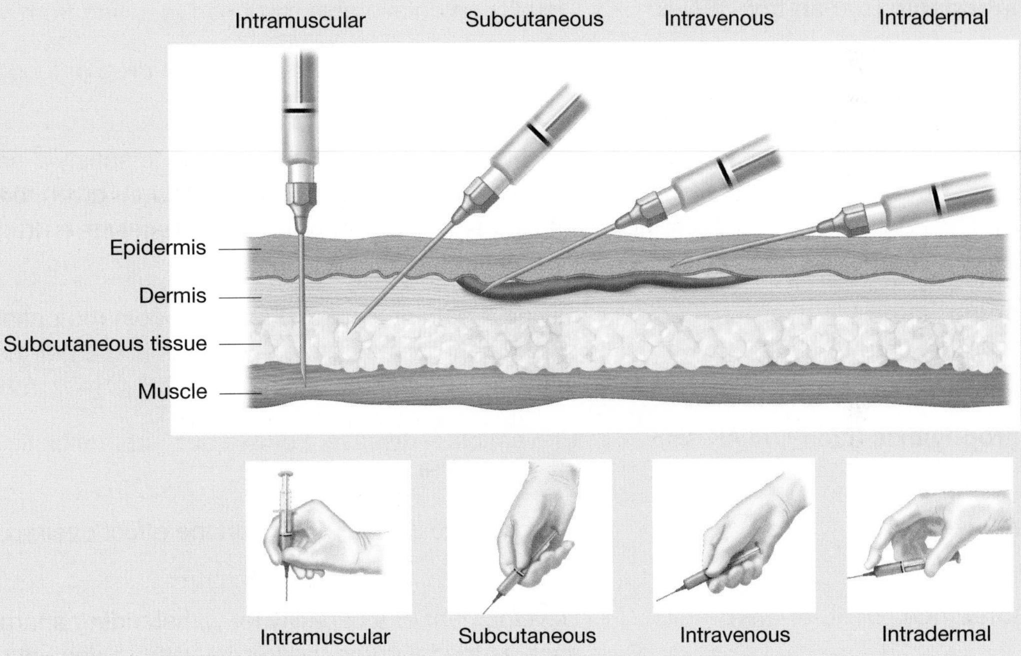

■ **Figure 14.4**
Parenteral medication administration. The angle of needle insertion for four different types of parenteral injections.

Intramuscular   Subcutaneous   Intravenous   Intradermal

Epidermis
Dermis
Subcutaneous tissue
Muscle

Intramuscular   Subcutaneous   Intravenous   Intradermal

Eardrops: Includes drops placed directly into the ear canal for the purpose of relieving pain or treating infection.

Buccal: Includes drugs that are placed under the lip or between the cheek and gum.

Vocabulary

TERM	DEFINITION
addiction (ah-DICK-shun)	Acquired dependence on a drug.
additive	Sum of the action of two (or more) drugs given. In this case, the total strength of the medications is equal to the sum of the strength of each individual drug.
antidote (AN-tih-doht)	Substance that will neutralize poisons or their side effects.

Vocabulary (continued)

TERM	DEFINITION
broad spectrum	Ability of a drug to be effective against a wide range of microorganisms.
contraindication (kon-trah-in-dih-KAY-shun)	Condition in which a particular drug should not be used.
cumulative action	Action that occurs in the body when a drug is allowed to accumulate or stay in the body.
drug interaction	Occurs when the effect of one drug is altered because it was taken at the same time as another drug.
drug tolerance	Decrease in susceptibility to a drug after continued use of the drug.
habituation (hah-bich-yoo-AY-shun)	Development of an emotional dependence on a drug due to repeated use.
iatrogenic (eye-ah-troh-JEN-ik)	Usually an unfavorable response resulting from taking a medication.
idiosyncrasy (id-ee-oh-SIN-krah-see)	Unusual or abnormal response to a drug or food.
placebo (plah-SEE-boh)	Inactive, harmless substance used to satisfy a patient's desire for medication. This is also used in research when given to a control group of patients in a study in which another group receives a drug. The effect of the placebo versus the drug is then observed.
potentiation (poe-ten-chee-A-shun)	Giving a patient a second drug to boost (potentiate) the effect of another drug. The total strength of the drugs is greater than the sum of the strength of the individual drugs.
prophylaxis (proh-fih-LAK-sis)	Prevention of disease. For example, an antibiotic can be used to prevent the occurrence of a disease.
side effect	Response to a drug other than the effect desired. Also called an *adverse reaction.*
tolerance (TAHL-er-ans)	Development of a capacity for withstanding a large amount of a substance, such as foods, drugs, or poison, without any adverse effect. A decreased sensitivity to further doses will develop.
toxicity (tok-SISS-ih-tee)	Extent or degree to which a substance is poisonous.
unit dose	Drug dosage system that provides prepackaged, prelabeled, individual medications that are ready for immediate use by the patient.

Abbreviations

@	at	**APAP**	acetaminophen (Tylenol™)
ā	before	**aq**	aqueous (water)
ac	before meals	**ASA**	aspirin
ad lib	as desired	**bid**	twice a day
ante	before	**c̄**	with

■ Abbreviations (continued)

cap(s)	capsule(s)	oz	ounce
cc	cubic centimeter	p̄	after
d	day	pc	after meals
d/c, DISC	discontinue	PCA	patient-controlled administration
DC, disc	discontinue	PDR	*Physician's Desk Reference*
DEA	Drug Enforcement Agency	per	with
dil	dilute	po	by mouth
disp	dispense	prn	as needed
dtd	give of such a dose	pt	patient
Dx	diagnosis	q	every
et	and	qam	every morning
FDA	Federal Drug Administration	qd	once a day/every day
gm	gram	qh	every hour
gr	grain	qhs	at bedtime
gt	drop	qid	four times a day
gtt	drops	qod	every other day
hs	at bedtime	qs	quantity sufficient
ī	one	Rx	take
ID	intradermal	s̄	without
īī	two	SC	subcutaneous
īīī	three	Sig	label as follows/directions
IM	intramuscular	sl	under the tongue
inj	injection	sol	solution
IU	international unit	s̄s̄	one-half
IV	intravenous	stat	at once/immediately
kg	kilogram	Subc, SubQ	subcutaneous
L	liter	suppos, supp	suppository
mcg	microgram	susp	suspension
mEq	milliequivalent	syr	syrup
mg	milligram	T, tbsp	tablespoon
mL	milliliter	t, tsp	teaspoon
noc	night	tab	tablet
no sub	no substitute	tid	three times a day
non rep	do not repeat	TO	telephone order
NPO	nothing by mouth	top	apply topically
NS	normal saline	u	unit
od	overdose	VO	verbal order
oint	ointment	wt	weight
OTC	over the counter	x	times

Med Term Tip

Many abbreviations have multiple meanings, such as od, which can mean overdose (od) or right eye (OD), depending on whether the letters are lower-case or uppercase. Care must be taken when reading abbreviations since some may be written too quickly, making them difficult to decipher. Never create your own abbreviations. Some of the most common abbreviations are listed above.

Combining Forms

anxi/o	anxiety
ment/o	mind
phren/o	mind
psych/o	mind
schiz/o	divided
somat/o	body
somn/o	sleep

Suffixes

-iatrist	physician
-mania	excessive preoccupation
-philia	affinity for, craving for
-phobia	irrational fear

Mental Health Disciplines

Psychology

abnormal psychology

clinical psychologist (sigh-KALL-oh-jist)

normal psychology

psychology (sigh-KALL-oh-jee)

Psychology is the study of human behavior and thought process. This behavioral science is primarily concerned with understanding how human beings interact with their physical environment and with each other. Behavior can be divided into two categories, normal and abnormal. The study of **normal psychology** includes how the personality develops, how people handle stress, and the stages of mental development. In contrast, **abnormal psychology** studies and treats behaviors that are outside of normal and that are detrimental to the person or society. These maladaptive behaviors range from occasional difficulty coping with stress, to bizarre actions and beliefs, to total withdrawal. A **clinical psychologist**, though not a physician, is a specialist in evaluating and treating persons with mental and emotional disorders.

> **Med Term Tip**
>
> All social interactions pose some problems for some people. These problems are not necessarily abnormal. One means of judging if behavior is abnormal is to compare one person's behavior with others in the community. Also, if a person's behavior interferes with the activities of daily living, it is often considered abnormal.

Psychiatry

psychiatric nurse (sigh-kee-AT-rik)

psychiatric social worker

psychiatrist (sigh-KIGH-ah-trist)

psychiatry (sigh-KIGH-ah-tree)

Psychiatry is the branch of medicine that deals with the diagnosis, treatment, and prevention of mental disorders. A **psychiatrist** is a medical physician specializing in the care of patients with mental, emotional, and behavioral disorders. Other health professions also have specialty areas in caring for clients with mental illness. Good examples are **psychiatric nurses** and **psychiatric social workers**.

Pathology

The legal definition of mental disorder is "impaired judgment and lack of self-control." The guide for terminology and classifications relating to psychiatric disorders is the *Diagnostic and Statistical Manual of Mental Disorders, Fourth Edition* (Text Revision) (DSM-IV-TR™, 2004), which is published by the American Psychiatric Association. The DSM organizes mental disorders into fourteen major diagnostic categories of mental disorders.

> **Med Term Tip**
>
> Mental disorders are sometimes more simply characterized by whether they are a *neurosis* or a *psychosis*. Neuroses are inappropriate coping mechanisms to handle stress, such as phobias and panic attacks. Psychoses involve extreme distortions of reality and disorganization of a person's thinking, including bizarre behaviors, hallucinations, and delusions. Schizophrenia is an example of a psychosis.

Anxiety disorders	Characterized by persistent worry and apprehension; include: • **panic attacks**—feeling of intense apprehension, terror, or sense of impending danger • **anxiety** (ang-ZY-eh-tee)—feeling of dread in the absence of a clearly identifiable stress trigger • **phobias** (FOH-bee-ahs)—irrational fear, such as *arachnophobia*, or fear of spiders • **obsessive-compulsive disorder** (OCD) (ob-SESS-iv kom-PUHL-siv)—performing repetitive rituals to reduce anxiety
Cognitive disorders	Deterioration of mental functions due to temporary brain or permanent brain dysfunction; also called **organic mental disease**; include: • **dementia** (dee-MEN-she-ah)—progressive confusion and disorientation • degenerative disorders such as **Alzheimer's disease** (ALTS-high-merz dih-ZEEZ)

Pathology *(continued)*

Disorders diagnosed in infancy and childhood	Mental disorders associated with childhood; include: • **mental retardation**—sub-average intellectual functioning • **attention deficit-hyperactivity disorder** (ADHD)—inattention and impulsive behavior • **autism** (AW-tizm)—extreme withdrawal
Dissociative disorders	Disorders in which severe emotional conflict is so repressed that a split in the personality occurs; include: • **amnesia** (am-NEE-zee-ah)—loss of memory • **multiple personality disorder**—having two or more distinct personalities
■ **Figure 14.5** Photograph of a young woman suffering from anorexia nervosa, posterior view.	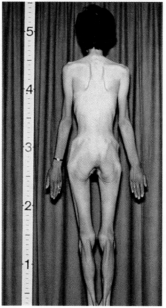 *(Custom Medical Stock Photo, Inc.)*
Eating disorders	Abnormal behaviors related to eating; include: • **anorexia nervosa** (an-oh-REK-see-ah ner-VOH-sah)—refusal to eat • **bulimia** (boo-LIM-ee-ah)—binge eating and intentional vomiting
Factitious disorders	Intentionally feigning illness symptoms in order to gain attention; include: • **malingering**—pretending to be ill or injured
Impulse control disorders	Inability to resist an impulse to perform some act that is harmful to the individual or others; include: • **kleptomania** (klep-toh-MAY-nee-ah)—stealing • **pyromania** (pie-roh-MAY-nee-ah)—setting fires • **explosive disorder**—violent rages • **pathological gambling** (path-ah-LOJ-ih-kal)—inability to stop gambling
Mood disorders	Characterized by instability in mood; include: • **major depression** with suicide potential • **mania** (MAY-nee-ah)—extreme elation • **bipolar disorder** (BPD)—alternation between periods of deep depression and mania **Med Term Tip** The healthcare professional must take all threats of suicide from patients seriously. Psychologists tell us that there is no clear suicide type, which means that we cannot predict who will actually take his or her own life. Always tell the physician about any discussion a patient has concerning suicide. If you believe a patient is in danger of suicide, do not be afraid to ask: "Are you thinking about suicide?"

Pathology (continued)

Personality disorders	Inflexible or maladaptive behavior patterns that affect person's ability to function in society; include: • **paranoid personality disorder**—exaggerated feelings of persecution • **narcissistic personality disorder** (nar-sis-SIST-ik)—abnormal sense of self-importance • **antisocial personality disorder**—behaviors that are against legal or social norms • **passive aggressive personality**—indirect expression of hostility or anger
Schizophrenia	Mental disorders characterized by distortions of reality such as: • **delusions** (dee-LOO-zhuns)—a false belief held even in the face of contrary evidence • **hallucinations** (hah-loo-sih-NAY-shuns)—perceiving something that is not there
Sexual disorders	Disorders include aberrant sexual activity and sexual dysfunction; include: • **pedophilia** (pee-doh-FILL-ee-ah)—sexual interest in children • **masochism** (MAS-oh-kizm)—gratification derived from being hurt or abused • **voyeurism** (VOY-er-izm)—gratification derived from observing others engaged in sexual acts
Sleeping disorders	Disorders relating to sleeping; include: • **insomnia** (in-SOM-nee-ah)—inability to sleep • **sleepwalking**—getting up and walking around unaware while sleeping
Somatoform disorder	Patient has physical symptoms for which no physical disease can be determined; include: • **hypochondria** (high-poh-KON-dree-ah)—a preoccupation with health concerns • **conversion reaction**—anxiety is transformed into physical symptoms such as heart palpitations, paralysis, or blindness
Substance-related disorders	Overindulgence or dependence on chemical substances including alcohol, illegal drugs, and prescription drugs

Therapeutic Procedures

TERM	DEFINITION
Electroconvulsive therapy (ECT) (ee-lek-troh-kon-VULL-siv)	Procedure occasionally used for cases of prolonged major depression. This controversial treatment involves placement of an electrode on one or both sides of the patient's head and a current is turned on briefly causing a convulsive seizure. A low level of voltage is used in modern electroconvulsive therapy, and the patient is administered a muscle relaxant and anesthesia. Advocates of this treatment state that it is a more effective way to treat severe depression than using drugs. It is not effective with disorders other than depression, such as schizophrenia and alcoholism.
Psychopharmacology (sigh-koh-far-mah-KALL-oh-jee)	Study of the effects of drugs on the mind and particularly the use of drugs in treating mental disorders. The main classes of drugs for the treatment of mental disorders are:

Therapeutic Procedures *(continued)*

TERM	DEFINITION
	• **antipsychotic drugs**—Major tranquilizers include chlorpromazine (Thorazine™), haloperidol (Haldol™), clozapine (Clozaril™), and risperidone. These drugs have transformed the treatment of patients with psychoses and schizophrenia by reducing patient agitation and panic and shortening schizophrenic episodes. One of the side effects of these drugs is involuntary muscle movements, which approximately one-fourth of all adults who take the drugs develop. • **antidepressant drugs**—Classified as stimulants and alter the patient's mood by affecting levels of neurotransmitters in the brain. Antidepressants, such as monoamine oxidase (MAO) inhibitors, are nonaddictive but they can produce unpleasant side effects such as dry mouth, weight gain, blurred vision, and nausea. • **minor tranquilizers**—Include Valium™ and Xanax™. These are also classified as central nervous system depressants and are prescribed for anxiety. • **lithium**—Special category of drug used successfully to calm patients who suffer from bipolar disorder (depression alternating with manic excitement).
Psychotherapy (sigh-koh-THAIR-ah-pee)	A method of treating mental disorders by mental rather than chemical or physical means. It includes: • **psychoanalysis**—Method of obtaining a detailed account of the past and present emotional and mental experiences from the patient to determine the source of the problem and eliminate the effects. It is a system developed by Sigmund Freud that encourages the patient to discuss repressed, painful, or hidden experiences with the hope of eliminating or minimizing the problem. • **humanistic psychotherapy**—Therapist does not delve into the patients' past when using these methods. Instead, it is believed that patients can learn how to use their own internal resources to deal with their problems. The therapist creates a therapeutic atmosphere, which builds patient self-esteem and encourages discussion of problems, thereby gaining insight in how to handle them. Also called *client-centered* or *nondirective psychotherapy.* • **family and group psychotherapy**—Often described as solution focused, the therapist places minimal emphasis on patient past history and strong emphasis on having patient state and discuss goals and then find a way to achieve them.

Abbreviations

AD	Alzheimer's disease	**ECT**	electroconvulsive therapy
ADD	attention deficit disorder	**MA**	mental age
ADHD	attention-deficit/hyperactivity disorder	**MAO**	monoamine oxidase
BPD	bipolar disorder	**MMPI**	Minnesota Multiphasic Personality Inventory
CA	chronological age	**OCD**	obsessive-compulsive disorder
DSM	*Diagnostic and Statistical Manual of Mental Disorders*	**SAD**	seasonal affective disorder

Section III: Diagnostic Imaging at a Glance

Combining Forms

fluor/o	fluorescence, luminous
radi/o	X-ray
roentgen/o	X-ray
son/o	sound
tom/o	to cut

Suffixes

-lucent	to shine through
-opaque	nontransparent

Diagnostic Imaging

roentgenology (rent-gen-ALL-oh-jee)   **X-rays**

Diagnostic imaging is the medical specialty that uses a variety of methods to produce images of the internal structures of the body. These images are then used to diagnose disease. This area of medicine began as **roentgenology**, named after German physicist Wilhelm Roentgen who discovered roentgen rays in 1895. This discovery, now commonly known as **X-rays**, revolutionized the diagnosis of disease.

Vocabulary

TERM	DEFINITION
anteroposterior view (AP view)	Positioning the patient so that the X-rays pass through the body from the anterior side to the posterior side.
barium (Ba) (BAH-ree-um)	Soft metallic element from the earth used as a radiopaque X-ray dye.
film	Thin sheet of cellulose material coated with a light-sensitive substance that is used in taking photographs. There is a special photographic film that is sensitive to X-rays.
film badge	Badge containing film that is sensitive to X-rays. This is worn by all personnel in radiology to measure the amount of X-rays to which they are exposed.
lateral view	Positioning of the patient so that the side of the body faces the X-ray machine.
oblique view (oh-BLEEK)	Positioning of the patient so that the X-rays pass through the body on an angle.
posteroanterior view (PA view)	Positioning of the patient so that the X-rays pass through the body from the posterior side to the anterior side.
radiography (ray-dee-OG-rah-fee)	Making of X-ray pictures.
radioisotope (ray-dee-oh-EYE-soh-tohp)	Radioactive form of an element.
radiologist (ray-dee-ALL-oh-jist)	Physician who uses images to diagnose abnormalities and radiant energy to treat various conditions such as cancer.
radiolucent (ray-dee-oh-LOO-cent)	Structures that allow X-rays to pass through; expose the photographic plate and appear as black areas on the X-ray.
radiopaque (ray-dee-oh-PAYK)	Structures that are impenetrable to X-rays, appearing as a light area on the radiograph (X-ray).
roentgen (RENT-gen)	Unit for describing an exposure dose of radiation.
scan	Recording on a photographic plate the emission of radioactive waves after a substance has been injected into the body (see Figure 14.6 ■).
shield	Protective device used to protect against radiation.

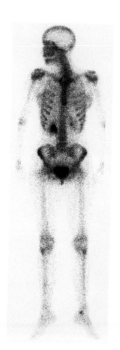

■Figure 14.6 Nuclear medicine. Bone scan produced after injection of radioactive substance into the body.

Vocabulary *(continued)*

TERM	DEFINITION
tagging	Attaching a radioactive material to a chemical, and tracing it as it moves through the body.
uptake	Absorption of radioactive material and medicines into an organ or tissue.
X-ray	High-energy wave that can penetrate most solid matter and present the image on photographic film.

Diagnostic Imaging Procedures

TERM	DEFINITION
computed tomography scan (CT scan) (toh-MOG-rah-fee)	An imaging technique that is able to produce a cross-sectional view of the body. X-ray pictures are taken at multiple angles through the body. A computer then uses all these images to construct a composite cross-section. Refer back to Figure 12.9 in Chapter 12 for an example of a computed tomography scan showing a brain tumor.
contrast studies	Radiopaque substance is injected or swallowed. X-rays are then taken that will outline the body structure containing the radiopaque substance. For example, angiograms and myelograms (see Figure 14.7 ■).
Doppler ultrasonography	Use of ultrasound to record the velocity of blood flowing through blood vessels. Used to detect blood clots and blood vessel obstructions.
fluoroscopy (floo-or-OS-koh-pee)	X-rays strike a fluorescing screen rather than a photographic plate, causing it to glow. The glowing screen changes from minute to minute, therefore movement, such as the heart beating or the digestive tract moving, can be seen.
magnetic resonance imaging (MRI) (REZ-oh-nence)	Use of electromagnetic energy to produce an image of soft tissues in any plane of the body. Atoms behave differently when placed in a strong magnetic field. When the body is exposed to this magnetic field the nuclei of the body's atoms emit radio-frequency signals that can be used to create an image (see Figure 14.8 ■).

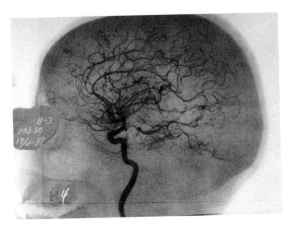

Figure 14.7 Contrast study. X-ray of cerebral blood vessels taken after injection of radiopaque substance into the bloodstream.

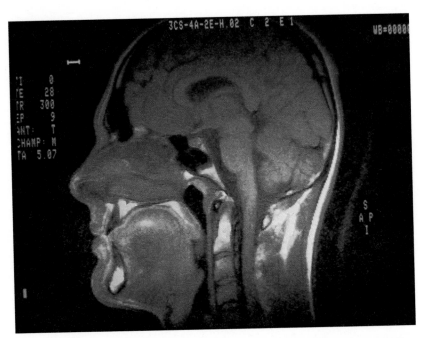

Figure 14.8 Color enhanced magnetic resonance image (MRI), showing a sagittal view of the head. *(Philippe Plailly/Science Photo Library/Photo Researchers, Inc.)*

Diagnostic Imaging Procedures *(continued)*

TERM	DEFINITION
nuclear medicine	Use of radioactive substances to diagnose diseases. A radioactive substance known to accumulate in certain body tissues is injected or inhaled. After waiting for the substance to travel to the body area of interest, the radioactivity level is recorded. Commonly referred to as a *scan* (see Figure 14.6). See Table 14.4 ▆ for examples of the radioactive substances used in nuclear medicine.

Table 14.4	Substances Used to Visualize Various Body Organs in Nuclear Medicine
ORGAN	**SUBSTANCE**
bone	technetium (^{99m}Tc) labeled phosphate
tumors	gallium (^{67}Ga)
lungs	xenon (^{133}Xe)
liver	technetium (^{99m}Tc) labeled sulfur
heart	thallium (^{201}Tl)
thyroid	iodine (^{131}I)

positron emission tomography (PET) (POS-ih-tron eh-MIS-shun toh-MOG-rah-fee)	Image is produced following the injection of radioactive glucose. The glucose will accumulate in areas of high metabolic activity. Therefore, this process will highlight areas that are consuming a large quantity of glucose. This may show an active area of the brain or a tumor (see Figure 14.9 ▆).
radiology (ray-dee-ALL-oh-jee)	Use of high-energy radiation, X-rays, to expose a photographic plate. The image is a black-and-white picture with radiopaque structures such as bone appearing white and radiolucent tissue such as muscles appearing dark.

Figure 14.9 Positron emission tomography (PET) image, showing the difference in the metabolic activity of the brain of a person with Alzheimer's disease and that of a normal person. *(Monte S. Buchsbaum, M.D., Mount Sinai School of Medicine, New York, N.Y.)*

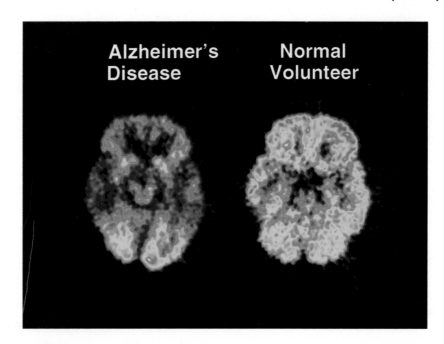

Diagnostic Imaging Procedures *(continued)*

TERM	DEFINITION
ultrasound (US) (ULL-trah-sound)	Use of high-frequency sound waves to produce an image. Sound waves directed into the body from a transducer will bounce off internal structures and echo back to the transducer. The speed of the echo is dependent on the density of the tissue. A computer is able to correlate speed of echo with density and produce an image. Used to visualize internal organs, heart valves, and fetuses.

Figure 14.10 Ultrasound, showing the outline of a fetus. *(Chad Ehlers/The Stock Connection)*

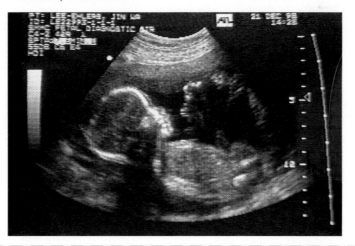

Abbreviations

^{67}**Ga**	radioactive gallium	**AP**	anteroposterior
^{99m}**Tc**	radioactive technetium	**Ba**	barium
^{131}**I**	radioactive iodine	**BaE**	barium enema
^{201}**Tl**	radioactive thallium	**CAT**	computerized axial tomography
^{133}**Xe**	radioactive xenon	**Ci**	curie
Angio	angiography	**CT**	computerized tomography

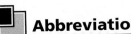

Abbreviations (continued)

CXR	chest x-ray	**mCi**	millicurie
decub	lying down	**MRA**	magnetic resonance angiography
DI	diagnostic imaging	**MRI**	magnetic resonance imaging
DSA	digital subtraction angiography	**NMR**	nuclear magnetic resonance
ERCP	endoscopic retrograde cholangiopancreatography	**PA**	posteroanterior
		PET	positive emission tomography
Fx	fracture	**PTC**	percutaneous transhepatic cholangiography
GB	gallbladder x-ray		
IVC	intravenous cholangiogram	**R**	roentgen
IVP	intravenous pyelogram	**Ra**	radium
KUB	kidneys, ureters, bladder	**rad**	radiation absorbed dose
LAT	lateral	**RL**	right lateral
LGI	lower gastrointestinal series	**RRT**	registered radiologic technologist
LL	left lateral	**UGI**	upper gastrointestinal series
mA	milliampere	**US**	ultrasound

Section IV: Rehabilitation Services at a Glance

Combining Forms

cry/o	cold
electr/o	electric current
erg/o	work
hydr/o	water
my/o	muscle
orth/o	straight, correct
phon/o	sound
prosth/o	addition
therm/o	heat

Suffixes

-phoresis	carrying
-therapy	treatment

Rehabilitation Services

occupational therapy   **physical therapy**

The goal of rehabilitation is to prevent disability and restore as much function as possible following disease, illness, or injury. Rehabilitation services include the healthcare specialties of **physical therapy** (PT) and **occupational therapy** (OT).

Physical Therapy

Physical therapy (PT) involves treating disorders using physical means and methods. Physical therapy personnel assess joint motion, muscle strength and endurance, function of heart and lungs, performance of activities required in daily living, and the ability to carry out other responsibilities. Physical therapy treatment includes gait training, therapeutic exercise, massage, joint and soft tissue mobilization, thermotherapy, cryotherapy, electrical stimulation, ultrasound, and hydrotherapy. These methods strengthen muscles, improve motion and circulation, reduce pain, and increase function.

Occupational Therapy

Occupational therapy (OT) assists patients to regain, develop, and improve skills that are important for independent functioning (activities of daily living). Occupational therapy personnel work with people who, because of illness, injury, or developmental or psychological impairments, require specialized training in skills that will enable them to lead independent, productive, and satisfying lives in regard to personal care, work, and leisure. Occupational therapists instruct patients in the use of adaptive equipment and techniques, body mechanics, and energy conservation. They also employ modalities such as heat, cold, and therapeutic exercise.

 # Vocabulary

TERM	DEFINITION
activities of daily living (ADL)	The activities usually performed in the course of a normal day, such as eating, dressing, and washing.

Figure 14.11 Photograph of an occupational therapist assisting a male patient with learning independence in activities of daily living (ADLs).

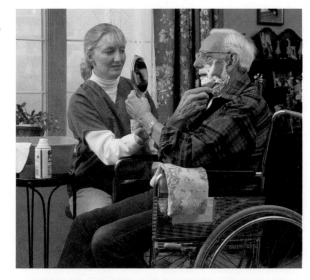

Vocabulary *(continued)*

TERM	DEFINITION
adaptive equipment	Modification of equipment or devices to improve the function and independence of a person with a disability.

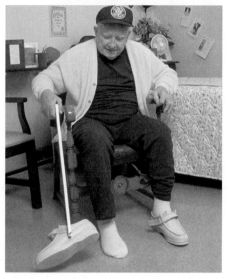 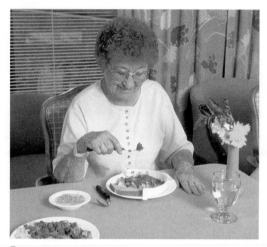

A   B

■**Figure 14.12** Using adaptive equipment. A) Male putting on shoe. B) Female eating one handed.

TERM	DEFINITION
body mechanics	Use of good posture and position while performing activities of daily living to prevent injury and stress on body parts.
ergonomics (er-goh-NOM-iks)	Study of human work including how the requirements for performing work and the work environment affect the musculoskeletal and nervous systems.
fine motor skills	Use of precise and coordinated movements in such activities such as writing, buttoning, and cutting.
gait (GAYT)	Manner of walking.
gross motor skills	Use of large muscle groups that coordinate body movements such as walking, running, jumping, and balance.
lower extremity (LE)	Refers to one of the legs.
mobility	State of having normal movement of all body parts.
orthotics (or-THOT-iks)	Use of equipment, such as splints and braces, to support a paralyzed muscle, promote a specific motion, or correct musculoskeletal deformities.
physical medicine	Branch of medicine focused on restoring function. Primarily cares for patients with musculoskeletal and nervous system disorders. Physician is a *physiatrist*.
prosthetics (pros-THET-iks)	Artificial devices, such as limbs and joints, that replace a missing body part (see Figure 14.13 ■).
range of motion (ROM)	Range of movement of a joint, from maximum flexion through maximum extension. It is measured as degrees of a circle.

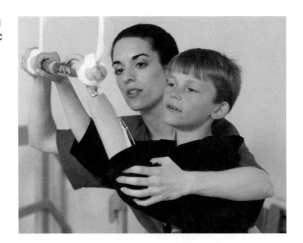

 ## Vocabulary *(continued)*

TERM	DEFINITION
rehabilitation	Process of treatment and exercise that can help a person with a disability attain maximum function and well-being.
upper extremity (UE)	Refers to one of the arms.

Therapeutic Procedures

TERM	DEFINITION
active exercises	Exercises that a patient performs without assistance.
active range of motion (AROM)	Range of motion for joints that a patient is able to perform without assistance from someone else.
active-resistive exercises	Exercises in which the patient works against resistance applied to a muscle, such as a weight. Used to increase strength.
cryotherapy (cry-oh-THAIR-ah-pee)	Using cold for therapeutic purposes.
debridement (day-breed-MON)	Removal of dead or damaged tissue from a wound. Commonly performed for burn therapy.
electromyogram (EMG) (ee-lek-troh-MY-oh-gram)	Graphic recording of the contraction of a muscle. The result of applying an electrical stimulation to the muscle.
gait training	Assisting a patient to learn to walk again or how to use an assistive device to walk (see Figure 14.14 ■).
hydrotherapy (high-droh-THAIR-ah-pee)	Application of warm water as a therapeutic treatment. Can be done in baths, swimming pools, and whirlpools.
massage	Kneading or applying pressure by hands to a part of the patient's body to promote muscle relaxation and reduce tension.
mobilization	Treatments such as exercise and massage to restore movement to joints and soft tissue.
moist hot packs	Applying moist warmth to a body part to produce the slight dilation of blood vessels in the skin. Causes muscle relaxation in the deeper regions of the body and increases circulation, which aids healing.

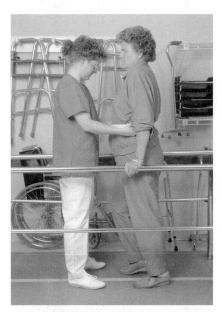

Figure 14.14 Physical therapist assisting a patient to walk in the parallel bars.

Therapeutic Procedures *(continued)*

TERM	DEFINITION
nerve conduction velocity	Test to determine if nerves have been damaged by recording the rate at which an electrical impulse travels along a nerve. If the nerve is damaged, the velocity will be decreased.
pain control	Managing pain through a variety of means, including medications, biofeedback, and mechanical devices.
passive range of motion (PROM)	Therapist putting a patient's joints through available range of motion without assistance from the patient.
phonophoresis (foh-noh-foh-REE-sis)	Use of ultrasound waves to introduce medication across the skin and into the subcutaneous tissues.
postural drainage with clapping	Draining secretions from the bronchi or a lung cavity by having the patient lie so that gravity allows drainage to occur. Clapping is using the hand in a cupped position to perform percussion on the chest. Assists in loosening secretions and mucus.
therapeutic exercise (thair-ah-PEW-tik)	Exercise planned and carried out to achieve a specific physical benefit, such as improved range of motion, muscle strength, or cardiovascular function.
thermotherapy (ther-moh-THAIR-ah-pee)	Applying heat to the body for therapeutic purposes.
traction	Process of pulling or drawing, usually with a mechanical device. Used in treating orthopedic (bone and joint) problems and injuries.
transcutaneous electrical nerve stimulation (TENS) (tranz-kyoo-TAY-nee-us)	Application of an electric current to a peripheral nerve to relieve pain.
ultrasound (US)	Use of high-frequency sound waves to create heat in soft tissues under the skin. It is particularly useful for treating injuries to muscles, tendons, and ligaments, as well as muscle spasms.
whirlpool	Bath in which there are continuous jets of hot water reaching the body surfaces.

Abbreviations

ADL	activities of daily living	**PROM**	passive range of motion
AAROM	active assistive range of motion	**PT**	physical therapy
AROM	active range of motion	**ROM**	range of motion
EMG	electromyogram	**TENS**	transcutaneous electrical stimulation
e-stim	electrical stimulation	**UE**	upper extremity
LE	lower extremity	**US**	ultrasound
OT	occupational therapy		

Section V: Surgery at a Glance

Combining Forms

cis/o	to cut
cry/o	cold
electr/o	electricity
esthesi/o	sensation, feeling
sect/o	cut

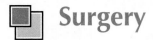 # Surgery

operative report   surgery
surgeon

Surgery is the branch of medicine dealing with operative procedures to correct deformities and defects, repair injuries, and diagnose and cure diseases. A **surgeon** is a physician who has completed additional training of five years or more in a surgical specialty area. These specialty areas include orthopedics; neurosurgery; gynecology; ophthalmology; urology; and thoracic, vascular, cardiac, plastic, and general surgery. The surgeon must complete an **operative report** for every procedure that he or she performs. This is a detailed description that includes the following:

- preoperative diagnosis
- indication for the procedure
- name of the procedure
- surgical techniques employed
- findings during surgery
- postoperative diagnosis
- name of the surgeon

This report also includes information pertaining to the patient such as name, address, age, patient number, and date of the procedure.

Surgical terminology includes terms related to anesthesiology, surgical instruments, surgical procedures, incisions, and suture materials. Specific surgical procedures are frequently named by using the combining form for the body part being operated on and adding a suffix that describes the procedure. For example, an incision into the chest is a *thoracotomy*, removal of the stomach is *gastrectomy*, and surgical repair of the skin is *dermatoplasty*. A list of the most frequently used surgical suffixes is found in Chapter 1 and common surgical procedures are defined in each system chapter.

Anesthesia

anesthesia (an-ess-THEE-zee-ah)   local anesthesia
anesthesiologist (an-es-thee-zee-OL-jist)   nurse anesthetist (ah-NES-the-tist)
general anesthesia   regional anesthesia
inhalation (in-hah-LAY-shun)   subcutaneous (sub-kyoo-TAY-nee-us)
intravenous (in-trah-VEE-nus)   topical anesthesia

An **anesthesiologist** is a physician who specializes in the practice of administering anesthetics. A **nurse anesthetist** is a registered nurse who has received additional training and education in the administration of anesthetic medications. **Anesthesia** results in the loss of feeling or sensation. The most common types of anesthesia are general, regional, local, and topical anesthesia.

- **General anesthesia** (GA) produces a loss of consciousness including an absence of pain sensation. It is administered to a patient by either an **intravenous** (IV) or **inhalation** method. The patient's vital signs (VS), heart rate, breathing rate, pulse, and blood pressure, are carefully monitored when using a general anesthetic.
- **Regional anesthesia** is also referred to as a *nerve block*. This anesthetic interrupts a patient's pain sensation in a particular region of the body, such as the arm. The anesthetic is injected near the nerve that will be blocked from sensation. The patient usually remains conscious.

- **Local anesthesia** produces a loss of sensation in one localized part of the body. The patient remains conscious. The anesthetic is administered either topically or via a **subcutaneous** route. For example, deadening the skin prior to suturing a laceration.
- **Topical anesthesia** uses an anesthetic liquid or gel placed directly into a specific area. The patient remains conscious. This type of anesthetic is used on the skin, the cornea, and the mucous membranes in dental work.

Surgical Instruments

Physicians have developed surgical instruments since the time of the early Egyptians. Instruments include surgical knives, saws, clamps, drills, and needles. Some of the more commonly used surgical instruments are listed in Table 14.5 ■ and shown in Figure 14.15 ■.

Surgical Positions

Patients are placed in specific positions so the surgeon is able to reach the area that is to be operated on. Table 14.6 ■ describes and Figure 14.16 ■ illustrates some common surgical positions.

Table 14.5	Common Surgical Instruments
INSTRUMENT	**USE**
aspirator (AS-pih-ray-tor)	suctions fluid
clamp	grasps tissue; controls bleeding
curette (kyoo-RET)	scrapes and removes tissue
dilator (dye-LAY-tor)	enlarges an opening by stretching
forceps (FOR-seps)	grasps tissue
hemostat (HEE-moh-stat)	forceps to grasp blood vessel to control bleeding
probe	explores tissue
scalpel	cuts and separates tissue
speculum (SPEK-yoo-lum)	spreads apart walls of a cavity
tenaculum (the-NAK-yoo-lum)	long-handled clamp
trephine (treh-FINE)	saw that removes disk-shaped piece of tissue or bone

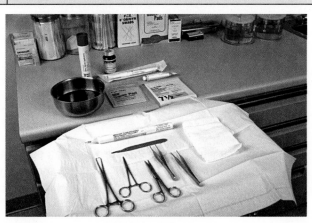

■ **Figure 14.15** Surgical instruments prepared for a procedure.

Figure 14.16 Examples of common surgical positions.

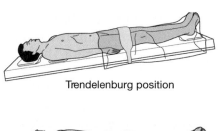
Trendelenburg position

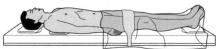

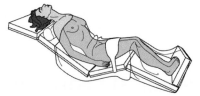
Fowler position

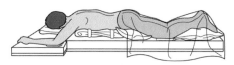
Supine position

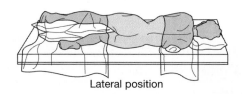
Prone position

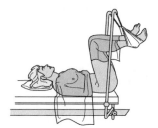
Lithotomy position

Lateral position

Table 14.6	Common Surgical Positions
SURGICAL POSITION	**DESCRIPTION**
Fowler	sitting with back positioned at a 45° angle
Lateral recumbent (ree-KUM-bent)	lying on either the left or right side
Lithotomy (lith-OT-oh-mee)	lying face up with hips and knees bent at 90° angles
Prone (PROHN)	lying horizontal with face down
Supine (soo-PINE)	lying horizontal and face up; also called dorsal recumbent
Trendelenburg (TREN-dee-len-berg)	lying face up and on an incline with head lower than legs

Vocabulary

TERM	DEFINITION
analgesic (an-al-JEE-zik)	Medication to relieve pain.
anesthetic (an-ess-THET-ik)	Medication to produce partial to complete loss of sensation.
cauterization (kaw-ter-ih-ZAY-shun)	Using heat, cold, electricity, or chemicals to scar, burn, or cut tissues.
circulating nurse	Nurse who assists the surgeon and scrub nurse by providing needed materials during the procedure and by handling the surgical specimen. This person does not wear sterile clothing and may enter and leave the operating room during the procedure.

Vocabulary *(continued)*

TERM	DEFINITION
cryosurgery (cry-oh-SER-jer-ee)	Technique of exposing tissues to extreme cold to produce cell injury and destruction. Used in the treatment of malignant tumors or to control pain and bleeding.
day surgery	Type of outpatient surgery in which the patient is discharged on the same day he or she is admitted; also called *ambulatory surgery.*
dissection (dih-SEK-shun)	Surgical cutting of parts for separation and study.
draping	Process of covering the patient with sterile cloths that allow only the operative site to be exposed to the surgeon.
electrocautery (ee-lek-troh-KAW-ter-ee)	Use of an electric current to stop bleeding by coagulating blood vessels.
endoscopic surgery (en-doh-SKOP-ik)	Use of a lighted instrument to examine the interior of a cavity.
hemostasis (hee-moh-STAY-sis)	Stopping the flow of blood using instruments, pressure, and/or medication.
intraoperative (in-trah-OP-er-ah-tiv)	Period of time during surgery.
laser surgery	Use of a controlled beam of light for cutting, hemostasis, or tissue destruction.
perioperative (per-ee-OP-er-ah-tiv)	Period of time that includes before, during, and after a surgical procedure.
postoperative (post-op) (post-OP-er-ah-tiv)	Period of time immediately following the surgery.
preoperative (preop, pre-op) (pree-OP-er-ah-tiv)	Period of time preceding surgery.
resection (ree-SEK-shun)	To surgically cut out or remove; excision.
scrub nurse	Surgical assistant who hands instruments to the surgeon. This person wears sterile clothing and maintains the sterile operative field.
suture material (SOO-cher)	Used to close a wound or incision. Examples are catgut, silk thread, or staples. They may or may not be removed when the wound heals, depending on the type of material that is used.

Abbreviations

D & C	dilation and curettage	**PARR**	postanesthetic recovery room
EUA	exam under anesthesia	**preop, pre-op**	preoperative
Endo	endoscopy	**prep**	preparation, prepared
GA	general anesthesia	**T & A**	tonsillectomy and adenoidectomy
I & D	incision and drainage	**TAH**	total abdominal hysterectomy
MUA	manipulation under anesthesia	**TURP**	transurethral resection of prostate
OR	operating room		

Section VI: Oncology at a Glance

Combining Forms

blast/o	primitive cell
carcin/o	cancerous
chem/o	chemical
mut/a	genetic change, mutation
onc/o	tumor
tox/o	poison

Suffixes

-plasia	-growth, formation
-plasm	growth, formation

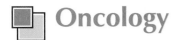

Oncology

benign (bee-NINE)

carcinoma (kar-sin-NOH-mah)

malignant (mah-LIG-nant)

oncology (ong-KALL-oh-jee)

protocol (PROH-toh-kall)

tumors

Oncology is the branch of medicine dealing with **tumors**. A tumor can be classified as **benign** or **malignant**. A benign tumor is one that is generally not progressive or recurring. Generally, a benign tumor will have the suffix *-oma* at the end of the term. However, a malignant tumor indicates that there is a cancerous growth present (see Figure 14.17 ■). These terms will usually have the word **carcinoma** added. The medical specialty of oncology primarily treats patients who have cancer.

The treatment for cancer can consist of a variety or a combination of treatments. The **protocol** (prot) for a particular patient will consist of the actual plan of care, including the medications, surgeries, and treatments such as chemotherapy and radiation therapy. Often, the entire healthcare team, including the physician, oncologist, radiologist, nurse, patient and family, will assist in designing the treatment plan.

> **Med Term Tip**
>
> Carcinoma or cancer (Ca) can affect almost every organ in the body. The medical term reflects the area of the body affected as well as the type of tumor cell. For example, there can be an esophageal carcinoma, gastric adenocarcinoma, or adenocarcinoma of the uterus.

Staging Tumors

grade

metastases (meh-TASS-tah-seez)

pathologist (path-ALL-oh-jist)

staging

The process of classifying tumors based on their degree of tissue invasion and the potential response to therapy is referred to as **staging**. The TNM staging system is frequently used. The *T* refers to the tumor's size and invasion, the *N* refers to lymph node involvement, and the *M* refers to the presence of **metastases** (mets) of the tumor cells (see Figure 14.18 ■).

In addition, a tumor can be graded from grade I through grade IV. The **grade** is based on the microscopic appearance of the tumor cells. The **pathologist** rates or grades the cells based on whether the tumor resembles the normal tissue. The classification system is illustrated in Table 14.7 ■. A grade I tumor is well differentiated and is easier to treat than the more advanced grades.

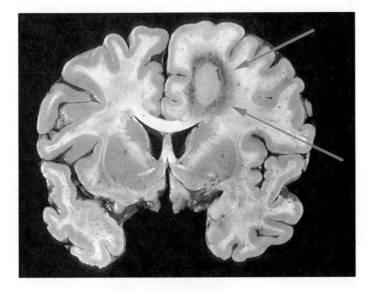

■ **Figure 14.17** Photograph of a brain specimen with a large malignant tumor. *(ISM/Phototake NYC)*

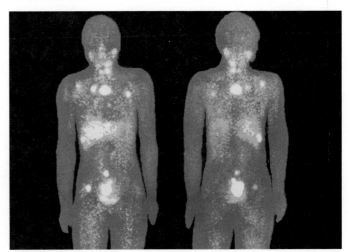

■ **Figure 14.18** Full body scan showing many areas of metastatic cancer. *(Collection CNRI/Phototake NYC)*

Table 14.7	Tumor Grade Classification
GRADE	**MEANING**
GX	The grade cannot be determined.
GI	The cells are well differentiated.
GII	The cells are moderately differentiated.
GIII	The cells are poorly differentiated.
GIV	The cells are undifferentiated.

Vocabulary

TERM	DEFINITION
carcinogen (kar-SIN-oh-jen)	Substance or chemical agent that produces or increases the risk of developing cancer. For example, cigarette smoke and insecticides are considered to be cancinogens.
	Med Term Tip
	The term *benign* comes from the Latin term *bene*, which means "kind or good." On the other hand, the term *malignant* comes from the Latin term *mal*, meaning "bad or malicious."
carcinoma in situ (CIS) (kar-sin-NOH-mah)	Malignant tumor that has not extended beyond the original site.
encapsulated (en-CAP-soo-lay-ted)	Growth enclosed in a sheath of tissue that prevents tumor cells from invading surrounding tissue.
hyperplasia (high-per-PLAY-zee-ah)	Excessive development of normal cells within an organ.
invasive disease (in-VAY-siv)	Tendency of a malignant tumor to spread to immediately surrounding tissue and organs.
metastasis (mets) (meh-TASS-tah-sis)	Movement and spread of cancer cells from one part of the body to another. Metastases is plural.

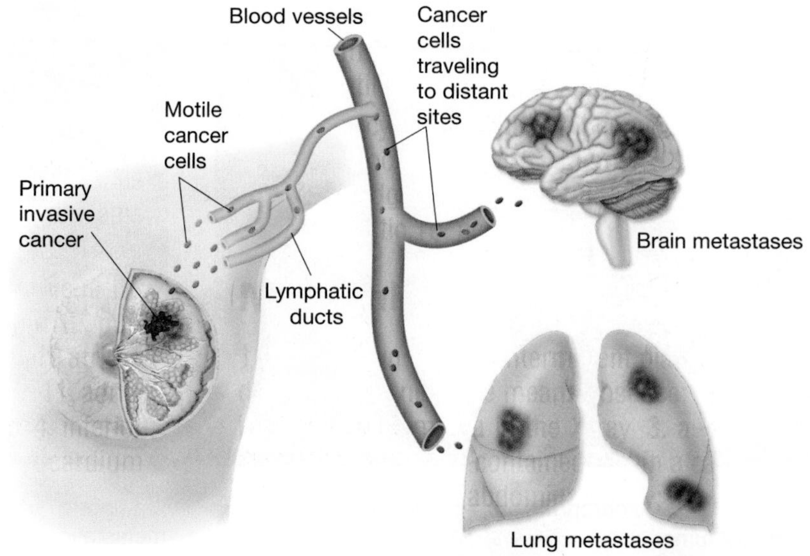

Figure 14.19 Illustration showing how the primary breast tumor metastasized through the lymphatic and blood vessels to secondary sites in the brain and lungs.

Vocabulary (continued)

TERM	DEFINITION
morbidity (mor-BID-ih-tee)	Number representing the sick persons in a particular population.
mortality (mor-TAL-ih-tee)	Number representing the deaths in a particular population.
mutation (mew-TAY-shun)	Change or transformation from the original.
neoplasm (NEE-oh-plazm)	New and abnormal growth or tumor. These can be benign or malignant.
oncogenic (ong-koh-JEN-ik)	Cancer causing.
primary site	Term used to designate where a malignant tumor first appeared.
relapse	Return of disease symptoms after a period of improvement.
remission (rih-MISH-un)	Period during which the symptoms of a disease or disorder leave. Can be temporary.

Diagnostic Procedures

TERM	DEFINITION
biopsy (bx) (BYE-op-see)	Excision of a small piece of tissue for microscopic examination to assist in determining a diagnosis.
cytologic testing (sigh-toh-LAH-jik)	Examination of cells to determine their structure and origin. Pap smears are considered a form of cytologic testing.
exploratory surgery	Surgery performed for the purpose of determining if cancer is present or if a known cancer has spread. Biopsies are generally performed.
staging laparotomy (lap-ah-ROT-oh-mee)	Surgical procedure in which the abdomen is entered to determine the extent and staging of a tumor.

Therapeutic Procedures

TERM	DEFINITION
chemotherapy (chemo) (kee-moh-THAIR-ah-pee)	Treating disease by using chemicals that have a toxic effect on the body, especially cancerous tissue.
hormone therapy	Treatment of cancer with natural hormones or with chemicals that produce hormonelike effects.
immunotherapy (im-yoo-noh-THAIR-ah-pee)	Strengthening the immune system to attack cancerous cells.
palliative therapy (PAL-ee-ah-tiv THAIR-ah-pee)	Treatment designed to reduce the intensity of painful symptoms, but does not produce a cure.
radiation therapy	Exposing tumors and surrounding tissues to X-rays or gamma rays to interfere with their ability to multiply.

Therapeutic Procedures *(continued)*

TERM	DEFINITION
radical surgery	Extensive surgery to remove as much tissue associated with a tumor as possible.
radioactive implant (ray-dee-oh-AK-tiv)	Embedding a radioactive source directly into tissue to provide a highly localized radiation dosage to damage nearby cancerous cells. Also called *brachytherapy*.

Abbreviations

bx	biopsy	**mets**	metastases
Ca	cancer	**MTX**	methotrexate
chemo	chemotherapy	**prot**	protocol
CIS	carcinoma in situ	**st**	stage
5-FU	5-fluorouracil	**TNM**	tumor, nodes, metastases
GA	gallium		

Chapter Review

Terminology Checklist

Below are all bolded key terms, Word Building, Vocabulary, Pathology, Diagnostic, and Therapeutic terms presented in this chapter. Use this list as a study tool by placing a check in the box in front of each term as you master its meaning.

- ☐ abnormal psychology
- ☐ active exercises
- ☐ active range of motion
- ☐ active-resistive exercises
- ☐ activities of daily living
- ☐ adaptive equipment
- ☐ addiction
- ☐ additive
- ☐ aerosol
- ☐ Alzheimer's disease
- ☐ amnesia
- ☐ analgesic
- ☐ anesthesia
- ☐ anesthesiologist
- ☐ anesthetic
- ☐ anorexia nervosa
- ☐ anteroposterior view
- ☐ antidepressant drugs
- ☐ antidote
- ☐ antipsychotic drugs
- ☐ antisocial personality disorder
- ☐ anxiety
- ☐ anxiety disorders
- ☐ aspirator
- ☐ attention deficit disorder
- ☐ autism
- ☐ barium
- ☐ benign
- ☐ biopsy
- ☐ bipolar disorder
- ☐ body mechanics
- ☐ brand name
- ☐ broad spectrum
- ☐ buccal
- ☐ bulimia
- ☐ carcinogen
- ☐ carcinoma
- ☐ carcinoma in situ
- ☐ cauterization

- ☐ chemical name
- ☐ chemotherapy
- ☐ circulating nurse
- ☐ clamp
- ☐ clinical psychologist
- ☐ cognitive disorders
- ☐ computed tomography scan
- ☐ contraindication
- ☐ contrast studies
- ☐ controlled substances
- ☐ conversion reaction
- ☐ cryosurgery
- ☐ cryotherapy
- ☐ cumulative action
- ☐ curette
- ☐ cytologic testing
- ☐ day surgery
- ☐ debridement
- ☐ delusions
- ☐ dementia
- ☐ dilator
- ☐ disorders diagnosed in infancy and childhood
- ☐ dissection
- ☐ dissociative disorders
- ☐ Doppler ultrasonography
- ☐ draping
- ☐ Drug Enforcement Agency
- ☐ drug interaction
- ☐ drug tolerance
- ☐ eardrops
- ☐ eating disorders
- ☐ electrocautery
- ☐ electroconvulsive therapy
- ☐ electromyogram
- ☐ encapsulated
- ☐ endoscopic surgery
- ☐ ergonomics
- ☐ exploratory surgery

- ☐ explosive disorder
- ☐ eyedrops
- ☐ factitious disorders
- ☐ family and group psychotherapy
- ☐ film
- ☐ film badge
- ☐ fine motor skills
- ☐ fluoroscopy
- ☐ forceps
- ☐ Fowler position
- ☐ gait
- ☐ gait training
- ☐ general anesthesia
- ☐ generic name
- ☐ grade
- ☐ gross motor skills
- ☐ habituation
- ☐ hallucinations
- ☐ hemostasis
- ☐ hemostat
- ☐ hormone therapy
- ☐ humanistic psychotherapy
- ☐ hydrotherapy
- ☐ hyperplasia
- ☐ hypochondria
- ☐ iatrogenic
- ☐ idiosyncrasy
- ☐ immunotherapy
- ☐ impulse control disorders
- ☐ inhalation
- ☐ insomnia
- ☐ intracavitary
- ☐ intradermal
- ☐ intramuscular
- ☐ intraoperative
- ☐ intrathecal
- ☐ intravenous
- ☐ invasive disease

- kleptomania
- laser surgery
- lateral recumbent position
- lateral view
- lithium
- lithotomy position
- local anesthesia
- lower extremity
- magnetic resonance imaging
- major depression
- malignant
- malingering
- mania
- masochism
- massage
- mental retardation
- metastases
- metastasis
- minor tranquilizers
- mobility
- mobilization
- moist hot packs
- mood disorders
- morbidity
- mortality
- multiple personality disorder
- mutation
- narcissistic personality disorder
- neoplasm
- nerve conduction velocity
- nonproprietary name
- normal psychology
- nuclear medicine
- nurse anesthetist
- oblique view
- obsessive-compulsive disorder
- occupational therapy
- oncogenic
- oncology
- operative report
- oral
- organic mental disease
- orthotics
- over-the-counter drug
- pain control

- palliative therapy
- panic attacks
- paranoid personality disorder
- parenteral
- passive aggressive personality
- passive range of motion
- pathological gambling
- pathologist
- pedophilia
- perioperative
- personality disorders
- pharmaceutical
- pharmacist
- pharmacology
- phobias
- phonophoresis
- physical medicine
- physical therapy
- placebo
- positron emission tomography
- posteroanterior view
- postoperative
- postural drainage with clapping
- potentiation
- preoperative
- prescription
- prescription drug
- primary site
- probe
- prone
- prophylaxis
- proprietary name
- prosthetics
- protocol
- psychiatric nurse
- psychiatric social worker
- psychiatrist
- psychiatry
- psychoanalysis
- psychology
- psychopharmacology
- psychotherapy
- pyromania
- radiation therapy

- radical surgery
- radioactive implant
- radiography
- radioisotope
- radiologist
- radiology
- radiolucent
- radiopaque
- range of motion
- rectal
- regional anesthesia
- rehabilitation
- relapse
- remission
- resection
- roentgen
- roentgenology
- scalpel
- scan
- Schedule I
- Schedule II
- Schedule III
- Schedule IV
- Schedule V
- schizophrenia
- scrub nurse
- sexual disorders
- shield
- side effect
- sleeping disorder
- sleepwalking
- somatoform disorders
- speculum
- staging
- staging laparotomy
- subcutaneous
- sublingual
- substance-related disorders
- supine
- suppositories
- surgeon
- surgery
- suture material
- tagging
- tenaculum

- [ ] therapeutic exercise
- [ ] thermotherapy
- [ ] tolerance
- [ ] topical
- [ ] topical anesthesia
- [ ] toxicity
- [ ] traction
- [ ] trademark
- [ ] transcutaneous electrical nerve stimulation
- [ ] transdermal
- [ ] Trendelenburg position
- [ ] trephine
- [ ] tumors
- [ ] ultrasound
- [ ] unit dose
- [ ] upper extremity
- [ ] uptake
- [ ] vaginal
- [ ] voyeurism
- [ ] whirlpool
- [ ] X-rays

Practice Exercises

A. Complete the following statements.

1. The reference book containing important information regarding medications is the _____.

2. A person specializing in the dispensing of medications is a _____.

3. The accepted official name for a drug is the _____ name.

4. The trade name for a drug is the _____ name.

5. What does the chemical name represent? _____

6. What federal agency enforces controls over the use of drugs causing dependency? _____

B. Name the route of drug administration for the following descriptions.

1. under the tongue _____

2. into the anus or rectum _____

3. applied to the skin _____

4. injected under the first layer of skin _____

5. injected into a muscle _____

6. injected into a vein _____

7. by mouth _____

C. Define the following terms in the space provided.

1. idiosyncrasy _____

2. parenteral _____

3. placebo _____

4. toxicity _____

5. side effect _____

6. unit dose _____

7. habituation _____

8. antidote _____

9. contraindication _____

10. prophylaxis _____

D. Give the meaning of the following abbreviations in the space provided.

1. gr _____

2. bid _____

3. tid _____

4. ad lib _____

5. prn _____

6. ante _____

7. OTC _____

8. gt _____

9. Sig _____

10. stat _____

11. mg _____

12. qd _____

13. noc _____

14. NPO _____

15. hs _____

16. IV _____

17. TO _____

18. gtt _____

19. pc _____

20. d/c _____

E. Write out the following prescription instructions in the space provided.

1. Pravachol, 20 mg., Sig. ī qd @ noc, 30, refill 3x, no sub. _____

2. Lanoxin 0.125 mg., Sig. iii stat, then ii q AM, 100, refills prn. _____

3. Synthroid 0.075 mg., Sig. ī qd, 100, refill x4. _____

4. Norvasc 5 mg., ī q am, 60, refillable. _____

F. Match each mental disorder to its example.

1. _____ cognitive disorders   a. hypochondria

2. _____ factitious disorders   b. kleptomania

3. _____ dissociative disorders   c. masochism

4. _____ eating disorders   d. narcissistic personality

5. _____ sleeping disorders   e. insomnia

6. _____ mood disorders   f. bipolar disease

7. _____ impulse control disorders   g. panic attacks

8. _____ somatoform disorders   h. amnesia

9. _____ personality disorders   i. dementia

10. _____ sexual disorders   j. anorexia nervosa

11. _____ anxiety disorders   k. malingering

G. Identify each mental health treatment from its description.

1. depressant drugs prescribed for anxiety _____

2. client-centered psychotherapy _____

3. drug used to calm patients with bipolar disorder _____

4. reduces patient agitation and panic and shortens schizophrenic episodes _____

5. obtains a detailed account of the past and present emotional and mental experiences _____

6. stimulants that alter the patient's mood by affecting neurotransmitter levels _____

H. Identify the following abbreviations.

1. MRI _____

2. Ba _____

3. AP _____

4. CT _____

5. RL _____

6. PA _____

7. LL _____

8. PET _____

9. UGI _____

10. KUB _____

I. Match each term to its definition.

1. _____ ultrasound

a. radiopaque substances used to outline hollow structures

2. _____ MRI

b. records velocity of blood flowing through vessels

3. _____ Doppler US

c. image created by electromagnetic energy

4. _____ nuclear medicine scan

d. glowing screen shows movement

5. _____ CT scan

e. making an X-ray

6. _____ contrast study

f. multiple-angle X-rays compiled into a cross-section

7. _____ fluoroscopy

g. uses radioactive substances

8. _____ radiography

h. image of internal organs using sound waves

9. _____ PET scan

i. indicates metabolic activity

J. Identify the following abbreviations.

1. ROM _____

2. OT _____

3. ADL _____

4. LE _____

5. EMG _____

6. TENS _____

7. PT _____

8. PROM _____

9. e-stim _____

10. US _____

K. Identify the rehabilitation procedure described by each phrase.

1. kneading or applying pressure by hands _____

2. removal of dead and damaged tissue from a wound _____

3. using water for treatment purposes _____

4. drainage of secretions from the bronchi _____

5. exercises performed by a patient without resistance _____

6. medication introduced by ultrasound waves _____

7. use of cold for therapeutic purposes _____

8. pulling with a mechanical device _____

L. Match each term to its definition.

1. _____ forceps
2. _____ tenaculum
3. _____ Trendelenburg
4. _____ lithotomy
5. _____ curette
6. _____ aspirator
7. _____ supine
8. _____ probe
9. _____ scalpel
10. _____ lateral recumbent

a. scrapes and removes tissue

b. cuts and separates tissue

c. lying horizontal and face up

d. lying on either the left or right side

e. long-handled clamp

f. explores tissue

g. lying face up with hips and knees bent at 90° angle

h. grasps tissue

i. suctions fluid

j. lying face up on an incline, head lower than legs

M. Identify the type of anesthesia for each description.

1. produces loss of consciousness and absence of pain _____

2. produces loss of sensation in one localized part of the body _____

3. anesthetic applied directly onto a specific skin area _____

4. also referred to as a nerve block _____

N. Match each term to its definition.

1. _____ oncogenic
2. _____ benign
3. _____ encapsulated
4. _____ relapse
5. _____ primary site
6. _____ protocol
7. _____ staging laparotomy
8. _____ cytologic testing
9. _____ radioactive implant
10. _____ bx

a. examine cells to determine their structure and origin

b. the plan for care for any individual patient

c. biopsy

d. growth that is not recurrent or progressive

e. placing a radioactive substance directly into the tissue

f. where the malignant tumor first appeared

g. growth is enclosed in a tissue sheath

h. cancer causing

i. abdominal surgery to determine extent of tumor

j. return of disease symptoms

Medical Record Analysis

Below is an item from a patient's medical record. Read it carefully, make sure you understand all the medical terms used, and then answer the questions that follow.

Oncology Consultation Report

Current Complaint:	Patient is a 72-year-old female complaining of increasing dyspnea with activity during the past six months. She now has a frequent harsh cough producing thick sputum and occasional hemoptysis.
History:	Patient had a hysterectomy for endometriosis at age 45, cholecystectomy for cholelithiasis at age 62, and recent compression fracture of the lumbar spine secondary to osteoporosis. Her only current medication is a calcium supplement for osteoporosis.
Physical Examination:	Patient is thin and short of stature. She has mild kyphosis. She is alert and answers all questions appropriately. She is not SOB sitting in examination room. Auscultation of chest reveals marked rales in her lower right lung, but no rhonchi. She has a persistent cough and sputum was collected for a sputum culture and sensitivity and a sputum cytologic testing.
Diagnostic Test Results:	Chest radiograph revealed a suspicious cloudy area in right lung. Follow-up with CT scan of the bronchial tree confirmed the presence of a mass in the right lung. Sputum specimen was negative for the presence of bacteria. Sputum cytologic testing revealed malignant cells, indicating presence of cancerous tumor in the lungs.
Diagnosis:	Bronchogenic carcinoma.
Treatment Plan:	Patient will be referred to thoracic surgeon for consultation regarding thoracotomy and lobectomy. Following recovery from this surgery she is to return to oncology clinic for chemotherapy and to determine if the tumor has metastasized.

Critical Thinking Questions

1. The patient had three complaints. List the three complaints and describe each in your own words.

   a. _____

   b. _____

   c. _____

2. This patient had two surgical procedures. Name them and explain why each was necessary.

   a. _____

   b. _____

3. The patient has mild kyphosis. What is kyphosis and which system is this pathology associated with?

   _____

4. What do the two abbreviations used in this case study stand for?

a. SOB _____

b. CT scan _____

5. The patient will have a surgical procedure before chemotherapy that is described by two words. List them and describe what each means.

a. _____

b. _____

6. What does the term *metastasized* mean? _____

_____

Chart Note Transcription

The chart note below contains eleven phrases that can be reworded with a medical term that you learned in this chapter. Each phrase is identified with an underline. Determine the medical term and write your answers in the space provided.

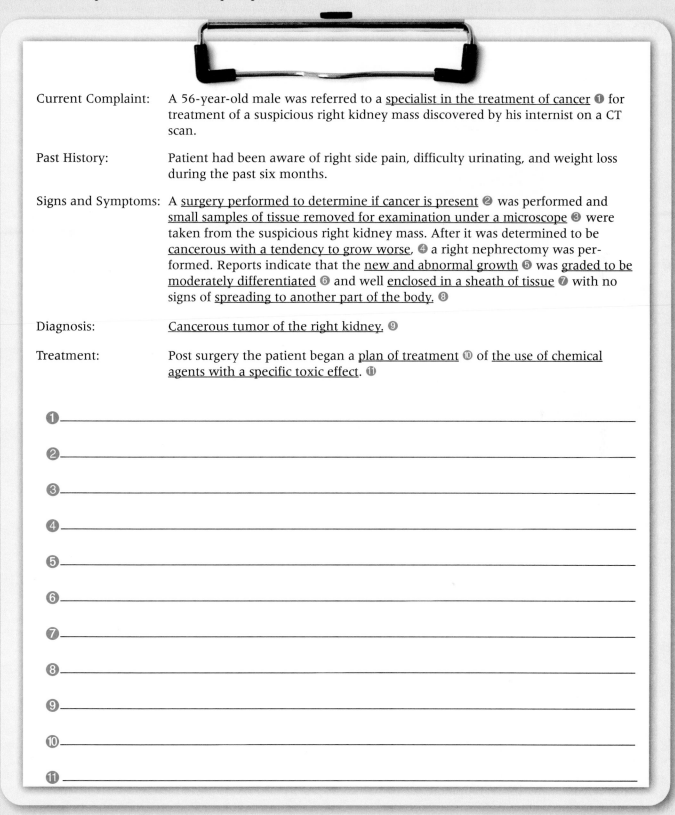

Current Complaint: A 56-year-old male was referred to a <u>specialist in the treatment of cancer</u> ❶ for treatment of a suspicious right kidney mass discovered by his internist on a CT scan.

Past History: Patient had been aware of right side pain, difficulty urinating, and weight loss during the past six months.

Signs and Symptoms: A <u>surgery performed to determine if cancer is present</u> ❷ was performed and <u>small samples of tissue removed for examination under a microscope</u> ❸ were taken from the suspicious right kidney mass. After it was determined to be <u>cancerous with a tendency to grow worse</u>, ❹ a right nephrectomy was performed. Reports indicate that the <u>new and abnormal growth</u> ❺ was <u>graded to be moderately differentiated</u> ❻ and well <u>enclosed in a sheath of tissue</u> ❼ with no signs of <u>spreading to another part of the body.</u> ❽

Diagnosis: <u>Cancerous tumor of the right kidney.</u> ❾

Treatment: Post surgery the patient began a <u>plan of treatment</u> ❿ of <u>the use of chemical agents with a specific toxic effect.</u> ⓫

❶ _____

❷ _____

❸ _____

❹ _____

❺ _____

❻ _____

❼ _____

❽ _____

❾ _____

❿ _____

⓫ _____

Multimedia Preview

Additional interactive resources and activities for this chapter can be found on the Companion Website. For videos, games, and pronunciations, please access the accompanying DVD-ROM that comes with this book.

DVD-ROM Highlights

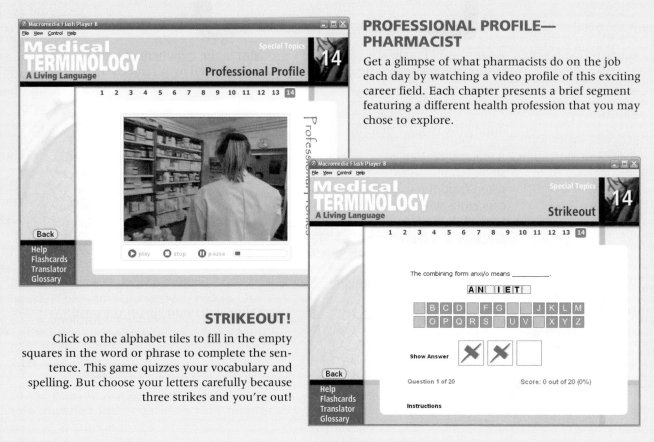

PROFESSIONAL PROFILE— PHARMACIST

Get a glimpse of what pharmacists do on the job each day by watching a video profile of this exciting career field. Each chapter presents a brief segment featuring a different health profession that you may chose to explore.

STRIKEOUT!

Click on the alphabet tiles to fill in the empty squares in the word or phrase to complete the sentence. This game quizzes your vocabulary and spelling. But choose your letters carefully because three strikes and you're out!

Website Highlights—www.prenhall.com/fremgen

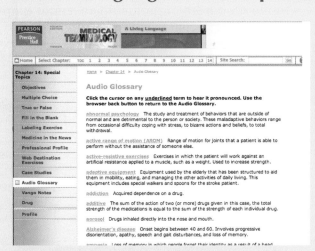

AUDIO GLOSSARY

Click here and take advantage of the free-access on-line study guide that accompanies your textbook. You'll find an audio glossary with definitions and audio pronunciations for every term in the book. By clicking on this URL you'll also access a variety of quizzes with instant feedback, links to download mp3 audio reviews, and current news articles.

Appendices

Appendix I

Abbreviations

Abbreviation	Meaning	Abbreviation	Meaning
@	at	ARF	acute renal failure
5-FU	5-fluorouracil	ARMD	age-related macular degeneration
^{67}Ga	radioactive gallium		
^{99m}Tc	radioactive technetium	AROM	active range of motion
^{131}I	radioactive iodine	AS	arteriosclerosis, left ear
^{133}Xe	radioactive xenon	ASA	aspirin
^{201}Tl	radioactive thallium	ASD	atrial septal defect
α	alpha	ASHD	arteriosclerotic heart disease
$\bar{a}$	before	ASL	American Sign Language
AAROM	active-assisted range of motion	AST	aspartate transaminase
AB	abortion	Astigm	astigmatism
ABGs	arterial blood gases	ATN	acute tubulor necrosis
ac	before meals	AU	both ears
ACTH	adrenocorticotropic hormone	AuD	doctor of audiology
AD	right ear, Alzheimer's disease	AV, A-V	atrioventricular
ad lib	as desired	β	beta
ADD	attention deficit disorder	Ba	barium
ADH	antidiuretic hormone	BaE	barium enema
ADHD	attention-deficit hyperactivity disorder	basos	basophil
		BBB	bundle branch block (L for left; R for right)
ADL	activities of daily living		
AE	above elbow	BC	bone conduction
AF	atrial fibrillation	BCC	basal cell carcinoma
AGN	acute glomerulonephritis	BDT	bone density testing
AI	artificial insemination	BE	barium enema, below elbow
AIDS	acquired immunodeficiency syndrome	bid	twice a day
		BK	below knee
AK	above knee	BM	bowel movement
ALL	acute lymphocytic leukemia	BMD	bone mineral density
ALS	amyotropic lateral sclerosis	BMR	basal metabolic rate
ALT	alanine transaminase	BMT	bone marrow transplant
AMI	acute myocardial infarction	BNO	bladder neck obstruction
AML	acute myelogenous leukemia	BP	blood pressure
Angio	angiography	BPD	bipolar disorder
ANS	autonomic nervous system	BPH	benign prostatic hypertrophy
ante	before	bpm	beats per minute
AP	anteroposterior	Bronch	bronchoscopy
APAP	acetaminophen (Tylenol)	BS	bowel sounds
aq	aqueous (water)	BSE	breast self-examination
ARC	AIDS-related complex	BSN	bachelor of science in nursing
ARDS	adult respiratory distress syndrome	BUN	blood urea nitrogen
		BX, bx	biopsy

Abbreviation	Meaning	Abbreviation	Meaning
$\bar{c}$	with	CV	cardiovascular
C1, C2, etc.	first cervical vertebra, second cervical vertebra, etc.	CVA	cerebrovascular accident
		CVD	cerebrovascular disease
Ca^{2+}	calcium	CVS	chorionic villus biopsy
CA	cancer, chronological age	Cx	cervix
CABG	coronary artery bypass graft	CXR	chest x-ray
CAD	coronary artery disease	cysto	cystoscopic exam
cap(s)	capsule(s)	d	day
CAPD	continuous ambulatory peritoneal dialysis	D	diopter (lens strength)
		D & C	dilation and curettage
CAT	computerized axial tomography	D/C, d/c	discontinue
		dB	decibel
cath	catheterization	DC	doctor of chiropractic
CBC	complete blood count	DDM	doctor of dental medicine
CBD	common bile duct	DDS	doctor of dental surgery
cc	cubic centimeter	DEA	Drug Enforcement Agency
CC	clean catch urine specimen, cardiac catheterization, chief complaint	decub	lying down, decubitus ulcer
		Derm, derm	dermatology
		DI	diabetes insipidus, diagnostic imaging
CCS	certified coding specialist		
CCU	cardiac care unit, coronary care unit	diff	differential
		dil	dilute
c.gl.	correction with glasses	disc	discontinue
chemo	chemotherapy	disp	dispense
CHF	congestive heart failure	DJD	degenerative joint disease
CIS	carcinoma in situ	DM	diabetes mellitus
Cl^-	chloride	DO	doctor of osteopathy
CLL	chronic lymphocytic leukemia	DOE	dyspnea on exertion
CLS	clinical laboratory scientist	DPT	diphtheria, pertussis, tetanus; doctor of physical therapy
CLT	clinical laboratory technician		
CMA	certified medical assistant	DRE	digital rectal exam
CML	chronic myelogenous leukemia	DSA	digital subtraction angiography
CNA	certified nurse aide	DSM-IV	*Diagnostic and Statistical Manual for Mental Disorders,* Fourth edition
CNS	central nervous system		
CO_2	carbon dioxide		
CoA	coarctation of the aorta	dtd	give of such a dose
COPD	chronic obstructive pulmonary disease	DTR	deep tendon reflex; dietetic technician, registered
COTA	certified occupational therapy assistant	DVA	distance visual acuity
		DVT	deep vein thrombosis
CP	cerebral palsy, chest pain	Dx	diagnosis
CPK	creatine phosphokinase	DXA	dual-energy absorptiometry
CPR	cardiopulmonary resuscitation	ECC	extracorporeal circulation
CRF	chronic renal failure	ECCE	extracapsular cataract extraction
crit	hematocrit		
CRT	certified respiratory therapist	ECG	electrocardiogram
C & S	culture and sensitivity test	Echo	echocardiogram
CS, CS-section	cesarean section	ECT	electroconvulsive therapy
CSD	congenital septal defect	ED	erectile dysfunction
CSF	cerebrospinal fluid	EDC	estimated date of confinement
CT	computerized tomography, cytotechnologist		
		EEG	electroencephalogram, electroencephalography
CTA	clear to auscultation		
CTS	carpal tunnel syndrome	EENT	eyes, ears, nose, throat

Abbreviation	Meaning	Abbreviation	Meaning
EGD	esophagogastroduodenoscopy	grav I	first pregnancy
EKG	electrocardiogram	gt	drop
ELISA	enzyme-linked immunosorbent assay	gtt	drops
		GTT	glucose tolerance test
EM	emmetropia	GU	genitourinary
EMB	endometrial biopsy	GVHD	graft vs. host disease
EMG	electromyogram	GYN, gyn	gynecology
EMT-B	emergency medical technician–basic	H_2O	water
		HA	headache
EMT-I	emergency medical technician–intermediate	HAV	hepatitis A virus
		Hb	hemoglobin
EMT-P	emergency medical technician–paramedic	HBV	hepatitis B virus
		HCG, hCG	human chorionic gonadotropin
Endo	endoscopy		
ENT	ear, nose, and throat	HCl	hydrochloric acid
EOM	extraocular movement	HCO_3^-	bicarbonate
eosins, eos	eosinophil	HCT, Hct	hematocrit
ER	emergency room	HCV	hepatitis C virus
ERCP	endoscopic retrograde cholangiopancreatography	HD	Hodgkin's disease, hemodialysis
ERT	estrogen replacement therapy	HDN	hemolytic disease of the newborn
ERV	expiratory reserve volume		
ESR	erythrocyte sedimentation rate	HDV	hepatitis D virus
		HEENT	head, ears, eyes, nose, throat
ESRD	end-stage renal disease	HEV	hepatitis E virus
e-stim	electrical stimulation	Hgb, HGB	hemoglobin
ESWL	extracorporeal shock-wave lithotripsy	HIV	human immunodeficieny virus
		HMD	hyaline membrane disease
et	and	HNP	herniated nucleus pulposus
EU	excretory urography	HPV	human papilloma virus
EUA	exam under anesthesia	HRT	hormone replacement therapy
FBS	fasting blood sugar	hs	at bed time
FDA	Federal Drug Administration	HSG	hysterosalpingography
FEKG	fetal electrocardiogram	HSV	*Herpes simplex* virus
FHR	fetal heart rate	HSV-1	*Herpes simplex* virus type 1
FHT	fetal heart tone	HTN	hypertension
FOBT	fecal occult blood test	Hz	hertz
FRC	functional residual capacity	ī	one
FS	frozen section	IBD	inflammatory bowel disease
FSH	follicle-stimulating hormone	IBS	irritable bowel syndrome
FTND	full-term normal delivery	IC	inspiratory capacity
FVC	forced vital capacity	ICCE	intracapsular cataract cryoextraction
Fx, FX	fracture		
GI	first pregnancy	ICP	intracranial pressure
GA	general anesthesia	ICU	intensive care unit
GB	gallbladder	I & D	incision and drainage
GC	gonorrhea	ID	intradermal
GERD	gastroesophageal reflux disease	IDDM	insulin-dependent diabetes mellitus
GH	growth hormone	Ig	immunoglobins (IgA, IgD, IgE, IgG, IgM)
GI	gastrointestinal		
gm	gram	ii	two
GOT	glutamic oxaloacetic transaminase	iii	three
		IM	intramuscular
gr	grain	inj	injection

Abbreviation	Meaning	Abbreviation	Meaning
I & O	intake and output	mL	milliliter
IOP	intraocular pressure	MLT	medical laboratory technician
IPD	intermittent peritoneal dialysis	MM	malignant melanoma
IPPB	intermittent positive pressure breathing	mm Hg	millimeters of mercury
		MMPI	Minnesota Multiphasic Personality Inventory
IRDS	infant respiratory distress syndrome	mono	mononucleosis
IRV	inspiratory reserve volume	monos	monocyte
IU	international unit	MR	mitral regurgitation
IUD	intrauterine device	MRA	magnetic resonance angiography
IV	intravenous		
IVC	intravenous cholangiogram	MRI	magnetic resonance imaging
IVF	*in vitro* fertilization	MS	mitral stenosis, multiple sclerosis, musculoskeletal
IVP	intravenous pyelogram		
JRA	juvenile rheumatoid arthritis	MSH	melanocyte-stimulating hormone
K⁺	potassium		
kg	kilogram	MSN	master of science in nursing
KS	Kaposi's sarcoma	MT	medical technologist
KUB	kidney, ureter, bladder	MTX	methotrexate
L	left, liter	MUA	manipulation under anesthesia
L1, L2, etc.	first lumbar vertebra, second lumbar vertebra, etc.	MVP	mitral valve prolapse
LASIK	laser-assisted in-situ keratomileusis	n & v	nausea and vomiting
		Na⁺	sodium
		NB	newborn
LAT, lat	lateral	NG	nasogastric (tube)
LBW	low birth weight	NHL	non-Hodgkin's lymphoma
LDH	lactate dehydrogenase	NIDDM	non–insulin-dependent diabetes mellitus
LE	lower extremity		
LGI	lower gastrointestinal series	NK	natural killer cells
LH	luteinizing hormone	NMR	nuclear magnetic resonance
LL	left lateral	no sub	no substitute
LLE	left lower extremity	noc	night
LLL	left lower lobe	non rep	do not repeat
LLQ	left lower quadrant	NP	nurse practitioner
LMP	last menstrual period	NPH	neutral protamine Hagedorn (insulin)
LP	lumbar puncture		
LPN	licensed practical nurse	NPO	nothing by mouth
LUE	left upper extremity	NS	normal saline, nephrotic syndrome
LUL	left upper lobe		
LUQ	left upper quadrant	NSAID	nonsteroidal anti-inflamma-tory drug
LVAD	left ventricular assist device		
LVH	left ventricular hypertrophy	O₂	oxygen
lymphs	lymphocyte	OA	osteoarthritis
LVN	licensed vocational nurse	OB	obstetrics
MA	mental age	OCD	obsessive-compulsive disorder
MAO	monoamine oxidase	OCPs	oral contraceptive pills
mcg	microgram	OD	overdose, right eye, doctor of optometry
MD	doctor of medicine, muscular dystrophy		
		oint	ointment
MDI	metered dose inhaler	OM	otitis media
mEq	milliequivalent	O & P	ova and parasites
mets	metastases	Ophth.	ophthalmology
mg	milligram	OR	operating room
MI	myocardial infarction, mitral insufficiency	ORIF	open reduction–internal fixation

Abbreviation	Meaning	Abbreviation	Meaning
Orth, ortho	orthopedics	pro-time	prothrombin time
OS	left eye	PROM	passive range of motion
OT	occupational therapy	prot	protocol
OTC	over the counter	PSA	prostate specific antigen
Oto	otology	pt	patient
OTR	occupational therapist	PT	prothrombin time, physical therapy, physical therapist
OU	each eye		
oz	ounce	PTA	physical therapy assistant
p̄	after	PTC	percutaneous transhepatic cholangiography
P	pulse		
PI	first delivery	PTCA	percutaneous transluminal coronary angioplasty
PA	posteroanterior, physician assistant, pernicious anemia		
		PTH	parathyroid hormone
PAC	premature atrial contraction	PUD	peptic ulcer disease
PAP	Papanicolaou test, pulmonary arterial pressure	PVC	premature ventricular contraction
para I	first delivery	q	every
PARR	postanesthetic recovery room	qam	every morning
PBI	protein-bound iodine	qd	once a day, every day
pc	after meals	qh	every hour
PCA	patient-controlled administration	qhs	every night
		qid	four times a day
PCP	Pneumocystis carinii pneumonia	qod	every other day
		qs	quantity sufficient
PCV	packed cell volume	R	respiration, right, roentgen
PDA	patent ductus arteriosus	Ra	radium
PDR	Physician's Desk Reference	RA	rheumatoid arthritis, room air
PE tube	pressure equalizing tube	rad	radiation absorbed dose
PEG	pneumoencephalogram, percutaneous endoscopic gastrostomy	RBC	red blood cell
		RD	registered dietitian
		RDH	registered dental hygienist
per	with	RDS	respiratory distress syndrome
PERRLA	pupils equal, round, react to light and accommodation	REEGT	registered electroencephalography technologist
PET	positron emission tomography	REM	rapid eye movement
PFT	pulmonary function test	REPT	registered evoked potential technologist
pH	acidity or alkalinity of urine		
PharmD	doctor of pharmacy	Rh–	Rh-negative
PID	pelvic inflammatory disease	Rh+	Rh-positive
PMNs	polymorphonuclear neutrophil	RHIA	registered health information administrator
PMS	premenstrual syndrome	RHIT	registered health information technician
PNS	peripheral nervous system		
PO, po	by mouth	RIA	radioimmunoassay
polys	polymorphonuclear neutrophil	RL	right lateral
		RLE	right lower extremity
PORP	partial ossicular replacement prosthesis	RLL	right lower lobe
		RLQ	right lower quadrant
pp	postprandial	RML	right mediolateral, right middle lobe
PPD	purified protein derivative (tuberculin test)		
		RN	registered nurse
preop, pre-op	preoperative	ROM	range of motion
prep	preparation, prepared	RP	retrograde pyelogram
PRK	photo refractive keratectomy	RPh	registered pharmacist
PRL	prolactin	RPR	rapid plasma reagin (test for syphilis)
prn	as needed		

Abbreviation	Meaning	Abbreviation	Meaning
RPSGT	registered polysomnographic technologist	susp	suspension
RRT	registered radiologic technologist, registered respiratory therapist	syr	syrup
		T	tablespoon
		t	teaspoon
RUE	right upper extremity	T & A	tonsillectomy and adenoidectomy
RUL	right upper lobe	T1, T2, etc.	first thoracic vertebra, second thoracic vertebra, etc.
RUQ	right upper quadrant		
RV	reserve volume	T_3	triiodothyronine
Rx	take	T_4	thyroxine
s̄	without	tab	tablet
S1	first heart sound	TAH	total abdominal hysterectomy
S2	second heart sound	TAH-BSO	total abdominal hysterectomy–bilateral salpingo-oophorectomy
SA, S-A	sinoatrial		
SAD	seasonal affective disorder		
SARS	severe acute respiratory syndrome	TB	tuberculosis
		tbsp	tablespoon
SC, sc	subcutaneous	TENS	transcutaneous electrical nerve stimulation
SCC	squamous cell carcinoma		
SCI	spinal cord injury	TFT	thyroid function test
SCIDS	severe combined immunodeficiency syndrome	THA	total hip arthroplasty
		THR	total hip replacement
sed-rate	erythrocyte sedimentation rate	TIA	transient ischemic attack
		tid	three times a day
segs	segmented neutrophils	TKA	total knee arthroplasty
SG	skin graft, specific gravity	TKR	total knee replacement
s.gl.	without correction or glasses	TLC	total lung capacity
SGOT	serum glutamic oxaloacetic transaminase	TNM	tumor, nodes, metastases
		TO	telephone order
SIDS	sudden infant death syndrome	top	apply topically
Sig	label as follows/directions	TORP	total ossicular replacement prosthesis
SK	streptokinase		
sl	under the tongue	tPA	tissue-type plasminogen activator
SLE	systemic lupus erythematosus		
SMAC	sequential multiple analyzer computer	TPN	total parenteral nutrition
		TPR	temperature, pulse, and respiration
SMD	senile macular degeneration		
SOB	shortness of breath	TSH	thyroid-stimulating hormone
sol	solution	tsp	teaspoon
SOM	serous otitis media	TSS	toxic shock syndrome
sp. gr.	specific gravity	TUR	transurethral resection
SPP	suprapubic prostatectomy	TURP	transurethral resection of prostate
SR	erythrocyte sedimentation rate		
		TV	tidal volume
ss̄	one-half	TX, Tx	traction, treatment
st	stage	u	unit
ST	esotropia	U/A, UA	urinalysis
stat, STAT	at once, immediately	UC	uterine contractions, urine culture
STD	skin test done, sexually transmitted disease		
		UE	upper extremity
STSG	split-thickness skin graft	UGI	upper gastrointestinal series
subcu	subcutaneous	ung	ointment
subq	subcutaneous	URI	upper respiratory infection
supp.	suppository	US	ultrasound
suppos	suppository	UTI	urinary tract infection

Abbreviation	Meaning
UV	ultraviolet
VA	visual acuity
VC	vital capacity
VCUG	voiding cystourethrography
VD	venereal disease
VF	visual field
VFib	ventricular fibrillation
VO	verbal order

Abbreviation	Meaning
VS	vital signs
VSD	ventricular septal defect
VT	ventricular tachycardia
WBC	white blood cell
wt	weight
x	times
XT	exotropia

Appendix II

Combining Forms

Combining Form	Meaning	Combining Form	Meaning
abdomin/o	abdomen	carcin/o	cancer
acous/o	hearing	cardi/o	heart
acr/o	extremities	carp/o	wrist
aden/o	gland	caud/o	tail
adenoid/o	adenoids	cec/o	cecum
adip/o	fat	cephal/o	head
adren/o	adrenal glands	cerebell/o	cerebellum
adrenal/o	adrenal glands	cerebr/o	cerebrum
aer/o	air	cerumin/o	cerumen
agglutin/o	clumping	cervic/o	neck, cervix
albin/o	white	chem/o	chemical, drug
alveol/o	alveolus; air sac	chol/e	bile, gall
ambly/o	dull or dim	cholangi/o	bile duct
amni/o	amnion	cholecyst/o	gallbladder
an/o	anus	choledoch/o	common bile duct
andr/o	male	chondr/o	cartilage
angi/o	vessel	chori/o	chorion
ankyl/o	stiff joint	chrom/o	color
anter/o	front	cis/o	to cut
anthrac/o	coal	clavicul/o	clavicle
anxi/o	anxiety	coagul/o	clotting
aort/o	aorta	coccyg/o	coccyx
append/o	appendix	cochle/o	cochlea
appendic/o	appendix	col/o	colon
aque/o	water	colon/o	colon
arteri/o	artery	colp/o	vagina
arthr/o	joint	coni/o	dust
articul/o	joint	conjunctiv/o	conjunctiva
atel/o	incomplete	core/o	pupil
ather/o	fatty substance, plaque	corne/o	cornea
atri/o	atrium	coron/o	heart
audi/o	hearing	cortic/o	outer portion
audit/o	hearing	cost/o	rib
aur/o	ear	crani/o	skull
auricul/o	ear	crin/o	secrete
azot/o	nitrogenous waste	crur/o	leg
bacteri/o	bacteria	cry/o	cold
balan/o	glans penis	crypt/o	hidden
bar/o	weight	culd/o	cul-de-sac
bas/o	base	cutane/o	skin
bi/o	life	cyan/o	blue
blast/o	primitive cell	cycl/o	ciliary muscle
blephar/o	eyelid	cyst/o	urinary bladder
brachi/o	arm	cyt/o	cell
bronch/o	bronchus	dacry/o	tear; tear duct
bronchi/o	bronchiole	dent/o	tooth
bronchiol/o	bronchiole	derm/o	skin
bucc/o	cheek	dermat/o	skin
burs/o	sac	diaphor/o	profuse sweating
calc/o	calcium	diaphragmat/o	diaphragm

Combining Form	Meaning	Combining Form	Meaning
dipl/o	double	ischi/o	ischium
dist/o	away from	jejun/o	jejunum
dors/o	back of body	kal/i	potassium
duoden/o	duodenum	kerat/o	cornea, hard, horny
electr/o	electricity	keton/o	ketone
embry/o	embryo	kinesi/o	movement
encephal/o	brain	kyph/o	hump
enter/o	small intestine	labi/o	lip
eosin/o	rosy red	labyrinth/o	labyrinth
epididym/o	epididymis	lacrim/o	tears
epiglott/o	epiglottis	lact/o	milk
episi/o	vulva	lamin/o	lamina, part of vertebra
epitheli/o	epithelium	lapar/o	abdomen
erg/o	work	laryng/o	larynx, voice box
erythr/o	red	later/o	side
esophag/o	esophagus	leuk/o	white
esthesi/o	feeling, sensation	lingu/o	tongue
estr/o	female	lip/o	fat
fasci/o	fibrous band	lith/o	stone
femor/o	femur	lob/o	lobe
fet/o	fetus	lord/o	bent backwards
fibr/o	fibers	lumb/o	loin
fibrin/o	fibers, fibrous	lymph/o	lymph
fibul/o	fibula	lymphaden/o	lymph node
fluor/o	fluorescence, luminous	lymphangi/o	lymph vessel
gastr/o	stomach	mamm/o	breast
gingiv/o	gums	mandibul/o	mandible
glauc/o	gray	mast/o	breast
gli/o	glue	maxill/o	maxilla
glomerul/o	glomerulus	meat/o	meatus
gloss/o	tongue	medi/o	middle
glute/o	buttock	medull/o	medulla oblongata, inner portion
glyc/o	sugar		
glycos/o	sugar, glucose	melan/o	black
gonad/o	sex glands	men/o	menses, menstruation
granul/o	granules	mening/o	meninges
gynec/o	female	meningi/o	meninges
hem/o	blood	ment/o	mind
hemangi/o	blood vessel	metacarp/o	metacarpals
hemat/o	blood	metatars/o	metatarsals
hepat/o	liver	metr/o	uterus
hidr/o	sweat	morph/o	shape
hist/o	tissue	muscul/o	muscle
home/o	sameness	mut/a	genetic change, mutation
humer/o	humerus	my/o	muscle
hydr/o	water	myc/o	fungus
hymen/o	hymen	myel/o	spinal cord, bone marrow
hyster/o	uterus	myocardi/o	heart muscle
ichthy/o	scaly, dry	myos/o	muscle
ile/o	ileum	myring/o	eardrum
ili/o	ilium	nas/o	nose
immun/o	immune, protection	nat/o	birth
infer/o	below	natr/o	sodium
ir/o	iris	necr/o	death
irid/o	iris	nephr/o	kidney

Combining Form	Meaning	Combining Form	Meaning
neur/o	nerve	poster/o	back
neutr/o	neutral	presby/o	old age
noct/i	night	proct/o	anus and rectum
nyctal/o	night	prostat/o	prostate
ocul/o	eye	prosth/o	addition
odont/o	tooth	proxim/o	near to
olig/o	scanty	psych/o	mind
onc/o	tumor	pub/o	pubis, genital region
onych/o	nail	pulmon/o	lung
oophor/o	ovary	pupill/o	pupil
ophthalm/o	eye	py/o	pus
opt/o	eye, vision	pyel/o	renal pelvis
optic/o	eye	pylor/o	pylorus
or/o	mouth	radi/o	x-ray, radius
orch/o	testes	radicul/o	nerve root
orchi/o	testes	rect/o	rectum
orchid/o	testes	ren/o	kidney
organ/o	organ	retin/o	retina
orth/o	straight, upright	rhin/o	nose
oste/o	bone	rhytid/o	wrinkle
ot/o	ear	roentgen/o	X-ray
ov/o	egg	sacr/o	sacrum
ovari/o	ovary	salping/o	fallopian tubes, uterine tubes, eustachian tubes
ox/i	oxygen		
ox/o	oxygen	sanguin/o	blood
palat/o	palate	scapul/o	scapula
pancreat/o	pancreas	schiz/o	divided
papill/o	optic disk	scler/o	hard, sclera
parathyroid/o	parathyroid gland	scoli/o	crooked, bent
patell/o	patella	seb/o	oil
path/o	disease	sect/o	cut
ped/o	foot, child	sialaden/o	salivary gland
pelv/o	pelvis	sigmoid/o	sigmoid colon
perine/o	perineum	sinus/o	sinus, cavity
peritone/o	peritoneum	somat/o	body
phac/o	lens	somn/o	sleep
phag/o	eat, swallow	son/o	sound
phalang/o	phalanges	spermat/o	sperm
pharmac/o	drug	sphygm/o	pulse
pharyng/o	throat, pharynx	spin/o	spine
phas/o	speech	spir/o	breathing
phleb/o	vein	splen/o	spleen
phon/o	sound	spondyl/o	vertebrae
phot/o	light	staped/o	stapes
phren/o	mind	stern/o	sternum
pil/o	hair	steth/o	chest
pineal/o	pineal gland	super/o	above
pituitar/o	pituitary gland	synovi/o	synovial membrane
plant/o	sole of the foot	synov/o	synovial membrane
pleur/o	pleura	system/o	system
pneum/o	lung, air	tars/o	ankle
pneumon/o	lung, air	ten/o	tendon
pod/o	foot	tend/o	tendon
poli/o	gray matter	tendin/o	tendon
pont/o	pons	testicul/o	testes

Combining Form	Meaning	Combining Form	Meaning
thalam/o	thalamus	urethr/o	urethra
thec/o	sheath (meninges)	urin/o	urine
therm/o	heat	uter/o	uterus
thorac/o	chest	uve/o	vascular
thromb/o	clot	vagin/o	vagina
thym/o	thymus	valv/o	valve
thyr/o	thyroid gland	valvul/o	valve
thyroid/o	thyroid gland	varic/o	varicose veins
tibi/o	tibia	vascul/o	blood vessel
tom/o	to cut	vas/o	vas deferens, vessel, duct
tonsill/o	tonsils	ven/o	vein
tox/o	poison	ventr/o	belly
toxic/o	poison	ventricul/o	ventricle
trache/o	trachea, windpipe	vertebr/o	vertebra
trich/o	hair	vesic/o	bladder
tympan/o	eardrum	vesicul/o	seminal vesicle
uln/o	ulna	viscer/o	internal organ
ungu/o	nail	vitre/o	glassy
ur/o	urine, urinary tract	vulv/o	vulva
ureter/o	ureter	xer/o	dry

Appendix III

Prefixes

Prefix	Meaning	Prefix	Meaning
a-	without, away from	micro-	small
ab-	away from	mono-	one
ad-	towards	multi-	many
allo-	other, different from usual	neo-	new
an-	without	nulli-	none
ante-	before, in front of	pan-	all
anti-	against	para-	beside, beyond, near
auto-	self	per-	through
bi-	two	peri-	around, about
brady-	slow	poly-	many
circum-	around	post-	behind, after
dys-	painful, difficult	pre-	before, in front of
endo-	within, inner	pseudo-	false
epi-	upon, over, above	quad-	four
eu-	normal, good	retro-	backward, behind
hemi-	half	semi-	partial, half
hetero-	different	sub-	below, under
homo-	same	super-	above, excess
hydro-	water	supra-	above
hyper-	over, above	tachy-	rapid, fast
hypo-	under, below	trans-	through, across
infra-	under, beneath, below	tri-	three
inter-	among, between	ultra-	beyond, excess
intra-	within, inside	uni-	one
macro-	large	xeno-	strange, foreign

Appendix IV

Suffixes

Suffix	Meaning	Suffix	Meaning
-ac	pertaining to	-ism	state of
-al	pertaining to	-itis	inflammation
-algesia	pain, sensitivity	-kinesia	movement
-algia	pain	-listhesis	slipping
-an	pertaining to	-lith	stone
-apheresis	removal, carry away	-lithiasis	condition of stones
-ar	pertaining to	-logist	one who studies
-arche	beginning	-logy	study of
-ary	pertaining to	-lucent	to shine through
-asthenia	weakness	-lysis	destruction
-blast	immature, embryonic	-malacia	abnormal softening
-capnia	carbon dioxide	-mania	excessive excitement
-cele	hernia, protrusion	-manometer	instrument to measure pressure
-centesis	puncture to withdraw fluid	-megaly	enlargement, large
-cise	cut	-meter	instrument for measuring
-clasia	to surgically break	-metrist	one who measures
-crine	to secrete	-metry	process of measuring
-cusis	hearing	-ole	small
-cyesis	state of pregnancy	-oma	tumor, mass
-cyte	cell	-opaque	nontransparent
-cytosis	more than the normal number of cells	-opia	vision
		-opsy	view of
-derma	skin	-orexia	appetite
-desis	stabilize, fuse	-ory	pertaining to
-dipsia	thirst	-ose	pertaining to
-dynia	pain	-osis	abnormal condition
-eal	pertaining to	-osmia	smell
-ectasia	dilation	-ostomy	surgically create an opening
-ectasis	dilation, expansion	-otia	ear condition
-ectomy	surgical removal, excision	-otomy	cutting into, incision
-emesis	vomit	-ous	pertaining to
-emia	blood condition	-para	to bear (offspring)
-esthesia	feeling, sensation	-paresis	weakness
-gen	that which produces	-partum	childbirth
-genesis	produces, generates	-pathy	disease
-genic	producing, produced by	-penia	abnormal decrease, too few
-globin	protein	-pepsia	digestion
-globulin	protein	-pexy	surgical fixation
-gram	record, picture	-phage	eat, swallow
-graph	instrument for recording	-phagia	eat, swallow
-graphy	process of recording	-phasia	speech
-gravida	pregnancy	-phil	attracted to
-ia	state, condition	-philia	to have an attraction for
-iac	pertaining to	-phobia	irrational fear
-iasis	abnormal condition	-phonia	voice
-iatrist	physician	-phoresis	carrying
-ic	pertaining to	-plasia	growth, formation, development
-ical	pertaining to		
-ile	pertaining to	-plasm	growth, formation, development
-ior	pertaining to		

Suffix	Meaning	Suffix	Meaning
-plasty	surgical repair	-stasis	standing still
-plegia	paralysis	-stenosis	narrowing
-pnea	breathing	-taxia	muscular coordination
-poiesis	formation	-tension	pressure
-porosis	porous	-therapy	treatment
-prandial	pertaining to a meal	-thorax	chest
-ptosis	drooping	-tic	pertaining to
-ptysis	spitting	-tocia	labor, childbirth
-rrhage	excessive, abnormal flow	-tome	instrument used to cut
-rrhaphy	suture	-tonia	tone
-rrhea	discharge, flow	-tripsy	surgical crushing
-rrhexis	rupture	-trophy	nourishment, development
-salpinx	fallopian tube	-tropia	to turn
-sclerosis	hardening	-tropin	stimulate
-scope	instrument for viewing	-ule	small
-scopy	process of visually examining	-uria	condition of the urine
-spermia	condition of sperm		

Chapter Review Answers

Chapter 1 Answers

Practice Exercises

A. 1. combining form 2. o 3. suffix 4. prefix 5. spelling 6. word root, combining vowel, prefix, suffix

B. 1. gland 2. cancer 3. heart 4. chemical 5. to cut 6. skin 7. small intestines 8. stomach 9. female 10. blood 11. water 12. immune 13. voice box 14. shape 15. kidney 16. nerve 17. eye 18. ear 19. lung 20. nose 21. urine, urinary tract

C. 1. surgical repair 2. narrowing 3. inflammation of 4. pertaining to 5. pain 6. cutting into 7. enlargement 8. surgical removal of 9. excessive, abnormal flow 10. puncture to remove fluid 11. record or picture 12. pertaining to 13. abnormal softening 14. state of 15. to suture 16. surgical creation of opening 17. surgical fixation 18. discharge or flow 19. process of visually examining 20. tumor, mass

D. 1. pulmonology 2. neuralgia or neurodynia 3. rhinorrhea 4. nephromalacia 5. cardiomegaly 6. gastrotomy 7. dermatitis 8. laryngectomy 9. arthroplasty 10. adenopathy

E. 1. intra-/endo- 2. macro- 3. pre-/ante- 4. peri- 5. neo- 6. a-/an- 7. hemi-/semi- 8. dys- 9. supra-/super-/hyper- 10. hyper-/super- 11. poly-/multi- 12. brady- 13. auto- 14. trans- 15. bi-

F. 1. tachy-, fast 2. pseudo-, false 3. hypo-, under/below 4. inter-, among/between 5. eu-, normal/good 6. post-, after 7. mono-, one 8. sub-, below/under

G. 1. metastases 2. ova 3. diverticula 4. atria 5. diagnoses 6. vertebrae

H. 1. cardiology 2. gastrology 3. dermatology 4. ophthalmology 5. urology 6. nephrology 7. hematology 8. gynecology 9. neurology 10. pathology

I. 1. cardiomalacia 2. gastrostomy 3. rhinoplasty 4. hypertrophy 5. pathology 6. adenoma 7. gastroenterology 8. otitis 9. hydrotherapy 10. carcinogen

J. 1. l 2. e 3. j 4. f 5. d 6. k 7. m 8. o 9. g 10. n 11. b 12. h 13. a 14. c 15. i

Chapter 2 Answers

Practice Exercises

A. 1. cells, tissues, organs, systems, body 2. cell membrane, cytoplasm, nucleus 3. histology 4. epithelial 5. anatomical 6. right lower 7. cranial, spinal 8. nine 9. right iliac 10. pleural, pericardial

B. 1. c 2. a 3. b

C. 1. n 2. f 3. k 4. d 5. a 6. e 7. m 8. i 9. b 10. j 11. h 12. l 13. c 14. g

D. 1. epi-; above 2. inter-; between 3. intra-; within 4. peri-; around or about 5. hypo-; under or below 6. retro-; behind or backward 7. sub-; under or below 8. trans-; through or across

E. 1. dorsal 2. thoracic 3. superior 4. caudal 5. visceral 6. lateral 7. distal 8. neural 9. systemic 10. muscular 11. ventral 12. anterior 13. cephalic 14. medial

F. 1. MS 2. lat 3. RUQ 4. CV 5. GI 6. AP 7. OB 8. LLQ

G. 1. internal organ 2. back 3. abdomen 4. chest 5. middle 6. belly 7. front 8. tissues 9. epithelium 10. skull 11. body 12. near to 13. head

H. 1. integumentary, d 2. cardiovascular, i 3. digestive, g 4. female reproductive, b 5. musculoskeletal (skeletal), a 6. respiratory, j 7. urinary, c 8. male reproductive, f 9. nervous, h 10. musculoskeletal (muscular), e

I. 1. a 2. c 3. f 4. e 5. a 6. d 7. b 8. e 9. c 10. b

J. 1. cephalic 2. pubic 3. crural 4. gluteal 5. cervical 6. brachial 7. dorsum 8. thoracic

K. 1. otorhinolaryngology 2. cardiology 3. gynecology 4. orthopedics 5. ophthalmology 6. urology 7. dermatology 8. gastroenterology

Labeling Exercise

A. 1. cell 2. tissue 3. organ 4. system 5. whole body

B1. 1. frontal or coronal plane 2. sagittal or median plane 3. transverse or horizontal plane

B2. 1. cephalic 2. cervical 3. thoracic 4. brachial 5. abdominal 6. pelvic 7. pubic 8. crural 9. trunk 10. vertebral 11. dorsum 12. gluteal

Chapter 3 Answers

Practice Exercises

A. 1. epidermis, dermis, subcutaneous layer 2. basal cell 3. adipose 4. dermis 5. keratin 6. melanin 7. corium 8. nail bed 9. sebaceous, sweat 10. apocrine

B. 1. dermatitis 2. dermatosis 3. dermatome 4. dermatologist 5. dermatoplasty 6. dermatology 7. melanoma 8. melanocyte 9. ichthyoderma 10. leukoderma 11. erythroderma 12. onychomalacia 13. paronychia 14. onychophagia 15. onychectomy

C. 1. cold 2. skin 3. profuse sweating 4. pus 5. blue 6. nail 7. fat 8. sweat 9. wrinkles 10. oil 11. hair 12. death

D. 1. flat, discolored area 2. small solid raised spot less than 0.5 cm 3. fluid filled sac 4. crack-like lesion 5. raised spot containing pus 6. small, round swollen area 7. fluid-filled blister 8. open sore 9. firm, solid mass larger than 0.5 cm 10. torn or jagged wound

E. 1. redness involving superficial layer of skin 2. burn damage through epidermis and into dermis causing vesicles 3. burn damage to full thickness of epidermis and dermis

F. 1. e 2. f 3. i 4. j 5. a 6. c 7. l 8. g 9. k 10. h 11. d 12. b

G. 1. h 2. i 3. j 4. e 5. c 6. a 7. f 8. g 9. b 10. d

H. 1. FS 2. I & D 3. ID 4. subq, subcu, SC, sc 5. UV 6. BX, bx

I. 1. culture and sensitivity 2. basal cell carcinoma 3. dermatology 4. skin graft 5. decubitus ulcer 6. malignant melanoma

J. 1. xeroderma 2. petechiae 3. tinea 4. scabies 5. paronychia 6. Kaposi's sarcoma 7. impetigo 8. keloid 9. exfoliative cytology 10. frozen section

K. 1. hypodermic, or subcutaneous 2. intradermal 3. epidermis

L. 1. graft from another human 2. graft from another species 3. graft from self 4. graft from another species

M. 1. antifungal, f 2. antipruritic, d 3. antiparasitic, a 4. anti-viral, c 5. corticosteroid cream, b 6. anesthetic, g 7. antibiotic, e

Medical Record Analysis

1. c—intense itching (urticaria) 2. translated into student's own words: size of 10 × 14 mm; left cheek 20 mm anterior to the ear; erythema; poorly defined borders, de-pigmentation, vesicles 3. wear sunscreen and a hat 4. congestive heart failure; CHF; dyspnea, lower extremity edema, cyanosis 5. biopsy 6. excision; dermatoplasty

Chart Note Transcription

1. ulcer 2. dermatologist 3. pruritus 4. erythema 5. pustules 6. dermis 7. necrosis 8. culture and sensitivity 9. cellulitis 10. debridement

Labeling Exercise

A. 1. epidermis 2. dermis 3. subcutaneous layer 4. sweat gland 5. sweat duct 6. hair 7. sebaceous gland 8. arrector pili muscle 9. sensory receptors

B1. 1. epidermis 2. dermis 3. subcutaneous layer 4. sebaceous gland 5. arrector pili muscle 6. hair shaft 7. hair follicle 8. hair root 9. papilla

B2. 1. free edge 2. lateral nail groove 3. lunula 4. nail bed 5. nail body 6. cuticle 7. nail root

Chapter 4 Answers

Practice Exercises

A. 1. axial, appendicular 2. smooth 3. frame, protect vital organs, work with muscles for movement, store minerals, red blood cell production 4. myoneural 5. short 6. periosteum 7. wrist 8. cancellous 9. synovial 10. skeletal, smooth, cardiac 11. foramen 12. diaphysis

B. 1. osteocyte 2. osteoblast 3. osteoporosis 4. osteopathy 5. osteotomy 6. osteotome 7. osteomyelitis 8. osteomalacia 9. osteochondroma 10. myopathy 11. myoplasty 12. myorrhaphy 13. electromyogram 14. myasthenia 15. tenodynia 16. tenorrhaphy 17. arthrodesis 18. arthroplasty 19. arthrotomy 20. arthritis 21. arthrocentesis 22. arthralgia 23. chondrectomy 24. chondroma 25. chondromalacia

C. 1. -desis 2. -asthenia 3. -listhesis 4. -clasia 5. -kinesia 6. -porosis

D. 1. femoral 2. sternal 3. clavicular 4. coccygeal 5. maxillary 6. tibial 7. patellar 8. phalangeal 9. humeral 10. pubic

E. 1. lamina, part of vertebra 2. stiff joint 3. cartilage 4. vertebrae 5. muscle 6. straight 7. hump 8. tendon 9. bone marrow 10. joint

F. 1. surgical repair of cartilage 2. slow movement 3. porous bone 4. abnormal increase in lumbar spine curve (swayback) 5. lack of development/nourishment 6. bone marrow tumor 7. artificial substitute for a body part 8. skull incision 9. puncture of a joint to withdraw fluid 10. bursa inflammation

G. 1. cervical, 7 2. thoracic, 12 3. lumbar, 5 4. sacrum, 1 (5 fused) 5. coccyx, 1 (3–5 fused)

H. 1. S = -scopy; visual examination of inside of a joint 2. P = inter-, S = -al; pertaining to between vertebrae 3. S = -malacia; softening of cartilage 4. S = -ectomy; surgical removal of disk 5. P = intra- S = -al; pertaining to inside the skull 6. P = sub-, -ar = pertaining to; pertaining to under the scapula

I. 1. e 2. d 3. b 4. c 5. a 6. h 7. g 8. f

J. 1. c 2. h 3. f 4. g 5. d 6. e 7. a 8. b

K. 1. medical doctor who treats musculoskeletal system 2. uses manipulation of vertebral column 3. specialty that treats disorders of feet 4. fitting of braces and splints 5. fabricates and fits artificial limbs

L. 1. patella 2. tarsals 3. clavicle 4. femur 5. phalanges 6. carpals 7. tibia 8. scapula 9. phalanges

M. 1. degenerative joint disease 2. electromyogram 3. first cervical vertebra 4. sixth thoracic vertebra 5. intramuscular 6. deep tendon reflex 7. juvenile rheumatoid arthritis 8. left lower extremity 9. orthopedics 10. carpal tunnel syndrome

N. 1. IM 2. TKR 3. HNP 4. DTR 5. UE 6. L5 7. BDT 8. AK 9. fx/FX 10. NSAID

O. 1. osteoporosis 2. rickets 3. lateral epicondylitis 4. herniated nucleus pulposus 5. osteogenic sarcoma 6. scoliosis 7. pseudotrophic muscular dystrophy 8. systemic lupus erythematosus 9. spondylolisthesis 10. carpal tunnel syndrome

P. 1. nonsteroidal anti-inflammatory drugs, b 2. corticosteroids, e 3. skeletal muscle relaxants, a 4. bone reabsorption inhibitors, c 5. calcium supplements, d

Medical Record Analysis

1. rehabilitation specialist; Motrin (a nonsteroidal anti-inflammatory medication), physical therapy for range of motion and strengthening exercises, and low-fat, low-calorie diet 2. arthroscopy; torn lateral meniscus and chondromalacia; arthroscopic meniscectomy 3. a—nonsurgical treatments, such as medicine and therapy; b—a patient who has not been admitted to the hospital 4. physical therapy for lower extremity ROM and strengthening exercises, and gait training with a walker; occupational therapy for ADL instruction, especially dressing and personal care 5. patient was able to bend knee to 90° but lacked 5° of being able to straighten it back out; 6. a—blockage of arteries to the heart muscle; b—high blood pressure

Chart Note Transcription

1. Colles' fracture (fx) 2. cast 3. fracture 4. orthopedist 5. osteoporosis 6. computerized axial tomography (CT or CAT scan) 7. flexion 8. extension 9. comminuted fracture (fx) 10. femur 11. total hip arthroplasty (THA)

Labeling Exercise

A. 1. skull 2. cervical vertebrae 3. sternum 4. ribs 5. thoracic vertebrae 6. lumbar vertebrae 7. ilium 8. pubis 9. ischium 10. femur 11. patella 12. tibia 13. fibula 14. tarsals 15. metatarsals 16. phalanges 17. maxilla 18. mandible 19. scapula 20. humerus 21. ulna 22. radius 23. sacrum 24. coccyx 25. carpals 26. metacarpals 27. phalanges

B1. 1. proximal epiphysis 2. diaphysis 3. distal epiphysis 4. articular cartilage 5. epiphyseal line 6. spongy or cancellous bone 7. compact or cortical bone 8. medullary cavity

B2. 1. periosteum 2. synovial membrane 3. articular cartilage 4. joint cavity 5. joint capsule

Chapter 5 Answers

Practice Exercises

A. 1. cardiology 2. endocardium, myocardium, epicardium 3. sinoatrial node 4. away from 5. tricuspid, pulmonary, mitral (bicuspid), aortic 6. atria, ventricles 7. pulmonary 8. apex 9. septum 10. systole, diastole

B. 1. cardiac 2. cardiomyopathy 3. cardiomegaly 4. tachycardia 5. bradycardia 6. cardiorrhexis 7. angiostenosis 8. angiitis 9. angiospasm 10. arterial 11. arteriosclerosis 12. arteriole

C. 1. endocarditis 2. epicarditis 3. myocarditis

D. 1. heart 2. valve 3. chest 4. artery 5. vein 6. vessel 7. ventricle 8. clot 9. atrium 10. fatty substance

E. 1. venous 2. cardiology 3. venogram 4. electrocardiography 5. hypertension 6. hypotension 7. valvoplasty 8. interventricular 9. atherectomy 10. arteriostenosis

F. 1. -tension 2. -stenosis 3. -manometer 4. -ule, -ole 5. –sclerosis

G. 1. blood pressure 2. congestive heart failure 3. myocardial infarction 4. coronary care unit 5. premature ventricular contraction 6. cardiopulmonary resuscitation 7. coronary artery disease 8. chest pain 9. electrocardiogram 10. first heart sound

H. 1. MVP 2. VSD 3. PTCA 4. Vfib 5. DVT 6. LDH 7. CoA 8. tPA 9. CV 10. ECC

I. 1. f 2. h 3. d 4. g 5. b 6. i 7. a 8. c 9. e 10. j

J. 1. thin flexible tube 2. an area of dead tissue 3. a blood clot 4. pounding heartbeat 5. backflow 6. weakened and ballooning arterial wall 7. complete stoppage of heart activity 8. serious cardiac arrhythmia 9. heart attack 10. varicose veins in anal region

K. 1. c 2. g 3. j 4. a 5. d 6. b 7. i 8. e 9. f 10. h

L. 1. antiarrhythmic, e 2. antilipidemic, g 3. cardiotonic, f 4. diuretic, h 5. anticoagulant, b 6. thrombolytic, a 7. vasodilator, d 8. calcium channel blocker, c

M. 1. murmur 2. defibrillation 3. hypertension 4. pacemaker 5. varicose veins 6. angina pectoris 7. CCU 8. MI 9. angiography 10. echocardiogram 11. Holter monitor 12. CHF

Medical Record Analysis

1. Lopressor to control blood pressure, Norpace to slow down the heart rate, Valium to reduce anxiety, Lasix to reduce swelling 2. EKG, cardiac enzymes blood test; myocardial infarction 3. patient developed dyspnea and cyanosis 4. b—dizziness 5. mitral valve replacement 6. compare: both conditions allow blood to flow backwards; contrast: prolapse—too floppy, valve droops down, and stenosis—too stiff, preventing it from opening all the way or closing all the way

Chart Note Transcription

1. angina pectoris 2. bradycardia 3. hypertension 4. myocardial infarction (MI) 5. electrocardiogram (EKG, ECG) 6. cardiac enzymes 7. coronary artery disease (CAD) 8. cardiac catheterization 9. stress test (treadmill test) 10. percutaneous transluminal coronary angioplasty (PTCA) 11. coronary artery bypass graft (CABG)

Labeling Exercise

A. 1. heart 2. artery 3. vein 4. capillary

B1. 1. right atrium 2. right ventricle 3. pulmonary arteries 4. capillary bed lungs 5. pulmonary veins 6. left atrium 7. left ventricle 8. aorta 9. systemic arteries 10. systemic capillary beds 11. systemic veins 12. vena cavae

B2. 1. right atrium 2. tricuspid valve 3. right ventricle 4. pulmonary valve 5. pulmonary trunk 6. pulmonary artery 7. pulmonary vein 8. left atrium 9. mitral or bicuspid valve 10. left ventricle 11. aortic valve 12. aorta 13. superior vena cava 14. inferior vena cava 15. endocardium 16. myocardium 17. pericardium

Chapter 6 Answers

Practice Exercises

A. 1. hematology 2. spleen, tonsils, thymus 3. thoracic duct, right lymphatic duct 4. axillary, cervical, mediastinal, inguinal 5. phagocytosis 6. erythrocytes (red blood cells), leukocytes (white blood cells), platelets (thrombocytes) 7. plasma 8. active acquired 9. antibody-mediated 10. hemostasis

B. 1. splenomegaly 2. splenectomy 3. splenotomy 4. lymphocytes 5. lymphoma 6. lymphadenopathy 7. lymphadenoma 8. lymphadenitis 9. immunologist 10. immunoglobulin 11. immunology 12. hematic 13. hematoma 14. hematopoiesis 15. hemolytic 16. hemoglobin

C. 1. leukopenia 2. erythropenia 3. thrombopenia 4. pancytopenia 5. leukocytosis 6. erythrocytosis 7. thrombocytosis 8. hemoglobin 9. immunoglobulin 10. erythrocyte 11. leukocyte 12. lymphocyte

D. 1. lymphaden/o 2. thromb/o 3. sanguin/o, hem/o, hemat/o 4. tonsill/o 5. tox/o 6. phag/o 7. lymphangi/o 8. path/o 9. splen/o 10. lymph/o

E. 1. basophil 2. complete blood count 3. hemoglobin 4. prothrombin time 5. graft vs. host disease 6. red blood count/red blood cell 7. packed cell volume 8. erythrocyte sedimentation rate 9. differential 10. lymphocyte

F. 1. AIDS 2. ARC 3. HIV 4. ALL 5. BMT 6. mono 7. KS 8. eosins, eos 9. IG 10. SCIDS

G. 1. g 2. i 3. e 4. a 5. h 6. d 7. c 8. j 9. b 10. f

H. 1. c 2. h 3. d 4. a 5. e 6. b 7. f 8. g 9. j 10. i

I. 1. d 2. f 3. b 4. g 5. a 6. e 7. c

J. 1. reverse transcriptase inhibitor, e 2. anticoagulant, a 3. antihemorrhagic, d 4. antihistamine, h 5. immunosuppresant, f 6. thrombolytic, b 7. hematinic, g 8. corticosteroid, c 9. antiplatelet, i

K. 1. polycythemia vera 2. mononucleosis 3. anaphylactic shock 4. HIV 5. Kaposi's sarcoma 6. AIDS 7. Hodgkin's disease 8. *Pneumocystis carinii* 9. aplastic 10. pernicious

Medical Record Analysis

1. feeling "run down," intermittent diarrhea, weight loss, dry cough 2. negative means absence; there was no evidence of pneumonia in the X-ray 3. a—the original or critical reaction; b—contained within a capsule; c—fluid collecting within the abdominal cavity; d—spread to a dis-

tant site 4. ultrasound 5. d—an enlarged spleen (splenomegaly) 6. magnetic resonance image (MRI); brain, liver 7. resolved: ascites, diarrhea; persisted: dry cough

Chart Note Transcription

1. hematologist 2. ELISA 3. prothrombin time 4. complete blood count (CBC) 5. erythropenia 6. thrombopenia 7. leukocytosis 8. bone marrow aspiration 9. leukemia 10. homologous transfusion

Labeling Exercise

A. 1. plasma 2. red blood cells or erythrocytes 3. platelets or thrombocytes 4. white blood cells or leukocytes

B1. 1. thymus gland 2. lymph node 3. tonsil 4. spleen 5. lymphatic vessels

B2. 1. cervical nodes 2. mediastinal nodes 3. axillary nodes 4. inguinal nodes

Chapter 7 Answers

Practice Exercises

A. 1. exchange of O_2 and CO_2 2. ventilation 3. exchange of O_2 and CO_2 in the lungs 4. exchange of O_2 and CO_2 at cellular level 5. nasal cavity, pharynx, larynx, trachea, bronchial tubes, lungs 6. pharynx 7. epiglottis 8. filter out dust 9. diaphragm 10. 12–20 11. 30–60 12. 3; 2 13. alveoli 14. pleura 15. palate 16. bronchioles

B. 1. rhinitis 2. rhinorrhagia 3. rhinorrhea 4. rhinoplasty 5. laryngitis 6. laryngospasm 7. laryngoscopy 8. laryngeal 9. laryngotomy 10. laryngectomy 11. laryngoplasty 12. laryngoplegia 13. bronchial 14. bronchitis 15. bronchoscopy 16. bronchogenic 17. bronchospasm 18. thoracoplasty 19. thoracotomy 20. thoracalgia 21. thoracic 22. tracheotomy 23. tracheoplasty 24. tracheostenosis 25. endotracheal 26. tracheitis 27. tracheostomy

C. 1. trachea or windpipe 2. larynx 3. bronchus 4. breathing 5. lung or air 6. nose 7. dust 8. pleura 9. epiglottis 10. alveolus or air sac 11. lung 12. oxygen 13. sinus 14. lobe 15. nose

D. 1. dilation 2. carbon dioxide 3. voice 4. chest 5. breathing 6. spitting 7. smell

E. 1. eupnea 2. dyspnea 3. tachypnea 4. orthopnea 5. apnea

F. 1. volume of air in the lungs after a maximal inhalation or inspiration 2. amount of air entering lungs in a single inspiration or leaving air in single expiration of quiet breathing 3. air remaining in the lungs after a forced expiration

G. 1. inhalation or inspiration 2. hemoptysis 3. pulmonary emboli 4. sinusitis 5. pharyngitis 6. pneumothorax 7. pertussis 8. pleurotomy 9. pleurisy 10. nasopharyngitis

H. 1. URI 2. PFT 3. LLL 4. O_2 5. CO_2 6. IPPB 7. COPD 8. Bronch 9. TLC 10. TB 11. IRDS

I. 1. chest X-ray 2. tidal volume 3. temperature, pulse, respirations 4. arterial blood gases 5. dyspnea on exertion 6. right upper lobe 7. sudden infant death syndrome 8. total lung capacity 9. adult respiratory distress syndrome 10. metered dose inhaler 11. clear to auscultation 12. severe acute respiratory syndrome

J. 1. e 2. k 3. h 4. a 5. j 6. l 7. c 8. g 9. f 10. b 11. d 12. i

K. 1. cardiopulmonary resuscitation 2. thoracentesis 3. respirator 4. supplemental oxygen 5. patent 6. ventilation-perfusion scan 7. sputum cytology 8. hyperventilation 9. rhonchi 10. anthracosis

L. 1. decongestant, f 2. antitussive, a 3. antibiotic, c 4. expectorant, g 5. mucolytic, h 6. bronchodilator, d 7. antihistamine, e 8. corticosteroid, b

Medical Record Analysis

1. sudden attack 2. intravenous, immediately, arterial blood gases 3. steroid to reduce inflammation; Alupent to relax bronchospasms 4. what triggers his attacks; referred patient to an allergist 5. hacking and producing thick, nonpurulent phlegm 6. a—crackling lung sounds

Chart Note Transcription

1. dyspnea 2. tachypnea 3. arterial blood gases (ABGs) 4. hypoxemia 5. auscultation 6. rales 7. purulent 8. sputum 9. CXR 10. pneumonia 11. endotracheal intubation

Labeling Exercise

A. 1. pharynx and larynx 2. trachea 3. nasal cavity 4. bronchial tubes 5. lungs

B1. 1. nares 2. paranasal sinuses 3. nasal cavity 4. pharyngeal tonsil 5. Eustachian tube 6. hard palate 7. soft palate 8. palatine tonsil 9. epiglottis 10. vocal cords 11. esophagus 12. trachea

B2. 1. trachea 2. right upper lobe 3. right middle lobe 4. right lower lobe 5. apex of lung 6. left upper lobe 7. left lower lobe 8. diaphragm

Chapter 8 Answers

Practice Exercises

A. 1. gastrointestinal 2. gut, alimentary canal, mouth, anus 3. salivary glands, liver, gallbladder, pancreas 4. digesting food, absorbing nutrients, eliminating waste 5. cutting, grinding 6. peristalsis 7. hydrochloric acid, chyme 8. duodenum, jejunum, ileum 9. sigmoid 10. bile, emulsification, gallbladder

B. 1. esophagus 2. liver 3. ileum 4. anus and rectum 5. tongue 6. lip 7. jejunum 8. sigmoid colon 9. rectum 10. gum 11. gallbladder 12. duodenum 13. anus 14. small intestine 15. teeth

C. 1. gastritis 2. gastroenterology 3. gastrectomy 4. gastroscopy 5. gastralgia 6. gastromegaly 7. gastrotomy 8. esophagitis 9. esophagoscopy 10. esophagoplasty 11. esophageal 12. esophagectasis 13. proctopexy 14. proctoptosis 15. proctitis 16. proctologist 17. cholecystectomy 18. cholecystolithiasis 19. cholecystolithotripsy 20. cholecystitis 21. laparoscope 22. laparotomy 23. laparoscopy 24. hepatoma 25. hepatomegaly 26. hepatic 27. hepatitis 28. pancreatitis 29. pancreatic 30. colostomy 31. colitis

D. 1. postprandial 2. cholelithiasis 3. anorexia 4. dysphagia 5. hematemesis 6. bradypepsia

E. 1. bowel movement 2. upper gastrointestinal series 3. barium enema 4. bowel sounds 5. nausea and vomiting 6. ova and parasites 7. by mouth 8. common bile duct 9. nothing by mouth 10. postprandial

F. 1. NG 2. GI 3. HBV 4. FOBT 5. IBD 6. HSV-1 7. AST 8. pc 9. PUD 10. GERD

G. 1. visual exam of the colon 2. tooth x-ray 3. bright red blood in the stools 4. blood test to determine amount of waste product in the bloodstream 5. weight loss and wasting from a chronic illness 6. use NG tube to wash out stomach 7. surgical repair of hernia 8. pulling teeth 9. surgical crushing of common bile duct stone 10. surgically create a connection between two organs

H. 1. h 2. i 3. f 4. c 5. a 6. j 7. l 8. e 9. b 10. k 11. d 12. g 13. o 14. p 15. n 16. m

I. 1. liver biopsy 2. colostomy 3. barium swallow 4. lower GI series 5. colectomy 6. fecal occult blood test 7. choledocholithotripsy 8. total parenteral nutrition 9. gastric stapling 10. intravenous cholecystography 11. colonoscopy 12. ileostomy

J. 1. d 2. g 3. h 4. e 5. f 6. b 7. c 8. a

K. 1. antidiarrheal, g 2. proton pump inhibitor, h 3. emetic, f 4. antiemetic, d 5. H_2-receptor antagonist, a 6. anorexiant, b 7. laxative, c 8. antacid, e

Medical Record Analysis

1. left upper quadrant, stomach, spleen 2. complete blood count (CBC), occult blood test 3. gastroscopy; a deep ulcer 1.5 cm in diameter, evidence of bleeding 4. gastric carcinoma 5. d—a blood transfusion 6. tonsillectomy, compound fracture, BPH, and TUR

Chart Note Transcription

1. gastroenterologist 2. constipation 3. cholelithiasis 4. cholecystectomy 5. gastroesophageal reflux disease 6. ascites 7. lower gastrointestinal series 8. polyposis 9. colonoscopy 10. sigmoid colon 11. colectomy 12. colostomy

Labeling Exercise

A. 1. salivary glands 2. esophagus 3. pancreas 4. small intestine 5. oral cavity 6. stomach 7. liver and gallbladder 8. colon

B1. 1. esophagus 2. cardiac or lower esophageal sphincter 3. pyloric sphincter 4. duodenum 5. antrum 6. fundus of stomach 7. rugae 8. body of stomach

B2. 1. cystic duct 2. common bile duct 3. gallbladder 4. duodenum 5. liver 6. hepatic duct 7. pancreas 8. pancreatic duct

Chapter 9 Answers

Practice Exercises

A. 1. nephrons 2. filtration, reabsorption, secretion 3. electrolytes 4. retroperitoneal 5. hilum 6. glomerulus 7. calyx 8. two, one 9. micturition, voiding 10. urinalysis

B. 1. nephropexy 2. nephrogram 3. nephrolithiasis 4. nephrectomy 5. nephritis 6. nephropathy 7. nephrosclerosis 8. cystitis 9. cystorrhagia 10. cystoplasty 11. cystoscope 12. cystalgia 13. pyeloplasty 14. pyelitis 15. pyelogram 16. ureterolith 17. ureterectasis 18. ureterostenosis 19. urethritis 20. urethroscope

C. 1. urine 2. meatus 3. urinary bladder 4. kidney 5. renal pelvis 6. sugar 7. night 8. scanty 9. ureter 10. glomerulus

D. 1. drooping 2. condition of the urine 3. stone 4. surgical crushing 5. condition of stones

E. 1. urination, voiding 2. increases urine production 3. pain associated with kidney stone 4. inserting a tube through urethra into the bladder 5. inflammation of renal pelvis 6. inflammation of glomeruli in the kidney 7. incision to remove stone

8. bedwetting 9. enlargement of uretheral opening 10. damage to glomerulus secondary to diabetes mellitus 11. lab test of chemical composition of urine 12. decrease in force of urine stream

F. 1. anuria 2. hematuria 3. calculus/nephrolith 4. lithotripsy 5. urethritis 6. pyuria 7. bacteriuria 8. dysuria 9. ketonuria 10. proteinuria 11. polyuria

G. 1. K^+ 2. Na^+ 3. UA 4. BUN 5. SG, sp.gr. 6. IVP 7. BNO 8. I & O 9. ATN 10. ESRD

H. 1. kidneys, ureters, bladder 2. catheter/catheterization 3. cystoscopy 4. genitourinary 5. extracorporeal shockwave lithotripsy 6. urinary tract infection 7. urine culture 8. retrograde pyelogram 9. acute renal failure 10. blood urea nitrogen 11. chronic renal failure 12. water

I. 1. c 2. g 3. h 4. i 5. f 6. e 7. d 8. b 9. a 10. j

J. 1. renal transplant 2. nephropexy 3. urinary tract infection 4. pyelolithectomy 5. renal biopsy 6. ureterectomy 7. cystostomy 8. cystoscopy 9. IVP

K. 1. antispasmodic, b 2. antibiotic, c 3. diuretic, a

Medical Record Analysis

1. bladder neck obstruction 2. severe right side pain, unable to stand fully erect, 101°F temperature, sweaty, and flushed skin 3. large enough to be visible with the naked eye 4. a—present from birth; b—of long duration; c—disease-causing; d—by mouth 5. a—protein 6. alike: both are infections of kidney tissue; different: glomerulonephritis—infection is in the glomerulus and it allows protein to leak into the urine; pyelonephritis—infection is in the renal pelvis portion of the kidney, more common, often caused by bladder infection moving up the ureters to the kidney

Chart Note Transcription

1. urologist 2. hematuria 3. cystitis 4. clean-catch specimen 5. urinalysis (U/A, UA) 6. pyuria 7. retrograde pyelogram 8. ureter 9. ureterolith 10. extracorporeal shockwave lithotripsy (ESWL) 11. calculi

Labeling Exercise

A. 1. kidney 2. urinary bladder 3. ureter 4. male urethra 5. female urethra

B1. 1. cortex 2. medulla 3. calyx 4. renal pelvis 5. renal papilla 6. renal pyramid 7. ureter

B2. 1. efferent arteriole 2. glomerular (Bowman's) capsule 3. glomerulus 4. afferent arteriole 5. proximal convoluted tubule 6. descending loop of Henle 7. distal convoluted tubule 8. collecting tubule 9. ascending loop of Henle 10. peritubular capillaries

Chapter 10 Answers

Practice Exercises

A. 1. gynecology 2. gynecologist 3. dilation, expulsion, placental 4. gestation 5. menopause 6. ovum 7. endometrium 8. uterus 9. fallopian tubes 10. total abdominal hysterectomy–bilateral salpingo-oophorectomy

B. 1. colposcopy 2. colposcope 3. cervicectomy 4. cervicitis 5. cervical 6. hysteropexy 7. hysterectomy 8. hysterorrhexis 9. oophoritis 10. oophorectomy 11. mammary 12. mammogram 13. mammoplasty 14. amniotic 15. amniotomy 16. amniorrhea

C. 1. cervix 2. last menstrual period 3. fetal heart rate 4. pelvic inflammatory disease 5. gynecology 6. cesarean section 7. newborn 8. premenstrual syndrome 9. toxic shock syndrome 10. low birth weight

D. 1. GI, grav I 2. AI 3. UC 4. FTND 5. IUD 6. D & C 7. HRT 8. gyn/GYN 9. AB 10. OCPs

E. 1. uterus 2. uterus 3. female 4. vulva 5. ovary 6. ovary 7. fallopian tube 8. menstruation or menses 9. vagina 10. breast

F. 1. b 2. e 3. h 4. c 5. i 6. j 7. d 8. n 9. l 10. f 11. o 12. g 13. k 14. m 15. a

G. 1. conization 2. stillbirth 3. puberty 4. premenstrual syndrome 5. laparoscopy 6. fibroid tumor 7. D & C 8. eclampsia 9. endometriosis 10. cesarean section

H. 1. labor, childbirth 2. pregnancy 3. beginning 4. pregnancy 5. childbirth 6. to bear (offspring) 7. fallopian tube 8. sperm condition

I. 1. e 2. i 3. h 4. c 5. a 6. d 7. g 8. b 9. f

J. 1. urinary, reproductive 2. testes, epididymis, penis 3. foreskin 4. testes 5. bulbourethral glands 6. testosterone 7. perineum

K. 1. prostatectomy 2. prostatic 3. prostatitis 4. orchiectomy 5. orchioplasty 6. orchiotomy 7. andropathy 8. androgen 9. spermatogenesis 10. spermatolysis

L. 1. suprapubic prostatectomy 2. transurethral resection 3. genitourinary 4. benign prostatic hypertrophy 5. digital rectal exam 6. prostate-specific antigen

M. 1. the formation of mature sperm 2. accumulation of fluid within the testes 3. surgical removal of the prostate gland by inserting a device through the urethra and removing prostate tissue 4. failure to produce sperm 5. surgical removal of the testes 6. surgical removal of part or all of the vas deferens 7. removal of testicles in male or ovaries in female

N. 1. androgen therapy, f 2. oxytocin, a 3. antiprostatic agent, b 4. birth control pills, g 5. kills sperm, d

6. erectile dysfunction agent, h 7. hormone replacement therapy, i 8. abortifacient, e 9. fertility drug, c

Medical Record Analysis

1. oophorectomy and chemotherapy; full body CT scan
2. menarche at 13, menorrhagia with chronic anemia
3. c—nullipara and d—multigravida 4. pelvic ultrasound; because the placenta overlies the cervix, it will detach before the baby can physically be born 5. size consistent with 25 weeks of gestation, turned head down, umbilical cord is not around the neck, fetal heart tones are strong, male, no evidence of developmental or genetic disorders
6. a—a greater than normal level of risk of problems developing or fetal death with this pregnancy; b—she looks like she is 8 months pregnant (her abdomen is not too small or too large)

Chart Note Transcription

1. ejaculation 2. cryptorchidism 3. orchidopexy
4. vasectomy 5. ejaculation 6. digital rectal exam (DRE)
7. prostate cancer 8. prostate-specific antigen (PSA)
9. benign prostatic hypertrophy (BPH) 10. transurethral resection (TUR)

Labeling Exercise

A1. 1. fallopian tube 2. ovary 3. fundus of uterus
    4. corpus (body) of uterus 5. cervix 6. vagina
    7. clitoris 8. labium majora 9. labia minora

A2. 1. seminal vesicles 2. vas deferens 3. prostate gland
    4. bulbourethral gland 5. urethra 6. epididymis
    7. glans penis 8. testis

B. 1. areola 2. nipple 3. lactiferous gland 4. lactiferous duct 5. fat

Chapter 11 Answers

Practice Exercises

A. 1. endocrinology 2. pituitary 3. gonads 4. corticosteroids 5. testosterone 6. estrogen, progesterone
    7. antidiuretic hormone (ADH) 8. thymus gland
    9. exophthalmos 10. adenocarcinoma

B. 1. thyroidectomy 2. thyroidal 3. hyperthyroidism
    4. pancreatic 5. pancreatitis 6. pancreatectomy
    7. pancreatotomy 8. adrenal 9. adrenomegaly
    10. adrenopathy 11. thymoma 12. thymectomy
    13. thymic 14. thymitis

C. 1. b 2. a 3. e 4. k 5. h 6. j 7. i 8. f 9. g 10. c
    11. d

D. 1. protein-bound iodine 2. potassium 3. thyroxine
    4. glucose tolerance test 5. diabetes mellitus 6. basal metabolic rate 7. sodium 8. antidiuretic hormone

E. 1. NIDDM 2. IDDM 3. ACTH 4. PTH 5. T_3 6. TSH
    7. FBS 8. PRL

F. 1. glycosuria 2. endocrine 3. polyuria 4. hypercalcemia 5. polydipsia 6. adrenocorticotropin
    7. postprandial

G. 1. hormone obtained from cortex of adrenal gland
    2. having excessive hair 3. a nerve condition characterized with spasms of extremities; can occur from imbalance of pH and calcium or disorder of parathyroid gland 4. disorder of the retina occurring with diabetes mellitus 5. increase in blood sugar level
    6. decrease in blood sugar level 7. another term for epinephrine; produced by inner portion of adrenal gland 8. hormone produced by pancreas; essential for metabolism of blood sugar 9. toxic condition due to hyperactivity of thyroid gland 10. a condition resulting when the endocrine gland secretes more hormone than is needed by the body

H. 1. sodium 2. female 3. pineal gland 4. pituitary gland 5. potassium 6. calcium 7. parathyroid glands 8. extremities 9. sugar 10. sex glands

I. 1. e 2. d 3. a 4. f 5. c 6. b

J. 1. insulinoma 2. ketoacidosis 3. panhypopituitarinism
    4. pheochromocytoma 5. Hashimoto's disease
    6. gynecomastia

K. 1. corticosteroids, e 2. human growth hormone therapy, a 3. oral hypoglycemic agent, d 4. antithyroid agent, c 5. insulin, f 6. vasopressin, b

Medical Record Analysis

1. hyperglycemia; ketoacidosis; glycosuria 2. student answers will vary 3. a—damage to the retina as a result of diabetes; b—a therapeutic plan; c—state of profound unconsciousness; d—twice a day 4. fasting blood sugar, serum glucose level, 2-hour postprandial glucose tolerance test 5. abdominal X-ray, pancreas CT scan 6. 2,000-calorie ADA diet with three meals and two snacks, may engage in any activity, return to school next Monday, check serum glucose level b.i.d., and call office for insulin dosage

Chart Note Transcription

1. endocrinologist 2. obesity 3. hirsutism 4. radioimmunoassay (RIA) 5. cortisol 6. adenoma 7. adrenal cortex 8. Cushing's syndrome 9. adenoma 10. adrenal cortex 11. adrenalectomy

Labeling Exercise

A. 1. pineal gland 2. thyroid and parathyroid glands 3. adrenal glands 4. pancreas 5. pituitary gland 6. thymus gland 7. ovary 8. testis

B1. 1. pituitary gland 2. bone and soft tissue 3. GH 4. testes 5. FSH, LH 6. ovary 7. FSH, LH 8. thyroid gland 9. TSH 10. adrenal cortex 11. ACTH 12. breast 13. PRL

B2. 1. liver 2. stomach 3. pancreas 4. beta cell 5. alpha cell 6. islet of Langerhans

Chapter 12 Answers

Practice Exercises

A. 1. neurology 2. brain, spinal cord, nerves 3. peripheral nervous system, central nervous system 4. efferent or motor 5. afferent or sensory 6. cerebrum 7. cerebellum 8. eyesight 9. hearing, smell 10. parasympathetic, sympathetic

B. 1. neuritis 2. neurologist 3. neuralgia 4. polyneuritis 5. neurectomy 6. neuroplasty 7. neuroma 8. neurorrhaphy 9. meningitis 10. meningocele 11. myelomeningocele 12. encephalogram 13. encephalopathy 14. encephalitis 15. encephalocele 16. cerebrospinal 17. cerebral

C. 1. b 2. f 3. g 4. h 5. i 6. a 7. e 8. c 9. d

D. 1. transient ischemic attack 2. multiple sclerosis 3. spinal cord injury 4. central nervous system 5. peripheral nervous system 6. headache 7. cerebral palsy 8. lumbar puncture 9. amyotrophic lateral sclerosis

E. 1. CSF 2. CVD 3. EEG 4. ICP 5. PET 6. CVA 7. SAH 8. ANS

F. 1. h 2. k 3. d 4. g 5. a 6. b 7. f 8. j 9. e 10. l 11. i 12. c

G. 1. injecting radiopaque dye into spinal canal to examine under X-ray the outlines made by the dye 2. X-ray of the blood vessels of the brain after the injection of radiopaque dye 3. reflex test on bottom of foot to detect lesion and abnormalities of nervous system 4. measures how fast an impulse travels along a nerve 5. laboratory examination of fluid taken from the brain and spinal cord 6. positron emission tomography to measure cerebral blood flow, blood volume, oxygen, and glucose uptake 7. recording the ultrasonic echoes of the brain 8. needle puncture into the spinal cavity to withdraw fluid

H. 1. paralysis 2. muscular coordination 3. pain, sensitivity 4. weakness 5. speech 6. feeling, sensation

I. 1. meninges 2. brain 3. cerebellum 4. spinal cord 5. head 6. thalamus 7. nerve 8. nerve root 9. cerebrum 10. pons

J. 1. tumor of astrocyte cells 2. seizure 3. without sensation 4. paralysis of one-half of body 5. physician that treats nervous system with surgery 6. without pain, sensitivity 7. localized seizure of one limb 8. paralysis of all four limbs 9. accumulation of blood in the subdural space 10. within the meninges

K. 1. d 2. e 3. f 4. g 5. b 6. a 7. c 8. j 9. h 10. i

L. 1. delirium 2. amyotrophic lateral sclerosis 3. Bell's palsy 4. cerebral aneurysm 5. Parkinson's disease 6. cerebrospinal fluid shunt 7. transient ischemic attack 8. subdural hematoma 9. cerebral palsy 10. nerve conduction velocity

M. 1. anesthetic, e 2. dopaminergic drugs, a 3. hypnotic, d 4. analgesic, g 5. sedative, b 6. narcotic analgesic, c 7. anticonvulsant, f

Medical Record Analysis

1. the muscles that receive nerve supply from or below the 2nd lumbar vertebra are paralyzed 2. no, the spinal cord was completely severed 3. a—comminuted—shattered bone; b—sanguinous—bloody; c—decubitus ulcer—pressure sore; d—catheterization—thin, flexible tube inserted into the bladder 4. d—leg strengthening 5. independent transfers, independent wheelchair mobility, independent ADLs 6. lumbar laminectomy with spinal fusion; stabilize the fracture and remove the epidural hematoma

Chart Note Transcription

1. neurologist 2. dysphasia 3. hemiparesis 4. convulsions 5. electroencephalography (EEG) 6. lumbar puncture (LP) 7. brain scan 8. cerebral cortex 9. astrocytoma 10. craniotomy 11. cryosurgery

Labeling Exercise

A. 1. brain 2. spinal nerves 3. spinal cord

B1. 1. dendrites 2. nerve cell body 3. unmyelinated region 4. myelinated axon 5. nucleus 6. axon 7. terminal end fibers

B2. 1. cerebrum 2. diencephalon 3. thalamus 4. hypothalamus 5. brain stem 6. midbrain 7. pons 8. cerebellum 9. medulla oblongata

Chapter 13 Answers

Practice Exercises

A.   1. ophthalmology 2. cilia 3. lacrimal 4. cornea 5. retina 6. iris 7. malleus, incus, stapes 8. otology 9. tympanic membrane 10. cerumen 11. eustachian or auditory 12. vestibulocochlear nerve

B.   1. blepharitis 2. blepharoplasty 3. blepharoptosis 4. retinopathy 5. retinopexy 6. ophthalmology 7. ophthalmic 8. ophthalmoscopy 9. iridoplegia 10. iridectomy 11. otoplasty 12. otopyorrhea 13. otalgia 14. otitis 15. tympanorrhexis 16. tympanotomy 17. tympanitis 18. audiogram 19. audiometer 20. audiology

C.   1. conductive—problem with outer or middle ear, muffles sound; sensorineural—damage of inner ear or nerve 2. cornea, pupil, lens, retina 3. mucous membrane that covers and protects front of eyeball 4. incus, malleus, stapes, vibrate to amplify and conduct sound waves from outer ear to inner ear

D.   1. -tropia 2. -opia 3. -itis 4. -logy 5. -otomy 6. -plasty 7. -pexy 8. -algia 9. -otia 10. -cusis

E.   1. tear or tear duct 2. choroid 3. water 4. light 5. cornea 6. glassy 7. double 8. gray 9. old age 10. dull or dim 11. ear 12. stapes 13. hearing 14. eustachian or auditory tube 15. eardrum or tympanic membrane

F.   1. dull/dim vision 2. double vision 3. enlarge or widen pupil 4. constrict pupil 5. diminished vision of old age 6. ringing in the ears 7. middle ear bone 8. measure movement in eardrum 9. auditory tube 10. inner ear 11. results of hearing test 12. middle ear infection

G.   1. h 2. g 3. a 4. d 5. b 6. i 7. c 8. f 9. e 10. j

H.   1. c 2. b 3. d 4. a 5. e 6. j 7. i 8. f 9. h 10. g

I.   1. otology 2. both eyes 3. rapid eye movement 4. hertz 5. senile macular degeneration 6. pupils equal, round, react to light and accommodation 7. intraocular pressure 8. decibel 9. right eye 10. visual field

J.   1. PE tube 2. EENT 3. BC 4. AU 5. OM 6. EM 7. XT 8. OS 9. EOM 10. VA

K.   1. tonometry 2. emmetropia 3. conjunctivitis 4. myopia 5. cataract 6. hordeolum 7. strabismus 8. hyperopia 9. presbycusis 10. otorhinolaryngologist 11. inner ear 12. Ménière's disease 13. acoustic neuroma

L.   1. artificial tears, h 2. antiglaucoma medication, c 3. antibiotic otic solution, i 4. mydriatic, a 5. antiemetic, g 6. antibiotic ophthalmic solution, j 7. anti-inflammatory otic solution, b 8. miotic, f 9. wax emulsifier, e 10. anesthetic ophthalmic solution, d

Medical Record Analysis

1. pupils open and close correctly when the physician shines a light into the eye; pupils become smaller in bright light and larger in dim light; it is important to prevent too much light from reaching the inside of the eyeball 2. eye muscles, conjunctiva, iris/pupil, retina, macular area of the retina, cornea 3. breast cancer with a mastectomy, cholelithiasis with a cholecystectomy 4. dilate the pupil, miotic drops 5. a—farsightedness (hyperopia) 6. cryoextraction

Chart Note Transcription

1. otorhinolaryngologist (ENT) 2. otitis media (OM) 3. AU, binaural 4. otoscopy 5. tympanic membrane 6. cerumen 7. tympanometry 8. audiometric test 9. conductive hearing loss 10. myringotomy

Labeling Exercise

A1. 1. iris 2. lens 3. conjunctiva 4. pupil 5. cornea 6. suspensory ligaments 7. ciliary body 8. fovea centralis 9. optic nerve 10. retina 11. choroid 12. sclera

A2. 1. pinna 2. external auditory meatus 3. auditory canal 4. tympanic membrane 5. malleus 6. incus 7. semicircular canals 8. vestibular nerve 9. cochlear nerve 10. cochlea 11. round window 12. stapes 13. Eustachian tube

B.   1. superior lacrimal gland 2. inferior lacrimal gland 3. lacrimal sac 4. lacrimal ducts 5. nasolacrimal duct

Chapter 14 Answers

Practice Exercises

A.   1. *Physician's Desk Reference* (PDR) 2. pharmacist 3. generic or nonproprietary 4. brand or proprietary 5. the chemical formula 6. Drug Enforcement Agency

B.   1. sublingual 2. rectal 3. topical 4. intradermal 5. intramuscular 6. intravenous 7. oral

C.   1. unusual or abnormal response to a drug 2. administration of a drug through a needle and syringe under the skin, or into a muscle, vein, or body cavity 3. harmless substance to satisfy patient's desire for medication 4. extent to which a substance is poisonous 5. response to drug other than the expected response 6. prepackaged and prelabeled method of medication distribution 7. emotional dependence on a drug 8. substance that neutralizes poisons 9. condition under which a particular drug should not be used 10. prevention of disease

D. 1. grain 2. two times a day 3. three times a day 4. as desired 5. as needed 6. before 7. over the counter 8. drop 9. label as follows/directions 10. immediately 11. milligrams 12. every day 13. night 14. nothing by mouth 15. at bedtime 16. intravenous 17. telephone order 18. drops 19. after meals 20. discontinue

E. 1. Pravachol, 20 milligrams each, take one every day at bedtime, supply with 30, refill three times with no substitutions 2. Lanoxin, 0.125 milligram each, take three now and then 2 every morning, supply with 100 and may refill as needed 3. Synthroid, 0. 075 milligram each, take 1 every day, supply with 100 and may refill four times 4. Norvasc, 5 milligram each, take 1 every morning, supply with 60 and may refill

F. 1. i 2. k 3. h 4. j 5. e 6. f 7. b 8. a 9. d 10. c 11. g

G. 1. minor tranquilizers 2. humanistic psychotherapy 3. lithium 4. antipsychotic drugs 5. psychoanalysis 6. antidepressant drugs

H. 1. magnetic resonance imaging 2. barium 3. anteroposterior 4. computerized tomography 5. right lateral 6. posteroanterior 7. left lateral 8. positive emission tomography 9. upper gastrointestinal series 10. kidneys, ureters, bladder

I. 1. h 2. c 3. b 4. g 5. f 6. a 7. d 8. e 9. i

J. 1. range of motion 2. occupational therapy 3. activities of daily living 4. lower extremity 5. electromyogram 6. transcutaneous electrical nerve stimulation 7. physical therapy 8. passive range of motion 9. electrical stimulation 10. ultrasound

K. 1. massage 2. debridement 3. hydrotherapy 4. postural drainage with clapping 5. active exercises 6. phonophoresis 7. cryotherapy 8. traction

L. 1. h 2. e 3. j 4. g 5. a 6. i 7. c 8. f 9. b 10. d

M. 1. general anesthesia 2. local anesthesia 3. topical anesthesia 4. regional anesthesia

N. 1. h 2. d 3. g 4. j 5. f 6. b 7. i 8. a 9. e 10. c

Medical Record Analysis

1. a—dyspnea—difficulty breathing; b—cough producing thick sputum—coughing up thick mucus material c—hemoptysis—coughing blood 2. a—uterus surgically removed due to endometrium becoming displaced in the pelvic cavity; b—gallbladder removed due to gallstones 3. increased thoracic curvature, musculoskeletal system 4. a—shortness of breath; b—computed tomography scan 5. a—incision into the chest; b—removal of a lobe of the lung 6. the tumor has spread to other areas of the body

Chart Note Transcription

1. oncologist 2. exploratory surgery 3. biopsies 4. malignant 5. neoplasm 6. Grade II 7. encapsulated 8. metastases 9. nephrocarcinoma 10. protocol 11. chemotherapy

Glossary/Index

Activities of daily living (ADL), the activities usually performed in the course of a normal day, such as eating, dressing, and washing, 484, 484f

Acute care hospitals, hospitals that typically provide services to diagnose (laboratory, diagnostic imaging) and treat (surgery, medications, therapy) diseases for a short period of time. In addition, they usually provide emergency and obstetrical care. Also called general hospital, 11

Acute respiratory distress syndrome, 221

Acute tubular necrosis (ATN), damage to the renal tubules due to presence of toxins in the urine or to ischemia; results in oliguria, 291

Adam's apple, 212, 366f

Adaptive equipment, equipment that has been structured to aid in mobility, eating, and managing the other activities of daily living. This equipment includes special walkers and spoons for the stroke patient, 485, 485f

Addiction, acquired dependence on a drug, 469

Addison's disease, disease that results from a deficiency in adrenocortical hormones. There may be an increased pigmentation of the skin, generalized weakness, and weight loss, 369

Additive, the sum of the action of two (or more) drugs given; in this case, the total strength of the medications is equal to the sum of the strength of each individual drug, 469

Adduction, directional term meaning to move toward the median or middle line of the body, 8, 108, 108f

Adenocarcinoma, malignant adenoma in a glandular organ, 371

Adenoidectomy, excision of the adenoids, 187

Adenoiditis, inflammation of the adenoid tissue, 187

Adenoids, another term for pharyngeal tonsils. The tonsils are a collection of lymphatic tissue found in the nasopharynx to combat microorganisms entering the body through the nose or mouth, 184, 211, 212

ADH, 373

Adhesion, scar tissue forming in the fascia surrounding a muscle making it difficult to stretch the muscle, 111

Adipose, a type of connective tissue. Also called fat. It stores energy and provides protective padding for underlying structures, 23

Adjective suffixes, 7

ADL, 488

Adrenal, pertaining to the adrenal gland, 366

Adrenal cortex, the outer portion of the adrenal glands; secretes several families of hormones: mineralocorticoids, glucocorticoids, and steroid sex hormones, 358t, 360, 360f

Adrenal feminization, development of female secondary sexual characteristics (such as breasts) in a male; often as a result of increased estrogen secretion by the adrenal cortex, 369

Adrenal glands, a pair of glands in the endocrine system located just above each kidney. These glands are composed of two sections, the cortex and the medulla, that function independently of each other. The cortex secretes steroids, such as aldosterone, cortisol, androgens, estrogens, and progestins. The medulla secretes epinephrine and norepinephrine. The adrenal glands are regulated by adrenocorticotropin hormone, which is secreted by the pituitary gland, 28t, 357f, 358, 358t, 360, 360f

Adrenal medulla, the inner portion of the adrenal gland. It secretes epinephrine and norepinephrine, 358t, 360, 360f

Adrenal virilism, development of male secondary sexual characteristics (such as deeper voice and facial hair) in a female; often as a result of increased androgen secretion by the adrenal cortex, 369

Adrenalectomy, excision of the adrenal gland, 367

Adrenaline, a hormone produced by the adrenal medulla. Also known as epinephrine. Some of its actions include increasing heart rate and force of contraction, bronchodilation, and relaxation of intestinal muscles, 358t, 360

Adrenalitis, inflammation of an adrenal gland, 367

Adrenocorticotropin hormone (ACTH), a hormone secreted by anterior pituitary. It regulates function of the adrenal gland cortex, 359t, 363–64

Adrenomegaly, enlarged adrenal gland, 366

Adrenopathy, adrenal gland disease, 366

Adult respiratory distress syndrome (ARDS), acute respiratory failure in adults characterized by tachypnea, dyspnea, cyanosis, tachycardia, and hypoxemia, 221

Aerosol, drugs inhaled directly into the nose and mouth, 467, 468

Aerosol therapy, medication suspended in a mist that is intended to be inhaled. Delivered by a *nebulizer*, which delivers the mist for a period of time while the patient breathes, or a *metered dose inhaler* (MDI), which delivers a single puff of mist, 225

Afferent, 283

Afferent arteriole, arteriole that carries blood into the glomerulus, 283, 284f, 286f

Afferent neurons, nerve that carries impulses to the brain and spinal cord from the skin and sense organs. Also called sensory neurons, 395, 396

Agglutinate, clumping together to form small clusters. Platelets agglutinate to start the clotting process, 172

Agranulocytes, nongranular leukocyte. This is one of the two types of leukocytes found in plasma that are classified as either monocytes or lymphocytes, 171, 171*t,* 173

AIDS, 192

AIDS-related complex (ARC), early stage of AIDS. There is a positive test for the virus but only mild symptoms of weight loss, fatigue, skin rash, and anorexia, 189

Alanine transaminase (ALT), an enzyme normally present in the blood. Blood levels are increased in persons with liver disease, 260

Albinism, a condition in which the person is not able to produce melanin. An albino person has white hair and skin and the pupils of the eye are red, 59

Albumin, a protein that is normally found circulating in the bloodstream. It is abnormal for albumin to be in the urine, 170, 286

Aldosterone, a hormone produced by the adrenal cortex. It regulates the levels of sodium and potassium in the body and as a side effect the volume of water lost in urine, 358*t,* 360

Alimentary canal, also known as the gastrointestinal system or digestive system. This system covers the area between the mouth and the anus and includes 30 feet of intestinal tubing. It has a wide range of functions. This system serves to store and digest food, absorb nutrients, and eliminate waste. The major organs of this system are the mouth, pharynx, esophagus, stomach, small intestine, colon, rectum, and anus, 244

Allergen, antigen capable of causing a hypersensitivity or allergy in the body, 187

Allergist, a physician who specializes in testing for and treating allergies, 187

Allergy, hypersensitivity to a substance in the environment or a medication, 187

Allograft, skin graft from one person to another; donor is usually a cadaver, 64

Alopecia, absence or loss of hair, especially of the head, 63

ALS, 408

ALT, 264

Alveoli, the tiny air sacs at the end of each bronchiole. The alveoli are surrounded by a capillary network. Gas exchange takes place as oxygen and carbon dioxide diffuse across the alveolar and capillary walls, 212, 213, 213*f*

Alzheimer's disease, chronic, organic mental disorder consisting of dementia that is more prevalent in adults between 40 and 60. Involves progressive disorientation, apathy, speech and gait disturbances, and loss of memory, 400, 473

Amblyopia, loss of vision not as a result of eye pathology; usually occurs in patients who see two images. In order to see only one image, the brain will no longer recognize the image being sent to it by one of the eyes; may occur if strabismus is not corrected; commonly referred to as lazy eye, 433

Ambulatory care center, a facility that provides services that do not require overnight hospitalization. The services range from simple surgeries, to diagnostic testing, to therapy. Also called a surgical center or an outpatient clinic, 11

Amenorrhea, absence of menstruation, which can be the result of many factors, including pregnancy, menopause, and dieting, 322

American Sign Language (ASL), nonverbal method of communicating in which the hands and fingers are used to indicate words and concepts. Used by people who are deaf and speech impaired, 445, 445*f*

Amino acids, organic substances found in plasma, used by cells to build proteins, 170

Amnesia, loss of memory in which people forget their identity as a result of a head injury or disorder, such as epilepsy, senility, and alcoholism. Can be either temporary or permanent, 474

Amniocentesis, puncturing of the amniotic sac using a needle and syringe for the purpose of withdrawing amniotic fluid for testing. Can assist in determining fetal maturity, development, and genetic disorders, 328

Amnion, the inner of two membranous sacs surrouding the fetus. The amniotic sac contains amniotic fluid in which the baby floats, 318, 320

Amniorrhea, discharge of amniotic fluid, 321

Amniotic, pertaining to the amnion, 321

Amniotic fluid, the fluid inside the amniotic sac, 318, 319*f,* 320

Amniotomy, incision into the amniotic sac, 321

Amplification device, 446

Amputation, partial or complete removal of a limb for a variety of reasons, including tumors, gangrene, intractable pain, crushing injury, or uncontrollable infection, 100

Amylase, digestive enzyme found in saliva that begins the digestion of carbohydrates, 250

Amyotrophic lateral sclerosis (ALS), disease with muscular weakness and atrophy due to degeneration of motor neurons of the spinal cord. Also called *Lou Gehrig's disease,* after the New York Yankees' baseball player who died from the disease, 403

Anacusis, total absence of hearing; unable to perceive sound. Also called *deafness,* 446

the uterus is abnormal. The forward bend is near the neck of the uterus. The position of cervix, or opening of the uterus, remains normal, 316

Antepartum, before birth, 323

Anterior, directional term meaning near or on the front or belly side of the body, 35f, 35t

Anterior lobe, the anterior portion of the pituitary gland. It secretes adrenocorticotropin hormone, follicle-stimulating hormone, growth hormone, luteinizing hormone, melanocyte-stimulating hormone, prolactin, and thyroid-stimulating hormone, 363

Anterior pituitary gland, 363f, 364f

Anterior tibial artery, 140f

Anterior tibial vein, 142f

Anteroposterior view (AP), positioning the patient so that the X-rays pass through the body from the anterior side to the posterior side, 478

Anthracosis, A type of pneumoconiosis that develops from the collection of coal dust in the lung. Also called black lung or miner's lung, 221

Anti-inflammatory otic solution, reduces inflammation, itching, and edema associated with otitis externa, 448

Anti-virals, substance that weakens a viral infection in the body, often by interfering with the virus's ability to replicate, 65

Antiarrhythmic, controls cardiac arrhythmias by altering nerve impulses within the heart, 151

Antibiotic, substance that destroys or prohibits the growth of microorganisms. Used to treat bacterial infections. Not found effective in treating viral infections. To be effective, it must be taken regularly for a specified period, 65, 227, 296

Antibiotic ophthalmic solution, eyedrops for the treatment of bacterial eye infections, 437

Antibiotic otic solution, Eardrops to treat otitis externa, 448

Antibody, protein material produced in the body as a response to the invasion of a foreign substance, 183f, 185–86

Antibody-mediated immunity, the production of antibodies by B cells in response to an antigen. Also called *humoral immunity.* 185

Anticoagulant, substance that prevents or delays the clotting or coagulation of blood, 151, 178

Anticonvulsant, prevents or relieves convulsions. Drugs such as phenobarbital reduce excessive stimulation in the brain to control seizures and other symptoms of epilepsy, 407

Antidepressant drugs, medications classified as stimulants that alter the patient's mood by affecting levels of neurotransmitters in the brain, 476

Antidiarrheal, prevents or relieves diarrhea, 264

Antidiuretic hormone (ADH), a hormone secreted by the posterior pituitary. It promotes water reabsorption by the kidney tubules, 359t, 363, 364

Antidote, substance that will neutralize poisons or their side effects, 469

Antiemetic, substance that controls nausea and vomiting, 264, 448

Antifungal, substance that kills fungi infecting the skin, 65

Antigen, substance that is capable of inducing the formation of an antibody. The antibody then intereacts with the antigen in the antigen–antibody reaction, 185

Antigen-antibody complex, combination of the antigen with its specific antibody; increases susceptibility to phagocytosis and immunity, 185, 186

Antiglaucoma medications, a group of drugs that reduce intraocular pressure by lowering the amount of aqueous humor in the eyeball; may achieve this by either reducing the production of aqueous humor or increasing its outflow, 437

Antihemorrhagic, substance that prevents or stops hemorrhaging, 178

Antihistamine, substance that acts to control allergic symptoms by counteracting histamine, which exists naturally in the body, and which is released in allergic reactions, 192, 227

Antilipidemic, substance that reduces amount of cholesterol and lipids in the bloodstream; treats hyperlipidemia, 151

Antiparasitic, substance that kills mites or lice, 65

Antiplatelet agent, substance that interferes with the action of platelets; prolongs bleeding time; commonly referred to as blood thinner. Used to prevent heart attacks and strokes, 178

Antiprostatic agents, medications to treat early cases of benign prostatic hypertrophy; may prevent surgery for mild cases, 340

Antipruritic, substance that reduces severe itching, 65

Antipsychotic drugs, major tranquilizer drugs that have transformed the treatment of patients with psychoses and schizophrenia by reducing patient agitation and panic and shortening schizophrenic episodes, 476

Antiseptic, substance used to kill bacteria in skin cuts and wounds or at a surgical site, 65

Antisocial personality disorder, a personality disorder in which the patient engages in behaviors that are illegal or outside of social norms, 475

Antispasmodic, medication to prevent or reduce bladder muscle spasms, 296

Antithyroid agents, medication given to block production of thyroid hormones in patients with hypersecretion disorders, 373

Benign, not cancerous. A benign tumor is generally not progressive or recurring, 495

Benign prostatic hypertrophy (BPH), enlargement of the prostate gland commonly seen in males over 50, 337

Beta blocker drugs, medication that treats hypertension and angina pectoris by lowering the heart rate, 152

Biceps, an arm muscle named for the number of attachment points. *Bi-* means two and biceps have two heads attached to the bone, 107

Bicuspid valve, a valve between the left atrium and ventricle. It prevents blood from flowing backwards into the atrium. It has two cusps or flaps. It is also called the mitral valve, 134*f*, 135, 135*f*, 137*f*

Bicuspids, premolar permanent teeth having two cusps or projections that assist in grinding food. Humans have eight bicuspids, 245*f*, 246, 246*f*

Bilateral, 4

Bile, substance produced by the liver and stored in the gallbladder. It is added to the chyme in the duodenum and functions to emulsify fats so they can be digested and absorbed. Cholesterol is essential to bile production, 250

Bile duct, 251*f*, 260*f*

Bilirubin, waste product produced from destruction of worn-out red blood cells; disposed of by the liver, 170

Binaural, referring to both ears, 445

Biopsy (Bx, bx), a piece of tissue is removed by syringe and needle, knife, punch, or brush to examine under a microscope. Used to aid in diagnosis, 63, 497

Bipolar disorder (BPD), a mental disorder in which the patient has alternating periods of depression and mania, 474

Bite-wing x-ray, x-ray taken with part of the film holder held between the teeth, and the film held parallel to the teeth, 261

Black lung, 221

Bladder, 317*f*

Bladder cancer, cancerous tumor that arises from the cells lining the bladder; major symptom is hematuria, 292

Bladder neck obstruction, blockage of the bladder outlet into the urethra, 292

Blepharectomy, excision of the eyelid, 430

Blepharitis, inflammatory condition of the eyelash follicles and glands of the eyelids that results in swelling, redness, and crusts of dried mucus on the lids. Can be the result of allergy or infection, 430

Blepharoplasty, surgical repair of the eyelid, 430

Blepharoptosis, drooping eyelid, 430

Blood, the major component of the hematic system. It consists of watery plasma, red blood cells, and white blood cells, 26*t*, 169–78, 169*f*, 287*t*

  abbreviations, 178

  ABO system, 172

  anatomy and physiology, 170–73

  diagnostic procedures, 176–77

  erythrocytes, 170

  leukocytes, 171

  pathology, 174–75

  pharmacology, 178

  plasma, 170

  platelets, 172

  Rh factor, 172–73

  therapeutic procedures, 177

  typing, 172–73

  vocabulary, 174

  word building, 173

Blood clot, the hard collection of fibrin, blood cells, and tissue debris that is the end result of hemostasis or the blood clotting process, 174, 174*f*

Blood culture and sensitivity (C&S), sample of blood is incubated in the laboratory to check for bacterial growth; if bacteria are present, they are identified and tested to determine which antibiotics they are sensitive to, 176

Blood poisoning, 175

Blood pressure (BP), measurement of the pressure that is exerted by blood against the walls of a blood vessel, 141

Blood serum test, blood test to measure the level of substances such as calcium, electrolytes, testosterone, insulin, and glucose. Used to assist in determining the function of various endocrine glands, 371

Blood sinuses, spread-out blood vessels within the spleen that result in slow-moving blood flow, 184

Blood thinners, 178

Blood transfusion, artificial transfer of blood into the bloodstream, 177

Blood tumor, 174

Blood typing, the blood of one person is different from another's due to the presence of antigens on the surface of the erythrocytes. The major method of typing blood is the ABO system and includes types A, B, O, and AB. The other major method of typing blood is the Rh factor, consisting of the two types, Rh+ and Rh–, 172–73

Blood urea nitrogen (BUN), blood test to measure kidney function by the level of nitrogenous waste, or urea, that is in the blood, 293

Blood vessels, the closed system of tubes that conducts blood throughout the body. It consists of arteries, veins, and capillaries, 132, 138–41, 496*f*

BMT, 178

Breech presentation, placement of the fetus in which the buttocks or feet are presented first for delivery rather than the head, 320, 321, 321*f*

Bridge, dental appliance that is attached to adjacent teeth for support to replace missing teeth, 254

Broad spectrum, ability of a drug to be effective against a wide range of microorganisms, 470

Bronch, 227

Bronchial, pertaining to the bronchi, 217

Bronchial tree, 213*f*

Bronchial tube, an organ of the respiratory system that carries air into each lung, 27*t*, 209*f*, 210, 212–13

Bronchiectasis, results from a dilation of a bronchus or the bronchi that can be the result of infection. This abnormal stretching can be irreversible and result in destruction of the bronchial walls. The major symptom is a large amount of purulent (pus-filled) sputum. Rales (bubbling chest sound) and hemoptysis may be present, 217, 221

Bronchioles, the narrowest air tubes in the lungs. Each bronchiole terminates in tiny air sacs called alveoli, 212, 213, 213*f*

Bronchitis, an acute or chronic inflammation of the lower respiratory tract that often occurs after other childhood infections such as measles, 217

Bronchodilator, dilates or opens the bronchi (airways in the lungs) to improve breathing, 227

Bronchogenic, originating in the bronchi, 217

Bronchogenic carcinoma, malignant lung tumor that originates in the bronchi. Usually associated with a history of cigarette smoking, 221, 221*f*

Bronchogram, an X-ray record of the lungs and bronchial tubes, 217, 223

Bronchography, process of taking an X-ray of the lung after a radiopaque substance has been placed into the trachea or bronchial tree, 223

Bronchoplasty, surgical repair of a bronchial defect, 217

Bronchoscope, an instrument to view inside a bronchus, 217, 224

Bronchoscopy (Broncho), using the bronchoscope to visualize the bronchi. The instrument can also be used to obtain tissue for biopsy and to remove foreign objects, 224, 224*f*

Bronchospasm, an involuntary muscle spasm in the bronchi, 217

Bronchus, the distal end of the trachea splits into a left and right main bronchi as it enters each lung. Each main bronchus is subdivided into smaller branches. The smallest bronchi are the bronchioles. Each bronchiole ends in tiny air sacs called alveoli, 212, 213

Bruit, 144

Buccal, (1) Pertaining to the cheeks. (2) Drugs that are placed under the lip or between the cheek and gum, 252, 467, 469

Buccolabial, pertaining to cheeks and lips, 252

Buffers, chemicals that neutralize acid, particularly stomach acid, 251

Bulbourethral gland, also called *Cowper's gland.* These two small male reproductive system glands are located on either side of the urethra just distal to the prostate. The secretion from these glands neutralizes the acidity in the urethra and the vagina, 28*t*, 332*f*, 333, 333*f*, 335

Bulimia, eating disorder that is characterized by recurrent binge eating and then purging of the food with laxatives and vomiting, 474

BUN, 297

Bundle branch block (BBB), occurs when the electrical impulse is blocked from travelling down the bundle of His or bundle branches. Results in the ventricles beating at a different rate than the atria. Also called a *heart block,* 145

Bundle branches, part of the conduction system of the heart; the electrical signal travels down the interventricular septum, 136, 137*f*, 138

Bundle of His, the bundle of His is located in the interventricular septum. It receives the electrical impulse from the atrioventricular node and distributes it through the ventricular walls, causing them to contract simultaneously, 136, 137*f*, 138

Bunion, inflammation of the bursa of the great toe, 99

Bunionectomy, removal of the bursa at the joint of the great toe, 100

Burn, a full-thickness burn exists when all the layers are burned; also called a *third-degree burn.* A partial-thickness burn exists when the first layer of skin, the epidermis, is burned, and the second layer of skin, dermis, is damaged; also called a *second-degree burn.* A *first-degree burn* damages only the epidermis, 60, 60*f*

Bursa, a saclike connective tissue structure found in some joints. It protects moving parts from friction. Some common bursa locations are the elbow, knee, and shoulder joints, 91, 92

Bursectomy, excision of a bursa, 93

Bursitis, inflammation of a bursa between bony prominences and muscles or tendons. Common in the shoulder and knee, 92, 93

Bx, bx, 65, 498

C

C&S, 65, 227, 297

CABG, 152

Cachexia, loss of weight and generalized wasting that occurs during a chronic disease, 254

CAD, 152

Calcitonin, a hormone secreted by the thyroid gland. It stimulates deposition of calcium into bone, 359t, 366

Calcium, an inorganic substance found in plasma. It is important for bones, muscles, and nerves, 170, 362

Calcium channel blocker drugs, medication that treats hypertension, angina pectoris, and congestive heart failure by causing the heart to beat less forcefully and less often, 152

Calcium supplements, maintaining high blood levels of calcium in association with vitamin D helps maintain bone density and treats osteomalacia, osteoporosis, and rickets, 101

Calculus, a stone formed within an organ by an accumulation of mineral salts. Found in the kidney, renal pelvis, bladder, or urethra. Plural is *calculi,* 290, 290f

Callus, the mass of bone tissue that forms at a fracture site during its healing, 95

Calyx, a duct that connects the renal papilla to the renal pelvis. Urine flows from the collecting tubule through the calyx and into the renal pelvis, 282, 283f

Cancellous bone, the bony tissue found inside a bone. It contains cavities that hold red bone marrow. Also called *spongy bone,* 82, 83, 83f

Cancerous tumors, malignant growths in the body, 184

Candidiasis, yeastlike infection of the skin and mucous membranes that can result in white plaques on the tongue and vagina, 325

Canines, also called the cuspid teeth or eyeteeth. Permanent teeth located between the incisors and the biscuspids that assist in biting and cutting food. Humans have four canine teeth, 246, 246f

Canker sores, 256

Capillaries, the smallest blood or lymphatic vessels. Blood capillaries are very thin to allow gas, nutrient, and waste exchange between the blood and the tissues. Lymph capillaries collect lymph fluid from the tissues and carry it to the larger lymph vessels, 131f, 132, 132f, 138–39, 139f, 182, 213f

Capillary bed, the network of capillaries found in a given tissue or organ, 138

Carbon dioxide, a waste product of cellular energy production. It is removed from the cells by the blood and eliminated from the body by the lungs, 132, 133, 210

Carbuncle, inflammation and infection of the skin and hair follicle that may result from several untreated boils. Most commonly found on neck, upper back, or head, 63

Carcinogen, substance or chemical agent that produces cancer or increases the risk of developing it. For example, cigarette smoke and insecticides are considered to be carcinogens, 496

Carcinoma, new growth or malignant tumor that occurs in epithelial tissue. Can spread to other organs through the blood or direct extension from the organ, 495

Carcinoma in situ (CIS), malignant tumor that has not extended beyond the original site, 496

Cardiac, pertaining to the heart, 143

Cardiac arrest, when the heart stops beating and circulation ceases, 145

Cardiac catheterization, passage of a thin tube (catheter) through an arm vein and the blood vessel leading into the heart. Done to detect abnormalities, to collect cardiac blood samples, and to determine the pressure within the cardiac area, 149

Cardiac enzymes, complex protein molecules found only in heart muscle. Cardiac enzymes are taken by blood sample to determine the amount of the heart disease or damage, 148

Cardiac muscle, the involuntary muscle found in the heart, 23, 105, 105f, 106, 106f, 133

Cardiac scan, patient is given radioactive thallium intravenously and then scanning equipment is used to visualize the heart; it is especially useful in determining myocardial damage, 149

Cardiac sphincter, also called the *lower esophageal sphincter.* Prevents food and gastric juices from backing up into the esophagus, 248, 248f

Cardiologist, a physician specializing in treating diseases and conditions of the cardiovascular system, 143

Cardiology, the branch of medicine specializing in conditions of the cardiovascular system, 26t, 143

Cardiomegaly, abnormally enlarged heart, 143

Cardiomyopathy, general term for a disease of the myocardium that may be caused by alcohol abuse, parasites, viral infection, and congestive heart failure, 145

Cardiopulmonary resuscitation (CPR), emergency treatment provided by persons trained in CPR and given to patients when their respirations and heart stop. CPR provides oxygen to the brain, heart, and other vital organs until medical treatment can restore a normal heart and pulmonary function, 150, 152, 226

Cardiorrhexis, ruptured heart, 143

Cardiotonic, substance that strengthens the heart muscle, 152

Cardiovascular system (CV), system that transports blood to all areas of the body. Organs of the

cardiovascular system include the heart and blood vessels (arteries, veins, and capillaries). Also called the *circulatory system,* 26*t,* 129–66
  abbreviations, 152
  anatomy and physiology, 132–41
  diagnostic procedures, 148–49
  pathology, 144–48
  pharmacology, 151–52
  therapeutic procedures, 150–51
  vocabulary, 143–44
  word building, 141, 143
Cardioversion, 150
Carditis, 6
Carotid artery, 140*f,* 441*f*
Carotid endarterectomy, surgical procedure for removing an obstruction within the carotid artery, a major artery in the neck that carries oxygenated blood to the brain. Developed to prevent strokes but found to be useful only in severe stenosis with TIA, 407
Carpal, pertaining to the wrist, 94
Carpal tunnel release, surgical cutting of the ligament in the wrist to relieve nerve pressure caused by carpal tunnel disease, which can be caused by repetitive motion such as typing, 112
Carpal tunnel syndrome, a painful disorder of the wrist and hand, induced by compression of the median nerve as it passes under ligaments on the palm side of the wrist. Symptoms include weakness, pain, burning, tingling, and aching in the forearm, wrist, and hand, 111
Carpals, the wrist bones in the upper extremity, 88, 89*f,* 90, 90*f*
Cartilage, strong, flexible connective tissue found in several locations in the body, such as covering the ends of bones in a synovial joint, nasal septum, external ear, eustachian tube, larynx, trachea, bronchi, and the intervertebral discs, 23, 82, 441*f*
Cartilaginous joints, a joint that allows slight movement but holds bones firmly in place by a solid piece of cartilage. The public symphysis is an example of a cartilaginous joint. The fetal skeleton is composed of cartilaginous tissue, 91, 92
Cast, application of a solid material to immobilize an extremity or portion of the body as a result of a fracture, dislocation, or severe injury. It is most often made of plaster of Paris, 95
Castration, excision of the testicles in the male or the ovaries in the female, 338
Cataract, diminished vision resulting from the lens of the eye becoming opaque or cloudy. Treatment is usually surgical removal of the cataract, 433, 433*f*

cath, 297
Catheter, a flexible tube inserted into the body for the purpose of moving fluids into or out of the body. In the cardiovascular system used to place dye into blood vessels so they may be visualized on X-rays. In the urinary system used to drain urine from the bladder, 143, 290, 290*f*
Catheterization, insertion of a tube through the urethra and into the urinary bladder for the purpose of withdrawing urine or inserting dye, 294
Caudal, directional term meaning toward the feet or tail, or below, 35*f,* 35*t*
Cauterization, destruction of tissue using an electric current, a caustic product, or a hot iron, or by freezing, 64, 492
CC, 297
Cecum, first portion of the colon. It is a blind pouch off the beginning of the large intestine. The appendix grows out of the end of the cecum, 249, 249*f,* 250*f*
Cell, the basic unit of all living things. All tissues and organs in the body are composed of cells. They perform survival functions such as reproduction, respiration, metabolism, and excretion. Some cells are also able to carry on specialized functions, such as contraction by muscle cells and electrical impulse transmission by nerve cells, 22
Cell membrane, the outermost boundary of the cell, 22
Cell-mediated immunity, immunity that results from the activation of sensitized T lymphocytes. The immune response causes antigens to be destroyed by the direct action of cells. Also called *cellular immunity,* 185
Cellular immunity, also called cell-mediated immunity. This process results in the production of T cells and natural killer, NK, cells that directly attach to foreign cells. This immune response fights invasion by viruses, bacteria, fungi, and cancer, 185
Cellulitis, inflammation of the cellular or connective tissues, 61
Cementum, anchors the root of a tooth into the socket of the jaw, 246, 247, 247*f*
Central canal, canal that extends down the length of the spinal cord; contains cerebrospinal fluid, 394
Central fissure, 393*f*
Central nervous system, the portion of the nervous system that consists of the brain and spinal cord. It receives impulses from all over the body, processes this information, and then responds with an action. It consists of both gray matter and white matter, 390–95

brain, 392–94

meninges, 395

spinal cord, 394

Centrifuge, 169*f*

Cephalalgia, a headache, 398

Cephalic, Directional term meaning toward the head, or above, 35*t*

Cephalic region, the head region of the body, 31, 32*f*

Cephalic vein, 142*f*

Cerebellar, pertaining to the cerebellum, 398

Cerebellitis, inflammation of the cerebellum, 398

Cerebellum, the second largest portion of the brain, located beneath the posterior portion of the cerebrum. This part of the brain aids in coordinating voluntary body movements and maintaining balance and equilibrium. It is attached to the brain stem by the pons. The cerebellum refines the muscular movement that is initiated in the cerebrum, 392, 392*f*, 393*f*

Cerebral, pertaining to the cerebrum, 398

Cerebral aneurysm, localized abnormal dilatation of a blood vessel, usually an artery; the result of a congenital defect or weakness in the wall of the vessel; a ruptured aneurysm is a common cause for a hemorrhagic CVA, 401, 401*f*

Cerebral angiography, x-ray of the blood vessels of the brain after the injection of a radiopaque dye, 405

Cerebral contusion, bruising of the brain from a blow or impact; symptoms last longer than 24 hours and include unconsciousness, dizziness, vomiting, unequal pupil size, and shock, 401

Cerebral cortex, the outer layer of the cerebrum. It is composed of folds of gray matter called gyri, which are separated by sulci, 392

Cerebral hemispheres, the division of the cerebrum into right and left halves, 392

Cerebral palsy (CP), a group of disabilities caused by injury to the brain either before or during birth or very early in infancy. This is the most common permanent disability in childhood, 401

Cerebrospinal, pertaining to the cerebrum and spine, 398

Cerebrospinal fluid (CSF), watery, clear fluid found in the ventricles of the brain. It provides protection from shock or sudden motion to the brain, 392, 394

Cerebrospinal fluid analysis, laboratory examination of the clear, watery, colorless fluid from within the brain and spinal cord. Infections and the abnormal presence of blood can be detected in this test, 405

Cerebrospinal fluid shunts, a surgical procedure in which a bypass is created to drain cerebrospinal fluid. It is used to treat hydrocephalus by draining the excess cerebrospinal fluid from the brain and diverting it to the abdominal cavity, 407

Cerebrovascular accident (CVA), also called a *stroke*. The development of an infarct due to loss in the blood supply to an area of the brain. Blood flow can be interrupted by a ruptured blood vessel (hemorrhage), a floating clot (embolus), a stationary clot (thrombosis), or compression. The extent of damage depends on the size and location of the infarct and often includes speech problems and muscle paralysis, 401, 402*f*

Cerebrum, the largest section of the brain. It is located in the upper portion and is the area that possesses our thoughts, judgment, memory, association skills, and the ability to discriminate between items. The outer layer of the cerebrum is the cerebral cortex, which is composed of folds of gray matter. The elevated portions of the cerebrum, or convolutions, are called gyri and are separated by fissures or sulci. The cerebrum has both a left and right division or hemisphere. Each hemisphere has four lobes: frontal, parietal, occipital, and temporal, 392, 392*f*

Cerumen, also called ear wax. A thick, waxy substance produced by oil glands in the auditory canal. This wax helps to protect and lubricate the ear, 441, 442

Ceruminoma, a hard accumulation of ear wax in the ear canal, 446

Cervical, (1) Pertaining to the neck. (2) Pertaining to the cervix, 94, 321

Cervical biopsy, taking a sample of tissue from the cervix to test for the presence of cancer cells, 328

Cervical cancer, malignant growth in the cervix. An especially difficult type of cancer to treat, it causes 5% of the cancer deaths in women. Pap tests have helped to detect early cervical cancer, 324

Cervical nerve, 397*f*

Cervical nodes, 182*t*, 183*f*

Cervical region, the neck region of the body, 31, 32*f*

Cervical vertebrae, the seven vertebrae in the neck region, 84, 85, 88*t*

Cervicectomy, excision of the cervix, 321

Cervix, the narrow, distal portion of the uterus that joins to the vagina, 314*f*, 316, 316*f*, 317*f*, 319*f*

Cesarean section (CS, C-section), surgical delivery of a baby through an incision into the abdominal and uterine walls. Legend has it that the Roman emperor Julius Caesar was the first person born by this method, 328

example, in the combining form *cardi/o, cardi* is the word root and */o* is the combining vowel, 4, 518–21

Combining vowel, a vowel inserted between word parts that makes it possible to pronounce long medical terms. It is usually the vowel *o*, 2, 3–4

Comedo, medical term for a blackhead. It is an accumulation of sebum in a sebaceous gland that has become blackened, 55

Comminuted fracture, a fracture in which the bone is shattered, splintered, or crushed into many pieces or fragments. The fracture is completely through the bone, 97

Common bile duct, a duct that carries bile from the gallbladder to the duodenum, 251

Common iliac artery, 140*f*

Common iliac vein, 142*f*

Compact bone, the hard exterior surface bone. Also called *cortical bone*, 82, 83*f*

Complemental air, 215*t*

Complete blood count (CBC), blood test that consists of five tests; red blood cell count (RBC), white blood count (WBC), hemoglobin (Hg), hematocrit (Hct), and white blood cell differential, 176

Compound fracture, an open fracture in which the skin has been broken through by the fracture, 96, 96*f*, 97

Compression fracture, fracture involving loss of height of a vertebral body, 97

Computed tomography scan (CT scan), an imaging technique that is able to produce a cross-sectional view of the body; X-ray pictures are taken at multiple angles through the body and a computer uses all these images to construct a composite cross-section, 479

Conception, fertilization of an ovum by a sperm, 315, 316

Concussion, injury to the brain that results from a blow or impact from an object. Can result in unconsciousness, dizziness, vomiting, unequal pupil size, and shock, 402

Conductive hearing loss, loss of hearing as a result of the blocking of sound transmission in the middle ear and outer ear, 443

Condyle, refers to the rounded portion at the end of a bone, 83, 84, 85*f*

Cones, the sensory receptors of the retina that are active in bright light and see in color, 427

Confidentiality, 12

Congenital anomalies, 319

Congenital septal defect (CSD), defect, present at birth, in the wall separating two chambers of the heart. Results in a mixture of oxygenated and deoxygenated blood being carried to the surrounding tissues. There can be an atrial sep-

tal defect (ASD) and a ventricular septal defect (VSD), 145

Congestive heart failure (CHF), pathological condition of the heart in which there is a reduced outflow of blood from the left side of the heart. Results in weakness, breathlessness, and edema, 145

Conization, surgical removal of a core of cervical tissue. Also refers to partial removal of the cervix, 328

Conjunctiva, a protective mucous membrane lining on the underside of each eyelid and across the anterior surface of each eyeball, 426, 426*f*, 428*f*, 429

Conjunctival, pertaining to the conjunctiva, 430

Conjunctivitis, also referred to as *pink eye* or an inflammation of the conjunctiva, 431

Conjunctivoplasty, surgical repair of the conjunctiva, 431

Connective tissue, the supporting and protecting tissue in body structures. Examples are fat or adipose tissue, cartilage, and bone, 23, 24*f*

Conscious, condition of being awake and aware of surroundings, 399

Constipation, experiencing difficulty in defecation or infrequent defecation, 254

Consultation reports, document in a patient's medical record. They are the reports given by specialists who the physician has requested to evaluate the patient, 11

Contracture, an abnormal shortening of a muscle, making it difficult to stretch the muscle, 99, 99*f*, 111

Contraindication, condition in which a particular drug should not be used, 470

Contrast studies, a radiopaque substance is injected or swallowed; X-rays are then taken that outline the body structure containing the radiopaque substance, 479, 480*f*

Controlled substances, drugs that have a potential for being addictive (habit forming) or can be abused, 465, 466, 466*t*

Contusion, injury caused by a blow to the body; causes swelling, pain, and bruising; the skin is not broken, 55

Conversion reaction, a somatoform disorder in which the patient unconsciously substitutes physical signs or symptoms for anxiety. The most common physical signs or symptoms are blindness, deafness, and paralysis, 475

Convulsions, severe involuntary muscle contractions and relaxations. These have a variety of causes, such as epilepsy, fever, and toxic conditions, 399

COPD, 227

Corium, the living layer of skin located between the epidermis and the subcutaneous tissue. Also referred to as the *dermis,* it contains hair follicles, sweat glands, sebaceous glands, blood vessels, lymph vessels, nerve fibers, and muscle fibers, 52

Cornea, a portion of the sclera that is clear and transparent and allows light to enter the interior of the eye. It also plays a role in bending light rays, 425*f,* 426*f,* 430*f*

Corneal, pertaining to the cornea, 431

Corneal abrasion, scraping injury to the cornea; if it does not heal, it may develop into an ulcer, 433

Coronal plane, a vertical plane that divides the body into front (anterior or ventral) and back (posterior or dorsal) sections. Also called the *frontal plane,* 30, 31

Coronal section, sectional view of the body produced by a cut along the frontal plane; also called a *frontal section.* 30, 31

Coronary, pertaining to the heart, 143

Coronary arteries, a group of three arteries that branch off the aorta and carry blood to the myocardium, 138, 139*f*

Coronary artery bypass graft (CABG), open-heart surgery in which a blood vessel is grafted to route blood around the point of constriction in a diseased coronary artery, 150

Coronary artery disease (CAD), insufficient blood supply to the heart muscle due to an obstruction of one or more coronary arteries; may be caused by atherosclerosis and may cause angina pectoris and myocardial infarction, 145

Corpus, the body or central portion of the uterus, 316

Corpus (uterus), 314*f*

Corpus albicans, 315*f*

Corpus luteum, 315*f*

Cortex, the outer layer of an organ. In the endocrine system, it refers to the outer layer of the adrenal glands; in the urinary system, the outer layer of the kidney, 282, 283*f*

Cortical, pertaining to the cortex, 93

Cortical bone, the hard exterior surface bone. Also called *compact bone,* 82, 83*f*

Corticosteroid cream, a powerful anti-inflammatory cream, 65

Corticosteroids, general term for the group of hormones secreted by the adrenal contex. They include mineralocorticoid hormones, glucocorticoid hormones, and steroid sex hormones. Used as a medication for its strong anti-inflammatory properties, 101, 192, 227, 360, 373

Cortisol, a steroid hormone secreted by the adrenal cortex. It regulates carbohydrate metabolism, 358*t,* 360

Costal, pertaining to the ribs, 94

Cowper's glands, also called *bulbourethral glands.* These two small male reproductive system glands are located on either side of the urethra just distal to the prostate. The secretion from these glands neutralizes the acidity in the urethra and the vagina, 335

CP, 408

CPK, 112, 152

CPR, 152, 227

Cranial, Pertaining to the skull, 94

Cranial bones, 87*t*

Cranial cavity, a dorsal body cavity. It is within the skull and contains the brain, 31, 32, 32*f,* 33*t*

Cranial nerves, nerves that arise from the brain, 390, 396*t*

Craniotomy, incision into the skull, 93

Cranium, the skull; bones that form a protective covering over the brain, 84, 85, 86*f*

Creatine phosphokinase (CPK), a muscle enzyme found in skeletal muscle and cardiac muscle; blood test becomes elevated in disorders such as heart attack, muscular dystrophy, and other skeletal muscle pathologies, 112, 148

Creatinine, a waste product of muscle metabolism, 170

Creatinine clearance, test of kidney function. Creatinine is a waste product cleared from the bloodstream by the kidneys. For this test, urine is collected for 24 hours and the amount of creatinine in the urine is compared to the amount of creatinine that remains in the bloodstream, 293

Crepitation, sound of broken bones rubbing together, 95

Cretinism, congenital condition due to a lack of thyroid that may result in arrested physical and mental development, 370

CRF, 297

Crick in the neck, 111

Cricoid cartilage, 211*f*

Crohn's disease, form of chronic inflammatory bowel disease affecting the ileum and/or colon. Also called *regional ileitis,* 257

Cross infection, occurs when a person, either a patient or healthcare worker, acquires a pathogen from another patient or healthcare worker, 186

Cross-eyed, 435

Cross-section, an internal view of the body produced by a slice perpendicular to the long axis of the structure, 30, 31

Croup, acute viral respiratory infection common in infants and young children and characterized by a hoarse cough, 220

Crown, portion of a tooth that is covered by enamel. Also an artificial covering for the

therapeutic procedures, 447–48

vocabulary, 445

word building, 444–45

Eardrops, substance placed directly into the ear canal for the purpose of relieving pain or treating infection, 467, 469

Eating disorders, abnormal behaviors related to eating; include anorexia nervosa and bulimia, 474

Ecchymosis, skin discoloration or bruise caused by blood collecting under the skin, 56, 56*f*

ECG, 152

Echocardiography (ECHO), noninvasive diagnostic method using ultrasound to visualize internal cardiac structures; cardiac valve activity can be evaluated using this method, 149

Echoencephalography, recording of the ultrasonic echoes of the brain; useful in determining abnormal patterns of shifting in the brain, 405

Eclampsia, convulsive seizures and coma that can occur in a woman between the twentieth week of pregnancy and the first week of postpartum. Often associated with hypertension, 326

ECT, 476

Ectopic pregnancy, 316

Eczema, superficial dermatitis accompanied by papules, vesicles, and crusting, 61

ED, 340

Edema, condition in which the body tissues contain excessive amounts of fluid, 368

EEG, 408

Effacement, the thinning of the cervix during labor, 320, 321

Efferent, 283

Efferent arteriole, arteriole that carries blood away from the glomerulus, 283, 284*f*, 286*f*

Efferent neurons, nerves that carry impulses away from the brain and spinal cord to the muscles and glands. Also called *motor neurons.* 395, 396, 397*f*

EGD, 264

Egg cell, 316*f*

Ejaculation, the impulse of forcing seminal fluid from the male urethra, 334

EKG, 152

Elastin fibers, 213*f*

Elbow, 83

Elective abortion, the legal termination of a pregnancy for nonmedical reasons, 329

Electrocardiogram (ECG,EKG), record of the electrical activity of the heart. Useful in the diagnosis of abnormal cardiac rhythm and heart muscle (myocardium) damage, 138*f*, 143

Electrocardiography, process of recording the electrical activity of the heart, 149

Electrocautery, to destroy tissue with an electric current, 64, 493

Electroconvulsive therapy (ECT), a procedure occasionally used for cases of prolonged major depression in which an electrode is placed on one or both sides of the patient's head and current is turned on briefly causing a convulsive seizure. A low level of voltage is used in modern ECT, and the patient is administered a muscle relaxant and an anesthesia. Advocates of this treatment state that it is a more effective way to treat severe depression than with the use of drugs. It is not effective with disorders other than depression, such as schizophrenia and alcoholism, 475

Electroencephalogram (EEG), a record of the brain's electrical activity, 398

Electroencephalography (EEG), recording the electrical activity of the brain by placing electrodes at various positions on the scalp. Also used in sleep studies to determine if there is a normal pattern of activity during sleep, 406

Electrolyte, chemical compound that separates into charged particles, or ionizes, in a solution. Sodium chloride (NaCl) and potassium (K) are examples of electrolytes, 286

Electromyogram (EMG), record of muscle electricity, 110, 486

Electromyography, recording of the electrical patterns of a muscle in order to diagnose diseases, 112

Elephantiasis, inflammation, obstruction, and destruction of the lymph vessels that results in enlarged tissues due to edema, 189

Elevation, a muscle action that raises a body part, as in shrug the shoulders, 109

ELISA, 192

Embolectomy, surgical removal of an embolus or clot from a blood vessel, 150

Embolus, obstruction of a blood vessel by a blood clot that moves from another area, 147, 148*f*

Embryo, the term to describe the developing infant from fertilization until the end of the eighth week, 318, 319, 319*f*

Embryonic, pertaining to the embryo, 322

Emesis, vomiting, usually with some force, 255

Emetic, substance that induces vomiting, 264

EMG, 112, 488

Emmetropia (EM), state of normal vision, 432

Emphysema, pulmonary condition that can occur as a result of long-term heavy smoking. Air pollution also worsens this disease. The patient may not be able to breathe except in a sitting or standing position, 221

Empyema, pus within the pleural space, usually the result of infection, 223

Emulsification, to make fats and lipids more soluble in water, 250

Enamel, the hardest substance in the body. Covers the outer surface of teeth, 246, 247, 247f

Encapsulated, growth enclosed in a sheath of tissue that prevents tumor cells from invading surrounding tissue, 496

Encephalitis, inflammation of the brain due to disease factors such as rabies, influenza, measles, or smallpox, 398

Endarterectomy, removal of the inside layer of an artery, 150

Endings

  plural, 9
  singular, 9

Endo, 493

Endocarditis, inflammation of the inner lining layer of the heart. May be due to microorganisms or to an abnormal immunological response, 134, 145

Endocardium, the inner layer of the heart, which is very smooth and lines the chambers of the heart, 133, 134, 134f

Endocervicitis, inflammation of the inner aspect of the cervix, 321

Endocrine glands, a glandular system that secretes hormones directly into the bloodstream rather than into a duct. Endocrine glands are frequently referred to as ductless glands. The endocrine system includes the thyroid gland, adrenal glands, parathyroid glands, pituitary gland, pancreas (islets of Langerhans), testes, ovaries, and thymus gland, 358, 358t–359t

Endocrine system, the body system that consists of glands that secrete hormones directly into the blood stream. The endocrine glands include the adrenal glands, parathyroid glands, pancreas, pituitary gland, testes, ovaries, thymus gland, and thyroid gland, 28t, 355–86, 357f, 358

  abbreviations, 373
  adrenal glands, 360
  anatomy and physiology, 358–66
  diagnostic procedures, 371–72
  ovaries, 360
  pancreas, 361–62
  parathyroid glands, 362
  pathology, 369–71
  pharmacology, 373
  pineal gland, 362–63
  pituitary gland, 363–64
  testes, 364
  therapeutic procedures, 372
  thymus gland, 364–66
  thyroid gland, 366
  vocabulary, 368
  word building, 366–68

Endocrinologist, physician who specializes in the treatment of endocrine glands, including diabetes, 367, 368

Endocrinology, the branch of medicine specializing in conditions of the endocrine system, 28t, 368

Endocrinopathy, a disease of the endocrine system, 367

Endometrial biopsy (EMB), taking a sample of tissue from the lining of the uterus to test for abnormalities, 328

Endometrial cancer, cancer of the endometrial lining of the uterus, 324

Endometriosis, abnormal condition of endometrium tissue appearing throughout the pelvis or on the abdominal wall. This tissue is usually found within the uterus, 322, 325

Endometritis, inflammation of the endometrial lining of the uterus, 325

Endometrium, the inner lining of the uterus. It contains a rich blood supply and reacts to hormonal changes every month, which results in menstruation. During a pregnancy, the lining of the uterus does not leave the body but remains to nourish the unborn child, 316, 316f

Endoscopic retrograde cholangiopancreatography (ERCP), using an endoscope to X-ray the bile and pancreatic ducts, 261

Endoscopic surgery, use of a lighted instrument to examine the interior of a cavity, 493

Endothelium, 139f

Endotracheal, pertaining to inside the trachea, 218

Endotracheal intubation, placing a tube through the mouth to create an airway, 225, 225f

ENT, 448

Enteric, pertaining to the small intestines, 252

Enteritis, inflammation of only the small intestine, 252

Enucleated, the loss of a cell's nucleus, 170

Enucleation, surgical removal of an eyeball, 436

Enuresis, involuntary discharge of urine after the age by which bladder control should have been established. This usually occurs by age 5. Also called bedwetting at night, 291

Enzyme-linked immunosorbent assay (ELISA), a blood test for an antibody to the AIDS virus. A positive test means that the person has been exposed to the virus. In the case of a false-positive reading, the Western blot test would be used to verify the results, 190

Eosinophils, granulocyte white blood cells that destroy parasites and increase during allergic reactions, 169f, 171f, 171t

eosins, eos, 178

Epicardium, the outer layer of the heart. It forms part of the pericardium, 133, 134

Epicondyle, a projection located above or on a condyle, 83, 84, 85*f*

Epidermal, pertaining to upon the skin, 54

Epidermis, the superficial layer of skin. It is composed of squamous epithelium cells. These are flat scalelike cells that are arranged in layers, called stratified squamous epithelium. The many layers of the epidermis create a barrier to infection. The epidermis does not have a blood supply, so it is dependent on the deeper layers of skin for nourishment. However, the deepest epidermis layer is called the basal layer. These cells are alive and constantly dividing. Older cells are pushed out toward the surface by new cells forming beneath. During this process, they shrink and die, becoming filled with a protein called keratin. The keratin-filled cells are sloughed off as dead cells, 50–51, 51*f*, 53*f*

Epididymal, pertaining to the epididymis, 335

Epididymectomy, surgical excision of the epididymis, 335

Epididymis, a coiled tubule that lies on top of the testes within the scrotum. This tube stores sperm as they are produced and turns into the vas deferens, 28*t*, 332*f*, 333, 334, 365*f*

Epididymitis, inflammation of the epididymis that causes pain and swelling in the inguinal area, 335

Epidural hematoma, mass of blood in the space outside the dura mater of the brain and spinal cord, 404

Epidural space, 395*f*

Epigastric, pertaining to above the stomach. An anatomical division of the abdomen, the middle section of the upper row, 34

Epigastric region, 34*t*

Epiglottis, a flap of cartilage that covers the larynx when a person swallows. This prevents food and drink from entering the larynx and trachea, 211*f*, 212, 245*f*, 247

Epilepsy, recurrent disorder of the brain in which convulsive seizures and loss of consciousness occur, 402

Epinephrine, a hormone produced by the adrenal medulla. Also known as *adrenaline.* Some of its actions include increased heart rate and force of contraction, bronchodilation, and relaxation of intestinal muscles, 358*t*, 360

Epiphyseal line, 83*f*

Epiphysis, the wide ends of a long bone, 82

Episiorrhaphy, suture the vulva, 322

Episiotomy, surgical incision of the perineum to facilitate the delivery process. Can prevent an irregular tearing of tissue during birth, 329

Epispadias, congenital opening of the urethra on the dorsal surface of the penis, 337

Epistaxis, nosebleed, 210, 219

Epithelial tissue, tissue found throughout the body as the skin, the outer covering of organs, and the inner lining for tubular or hollow structures, 23, 24*f*

Epithelium, epithelial tissue composed of close-packed cells that form the covering for and lining of body structures, 23

Equilibrium, The sense of balance, 441, 441*f*

ERCP, 264

Erectile dysfunction (ED), inability to copulate due to inability to maintain an erection; also called *impotence,* 336

Erectile dysfunction agents, medications that temporarily produce an erection in patients with erectile dysfunction, 340

Erectile tissue, tissue with numerous blood vessels and nerve endings. It becomes filled with blood and enlarges in size in response to sexual stimulation, 317, 334

Ergonomics, the study of human work including how the requirements for performing work and the work environment affect the musculoskeletal and nervous system, 485

ERT, 330

Erythema, redness or flushing of the skin, 56

Erythroblastosis fetalis, 326

Erythrocyte sedimentation rate (ESR, sed rate), blood test to determine the rate at which mature red blood cells settle out of the blood after the addition of an anticoagulant. An indicator of the presence of an inflammatory disease, 176

Erythrocytes, also called red blood cells or RBCs. Cells that contain hemoglobin, an iron-containing pigment that binds oxygen in order to transport it to the cells of the body, 26*t*, 170, 171*f*, 173, 175

Erythrocytosis, too many red cells, 173

Erythroderma, red skin, 55

Erythropenia, too few red cells, 173

Erythropoiesis, the process of forming erythrocytes, 173

Eschar, a thick layer of dead tissue and tissue fluid that develops over a deep burn area, 56

Esophageal, pertaining to the esophagus, 252

Esophageal varices, enlarged and swollen varicose veins in the lower end of the esophagus; they can rupture and result in serious hemorrhage, 256

Esophagectasis, stretched out or dilated esophagus, 252

Esophagogastroduodenoscopy (EGD), use of a flexible fiberoptic scope to visually examine the esophagus, stomach, and beginning of the duodenum, 262

vocabulary, 432
word building, 430–32
Eye muscles, there are six muscles that connect the eyeball to the orbit cavity. These muscles allow for rotation of the eyeball, 426
Eyeball, the eye by itself, without any appendages such as the eye muscles or tear ducts, 426–27
Eyedrops, substance placed into the eye to control eye pressure in glaucoma. Also used during eye examinations to dilate the pupil of the eye for better examination of the interior of the eye, 467, 468
Eyelashes, along the upper and lower edges of the eyelids; protect the eye from foreign particles; also called *cilia.* 429
Eyelids, an upper and lower fold of skin that provides protection from foreign particles, injury from the sun and intense light, and trauma. Both the upper and lower edges of the eyelids have small hairs or cilia. In addition, sebaceous or oil glands are located in the eyelids. These secrete a lubricating oil, 426, 426f, 429

F
Facial bones, the skull bones that surround the mouth, nose, and eyes; muscles for chewing are attached to the facial bones, 84, 85, 86f, 87t
Facial nerve, 396t
Factitious disorders, intentionally feigning illness symptoms in order to gain attention such as malingering, 474
Falling test, test used to observe balance and equilibrium. The patient is observed balancing on one foot, then with one foot in front of the other, and then walking forward with eyes open. The same test is conducted with the patient's eyes closed. Swaying and falling with the eyes closed can indicate an ear and equilibrium malfunction, 447
Fallopian tubes, organs in the female reproductive system that transport eggs from the ovary to the uterus, 28t, 33t, 34t, 313f, 314, 314f, 315–16, 315f, 316f, 361f
Family and group psychotherapy, form of psychological counseling in which the therapist places minimal emphasis on patient past history and strong emphasis on having patient state and discuss goals and then find a way to achieve them, 476
Farsightedness, 433
Fascia, connective tissue that wraps muscles. It tapers at each end of a skeletal muscle to form tendons, 106
Fascial, pertaining to fascia, 110
Fasciitis, inflammation of fascia, 110

Fasciotomy, incision into fascia, 110
Fasting blood sugar (FBS), blood test to measure the amount of sugar circulating throughout the body after a 12-hour fast, 371
Fats, lipid molecules transported throughout the body dissolved in the blood, 170
FBS, 373
FDA, 471
Fecal occult blood test (FOBT), laboratory test on the feces to determine if microscopic amounts of blood are present; also called *hemoccult* or *stool guaiac.* 260
Feces, food that cannot be digested becomes a waste product and is expelled or defecated as feces, 249
Federal Drug Administration (FDA), 471
Female reproductive system, system responsible for producing eggs for reproduction and provides place for growing baby. Organs include ovaries, fallopian tubes, uterus, vagina, and mammary glands, 28t, 313f, 314f
abbreviations, 330
anatomy and physiology, 314–21
breast, 318
diagnostic procedures, 327–28
internal genitalia, 314–17
pathology, 324–27
pharmacology, 329
therapeutic procedures, 328–29
vocabulary, 323–24
vulva, 317
word building, 321–23
Female urethra, 281f
Femoral, pertaining to the femur or thigh bone, 94
Femoral artery, 140f
Femoral vein, 142f
Femur, also called the *thigh bone.* It is a lower extremity bone, 82, 85f, 88, 89f, 90, 91f, 91t
Fertility drug, medication that triggers ovulation. Also called *ovulation stimulant,* 329
Fertilization, also called *impregnation.* The fusion of an ova and sperm to produce an embryo, 314
Fetal, pertaining to the fetus, 322
Fetal monitoring, using electronic equipment placed on the mother's abdomen to check the baby's heart rate and strength during labor, 328
Fetus, the term to describe the developing newborn from the end of the eighth week until birth, 318, 319, 319f
Fever blisters, 256
Fibrillation, abnormal quivering or contractions of heart fibers. When this occurs within the fibers of the ventricle of the heart, arrest and death can occur. Emergency equipment to defibrillate, or convert the heart to a normal beat, is necessary, 145

Fibrin, whitish protein formed by the action of thrombin and fibrinogen, which is the basis for the clotting of blood, 172

Fibrinogen, blood protein that is essential for clotting to take place, 170, 173

Fibrinolysis, destruction of fibers, 173

Fibrinous, pertaining to being fibrous, 173

Fibrocystic breast disease, benign cysts forming in the breast, 326, 326f

Fibroid tumor, benign tumor or growth that contains fiberlike tissue. Uterine fibroid tumors are the most common tumors in women, 325, 325f

Fibromyalgia, a condition with widespread aching and pain in the muscles and soft tissue, 111

Fibrous joints, a joint that has almost no movement because the ends of the bones are joined together by thick fibrous tissue. The sutures of the skull are an example of a fibrous joint, 91, 92

Fibula, one of the lower leg bones in the lower extremity, 89f, 90, 91f, 91t

Fibular, pertaining to the fibula, a lower leg bone, 94

Fibular vein, 142f

Film, thin sheet of cellulose material coated with a light-sensitive substance that is used in taking photographs. There is a special photographic film that is sensitive to X-rays, 478

Film badge, badge containing film that is sensitive to X-rays. This is worn by all personnel in radiology to measure the amount of X-rays to which they are exposed, 478

Filtration, first stage of urine production during which waste products are filtered from the blood, 286, 287

Fimbriae, the fingerlike extensions on the end of the fallopian tubes. The fimbriae drape over each ovary in order to direct the ovum into the fallopian tube after it is expelled by the ovary, 315, 316, 316f, 361f

Fine motor skills, the use of precise and coordinated movements in such activities as writing, buttoning, and cutting, 485

First-degree burn, 60, 60f

Fissure, a deep groove or slit-type opening, 58, 58f, 83, 84

Fistulectomy, excision of a fistula, 263

Fixation, a procedure to stabilize a fractured bone while it heals. *External fixation* includes casts, splints, and pins inserted through the skin. *Internal fixation* includes pins, plates, rods, screws, and wires that are applied during an *open reduction*, 101

Flat bone, a type of bone with a thin flattened shape. Examples include the scapula, ribs, and pelvic bones, 82, 83

Flexion, act of bending or being bent, 108, 108f

Flexor carpi, a muscle named for its action, flexion, 107

Floating kidney, 292

Fluorescein angiography, process of injecting a dye (fluorescein) to observe the movement of blood for detecting lesions in the macular area of the retina. Used to determine if there is a detachment of the retina, 434

Fluorescein staining, applying dye eyedrops that are a bright green fluorescent color; used to look for corneal abrasions or ulcers, 434

Fluoroscopy, x-rays strike a glowing screen which can change from minute to minute, therefore able to show movement such as the digestive tract moving, 479

Flutter, an arrhythmia in which the atria beat too rapidly, but in a regular pattern, 146

Focal seizure, a localized epileptic seizure often affecting one limb, 400

Follicle-stimulating hormone (FSH), a hormone secreted by the anterior pituitary gland. It stimulates growth of eggs in females and sperm in males, 314, 359t, 363

Foramen, a passage or opening through a bone for nerves and blood vessels, 83, 84

Forceps, a surgical instrument used to grasp tissues, 491t

Formed elements, the solid, cellular portion of blood. It consists of erythrocytes, leukocytes, and platelets, 170

Fossa, a shallow cavity or depression within or on the surface of a bone, 83, 84

Fovea capitis, 85f

Fovea centralis, the area of the retina that has the sharpest vision, 427

Fowler position, surgical position in which the patient is sitting with back positioned at a 45° angle, 492f, 492t

Fracture, an injury to a bone that causes it to break. Fractures are named to describe the type of damage to the bone, 96–98, 97

Fraternal twins, twins that develop from two different ova fertilized by two different sperm; although twins, these siblings do not have identical DNA, 323

Free edge, the exposed edge of a nail that is trimmed when nails become too long, 52

Frequency, a greater than normal occurrence in the urge to urinate, without an increase in the total daily volume of urine. Frequency is an indication of inflammation of the bladder or urethra, 291

Frontal bone, the forehead bone of the skull, 84, 85, 87f, 87t

Frontal lobe, one of the four cerebral hemisphere lobes. It controls motor functions, 392, 393, 393f

Frontal plane, a vertical plane that divides the body into front (anterior or ventral) and back (posterior or dorsal) sections. Also called the *coronal plane,* 30, 30*f,* 31

Frontal section, sectional view of the body produced by a cut along the frontal plane; also called a *coronal section.* 30, 31

Frozen section (FS), a thin piece of tissue is cut from a frozen specimen for rapid examination under a microscope, 63

FS, 65

FSH, 373

Full-term pregnancy, 319*f*

Functional bowel syndrome, 259

Functional residual capacity (FRC), the air that remains in the lungs after a normal exhalation has taken place, 215*t*

Fundus, the domed upper portion of an organ such as the stomach or uterus, 248, 248*f*

Fundus (uterus), 314*f,* 316, 316*f,* 319*f*

Fungal scrapings, scrapings, taken with a curette or scraper, of tissue from lesions are placed on a growth medium and examined under a microscope to identify fungal growth, 63

Fungi, organisms found in the Kingdom Fungi. Some are capable of causing disease in humans, such as yeast infections or histoplasmosis, 184

Funny bone, 83

Furuncle, staphylococcal skin abscess with redness, pain, and swelling. Also called a *boil,* 63

G

Gait, manner of walking, 486

Gait training, assisting a person to learn to walk again or how to use an assistive device to walk, 486

Gallbladder (GB), small organ located just under the liver. It functions to store the bile produced by the liver. The gallbladder releases bile into the duodenum through the common bile duct, 27*t,* 33*t,* 34*t,* 243*f,* 244, 251, 251*f,* 260*f*

Gametes, the reproductive sex cells—ova and sperm, 360

Gamma globulin, protein component of blood containing antibodies that help to resist infection, 170

Ganglion, knotlike mass of nerve tissue located outside the brain and spinal cord, 395, 396

Ganglion cyst, cyst that forms on tendon sheath, usually on hand, wrist, or ankle, 111

Gangrene, necrosis of the skin usually due to deficient blood supply, 61

Gastralgia, stomach pain, 252

Gastrectomy, surgical removal of the stomach, 253

Gastric, pertaining to the stomach, 252

Gastric carcinoma, cancerous tumor of the stomach, 256

Gastric stapling, procedure that closes off a large section of the stomach with rows of staples. Results in a much smaller stomach to assist very obese patients to lose weight, 263

Gastritis, inflammation of the stomach that can result in pain, tenderness, nausea, and vomiting, 253

Gastroenteritis, inflammation of the stomach and small intestines, 3, 252

Gastroenterologist, a physician specialized in treating diseases and conditions of the gastrointestinal tract, 252

Gastroenterology, branch of medicine specializing in conditions of the gastrointestinal system, 27*t,* 255

Gastroesophageal reflux disease (GERD), acid from the stomach backs up into the esophagus, causing inflammation and pain, 256

Gastrointestinal, 27*t*

Gastrointestinal system (GI), system that digests food and absorbs nutrients. Organs include the mouth, pharynx, esophagus, stomach, small and large intestines, liver, gallbladder, and anus. Also called the digestive system, 244

Gastrointestinal tract, the continuous tube that extends from mouth to anus; also called *gut* or *alimentary canal,* 244

Gastromalacia, softening of the stomach, 252

Gastroscope, instrument to view inside the stomach, 253, 262

Gastroscopy, a flexible gastroscope is passed through the mouth and down the esophagus in order to visualize inside the stomach; used to diagnose peptic ulcers and gastric carcinoma, 262

Gastrostomy, surgical creation of a gastric fistula or opening through the abdominal wall. The opening is used to place food into the stomach when the esophagus is not entirely open (esophageal stricture), 252

Gavage, using a nasogastric tube to place liquid nourishment directly into the stomach, 262

General anesthesia (GA), general anesthesia produces a loss of consciousness including an absence of pain sensation. It is administered to a patient by either an intravenous or inhalation method. The patient's vital signs are carefully monitored when using a general anesthetic, 490

General hospital, hospitals that typically provide services to diagnose (laboratory, diagnostic imaging) and treat (surgery, medications, therapy) diseases for a short period of time. In addition, they usually provide emergency and obstetrical care. Also called an *acute care hospital,* 11

Generic name, the recognized and accepted official name for a drug. Each drug has only one generic name. This name is not subject to trademark, so any pharmaceutical manufacturer may use it. Also called *nonproprietary name,* 465

Genital herpes, creeping skin disease that can appear like a blister or vesicle, caused by a sexually transmitted virus, 337

Genital warts, growths and elevations of warts on the genitalia of both males and females that can lead to cancer of the cervix in females, 338

Genitalia, the male and female reproductive organs, 314

Genitourinary system (GU), the organs of the urinary system and the female or male sexual organs, 282, 333

GERD, 264

Gestation, length of time from conception to birth, generally nine months. Calculated from the first day of the last menstrual period, with a range of from 259 days to 280 days, 318

GH, 373

Gigantism, excessive development of the body due to the overproduction of the growth hormone by the pituitary gland. The opposite of dwarfism, 370

Gingiva, the tissue around the teeth; also called *gums.* 244, 245f, 246, 247f

Gingival, pertaining to the gums, 253

Gingivitis, inflammation of the gums characterized by swelling, redness, and a tendency to bleed, 253

Girdle, 88

Glands, the organs of the body that release secretions. Exocrine glands, like sweat glands, release their secretions into ducts. Endocrine glands, such as the thyroid gland, release their hormones directly into the blood stream, 358, 390
adrenal, 28t
apocrine, 53, 54
bulbourethral, 28t
lymph, 182
parathyroid, 28t
pineal, 28t
pituitary, 28t
prostate, 28t, 33t
salivary, 27t
sebaceous, 25t, 50, 51f, 52–53
sudoriferous, 53
sweat, 25t, 50, 51f, 53–54
thymus, 26t, 28t, 33t, 181, 184
thyroid, 28t, 211f

Glans penis, the larger and softer tip of the penis. It is protected by a covering called the prepuce or foreskin, 333f, 334

Glaucoma, increase in intraocular pressure that, if untreated, may result in atrophy (wasting away) of the optic nerve and blindness. Glaucoma is treated with medication and surgery. There is an increased risk of developing glaucoma in persons over 60 years of age, people of African ancestry, persons who have sustained a serious eye injury, and anyone with a family history of diabetes or glaucoma, 433

Globulins, one type of protein found dissolved in the plasma, 170

Glomerular, 284f

Glomerular capsule, also called Bowman's capsule. Part of the renal corpuscle. It is a double-walled cuplike structure that encircles the glomerulus. In the filtration stage of urine production, waste products filtered from the blood enter Bowman's capsule as the glomerular filtrate, 283, 286f

Glomerular filtrate, the product of the filtration stage of urine production. Water, electrolytes, nutrients, wastes, and toxins that are filtered from blood passing through the glomerulus. The filtrate enters Bowman's capsule, 286

Glomerulonephritis, inflammation of the kidney (primarily of the glomerulus). Since the glomerular membrane is inflamed, it becomes more permeable and will allow protein and blood cells to enter the filtrate. Results in protein in the urine (proteinuria) and hematuria, 292

Glomerulus, ball of capillaries encased by Bowman's capsule. In the filtration stage of urine production, wastes filtered from the blood leave the glomerulus capillaries and enter Bowman's capsule, 283, 284f, 286f

Glossal, pertaining to the tongue, 253

Glossopharyngeal nerve, 396t

Glottis, the opening between the vocal cords. Air passes through the glottis as it moves through the larynx. Changing the tension of the vocal cords changes the size of the opening, 212

Glucagon, a hormone secreted by the pancreas. It stimulates the liver to release glucose into the blood, 359t, 361

Glucocorticoids, a group of hormones secreted by the adrenal cortex. They regulate carbohydrate levels in the body. Cortisol is an example of a glucocorticoid, 358t, 360

Glucose, the form of sugar used by the cells of the body to make energy. It is transported to the cells in the blood, 170

Glucose tolerance test (GTT), test to determine the blood sugar level. A measured dose of glucose is given to a patient either orally or intravenously. Blood samples are then drawn at certain intervals to determine the ability of the patient to utilize glucose. Used for diabetic patients to determine their insulin response to glucose, 372

Glutamic oxaloacetic transaminase (GOT), 148

Gluteal, pertaining to the buttocks, 31, 36

Gluteal region, refers to the buttock region of the body, 31, 32*f*

Gluteus maximus, a muscle named for its size and location: Gluteus means *rump area* and maximus means *large.* 107

Glycosuria, presence of an excess of sugar in the urine, 290, 368

Goiter, enlargement of the thyroid gland, 371, 371*f*

Gonadotropins, common name for follicle-stimulating hormone and luteinizing hormone, 363

Gonads, the organs responsible for producing sex cells. The female gonads are the ovaries, and they produce ova. The male gonads are the testes, and they produce sperm, 360

Gonorrhea, sexually transmitted inflammation of the mucous membranes of either sex. Can be passed on to an infant during the birth process, 338

GOT, 152

Grade, a tumor can be graded from grade I through grade IV. The grade is based on the microscopic appearance of the tumor cells. A grade I tumor is well differentiated and is easier to treat than the more advanced grades, 495, 496*t*

Graft *versus* host disease (GVHD), serious complication of bone marrow transplant; immune cells from the donor bone marrow (graft) attack the recipient's (host's) tissues. 189

Grand mal seizure, 403

Granulocytes, granular polymorphonuclear leukocyte. There are three types: neutrophil, eosinophil, and basophil, 171, 171*t*, 173

Graves' disease, condition, named for Robert Graves, an Irish physician, that results in overactivity of the thyroid gland and can result in a crisis situation. Also called *hyperthyroidism,* 368, 371

Gray matter, tissue within the central nervous system. It consists of unsheathed or uncovered nerve cell bodies and dendrites, 390, 391

Great saphenous vein, 142*f*

Greenstick fracture, fracture in which there is an incomplete break; one side of the bone is broken and the other side is bent. This type of fracture is commonly found in children due to their softer and more pliable bone structure, 97

Gross motor skills, the use of large muscle groups that coordinate body movements such as walking, running, jumping, and balance, 485

Growth hormone (GH), a hormone secreted by the anterior pituitary that stimulates growth of the body, 359*t*, 363

GTT, 373

Guillain-Barré syndrome, disease of the nervous system in which nerves lose their myelin covering; may be caused by an autoimmune reaction; characterized by loss of sensation and/or muscle control in the arms and legs; symptoms then move toward the trunk and may even result in paralysis of the diaphragm, 404

Gums, the tissue around the teeth; also called *gingiva.* 244, 246

Gut, name for the continuous muscular tube that stretches between the mouth and anus; also called the *alimentary canal,* 244

GVHD, 192

GYN, gyn, 330

Gynecologist, a physician specialized in treating conditions and diseases of the female reproductive system, 322, 323

Gynecology, branch of medicine specializing in conditions of the female reproductive system, 28*t*, 323

Gynecomastia, the development of breast tissue in males; may be a symptom of adrenal feminization, 368

Gyri, the convoluted, elevated portions of the cerebral cortex. They are separated by fissures or sulci. Singular is gyrus, 392

H

H₂-receptor antagonist, blocks the production of stomach acids, 264

Habituation, development of an emotional dependence on a drug due to repeated use, 470

Hair, a structure in the integumentary system, 25*t*, 49, 50, 51*f*, 52

Hair follicle, cavities in the dermis that contain the hair root. Hair grows longer from the root, 52, 53*f*

Hair root, deeper cells that divide to grow a hair longer, 52, 53*f*

Hair shaft, older keratinized cells that form most of the length of a hair, 52, 53*f*

Hallucinations, the perception of an object that is not there or event that has not happened. Hallucinations may be visual, auditory, olfactory, gustatory, or tactile, 475

Hammer, 441*f*, 442

Hand, 92*f*

Hard palate, 211*f*, 245*f*

Hashimoto's disease, chronic form of thyroiditis, named for a Japanese surgeon, 371

HCT, Hct, crit, 178

HD, 192, 297

Hemophilia, hereditary blood disease in which there is a prolonged blood clotting time. It is transmitted by a sex-linked trait from females to males. It appears almost exclusively in males, 174

Hemoptysis, coughing up blood or blood-stained sputum, 219

Hemorrhage, blood flow, the escape of blood from a blood vessel, 173

Hemorrhoid, varicose veins in the rectum, 147, 258

Hemorrhoidectomy, surgical excision of hemorrhoids from the anorectal area, 263

Hemostasis, to stop bleeding or the stagnation of the circulating blood, 172, 174, 493

Hemostat, a surgical instrument used to grasp blood vessels to control bleeding, 491*t*

Hemostatic agent, 178

Hemothorax, condition of having blood in the chest cavity, 218

Hepatic, pertaining to the liver, 253

Hepatic duct, the duct that leads from the liver to the common bile duct; transports bile, 251, 251*f*, 260*f*

Hepatic portal vein, 142*f*

Hepatitis, infectious, inflammatory disease of the liver. Hepatitis B and C types are spread by contact with blood and bodily fluids of an infected person, 253, 260

Hepatoma, liver tumor, 253

Herniated nucleus pulposus (HNP), a rupture of the fibrocartilage disk between two vertebrae. This results in pressure on a spinal nerve and causes pain, weakness, and nerve damage. Also called a slipped disk, 98, 98*f*

Hernioplasty, surgical repair of a hernia; also called herniorrhaphy, 263

Herniorrhaphy, 263

Herpes labialis, infection of the lip by the herpes simplex virus type 1 (HSV-1). Also called *fever blisters* or *cold sores,* 256

Herpes simplex virus (HSV), 65

Herpes zoster virus, 404

Hertz (Hz), measurement of the frequency or pitch of sound. The lowest pitch on an audiogram is 250 Hz. The measurement can go as high as 8000 Hz, which is the highest pitch measured, 445

Hesitancy, a decrease in the force of the urine stream, often with difficulty initiating the flow. It is often a symptom of a blockage along the urethra, such as an enlarged prostate gland, 291

Heterograft, skin graft from an animal of another species (usually a pig) to a human; also called a *xenograft,* 64

Hiatal hernia, protrusion of the stomach through the diaphragm and extending into the thoracic cavity; gastroesophageal reflux disease is a common symptom, 256, 256*f*

Hilum, the controlled entry/exit point of an organ such as the kidney or lung, 214, 282, 283*f*

Hipbone, 90

Hirsutism, excessive hair growth over the body, 56, 368

Histology, the study of tissues, 23

Histoplasma capsulatum, 222

Histoplasmosis, pulmonary disease caused by a fungus found in dust in the droppings of pigeons and chickens, 222

History and physical, medical record document written by the admitting physician. It details the patient's history, results of the physician's examination, initial diagnoses, and physician's plan of treatment, 10

HIV, 192

Hives, appearance of wheals as part of an allergic reaction, 57, 187

Hodgkin's disease (HD), also called Hodgkin's lymphoma. Cancer of the lymphatic cells found in concentration in the lymph nodes, 189, 189*f*

Hodgkin's lymphoma, 189, 189*f*

Holter monitor, portable ECG monitor worn by the patient for a period of a few hours to a few days to assess the heart and pulse activity as the person goes through the activities of daily living, 149

Home health care, agencies that provide nursing, therapy, personal care, or housekeeping services in the patient's own home, 12

Homeostasis, steady state or state of balance within the body. The kidneys assist in maintaining this regulatory, steady state, 285, 358

Homologous transfusion, replacement of blood by transfusion of blood received from another person, 177

Hordeolum, a *stye* (or sty), a small purulent inflammatory infection of a sebaceous gland of the eye, treated with hot compresses and surgical incision, 434

Horizontal plane, a horizontal plane that divides the body into upper (superior) and lower (inferior) sections. Also called the *transverse plane,* 30, 31

Hormonal contraception, use of hormones to block ovulation and prevent contraception. May be in the form of a pill, a patch, an implant under the skin, or injection, 323

Hormone, a chemical substance secreted by an endocrine gland. It enters the blood stream and is carried to target tissue. Hormones work to control the functioning of the target tissue. Given to replace the loss of natural hormones or to treat disease by stimulating hormonal effects, 358

Hormone replacement therapy (HRT), artificial replacement of hormones in a patient who is unable to produce sufficient hormones. Example is estrogen replacement in menopausal women, 329, 372

Hormone therapy, treatment of cancer with natural hormones or with chemicals that produce hormonelike effects, 497

Hospice, an organized group of healthcare workers who provide supportive treatment to dying patients and their families, 12

HPV, 330

HRT, 330

HSG, 330

HSV, 65

Human growth hormone therapy, therapy with human growth hormone in order to stimulate skeletal growth; used to treat children with abnormally short stature, 373

Human immunodeficiency virus (HIV), virus that causes AIDS; also known as a retrovirus, 188, 188f, 338

Human papilloma virus (HPV), 324

Humanistic psychotherapy, form of psychological counseling in which the therapist does not delve into the patients' past; it is believed that patients can learn how to use their own internal resources to deal with their problems, 476

Humeral, pertaining to the humerus or upper arm bone, 94

Humerus, the upper arm bone in the upper extremity, 82, 88, 89f, 90, 90f

Humoral immunity, immunity that responds to antigens, such as bacteria and foreign agents, by producing antibodies. Also called *antibody-mediated immunity,* 185

Humpback, 95

Hunchback, 95

Hyaline membrane disease (HMD), 222

Hydrocele, accumulation of fluid within the testes, 336

Hydrocephalus, accumulation of cerebrospinal fluid within the ventricles of the brain, causing the head to be enlarged. It is treated by creating an artificial shunt for the fluid to leave the brain, 402, 402f

Hydrochloric acid (HCl), acid secreted by the stomach lining. Aids in digestion, 248

Hydronephrosis, distention of the pelvis due to urine collecting in the kidney resulting from an obstruction, 292

Hydrotherapy, using water for treatment purposes, 486

Hymen, a thin membranous tissue that covers the external vaginal opening or orifice. The membrane is broken during the first sexual encounter of the female. It can also be broken prematurely by the use of tampons or during some sports activities, 317

Hymenectomy, surgical removal of the hymen. Performed when the hymen tissue is particularly tough, 322

Hyoid bone, a single, U-shaped bone suspended in the neck between the mandible and larynx. It is a point of attachment for swallowing and speech muscles, 84, 85, 211f

Hypercalcemia, condition of having an excessive amount of calcium in the blood, 367

Hypercapnia, excessive carbon dioxide, 218

Hyperemesis, excessive vomiting, 254

Hyperemia, redness of the skin caused by increased blood flow to the skin, 56

Hyperesthesia, having excessive sensation, 399

Hyperglycemia, having an excessive amount of glucose (sugar) in the blood, 367

Hyperhidrosis, abnormal condition of excessive sweat, 54

Hyperkalemia, condition of having an excessive amount of potassium in the blood, 367

Hyperkinesia, an excessive amount of movement, 110

Hyperlipidemia, condition of having too high a level of lipids such as cholesterol in the bloodstream; a risk factor for developing atherosclerosis and coronary artery disease, 174

Hyperopia, with this condition a person can see things in the distance but has trouble reading material at close vision. Also known as *farsightedness,* 433, 433f

Hyperparathyroidism, state of excessive thyroid, 367

Hyperpigmentation, abnormal amount of pigmentation in the skin, which is seen in diseases such as acromegaly and adrenal insufficiency, 56

Hyperpituitarism, state of excessive pituitary gland, 367

Hyperplasia, excessive development of normal cells within an organ, 496

Hyperpnea, excessive deep breathing, 218

Hypersecretion, excessive hormone production by an endocrine gland, 368

Hypertension, high blood pressure, 148

Hyperthyroidism, condition resulting from overactivity of the thyroid gland that can result in a crisis situation. Also called *Graves' disease,* 368, 371

Hypertonia, excessive tone, 110

Hypertrophy, an increase in the bulk or size of a tissue or structure, 111

Hyperventilation, to breathe both fast (tachypnea) and deep (hyperpnea), 219

Hypnotic, substance used to produce sleep or hypnosis, 407

Hypocalcemia, condition of having a low calcium level in the blood, 367

Hypochondria, a somatoform disorder involving a preoccupation with health concerns, 475

Hypochondriac, 34*t*

Hypochromic anemia, anemia resulting from having insufficient hemoglobin in the erythrocytes; named because the hemoglobin molecule is responsible for the dark red color of the erythrocytes, 175

Hypodermic, pertaining to under the skin, 54

Hypodermis, the deepest layer of skin; composed primarily of adipose, 52

Hypogastric, pertaining to below the stomach. An anatomical division of the abdomen, the middle section of the bottom row, 34*t*

Hypogastric region, 34*t*

Hypoglossal, pertaining to under the tongue, 253

Hypoglossal nerve, 396*t*

Hypoglycemia, condition of having a low sugar level in the blood, 367

Hypokinesia, insufficient movement, 110

Hyponatremia, condition of having a low sodium level in the blood, 367

Hypoparathyroidism, state of insufficient thyroid, 367

Hypopituitarism, state of insufficient pituitary gland, 367

Hypopnea, insufficient or shallow breathing, 218

Hyposecretion, deficient hormone production by an endocrine gland, 368

Hypospadias, congenital opening of the male urethra on the underside of the penis, 337

Hypotension, low blood pressure, 148

Hypothalamus, a portion of the diencephalon that lies just below the thalamus. It controls body temperature, appetite, sleep, sexual desire, and emotions such as fear. It also regulates the release of hormones from the pituitary gland and regulates the parasympathetic and sympathetic nervous systems, 363, 363*f,* 392, 392*f,* 393

Hypothyroidism, result of a deficiency in secretion by the thyroid gland. This results in a lowered basal metabolism rate with obesity, dry skin, slow pulse, low blood pressure, sluggishness, and goiter. Treatment is replacement with synthetic thyroid hormone, 368

Hypotonia, insufficient tone, 110

Hypoventilation, to breathe both slow (bradypnea) and shallow (hypopnea), 219

Hypoxemia, deficiency of oxygen in the blood, 217

Hypoxia, absence of oxygen in the tissues, 217

Hysterectomy, removal of the uterus, 322

Hysteropexy, surgical fixation of the uterus, 322

Hysterorrhexis, rupture of the uterus, 322

Hysterosalpingectomy, 8

Hysterosalpingography, process of taking an X-ray of the uterus and oviducts after a radiopaque material is injected into the organs, 327

Hz, 448

I

I&D, 65

Iatrogenic, usually an unfavorable response that results from taking a medication, 470

Ichthyoderma, dry and scaly skin condition, 55

Ichthyosis, condition in which the skin becomes dry, scaly, and keratinized, 61

ID, 65

IDDM, 373

Identical twins, twins that develop from the splitting of one fertilized ovum; these siblings have identical DNA, 323

Idiosyncrasy, unusual or abnormal response to a drug or food, 470

Ileal, pertaining to the ileum, 253

Ileocecal valve, sphincter between the ileum and the cecum, 248, 249, 250*f*

Ileostomy, surgical creation of a passage through the abdominal wall into the ileum, 253

Ileum, the third portion of the small intestines. Joins the colon at the cecum. The ileum and cecum are separated by the ileocecal valve, 9, 248, 249, 249*f*

Ileus, severe abdominal pain, inability to pass stools, vomiting, and abdominal distention as a result of an intestinal blockage; may require surgery to reverse the blockage, 258

Iliac, pertaining to the ilium; one of the pelvic bones, 94

Ilium, one of three bones that form the os coxae or innominate bone of the pelvis, 9, 88, 89*f,* 90, 91*f,* 91*t*

IM, 112

Immune response, ability of lymphocytes to respond to specific antigens, 184, 185–86

Immunity, the body's ability to defend itself against pathogens, 184–86

immune response, 185–86

standard precautions, 186

Immunization, providing protection against communicable diseases by stimulating the immune system to produce antibodies against that disease. Children can now be immunized for the following diseases; hepatitis B, diphtheria, tetanus, pertussis, tetanus, *Haemophilus influenzae* type b, polio, measles, mumps, rubella, and chickenpox. Also called *vaccination,* 184, 185, 192

Immunocompromised, having an immune system that is unable to respond properly to pathogens, 188

Immunodeficiency disorder, 188

Immunoglobulins (Ig), antibodies secreted by the B cells. All antibodies are immunoglobulins. They assist in protecting the body and its surfaces from the invasion of bacteria. For example, the immunoglobulin IgA in colostrum, the first milk from the mother, helps to protect the newborn from infection, 188

Immunologist, a physician who specializes in treating infectious diseases and other disorders of the immune system, 187, 188

Immunology, branch of medicine specializing in conditions of the lymphatic and immune systems, 26*t*, 188

Immunosuppressants, substances that block certain actions of the immune system; required to prevent rejection of a transplanted organ, 192

Immunotherapy, the production or strengthening of a patient's immune system in order to treat a disease, 192, 497

Impacted fracture, fracture in which bone fragments are pushed into each other, 97

Impetigo, a highly contagious staphylococcal skin infection, most commonly occurring on the faces of children. It begins as blisters that then rupture and dry into a thick, yellow crust, 61, 61*f*

Implant, prosthetic device placed in the jaw to which a tooth or denture may be anchored, 255

Implantable cardiovert-defibrillator, a device implanted in the heart that delivers an electrical shock to restore a normal heart rhythm. Particularly useful for persons who experience ventricular fibrillation, 150

Impulse control disorders, inability to resist an impulse to perform some act that is harmful to the individual or others; includes kleptomania, pyromania, explosive disorder, and pathological gambling, 474

Incision and drainage (I&D), making an incision to create an opening for the drainage of material such as pus, 64

Incisors, biting teeth in the very front of the mouth that function to cut food into smaller pieces. Humans have eight incisors, 245*f*, 246, 246*f*

Incus, one of the three ossicles of the middle ear. Also called the *anvil*, 441*f*, 442, 442*f*

Infant respiratory distress syndrome (IRDS), a lung condition most commonly found in premature infants that is characterized by tachypnea and respiratory grunting. Also called *hyaline membrane disease* (HMD) and *respiratory distress syndrome of the newborn,* 222

Infarct, area of tissue within an organ that undergoes necrosis (death) following the loss of blood supply, 143

Inferior, directional term meaning toward the feet or tail, or below, 35*f*, 35*t*

Inferior vena cava, the branch of the vena cava that drains blood from the abdomen and lower body, 134*f*, 135, 136, 137*f*, 142*f*, 360*f*

Infertility, inability to produce children; generally defined as no pregnancy after properly timed intercourse for one year, 324

Inflammation, the tissue response to injury from pathogens or physical agents; characterized by redness, pain, swelling, and feeling hot to touch, 188, 188*f*

Inflammatory bowel disease (IBD), 259

Influenza, viral infection of the respiratory system characterized by chills, fever, body aches, and fatigue. Commonly called the *flu,* 222

Informed consent, a medical record document, voluntarily signed by the patient or a responsible party, that clearly describes the purpose, methods, procedures, benefits, and risks of a diagnostic or treatment procedure, 11

Inguinal, pertaining to the groin area. There is a collection of lymph nodes in this region that drain each leg, 182

Inguinal hernia, hernia or outpouching of intestines into the inguinal region of the body, 258, 258*f*

Inguinal nodes, 182*t*, 183*f*

Inhalation, (1) To breathe air into the lungs. Also called *inspiration.* (2) To introduce drugs into the body by inhaling them, 210, 467, 468, 468*f*, 490

Innate immunity, 184

Inner ear, the innermost section of the ear. It contains the cochlea, semicircular canals, saccule, and utricle, 440*f*, 441, 441*f*, 442, 443*f*

Inner ear infection, 446

Innominate bone, also called the os coxae or hip bone. It is the pelvis portion of the lower extremity. It consists of the ilium, ischium, and pubis and unites with the sacrum and coccyx to form the pelvis, 88, 90

Insertion, the attachment of a skeletal muscle to the more movable bone in the joint, 107

Insomnia, a sleeping disorder characterized by a marked inability to fall asleep, 475

Inspiration, 210, 216*f*

Inspiratory capacity (IC), the volume of air inhaled after a normal exhale, 215*t*

Inspiratory reserve volume (IRV), the air that can be forcibly inhaled after a normal respiration has taken place. Also called *complemental air,* 215*t*

Insulin, the hormone secreted by the pancreas. It regulates the level of sugar in the blood stream. The more insulin present in the blood, the lower the blood sugar will be, 359t, 361, 373

Insulin-dependent diabetes mellitus (IDDM), also called type 1 diabetes mellitus; it develops early in life when the pancreas stops insulin production. Persons with IDDM must take daily insulin injections, 369

Insulinoma, tumor of the islets of Langerhans cells of the pancreas that secretes an excessive amount of insulin, 369

Integument, another term for skin, 50

Integumentary system, the skin and its appendages including sweat glands, oil glands, hair, and nails. Sense organs that allow us to respond to changes in temperature, pain, touch, and pressure are located in the skin. It is the largest organ in the body, 25t, 48–77
  abbreviations, 65
  accessory organs, 52–54
  anatomy and physiology of, 50
  diagnostic procedures, 63
  pathology, 58–63
  pharmacology, 65
  skin, 50–52
  therapeutic procedures, 64
  vocabulary, 55–57
  word building, 54–55

Interatrial, pertaining to between the atria, 143

Interatrial septum, the wall or septum that divides the left and right atria, 134

Intercostal muscles, muscles between the ribs. When they contract, they raise the ribs, which helps to enlarge the thoracic cavity, 215

Intercostal nerve, 397f

Intermittent claudication, attacks of severe pain and lameness caused by ischemia of the muscles, typically the calf muscles; brought on by walking even very short distances, 111

Intermittent positive pressure breathing (IPPB), method for assisting patients to breathe using a mask connected to a machine that produces an increased pressure, 225

Internal genitalia, 314–17

Internal iliac artery, 140f

Internal iliac vein, 142f

Internal medicine, branch of medicine involving the diagnosis and treatment of diseases and conditions of internal organs such as the respiratory system. The physician is an *internist*, 219, 255

Internal respiration, the process of oxygen and carbon dioxide exchange at the cellular level when oxygen leaves the bloodstream and is delivered to the tissues, 210

Internal sphincter, ring of involuntary muscle that keeps urine within the bladder, 284

Internist, a physician specialized in treating diseases and conditions of internal organs such as the respiratory system, 219, 255

Internodal pathway, 137f

Interstitial cystitis, disease of unknown cause in which there is inflammation and irritation of the bladder. Most commonly seen in middle-aged women, 293

Interventricular, pertaining to between the ventricles, 143

Interventricular septum, the wall or septum that divides the left and right ventricles, 134, 135f, 137f

Intervertebral, pertaining to between vertebrae, 93

Intervertebral disk, fibrous cartilage cushion between vertebrae, 84, 85

Intracavitary, injection into a body cavity such as the peritoneal and chest cavity, 469t

Intracoronary artery stent, placing a stent within a coronary artery to treat coronary ischemia due to atherosclerosis, 151

Intracranial, pertaining to inside the skull, 93

Intradermal (ID), (1) Pertaining to within the skin. (2) Injection of medication into the skin, 54, 65, 469t

Intramuscular (IM), injection of medication into the muscle, 112, 469t

Intraocular, pertaining to within the eye, 431

Intraoperative, period of time during an operation, 493

Intrathecal, (1) Pertaining to within the meninges. (2) Injection into the meninges space surrounding the brain and spinal cord, 399, 469t

Intrauterine device (IUD), device that is inserted into the uterus by a physician for the purpose of contraception, 324, 324f

Intravenous (IV), injection into the veins. This route can be set up so that there is a continuous administration of medication, 469t, 490

Intravenous cholecystography, a dye is administered intravenously to the patient that allows for X-ray visualization of the gallbladder, 261

Intravenous pyelogram (IVP), injecting a contrast medium into a vein and then taking an X-ray to visualize the renal pelvis, 293

Intussusception, an intestinal condition in which one portion of the intestine telescopes into an adjacent portion causing an obstruction and gangrene if untreated, 258, 258f

Invasive disease, tendency of a malignant tumor to spread to immediately surrounding tissue and organs, 496

Inversion, directional term meaning turning inward or inside out, 109, 109f

Involuntary muscles, muscles under the control of the subconscious regions of the brain. The smooth muscles found in internal organs and cardiac muscles are examples of involuntary muscle tissue, 105

Iodine, a mineral required by the thyroid to produce its hormones, 366

IPPB, 227

IRDS, 227

Iridal, pertaining to the iris, 431

Iridectomy, excision of the iris, 431

Iridoplegia, paralysis of the iris, 431

Iridosclerotomy, incision into the iris and sclera, 431

Iris, the colored portion of the eye. It can dilate or constrict to change the size of the pupil and control the amount of light entering the interior of the eye, 425f, 426f, 427, 430f

Iritis, inflammation of the iris, 431

Iron-deficiency anemia, anemia that results from having insufficient iron to manufacture hemoglobin, 175

Irregular bones, a type of bone having an irregular shape. Vertebrae are irregular bones, 82

Irritable bowel syndrome (IBS), disturbance in the functions of the intestine from unknown causes. Symptoms generally include abdominal discomfort and an alteration in bowel activity. Also called *functional bowel syndrome* or *spastic colon,* 259

Ischemia, localized and temporary deficiency of blood supply due to an obstruction of the circulation, 143

Ischial, pertaining to the ischium, one of the pelvic bones, 94

Ischium, one of the three bones that form the os coxae or innominate bone of the pelvis, 88, 89f, 90, 91f, 91t

Islets of Langerhans, the regions within the pancreas that secrete insulin and glucagon, 361, 361f

Isthmus, 366f

IVF, 330

IVP, 297

J

Jaundice, yellow cast to the skin, mucous membranes, and the whites of the eyes caused by the deposit of bile pigment from too much bilirubin in the blood. Bilirubin is a waste product produced when worn-out red blood cells are broken down. May be a symptom of disorders such as gallstones blocking the common bile duct or carcinoma of the liver, 255

Jaw bone, 247f

Jejunal, pertaining to the jejunum, 253

Jejunostomy, 249

Jejunum, the middle portion of the small intestines. Site of nutrient absorption, 248, 249, 249f

Joint, the point at which two bones meet. It provides flexibility, 25t, 82, 91–92

Joint capsule, elastic capsule that encloses synovial joints, 91, 92

Jugular vein, 142f, 441f

K

Kaposi's sarcoma (KS), form of skin cancer frequently seen in acquired immunodeficiency syndrome (AIDS) patients. Consists of brownish-purple papules that spread from the skin and metastasize to internal organs, 62, 189

Keloid, formation of a scar after an injury or surgery that results in a raised, thickened red area, 56

Keratin, a hard protein substance produced by the body. It is found in hair and nails, and filling the inside of epidermal cells, 50, 51

Keratitis, inflammation of the cornea, 431

Keratometer, instrument to measure the cornea, 431, 435

Keratometry, measurement of the curvature of the cornea using an instrument called a keratometer, 435

Keratoplasty, surgical repair of the cornea (corneal transplant), 436

Keratosis, overgrowth and thickening of the epithelium, 56

Keratotomy, incision into the cornea, 431

Ketoacidosis, acidosis due to an excess of ketone bodies (waste products). A serious condition that requires immediate treatment and can result in death for the diabetic patient if not reversed, 369

Ketones, 287t

Ketonuria, ketones in the urine, 290

Kidneys, the two kidneys are located in the lumbar region of the back behind the parietal peritoneum. They are under the muscles of the back, just a little above the waist. The kidneys have a concave or depressed area that gives them a bean-shaped appearance. The center of this concavity is called the hilum, 27t, 33, 34t, 281f, 282–83, 283f, 284f, 360f

Kidneys, ureters, bladder (KUD), x-ray taken of the abdomen demonstrating the kidneys, ureters, and bladder without using any contrast dye; also called a flat-plate abdomen, 293

Kinesiology, the study of movement, 110

Kleptomania, an impulse control disorder in which the patient is unable to refrain from stealing. The items are often trivial and unneeded, 474

KS, 192

KUB, 297, 483

Kyphosis, abnormal increase in the outward curvature of the thoracic spine. Also known as hunchback or humpback, 95, 95f

Medical terms, interpreting, 8–9
    pronunciation, 8–9
    spelling, 9
Medication, 465
Medulla, the central area of an organ. In the endocrine system it refers to the adrenal medulla; in the urinary system, it refers to the inner portion of the kidney, 282, 283f, 393f
Medulla oblongata, a portion of the brain stem that connects the spinal cord with the brain. It contains the respiratory, cardiac, and blood pressure control centers, 392, 392f, 393
Medullary, pertaining to the medulla, 93
Medullary cavity, the large open cavity that extends the length of the shaft of a long bone; contains yellow bone marrow, 82, 83
Melanin, the black color pigment in the skin. It helps to prevent the sun's ultraviolet rays from entering the body, 50, 51
Melanocyte-stimulating hormone (MSH), a hormone secreted by the anterior pituitary. It stimulates pigment production in the skin, 359t, 363–64
Melanocytes, special cells in the basal layer of the epidermis. They contain the black pigment melanin that gives skin its color and protects against the ultraviolet rays of the sun, 50, 51, 54
Melanoma, also called *malignant melanoma.* A dangerous form of skin cancer caused by an overgrowth of melanin in a melanocyte. It may metastasize or spread. Exposure to ultraviolet light is a risk factor for developing melanoma, 54
Melatonin, hormone secreted by the pineal gland; plays a role in regulating the body's circadian rhythm, 362
Melena, passage of dark tarry stools; color is the result of digestive enzymes working on blood in the stool, 255
Menarche, the first menstrual period, 316, 317
Ménière's disease, abnormal condition within the labyrinth of the inner ear that can lead to a progressive loss of hearing. The symptoms are dizziness or vertigo, hearing loss, and tinnitus (ringing in the ears), 446
Meningeal, pertaining to the meninges, 398
Meninges, three connective tissue membrane layers that surround the brain and spinal cord. The three layers are dura mater, arachnoid layer, and pia mater. The dura mater and arachnoid layer are separated by the subdural space. The arachnoid layer and pia mater are separated by the subarachnoid space, 390, 392, 395
Meningioma, slow-growing tumor in the meninges of the brain, 398

Meningitis, inflammation of the membranes of the spinal cord and brain that is caused by a microorganism, 398
Meningocele, congenital hernia in which the meninges, or membranes, protrude through an opening in the spinal column or brain, 403, 403f
Menometrorrhagia, excessive bleeding during the menstrual period and at intervals between menstrual periods, 325
Menopause, cessation or ending of menstrual activity. This is generally between the ages of 40 and 55, 316, 317
Menorrhagia, excessive bleeding during the menstrual period. Can be either in the total number of days or the amount of blood or both, 322
Menstrual cycle, the 28-day fertility cycle in women; includes ovulation and sloughing off the endometrium if a pregnancy does not occur, 360
Menstrual period, another name for the menstrual cycle, 316, 317
Menstruation, the loss of blood and tissue as the endometrium is shed by the uterus. The flow exits the body through the cervix and vagina. The flow occurs approximately every 28 days, 316, 317
Mental health disciplines, 473–76
    abbreviations, 476
    pathology, 473–75
    psychiatry, 473
    psychology, 473
    therapeutic procedures, 475–76
Mental retardation, a disorder characterized by a diminished ability to process intellectual functions, 474
Metacarpal, pertaining to the hand bones, 94
Metacarpals, the hand bones in the upper extremity, 88, 89f, 90, 90f
Metastacized, 182
Metastases (mets), the spreading of a cancerous tumor from its original site to different locations of the body. Singular is metastasis, 495, 495f
Metastasis (mets), movement and spread of cancer cells from one part of the body to another. Metastases is plural, 496, 496f
Metastasize, when cancerous cells migrate away from a tumor site. They commonly move through the lymphatic system and become trapped in lymph nodes, 182
Metatarsal, pertaining to the foot bones, 94
Metatarsals, the ankle bones in the lower extremity, 88, 89f, 90, 91f, 91t
Metered dose inhaler (MDI), 225
Metrorrhagia, rapid (menstrual) blood flow from the uterus, 322

Metrorrhea, discharge from the uterus, 322

mets, 498

MI, 152

Microtia, abnormally small ears, 445

Micturition, another term for urination, 291

Midbrain, a portion of the brain stem, 363*f*, 392, 392*f*, 393

Middle ear, the middle section of the ear. It contains the ossicles, 440*f*, 441, 441*f*, 442, 443*f*

Middle ear infection, 446

Midline organs, 34*t*

Migraine, a specific type of headache characterized by severe head pain, photophobia, vertigo, and nausea, 403

Miner's lung, 221

Mineralocorticoids, a group of hormones secreted by the adrenal cortex. They regulate electrolytes and fluid volume in the body. Aldosterone is an example of a mineralocorticoid, 358*t*, 360

Minnesota Multiphasic Personality Inventory (MMPI), 476

Minor tranquilizers, medications that are central nervous system depressants and are prescribed for anxiety, 476

Miotic, substance that causes the pupil to constrict, 438

Miscarriage, 327

Mitral valve, a valve between the left atrium and ventricle in the heart. It prevents blood from flowing backwards into the atrium. It is also called the bicuspid valve because it has two cusps or flaps, 134*f*, 135, 136*f*, 137*f*

MM, 65

MMPI, 476

Mobility, state of having normal movement of all body parts, 485

Mobilization, treatments such as exercise and massage to restore movement to joints and soft tissue, 486

Moist hot packs, applying moist warmth to a body part to produce the slight dilation of blood vessels in the skin; causes muscle relaxation in the deeper regions of the body and increases circulation, which aids healing, 486

Molars, large somewhat flat-topped back teeth. Function to grind food. Humans have up to twelve molars, 245*f*, 246, 246*f*

mono, 192

Monoaural, referring to one ear, 445

Monochromatism, unable to perceive one color, 434

Monocytes (monos), an agranulocyte white blood cell that is important for phagocytosis, 169*f*, 171*f*, 171*t*

Mononucleosis (Mono), acute infectious disease with a large number of atypical lymphocytes. Caused by the Epstein–Barr virus. There may be abnormal liver function, 189

Monoparesis, weakness of one extremity, 399

Monoplegia, paralysis of one extremity, 399

monos, 178

Monospot, test of infectious mononucleosis in which there is a nonspecific antibody called heterophile antibody, 190

Mood disorders, characterized by instability in mood; includes major depression, mania, and bipolar disorder, 475

Morbid obesity, 255

Morbidity, number that represents the number of sick persons in a particular population, 497

Mortality, number that represents the number of deaths in a particular population, 497

Motor neurons, nerves that carry activity instruction from the CNS to muscles or glands out in the body; also called *efferent neurons.* 106, 395, 396, 397*f*

MRI, 482

MS, 152, 408

MSH, 373

Mucolytic, substance that liquefies mucus so it is easier to cough and clear it from the respiratory tract, 227

Mucous membrane, membrane that lines body passages that open directly to the exterior of the body, such as the mouth and reproductive tract, and secretes a thick substance, or mucus, 210

Mucus, sticky fluid secreted by mucous membrane lining of the respiratory tract. Assists in cleansing air by trapping dust and bacteria, 210

Multigravida, woman who has had more than one pregnancy, 323

Multipara, woman who has given birth to more than one child, 323

Multiple personality disorder, a type of dissociative disorder in which the person displays two or more distinct conscious personalities that alternate in controlling the body. The alternate personalities may or may not be aware of each other, 474

Multiple sclerosis (MS), inflammatory disease of the central nervous system. Rare in children. Generally strikes adults between the ages of 20 and 40. There is progressive weakness and numbness, 404

Murmur, an abnormal heart sound as a soft blowing sound or a harsh click. It may be soft and heard only with a stethoscope, or so loud it can be heard several feet away. Also called a *bruit,* 144

Muscle actions, 107, 108*t*–109*t*

Muscle biopsy, removal of muscle tissue for pathological examination, 112

Muscle cells, 22*f*

Muscle tissue, tissue that is able to contract and shorten its length, thereby producing movement. Muscle tissue may be under voluntary control (attached to the bones) or involuntary control (heart and digestive organs), 23, 24*f*

Muscle tissue fibers, the bundles of muscle tissue that form a muscle, 23, 53*f*, 105

Muscle wasting, 111

Muscles, muscles are bundles of parallel muscle tissue fibers. As the fibers contract (shorten in length) they pull whatever they are attached to closer together. This may move two bones closer together or make an opening more narrow. A muscle contraction occurs when a message is transmitted from the brain through the nervous system to the muscles, 25*t*, 105, 390. *See also* Muscular system

Muscular, pertaining to muscles, 110

Muscular dystrophy (MD), inherited disease causing a progressive muscle weakness and atrophy, 111

Muscular system, 104–27
  abbreviations, 112
  anatomy and physiology, 105–9
  combining forms, 110
  diagnostic procedures, 111–12
  muscle types, 105–6
  pathology, 111
  pharmacology, 112
  suffixes, 110
  terminology for muscle actions, 107, 108*t*–109*t*
  treatment procedures, 112
  vocabulary, 111
  word building, 110

Musculoskeletal system. system that provides support for the body and produces movement. Organs of the musculoskeletal system includes muscles, tendons, bones, joints, and cartilage. *See* Muscular system; Skeletal system

Mutation, change or transformation from the original, 497

Myalgia, muscle pain, 110

Myasthenia, lack of muscle strength, 110

Myasthenia gravis, disorder causing loss of muscle strength and paralysis. This is an autoimmune disease, 404

Mycoplasma **pneumonia,** a less severe but longer lasting form of pneumonia caused by the *Mycoplasma pneumoniae* bacteria. Also called *walking pneumonia,* 222

Mydriatic, substance that causes the pupil to dilate, 438

Myelin, tissue that wraps around many of the nerve fibers. It is composed of fatty material and functions as an insulator, 390, 391*f*, 392

Myelinated, nerve fibers covered with a layer of myelin, 390

Myelitis, inflammation of the spinal cord, 398

Myelogram, x-ray record of the spinal cord following injection of meninges with radiopaque dye, 398

Myelography, injection of a radiopaque dye into the spinal canal. An X-ray is then taken to examine the normal and abnormal outlines made by the dye, 100, 405

Myeloma, malignant neoplasm originating in plasma cells in the bone, 93

Myelomeningocele, a hernia composed of meninges and spinal cord, 403*f*, 404

Myocardial, pertaining to heart muscle, 110, 143

Myocardial infarction (MI), condition caused by the partial or complete occlusion or closing of one or more of the coronary arteries. Symptoms include severe chest pain or heavy pressure in the middle of the chest. A delay in treatment could result in death. Also referred to as *MI* or *heart attack,* 145*f*, 146, 146*f*

Myocarditis, inflammation of heart muscle, 146

Myocardium, the middle layer of the muscle. It is thick and composed of cardiac muscle. This layer produces the heart contraction, 106, 133, 134, 134*f*, 137*f*

Myometrium, the middle muscle layer of the uterus, 316, 316*f*

Myoneural junction, the point at which a nerve contacts a muscle fiber, 106

Myopathy, any disease of muscles, 110

Myopia, with this condition a person can see things that are close up but distance vision is blurred. Also known as *nearsightedness,* 434, 434*f*

Myoplasty, surgical repair of muscle, 110

Myorrhaphy, suture a muscle, 110

Myorrhexis, muscle ruptured, 110

Myotonia, muscle tone, 110

Myringectomy, excision of the eardrum, 444

Myringitis, eardrum inflammation, 444

Myringoplasty, surgical reconstruction of the eardrum. Also called *tympanoplasty,* 444

Myringotomy, surgical puncture of the eardrum with removal of fluid and pus from the middle ear, to eliminate a persistent ear infection and excessive pressure on the tympanic membrane. A polyethylene tube is placed in the tympanic membrane to allow for drainage of the middle ear cavity, 448

Myxedema, condition resulting from a hypofunction of the thyroid gland. Symptoms can include anemia, slow speech, enlarged tongue and facial features, edematous skin, drowsiness, and mental apathy, 371

N

Nail bed, connects nail body to connective tissue underneath, 52

Nerves, structures in the nervous system that conduct electrical impulses from the brain and spinal cord to muscles and other organs, 23, 29*t*, 51*f*, 389*f*, 390

Nervous system, system that coordinates all the conscious and subconscious activities of the body. Organs include the brain, spinal cord, and nerves, 29*t*, 387–421, 389*f*
   abbreviations, 408
   anatomy and physiology, 390–98
   central, 390–95
   diagnostic procedures, 405–6
   nervous tissue, 390
   pathology, 400–405
   peripheral, 395–98
   pharmacology, 407
   therapeutic procedures, 407
   vocabulary, 399–400
   word building, 398–99

Nervous tissue, nervous tissue conducts electrical impulses to and from the brain and the rest of the body, 23, 24*f*, 390

Neural, pertaining to nerves, 398

Neuralgia, nerve pain, 398

Neurectomy, excision of a nerve, 398

Neurogenic bladder, loss of nervous control that leads to retention; may be caused by spinal cord injury or multiple sclerosis, 293

Neuroglial cells, cells that perform support functions for neurons, 390

Neurologist, physician who specializes in disorders of the nervous system, 398, 400

Neurology, branch of medicine specializing in conditions of the nervous system, 29*t*, 400

Neuroma, nerve tumor, 398

Neuron, the name for an individual nerve cell. Neurons group together to form nerves and other nervous tissue, 23, 390

Neuropathy, disease of the nerves, 398

Neuroplasty, surgical repair of nerves, 398

Neurorrhaphy, suture a nerve, 399

Neurosurgery, branch of medicine specializing in surgery on the nervous system, 29*t*, 400

Neurotransmitter, chemical messenger that carries an electrical impulse across the gap between two neurons, 390

Neutrophils, granulocyte white blood cells that are important for phagocytosis. They are also the most numerous of the leukocytes, 169*f*, 171*f*, 171*t*

Nevus, pigmented (colored) congenital skin blemish, birthmark, or mole. Usually benign but may become cancerous, 56

NHL, 192

NIDDM, 373

Night-blindness, 432

Nipple, point at which milk is released from the breast, 318, 318*f*

Nitrogenous wastes, waste products that contain nitrogen. These products, such as ammonia and urea, are produced during protein metabolism, 286

NK, 192

Nocturia, excessive urination during the night. May or may not be abnormal, 290

Nocturnal enuresis, 291

Nodule, solid, raised group of cells, 58, 58*f*

Non-Hodgkins's lymphoma (NHL), cancer of the lymphatic tissues other than Hodgkin's lymphoma, 189

Non-insulin-dependent diabetes mellitus (NIDDM), also called type 2 diabetes mellitus. It develops later in life when the pancreas produces insufficient insulin; persons may take oral hypoglycemics to stimulate insulin secretion, or may eventually have to take insulin, 369, 370

Nonproprietary name, the recognized and accepted official name for a drug. Each drug has only one generic name, which is not subject to trademark, so any pharmaceutical manufacturer may use it. Also called *generic name*, 465

Nonsteroidal antiinflammatory drugs (NSAIDs), a large group of drugs including aspirin and ibuprofen that provide mild pain relief and anti-inflammatory benefits for conditions such as arthritis, 101

Norepinephrine, a hormone secreted by the adrenal medulla. It is a strong vasoconstrictor, 358*t*, 360

Normal psychology, behaviors that include how the personality develops, how people handle stress, and the stages of mental development, 473

Nosocomial infection, an infection acquired as a result of hospital exposure, 186

Nuclear medicine, use of radioactive substances to diagnose diseases. A radioactive substance known to accumulate in certain body tissues is injected or inhaled. After waiting for the substance to travel to the body area of interest the radioactivity level is recorded. Commonly referred to as a *scan*, 480

Nucleus, organelle of the cell that contains the DNA, 22, 391*f*

Nulligravida, woman who has never been pregnant, 323

Nullipara, woman who has never produced a viable baby, 323

Number prefixes, 5–6

Nurse, to breastfeed a baby, 318

Nurse anesthetist, a registered nurse who has received additional training and education in the administration of anesthetic medications, 490

Nurse's notes, medical record document that records the patient's care throughout the day. It includes vital signs, treatment specifics, patient's response to treatment, and patient's condition, 10

Nursing home, a facility that provides long-term care for patients who need extra time to recover from all illness or accident before they return home or for persons who can no longer care for themselves. Also called a *long-term care facility,* 11

Nyctalopia, difficulty seeing in dim light; usually due to damaged rods, 432

Nystagmus, jerky-appearing involuntary eye movement, 435

O

O&P, 264

Obesity, having an abnormal amount of fat in the body, 255, 368

Oblique fracture, fracture at an angle to the bone, 97, 97f

Oblique muscles, oblique means slanted. Two of the eye muscles are oblique muscles, 428, 428f

Oblique view, positioning the patient so that the X-rays pass through the body on an angle, 478

Obsessive-compulsive disorder (OCD), a type of anxiety disorder in which the person performs repetitive rituals in order to reduce anxiety, 473

Obstetrician, 324

Obstetrics (OB), branch of medicine that treats women during pregnancy and childbirth, and immediately after childbirth, 28t, 324

Occipital bone, a cranial bone, 84, 85, 87f, 87t

Occipital lobe, one of the four cerebral hemisphere lobes. It controls eyesight, 392, 393, 393f

Occupational Safety and Health Administration (OSHA), federal agency that issued mandatory guidelines to ensure that all employees at risk of exposure to body fluids are provided with personal protective equipment, 186

Occupational therapy (OT), assists patients to regain, develop, and improve skills that are important for independent functioning. Occupational therapy personnel work with people who, because of illness, injury, developmental, or psychological impairments, require specialized training in skills that will enable them to lead independent, productive, and satisfying lives. Occupational therapists instruct patients in the use of adaptive equipment and techniques, body mechanics, and energy conservation. They also employ modalities such as heat, cold, and therapeutic exercise, 484

OCD, 476

Ocular, pertaining to the eye, 431

Oculomotor nerve, 396t

Oculomycosis, condition of eye fungus, 431

Olfactory nerve, 396t

Oligomenorrhea, scanty menstrual flow, 322

Oligospermia, condition of having few sperm, 336

Oliguria, condition of scanty amount of urine, 290

OM, 448

Oncogenic, cancer causing, 497

Oncology, the branch of medicine dealing with tumors, 495–98

abbreviations, 498

diagnostic procedures, 497

staging tumors, 495

therapeutic procedures, 497–98

vocabulary, 496–97

Onychectomy, excision of a nail, 54

Onychia, infected nailbed, 63

Onychomalacia, softening of nails, 54

Onychomycosis, abnormal condition of nail fungus, 54

Onychophagia, nail biting, 54

Oophorectomy, removal of an ovary, 322

Oophoritis, inflammation of an ovary, 322

Open fracture, 96, 96f

Operative report, a medical record report from the surgeon detailing an operation. It includes a pre- and postprocedure itself, and how the patient tolerated the procedure, 11, 490

Ophthalmalgia, eye pain, 431

Ophthalmic, pertaining to the eyes, 431

Ophthalmic decongestants, over-the-counter medications that constrict the arterioles of the eye, reduce redness and itching of the conjunctiva, 438

Ophthalmologist, a physician specialized in treating conditions and diseases of the eye, 431, 432

Ophthalmology (Ophth), branch of medicine specializing in condition of the eye, 29t, 426, 432

Ophthalmoplegia, paralysis of the eye, 431

Ophthalmorrhagia, rapid bleeding from the eye, 431

Ophthalmoscope, instrument to view inside the eye, 431, 435, 436f

Ophthalmoscopy, examination of the interior of the eyes using an instrument called an ophthalmoscope. The physician will dilate the pupil in order to see the cornea, lens, and retina. Identifies abnormalities in the blood vessels of the eye and some systemic diseases, 435

Opiates, 407

Opportunistic infections, infectious diseases that are associated with AIDS since they occur as a result of the lowered immune system and resistance of the body to infections and parasites, 188

Opposition, moves thumb away from palm; the ability to move the thumb into contact with the other fingers, 109

Optic, pertaining to the eye, 431

Optic disk, the area of the retina associated with the optic nerve. Also called the blind spot, 427

Optic nerve, the second cranial nerve that carries impulses from the retinas to the brain, 396*t*, 426, 426*f*, 430*f*

Optician, grinds and fits prescription lenses and contacts as prescribed by a physician or optometrist, 432

Optometer, instrument to measure vision, 431

Optometrist (OD), doctor of optometry; provides care for the eyes including examining the eyes for diseases, assessing visual acuity, prescribing corrective lenses and eye treatments, and educating patients, 431, 432

Optometry, process of measuring vision, 432

OR, 494

Oral, (1) Pertaining to the mouth. (2) Administration of medication through the mouth, 253, 467, 468

Oral cavity, the mouth, 27*t*, 243*f*, 244–47, 245*f*

Oral contraceptive pills (OCPs), birth control medication that uses low doses of female hormones to prevent conception by blocking ovulation, 329

Oral hypoglycemic agents, medication taken by mouth that causes a decrease in blood sugar. This is not used for insulin-dependent patients. There is no proof that this medication will prevent the long-term complications of diabetes mellitus, 373

Oral surgeon, 254

Orbit, 87*f*

Orchidectomy, excision of the testes, 336

Orchidopexy, surgical fixation to move undescended testes into the scrotum and attaching to prevent retraction, 336, 339

Orchiectomy, surgical removal of the testes, 336

Orchioplasty, surgical repair of the testes, 336

Orchiotomy, incision into the testes, 336

Organic, pertaining to organs, 37

Organic mental disease, deterioration of mental functions due to temporary brain or permanent brain dysfunction; includes dementia and Alzheimer's disease; also called *cognitive disorders.* 473

Organs, group of different types of tissue coming together to perform special functions. For example, the heart contains muscular fibers, nerve tissue, and blood vessels, 25–29, 33*t*–36*t*

Organs of Corti, the sensory receptor hair cells lining the cochlea. These cells change the sound vibrations to electrical impulses and send the impulses to the brain via the vestibulocochlear nerve, 442

Origin, the attachment of a skeletal muscle to the less movable bone in the joint, 107

Oropharynx, the middle section of the pharynx that receives food and drink from the mouth, 211, 211*f*, 247

Orthodontic, pertaining to straight teeth, 253

Orthodontics, the dental specialty concerned with straightening teeth, 247, 255

Orthodontist, 255

Orthopedic surgeon, 96

Orthopedic surgery, the branch of medicine specializing in surgical treatments of the musculoskeletal system, 25*t*, 96

Orthopedics (Ortho), branch of medicine specializing in the diagnosis and treatment of conditions of the musculoskeletal system, 25*t*, 96

Orthopedist, 96

Orthopnea, term to describe a patient who needs to sit up straight in order to breathe comfortably, 218, 219

Orthostatic hypotension, the sudden drop in blood pressure a person experiences when standing up suddenly, 144

Orthotics, the use of equipment, such as splints and braces, to support a paralyzed muscle, promote a specific motion, or correct musculoskeletal deformities, 96, 485

Os coxae, also called the innominate bone or hip bone. It is the pelvis portion of the lower extremity. It consists of the ilium, ischium, and pubis and unites with the sacrum and coccyx to form the pelvis, 88, 90, 91*t*

Osseous tissue, bony tissue. One of the hardest tissues in the body, 82

Ossicles, the three small bones in the middle ear. The bones are the incus, malleus, and stapes. The ossicles amplify and conduct the sound waves to the inner ear, 442, 442*f*

Ossification, the process of bone formation, 82

Ostealgia, bone pain, 93

Osteoarthritis (OA), noninflammatory type of arthritis resulting in degeneration of the bones and joints, especially those bearing weight, 3, 99

Osteoblast, an embryonic bone cell, 82

Osteochondroma, tumor composed of both cartilage and bony substance, 93

Osteoclasia, intentional breaking of a bone in order to correct a deformity, 93

Osteocyte, mature bone cells, 82

Osteogenic sarcoma, the most common type of bone cancer; usually begins in osteocytes found at the ends of long bones, 98

Osteomalacia, softening of the bones caused by a deficiency of phosphorus or calcium. It is thought that in children the cause is insufficient sunlight and vitamin D, 98

Placebo, inactive, harmless substance used to satisfy a patient's desire for medication. It is also given to control groups of patients in research studies in which another group receives a drug. The effect of the placebo versus the drug is then observed, 471

Placenta, also called afterbirth. An organ attached to the uterine wall that is composed of maternal and fetal tissues. Oxygen, nutrients, carbon dioxide, and wastes are exchanged between the mother and baby through the placenta. The baby is attached to the placenta by way of the umbilical cord, 318, 319, 319*f*

Placenta previa, occurs when the placenta is in the lower portion of the uterus and thus blocks the birth canal, 326, 326*f*

Placental stage, the third stage of labor, which takes place after delivery of the infant. The uterus resumes strong contractions and the placenta detaches from the uterine wall and is delivered through the vagina, 320, 320*f*, 321

Plantar flexion, bend sole of foot; point toes downward, 108, 108*f*

Plaque, a yellow, fatty deposit of lipids in an artery, 144, 145*f*, 147*f*

Plasma, the liquid portion of blood containing 90% water. The remaining 10% consists of plasma proteins (serum albumin, serum globulin, fibrinogen, and prothrombin), inorganic substances (calcium, potassium, and sodium), organic components (glucose, amino acids, cholesterol), and waste products (urea, uric acid, ammonia, and creatinine), 26*t*, 169*f*, 170

Plasma proteins, proteins that are found in plasma. Includes serum albumin, serum globulin, fibrinogen, and prothrombin, 170

Plasmapheresis, method of removing plasma from the body without depleting the formed elements; whole blood is removed and the cells and plasma are separated; the cells are returned to the patient along with a donor plasma transfusion, 177

Plastic surgery, surgical specialty involved in repair, reconstruction, or improvement of body structures such as the skin that are damaged, missing, or misshapen. Physician is a plastic surgeon, 57

Platelet count, blood test to determine the number of platelets in a given volume of blood, 176

Platelets, cells responsible for the coagulation of blood. These are also called thrombocytes and contain no hemoglobin, 26*t*, 169*f*, 170, 172*f*

Pleura, a protective double layer of serous membrane around the lungs. The parietal membrane is the outer layer and the visceral layer is the inner membrane. It secretes a thin, watery fluid to reduce friction associated with lung movement, 31, 33, 214

Pleural, pertaining to the pleura, 37

Pleural cavity, cavity formed by the serous membrane sac surrounding the lungs, 31, 33, 33*t*, 214

Pleural effusion, abnormal presence of fluid or gas in the pleural cavity. Physicians can detect the presence of fluid by tapping the chest (percussion) or listening with a stethoscope (auscultation), 223

Pleural rub, grating sound made when two surfaces, such as the pleural surfaces, rub together during respiration. It is caused when one of the surfaces becomes thicker as a result of inflammation or other disease conditions. This rub can be felt through the fingertips when they are placed on the chest wall or heard through the stethoscope, 219

Pleurectomy, excision of the pleura, 217

Pleurisy, inflammation of the pleura, 223

Pleuritis, 223

Pleurocentesis, a puncture of the pleura to withdraw fluid from the thoracic cavity in order to diagnose disease, 217

Pleurodynia, Pleural pain, 217

Plural endings, 9

Pneumoconiosis, condition resulting from inhaling environmental particles that become toxic, such as coal dust (anthracosis) or asbestos (asbestosis), 222

***Pneumocystis carinii* pneumonia (PCP),** pneumonia with a nonproductive cough, very little fever, and dyspnea. Seen in persons with weakened immune systems, such as patients with AIDS, 189, 222

Pneumonia, inflammatory condition of the lung, which can be caused by bacterial and viral infections, diseases, and chemicals, 222

Pneumothorax, collection of air or gas in the pleural cavity, which can result in the collapse of a lung, 218, 223, 223*f*

PNS, 408

Podiatrist, 96

Podiatry, healthcare profession specializing in diagnosis and treatment of disorders of the feet and lower legs. Healthcare professional is a *podiatrist*, 96

Poliomyelitis, acute viral disease that causes an inflammation of the gray matter of the spinal cord, resulting in paralysis in some cases. Has been brought under almost total control through vaccinations, 404

Polyarteritis, inflammation of many arteries, 148

Polycystic kidneys, formation of multiple cysts within the kidney tissue; results in the destruction of normal kidney tissue and uremia, 292, 292f

Polycythemia vera, production of too many red blood cells in the bone marrow, 175

Polydipsia, condition of having an excessive amount of thirst, such as in diabetes, 368

Polymyositis, disease involving muscle inflammation and weakness from an unknown cause, 110

Polyneuritis, inflammation of many nerves, 398

Polyp, small tumor with a pedicle or stem attachment. Commonly found in vascular organs such as the nose, uterus, and rectum, 255

Polyphagia, to eat excessively, 254

Polyposis, small tumors that contain a pedicle or footlike attachment in the mucous membranes of the large intestine (colon), 259, 259f

Polysomnography, monitoring a patient while sleeping to identify sleep apnea. Also called *sleep apnea study,* 224

Polyuria, condition of having excessive urine production. This can be a symptom of disease conditions such as diabetes, 290, 368

Pons, this portion of the brain stem forms a bridge between the cerebellum and cerebrum. It is also where nerve fibers cross from one side of the brain to control functions and movement on the other side of the brain, 392, 392f, 393, 393f

Pontine, pertaining to the pons, 399

Popliteal artery, 140f

Popliteal vein, 142f

Positron emission tomography (PET), use of positive radionuclides to reconstruct brain sections. Measurements can be taken of oxygen and glucose uptake, cerebral blood flow, and blood volume, 406, 480, 481f

Posterior, directional term meaning near or on the back or spinal cord side of the body, 35f, 35t

Posterior lobe, the posterior portion of the pituitary gland. It secretes antidiuretic hormone and oxytocin, 363

Posterior pituitary gland, 363f

Posterior tibial artery, 140f

Posterior tibial vein, 142f

Posteroanterior (PA) view, positioning patient so that X-rays pass through the body from back to front, 478

Postoperative, the period of time immediately following the surgery, 493

Postpartum, period immediately after delivery or childbirth, 323

Postprandial, pertaining to after a meal, 254

Postural drainage, draining secretions from the bronchi by placing the patient in a position that uses gravity to promote drainage. Used for the treatment of cystic fibrosis and bronchiectasis, and before lobectomy surgery, 225

Postural drainage with clapping, drainage of secretions from the bronchi or a lung cavity by having the patient lie so that gravity allows drainage to occur. Clapping is using the hand in a cupped position to perform percussion on the chest. Assists in loosening secretions and mucus, 487

Potassium (K+), an inorganic substance found in plasma. It is important for bones and muscles, 170

Potentiation, giving a patient a second drug to boost (potentiate) the effect of another drug; the total strength of the drugs is greater than the sum of the strength of the individual drugs, 470

PPD, 227

Preeclampsia, toxemia of pregnancy that, if untreated, can result in true eclampsia. Symptoms include hypertension, headaches, albumin in the urine, and edema, 327

Prefix, a word part added in front of the word root. It frequently gives information about the location of the organ, the number of parts or the time (frequency). Not all medical terms have a prefix, 2, 3, 4–6, 524

number, 5–6

Pregnancy, the time from fertilization of an ovum to the birth of the newborn, 314, 318–21

labor and delivery, 320–21

Pregnancy test, chemical test that can determine a pregnancy during the first few weeks. Can be performed in a physician's office or with a home-testing kit, 327

Premature, infant born prior to thirty-seven weeks of gestation, 318

Premenstrual syndrome (PMS), symptoms that develop just prior to the onset of a menstrual period, which can include irritability, headache, tender breasts, and anxiety, 324

Premolar, another term for the bicuspid teeth, 246, 246f

preop, pre-op, 493

Preoperative (preop, pre-op), the period of time preceding surgery, 493

Prepatellar bursitis, 92

Prepuce, also called the foreskin. A protective covering over the glans penis. It is this covering of the skin that is removed during circumcision, 334

Presbycusis, loss of hearing that can accompany the aging process, 445

Presbyopia, visual loss due to old age, resulting in difficulty in focusing for near vision (such as reading), 432

Prescription, a written explanation to the pharmacist regarding the name of the medication, the dosage, and the times of administration, 465, 467, 467f

Prescription drug, a drug that can only be ordered by a licensed physician, dentist, or veterinarian, 465

Pressure equalizing tube (PE tube), small tube surgically placed in a child's ear to assist in drainage of infection, 448

Priapism, a persistent and painful erection due to pathological causes, not sexual arousal, 337

Primary site, designates where a malignant tumor first appeared, 497

Primigravida, woman who has been pregnant once, 323

Primipara, woman who has given birth once, 323

PRK, 438

PRL, 373

Probe, a surgical instrument used to explore tissue, 491t

Procedural suffixes, 8

Process, a projection from the surface of a bone, 83, 84

Proctologist, specialist in the rectum, 253, 255

Proctology, branch of medicine specializing in conditions of the lower gastrointestinal system, 27t, 255

Proctopexy, surgical fixation of the rectum, 253

Proctoptosis, drooping rectum, 253

Progesterone, one of the hormones produced by the ovaries. It works with estrogen to control the menstrual cycle, 314, 358t, 359t, 360

Prolactin (PRL), a hormone secreted by the anterior pituitary. It stimulates milk production, 359t, 363

Prolapsed umbilical cord, when the umbilical cord of the baby is expelled first during delivery and is squeezed between the baby's head and the vaginal wall. This presents an emergency situation since the baby's circulation is compromised, 327

Prolapsed uterus, fallen uterus that can cause the cervix to protrude through the vaginal opening. Generally caused by weakened muscles from vaginal delivery or as the result of pelvic tumors pressing down, 325

PROM, 489

Pronation, to turn downward or backward, as with the hand or foot, 109, 109f

Prone, directional term meaning lying horizontally facing downward, 36f, 36t

Prone position, 492f, 492t

Pronunciation, of medical terms, 8–9

Prophylaxis, prevention of disease. For example, an antibiotic can be used to prevent the occurrence of a disease, 470

Proprietary name, the name a pharmaceutical company chooses as the trademark or market name for its drug. Also called *brand* or *trade name*, 465

Prostate cancer, slow-growing cancer that affects a large number of males after age 50. The PSA (prostate-specific antigen) test is used to assist in early detection of this disease, 337

Prostate gland, a gland in the male reproductive system that produces fluids that nourish the sperm, 28t, 33t, 284f, 286f, 332f, 333, 333f, 335

Prostate-specific antigen (PSA), a blood test to screen for prostate cancer. Elevated blood levels of PSA are associated with prostate cancer, 338

Prostatectomy, surgical removal of the prostate gland, 336

Prostatic, pertaining to the prostate gland, 336

Prostatitis, inflamed condition of the prostate gland that may be a result of an infection, 336

Prosthesis, artificial device used as a substitute for a body part that is either congenitally missing or absent as a result of accident or disease; for instance, an artificial leg or hip prosthesis, 96

Prosthetic hip joint, 101f

Prosthetics, artificial devices, such as limbs and joints, that replace a missing body part, 96, 485, 486f

Prosthetist, 96

Protease inhibitor drugs, medications that inhibit protease, an enzyme viruses need to reproduce, 192

Protein-bound iodine test (PBI), blood test to measure the concentration of thyroxine (T$_4$) circulating in the blood stream. The iodine becomes bound to the protein in the blood and can be measured. Useful in establishing thyroid function, 372

Proteinuria, protein in the urine, 290

Prothrombin, protein element within the blood that interacts with calcium salts to form thrombin, 172

Prothrombin time (Pro time), measurement of the time it takes for a sample of blood to coagulate, 176

Protocol (prot), the actual plan of care, including the medications, surgeries, and treatments for the care of a patient. Often, the entire healthcare team, including the physician, oncologist, radiologist, nurse, and patient, will assist in designing the treatment plan, 495

Proton pump inhibitor, blocks the stomach's ability to secrete acid. Used to treat peptic ulcers and gastroesophageal reflux disease, 264

Protozoans, single-celled organisms that can infect the body, 184

Proximal, directional term meaning located closest to the point of attachment to the body, 35f, 35t

Proximal convoluted tubule, a portion of the renal tubule, 283, 284f, 286f

Pruritus, severe itching, 57

PSA, 340

Pseudocyesis, false pregnancy, 323

Pseudohypertrophic muscular dystrophy, one type of inherited muscular dystrophy in which the muscle tissue is gradually replaced by fatty tissue, making the muscle look strong, 111

Psoriasis, chronic inflammatory condition consisting of crusty papules forming patches with circular borders, 62, 62f

Psychiatric nurse, a nurse with additional training in the care of patients with mental, emotional, and behavioral disorders, 473

Psychiatric social work, a social worker with additional training in the care of patients with mental, emotional, or behavioral disorders, 473

Psychiatrist (MD or DO), a physician with specialized training in diagnosing and treating mental disorders; prescribes medication and conducts counseling, 473

Psychiatry, the branch of medicine that deals with the diagnosis, treatment, and prevention of mental disorders, 473

Psychoanalysis, method of obtaining a detailed account of the past and present emotional and mental experiences from the patient to determine the source of the problem and eliminate the effects, 476

Psychology, the study of human behavior and thought process. This behavioral science is primarily concerned with understanding how human beings interact with their physical environment and with each other, 473

Psychopharmacology, the study of the effects of drugs on the mind and particularly the use of drugs in treating mental disorders. The main classes of drugs for the treatment of mental disorders are antipsychotic drugs, antidepressant drugs, minor tranquilizers, and lithium, 475–76

Psychotherapy, a method of treating mental disorders by mental rather than chemical or physical means. It includes psychoanalysis, humanistic therapies, and family and group therapy, 476

PT, 488

PTCA, 152

Pterygium, hypertrophied conjunctival tissue in the inner corner of the eye, 434

PTH, 373

Puberty, beginning of menstruation and the ability to reproduce. Usually occurs around 16 years of age, 324

Pubic, pertaining to the pubis; one of the pelvic bones, 94

Pubic region, the genital region of the body, 31, 32f

Pubis, one of the three bones that form the os coxae or innominate bone, 88, 89f, 90, 91f, 91t

PUD, 264

Pulmonary, pertaining to the lung, 217, 220

Pulmonary angiography, injecting dye into a blood vessel for the purpose of taking an X-ray of the arteries and veins of the lungs, 224

Pulmonary artery, the large artery that carries deoxygenated blood from the right ventricle to the lung, 132f, 135, 136, 137f

Pulmonary capillaries, network of capillaries in the lungs that tightly encase each alveolus; site of gas exchange, 212, 213

Pulmonary circulation, the pulmonary circulation transports deoxygenated blood from the right side of the heart to the lungs where oxygen and carbon dioxide are exchanged. Then it carries oxygenated blood back to the left side of the heart, 132

Pulmonary edema, condition in which lung tissue retains an excessive amount of fluid. Results in labored breathing, 222

Pulmonary embolism, blood clot or air bubble in the pulmonary artery or one of its branches, 222

Pulmonary fibrosis, formation of fibrous scar tissue in the lungs, which leads to decreased ability to expand the lungs. May be caused by infections, pneumoconiosis, autoimmune diseases, and toxin exposure, 222

Pulmonary function test (PFT), breathing equipment used to determine respiratory function and measure lung volumes and gas exchange, 214, 215, 224

Pulmonary semilunar valve, 135f

Pulmonary trunk, 133f, 134f

Pulmonary valve, the semilunar valve between the right ventricle and pulmonary artery in the heart. It prevents blood from flowing backwards into the ventricle, 134f, 135, 136f, 137f

Pulmonary vein, large vein that returns oxygenated blood from the lungs to the left atrium, 132f, 135, 136, 137f

Pulmonologist, a physician specialized in treating diseases and disorders of the respiratory system, 217, 220

Pulmonology, branch of medicine specializing in conditions of the respiratory system, 27t

Pulp cavity, the hollow interior of a tooth; contains soft tissue made up of blood vessels, nerves, and lymph vessels, 246, 247, 247f

Pulse (P), expansion and contraction produced by blood as it moves through an artery. The pulse can be taken at several pulse points throughout the body where an artery is close to the surface, 141

Pupil, the hole in the center of the iris. The size of the pupil is changed by the iris dilating or constricting, 425*f*, 426*f*, 427, 430*f*

Pupillary, pertaining to the pupil, 432

Purified protein derivative (PPD), 224

Purkinje fibers, part of the conduction system of the heart; found in the ventricular myocardium, 136, 137*f*, 138

Purpura, hemorrhages into the skin and mucous membranes, 56*f*, 57

Purulent, pus-filled sputum, which can be the result of infection, 57

Pustule, raised spot on the skin containing pus, 58, 58*f*

Pyelitis, inflammation of the renal pelvis, 289

Pyelogram, x-ray record of the renal pelvis after injection of a radiopaque dye, 289

Pyelonephritis, inflammation of the renal pelvis and the kidney. One of the most common types of kidney disease. It may be the result of a lower urinary tract infection that moved up to the kidney by way of the ureters. There may be large quantities of white blood cells and bacteria in the urine, and blood (hematuria) may even be present in the urine in this condition. Can occur with any untreated or persistent case of cystitis, 292

Pyeloplasty, surgical repair of the renal pelvis, 289

Pyloric, pertaining to the pylorus, 253

Pyloric sphincter, sphincter at the distal end of the stomach. Controls the passage of food into the duodenum, 248, 248*f*, 249*f*, 251*f*

Pyoderma, pus producing skin infection, 55

Pyogenic, pus-forming, 54

Pyosalpinx, condition of having pus in the fallopian tubes, 323

Pyothorax, condition of having pus in the chest cavity, 218, 223

Pyromania, an impulse control disorder in which the patient is unable to control the impulse to start fires, 474

Pyrosis, heartburn, 255

Pyuria, presence of pus in the urine, 290

Q

Quadriplegia, paralysis of all four extremities. Same as tetraplegia, 399

R

Radial, pertaining to the radius; a lower arm bone, 94

Radial artery, 140*f*

Radial keratotomy, spokelike incisions around the cornea that result in it becoming flatter; a surgical treatment for myopia, 437

Radial nerve, 397*f*

Radial vein, 142*f*

Radiation therapy, use of X-rays to treat disease, especially cancer, 497

Radical mastectomy, surgical removal of the breast tissue plus chest muscles and axillary lymph nodes, 329

Radical surgery, extensive surgery to remove as much tissue associated with a tumor as possible, 498

Radiculitis, nerve root inflammation, 399

Radiculopathy, disease of the nerve root, 399

Radioactive implant, embedding a radioactive source directly into tissue to provide a highly localized radiation dosage to damage nearby cancerous cells. Also called *brachytherapy.* 498

Radiography, making of X-ray pictures, 100, 478

Radioimmunoassay (RIA), test used to measure the levels of hormones in the plasma of the blood, 372

Radioisotope, radioactive form of an element, 478

Radiologist, physician who practices diagnosis and treatment by the use of radiant energy. He or she is responsible for interpreting X-ray films, 478

Radiology, the branch of medicine that uses radioactive substances such as X-rays, isotopes, and radiation to prevent, diagnose, and treat diseases, 480

Radiolucent, structures that allow X-rays to pass through and expose the photographic plate, making it appear as a black area on the X-ray, are termed radiolucent, 478

Radiopaque, structures that are impenetrable to X-rays, appearing as a light area on the radiograph (X-ray), 478

Radius, one of the forearm bones in the upper extermity, 88, 89*f*, 90, 90*f*

Rales, abnormal crackling sound made during inspiration. Usually indicates the presence of moisture and can indicate a pneumonia condition, 220

Range of motion, the range of movement of a joint, from maximum flexion through maximum extension. It is measured as degrees of a circle, 485

Raynaud's phenomenon, periodic ischemic attacks affecting the extremities of the body, especially the fingers, toes, ears, and nose. The affected extremities become cyanotic and very painful. These attacks are brought on by arterial constriction due to extreme cold or emotional stress, 148

RBC, 178

RDS, 227

Reabsorption, second phase of urine production; substances needed by the body are reabsorbed as the filtrate passes through the kidney tubules, 286, 287

Recklinghausen disease, excessive production of parathyroid hormone, which results in degeneration of the bones, 370

Reaction, 470

Rectal, (1) Pertaining to the rectum. (2) Substances introduced directly into the rectal cavity in the form of suppositories or solution. Drugs may have to be administered by this route if the patient is unable to take them by mouth due to nausea, vomiting, and surgery, 253, 467, 468

Rectocele, protrusion or herniation of the rectum into the vagina, 325

Rectum, an area at the end of the digestive tube for storage of feces that leads to the anus, 249, 249f, 250, 250f, 314f, 317f, 319f, 333f

Rectus abdominis, a muscle named for its location and the direction of its fibers: rectus means straight and abdominis means abdominal, 107

Rectus muscles, rectus means straight. Four of the eye muscles are rectus muscles, 428, 428f

Red blood cell count (RBC), blood test to determine the number of erythrocytes in a volume of blood; a decrease in red blood cells may indicate anemia; an increase may indicate polycythemia, 176

Red blood cell morphology, examination of blood for abnormalities in the shape (morphology) of the erythrocytes. Used to determine diseases like sickle-cell anemia, 176

Red blood cells (RBC), also called erythrocytes or RBCs. Cells that contain hemoglobin and iron-containing pigment that binds oxygen in order to transport it to the cells of the body, 169f, 170

Red bone marrow, tissue that manufactures most of the blood cells. It is found in cancellous bone cavities, 82, 83

Reduction, correcting a fracture by realigning the bone fragments. *Closed reduction* is doing this without entering the body. *Open reduction* is making a surgical incision at the site of the fracture to do the reduction, often necessary where there are bony fragments to be removed, 101

Refractive error test, eye examination performed by a physician to determine and correct refractive errors in the eye, 436

Refracts, the bending of light rays as they enter the eye, 426

Regional anesthesia, regional anesthesia is also referred to as a nerve block. This anesthetic interrupts a patient's pain sensation in a particular region of the body. The anesthetic is injected near the nerve that will be blocked

from sensation. The patient usually remains conscious, 490

Regional ileitis, 257

Regurgitation, to flow backwards. In cardiovascular system refers to blood flowing backwards through valve. In digestive system refers to food flowing backwards from stomach to mouth, 144, 255

Rehabilitation, process of treatment and exercise that can help a person with a disability attain maximum function and well-being, 486

Rehabilitation centers, facilities that provide intensive physical and occupational therapy. They include inpatient and outpatient treatment, 12

Rehabilitation services, 484–88
    abbreviations, 488
    occupational therapy, 484
    physical therapy, 484
    therapeutic procedures, 486–87
    vocabulary, 484–86

Reinfection, an infection that occurs when a person becomes infected again with the same pathogen that originally brought him or her to the hospital, 186

Relapse, return of disease symptoms after period of improvement, 497

Remission, period during which the symptoms of a disease or disorder leave. Can be temporary, 497

Renal, pertaining to the kidney, 289

Renal artery, artery that originates from the abdominal aorta and carries blood to the nephrons of the kidney, 140f, 282, 283f, 286f

Renal cell carcinoma, cancerous tumor that arises from kidney tubule cells, 292

Renal colic, pain caused by a kidney stone, which can be excruciating and generally requires medical treatment, 291

Renal corpuscle, part of a nephron. It is a double-walled cuplike structure called the glomerular capsule or Bowman's capsule and contains a capillary network called the glomerulus. An afferent arteriole carries blood to the glomerulus and an efferent arteriole carries blood away from the glomerulus. The filtration stage of urine production occurs in the renal corpuscle as wastes are filtered from the blood in the glomerulus and enter Bowman's capsule, 283

Renal failure, inability of the kidneys to filter wastes from the blood resulting in uremia; may be acute or chronic; major reason for a patient being placed on dialysis, 292

Renal papilla, tip of a renal pyramid, 282, 283f

Renal pelvis, large collecting site for urine within the kidney. Collects urine from each calyx. Urine leaves the renal pelvis via the ureter, 282, 283f

Renal pyramid, triangular-shaped region of the renal medulla, 282, 283*f*

Renal transplant, surgical replacement with a donor kidney, 296, 296*f*

Renal tubule, network of tubes found in a nephron. It consists of the proximal convoluted tubule, the loop of Henle, the distal tubule, and the collecting tubule. The reabsorption and secretion stages of urine production occur within the renal tubule. As the glomerular filtrate passes through the renal tubule, most of the water and some of the dissolved substances, such as amino acids and electrolytes, are reabsorbed. At the same time, substances that are too large to filter into Bowman's capsule, such as urea, are secreted directly from the bloodstream into the renal tubule. The filtrate that reaches the collecting tubule becomes urine, 283

Renal vein, vein that carries blood away from the kidneys, 142*f*, 282, 283*f*, 286*f*

Repetitive motion disorder, group of chronic disorders involving the tendon, muscle, joint, and nerve damage, resulting from the tissue being subjected to pressure, vibration, or repetitive movements for prolonged periods, 111

Reproductive system, 311–54

Resection, to surgically cut out; excision, 493

Residual hearing, amount of hearing that is still present after damage has occurred to the auditory mechanism, 445

Residual volume (RV), the air remaining in the lungs after a forced exhalation, 215*t*

Respirator, 225, 225*f*

Respiratory membrane, formed by the tight association of the walls of alveoli and capillaries; gas exchange between lungs and blood occurs across this membrane, 212, 213

Respiratory muscles, 215

Respiratory rate, 215–16, 216*t*

Respiratory system, system that brings oxygen into the lungs and expels carbon dioxide. Organs include the nose, pharynx, larynx, trachea, bronchial tubes, and lungs, 27*t*, 207–40, 209*f*

    abbreviations, 227

    anatomy and physiology, 210–16

    bronchial tubes, 212–13

    diagnostic procedures, 223–24

    larynx, 212

    lung volumes/capacities, 214–15

    lungs, 214

    muscles, 215

    nasal cavity, 210–11

    pathology, 220–23

    pharmacology, 227

    pharynx, 211–12

    rate, 215–16

    therapeutic procedures, 225–26

    trachea, 212

    vocabulary, 218–20

    word building, 217–18

Respiratory therapist (RT), allied health professional whose duties include conducting pulmonary function tests, monitoring oxygen and carbon dioxide levels in the blood, and administering breathing treatments, 214, 215, 220

Respiratory therapy, allied health specialty that assists patients with respiratory and cardiopulmonary disorders, 220

Retina, the innermost layer of the eye. It contains the visual receptors called rods and cones. The rods and cones receive the light impulses and transmit them to the brain via the optic nerve, 425*f*, 426, 426*f*, 427, 427*f*, 430*f*

Retinal, pertaining to the retina, 432

Retinal arteries, 430*f*

Retinal blood vessels, the blood vessels that supply oxygen to the rods and cones of the retina, 427

Retinal detachment, occurs when the retina becomes separated from the choroid layer. This separation seriously damages blood vessels and nerves, resulting in blindness, 434

Retinal veins, 430*f*

Retinitis pigmentosa, progressive disease of the eye that results in the retina becoming hard (sclerosed), pigmented (colored), and atrophied (wasting away). There is no known cure for this condition, 434

Retinoblastoma, malignant glioma of the retina, 434

Retinopathy, retinal disease, 432

Retinopexy, surgical fixation of the retina, 432

Retrograde pyelogram (RP), a diagnostic X-ray in which dye is inserted through the urethra to outline the bladder, ureters, and renal pelvis, 294, 294*f*

Retroperitoneal, pertaining to behind the peritoneum. Used to describe the position of the kidneys, which is outside of the peritoneal sac alongside the spine, 33, 282

Retrovirus, 188

Reverse transcriptase inhibitor drugs, medication that inhibits reverse transcriptase, an enzyme needed to viruses to reproduce, 192

Reye's syndrome, a brain inflammation that occurs in children following a viral infection, usually the flu or chickenpox. It is characterized by vomiting and lethargy and may lead to coma and death, 403

Rh factor, an antigen marker found on erythrocytes of persons with Rh+ blood, 172–73

Rh-negative (Rh-), a person with Rh– blood type. The person's RBCs do not have the Rh marker and will make antibodies against Rh+ blood, 172, 173

Rh-positive (Rh+), a person with Rh+ blood type. The person's RBCs have the Rh marker, 172

Rheumatoid arthritis (RA), chronic form of arthritis with inflammation of the joints, swelling, stiffness, pain, and changes in the cartilage that can result in crippling deformities, 99, 99f

Rhinitis, inflammation of the nose, 217

Rhinomycosis, condition of having a fungal infection in the nose, 217

Rhinoplasty, plastic surgery of the nose, 217

Rhinorrhagia, rapid and excessive flow of blood from the nose, 218

Rhinorrhea, watery discharge from the nose, especially with allergies or a cold, runny nose, 218

Rhonchi, somewhat musical sound during expiration, often found in asthma or infection, and caused by spasms of the bronchial tubes. Also called *wheezing,* 220

Rhytidectomy, surgical removal of excess skin to eliminate wrinkles. Commonly referred to as a *facelift,* 54, 64

Rhytidoplasty, excision of wrinkles, 54

RIA, 373

Rib cage, also called the chest cavity. It is the cavity formed by the curved ribs extending from the vertebral column around the sides and attaching to the sternum. The ribs are part of the axial skeleton, 84, 85, 88f

Ribs, 86f

Rickets, deficiency in calcium and vitamin D found in early childhood that results in bone deformities, especially bowed legs, 98

Right atrium, 132f, 134f, 135f, 137f

Right coronary artery, 139f

Right hypochondriac, an anatomical division of the abdomen; the right upper row, 34t

Right iliac, an anatomical division of the abdomen; the right lower row. Also called the *right inguinal,* 34t

Right lower quadrant (RLQ), a clinical division of the abdomen. It contains portions of small and large intestines, right ovary and fallopian tube, appendix, right ureter, 34t

Right lumbar, an anatomical division of the abdomen, the right middle row, 34t

Right lymphatic duct, one of two large lymphatic ducts. It drains right arm and the right side of the neck and chest; empties lymph into the right subclavian vein, 181, 182

Right upper quadrant (RUQ), a clinical division of the abdomen. It contains the right lobe of the liver, the gallbladder, a portion of the pancreas, and portions of small and large intestine, 34t

Right ventricle, 132f, 134f, 135f, 137f

Rinne and Weber tuning-fork tests, the physician holds a tuning fork, an instrument that produces a constant pitch when it is struck against or near the bones on the side of the head. These tests assess both nerve and bone conduction of sound, 447

RLQ, 34t

Rods, the sensory receptors of the retina that are active in dim light and do not perceive color, 427

Roentgen (r), unit for describing an exposure dose of radiation, 478

Roentgenology, X-rays, 478

ROM, 488

Root, the portion of a tooth below the gum line, 246, 247f

Root canal, dental treatment involving the pulp cavity of the root of a tooth. Procedure is used to save a tooth that is badly infected or abscessed, 246, 247, 247f, 262

Rotation, moving around a central axis, 109

Rotator cuff injury, the rotator cuff consists of the joint capsule of the shoulder joint that is reinforced by the tendons from several shoulder muscles; at high risk for strain or tearing injuries, 111

Round window, 441f

Route of administration, 467

Rubella, contagious viral skin infection; commonly called *German measles.* 62

Rugae, the prominent folds in the mucosa of the stomach. They smooth out and almost disappear allowing the stomach to expand when it is full of food. Also found in the urinary bladder, 248, 248f, 284

Rule of nines, 61f

RUQ, 34t

S

Saccule, found in the inner ear. It plays a role in equilibrium, 442

Sacral, pertaining to the sacrum, 94

Sacrum, the five fused vertebrae that form a large flat bone in the upper buttock region, 84, 85, 86f, 88t

Sagittal plane, a vertical plane that divides the body into left and right sections, 30, 30f, 31

Sagittal section, sectional view of the body produced by a cut along the sagittal plane, 30, 31

Saliva, watery fluid secreted into the mouth from the salivary glands; contains digestive enzymes that break down carbohydrates and lubricants that make it easier to swallow food, 244

Salivary glands, exocrine glands with ducts that open into the mouth. They produce saliva, which makes the bolus of food easier to swallow and begins the digestive process. There

arteries, veins, nerves, and lymph vessels. The spermatic cord suspends the testes within the scrotum, 335

Spermatocide, substance that kills sperm, 340

Spermatogenesis, formation of mature sperm, 333

Spermatolysis, destruction of sperm, 336

Spermatozoon, 334

Sphenoid bone, a cranial bone, 84, 85, 87*f*, 87*t*

Sphincter, a ring of muscle around a tubular organ. It can contract to control the opening of the tube, 248, 334

Sphygmomanometer, instrument for measuring blood pressure. Also referred to as a *blood pressure cuff,* 141, 144, 144*f*

Spina bifida, congenital defect in the walls of the spinal canal in which the laminae of the vertebra do not meet or close. Results in membranes of the spinal cord being pushed through the opening. Can also result in other defects, such as hydrocephalus, 99, 403*f*, 404

Spinal, pertaining to the spine, 37

Spinal cavity, a dorsal body cavity within the spinal column that contains the spinal cord, 31, 32, 32*f*, 33*t*, 394

Spinal column, 88*t*

Spinal cord, the spinal cord provides a pathway for impulses traveling to and from the brain. It is a column of nerve fibers that extends from the medulla oblongata of the brain down to the level of the second lumbar vertebra, 23, 29*t*, 33*t*, 389*f*, 390, 393*f*, 394, 394*f*, 397*f*

Spinal cord injury (SCI), bruising or severing of the spinal cord from a blow to the vertebral column resulting in muscle paralysis and sensory impairment below the injury level, 404

Spinal fusion, surgical immobilization of adjacent vertebrae. This may be done for several reasons, including correction for a herniated disk, 100

Spinal nerves, the nerves that arise from the spinal cord, 390, 397*f*

Spinal puncture, 406, 406*f*

Spinal stenosis, narrowing of the spinal canal causing pressure on the cord and nerves, 99

Spinal tap, 406, 406*f*

Spiral fracture, fracture in an S-shaped spiral. It can be caused by a twisting injury, 97

Spirometer, instrument consisting of a container into which a patient can exhale for the purpose of measuring the air capacity of the lungs, 224

Spirometry, using a device to measure the breathing capacity of the lungs, 224

Spleen, organ in the lymphatic system that filters microorganisms and old red blood cells from the blood, 26*t*, 33*t*, 34*t*, 180*f*, 181, 184, 184*f*

Splenectomy, excision of the spleen, 187

Splenomegaly, enlargement of the spleen, 187

Split-thickness skin graft (STSG), 65

Spondylolisthesis, the forward sliding of a lumbar vertebra over the vertebra below it, 99

Spondylosis, 99

Spongy bone, the bony tissue found inside a bone. It contains cavities that hold red bone marrow. Also called *cancellous bone,* 82, 83, 83*f*

Spontaneous abortion, loss of a fetus without any artificial aid. Also called a *miscarriage,* 327

Sprain, pain and disability caused by trauma to a joint. A ligament may be torn in severe sprains, 99

Sputum, mucus or phlegm that is coughed up from the lining of the respiratory tract. Tested to determine what type of bacteria of virus is present as an aid in selecting the proper antibiotic treatment, 219, 220

Sputum culture and sensitivity (C&S), testing sputum by placing it on a culture medium and observing any bacterial growth. The specimen is then tested to determine antibiotic effectiveness, 223

Sputum cytology, testing for malignant cells in sputum, 223

Squamous cell carcinoma (SCC), epidermal cancer that may go into deeper tissue but does not generally metastasize, 62

Staging, the process of classifying tumors based on their degree of tissue invasion and the potential response to therapy. The TNM staging system is frequently used. The T refers to the tumor's size and invasion, the N refers to lymph node involvement, and the M refers to the presence of metastases of the tumor cells, 495

Staging laparotomy, surgical procedure in which the abdomen is entered to determine the extent and staging of a tumor, 497

Staging tumors, 495

Standard precautions, 186

Stapedectomy, removal of the stapes bone to treat otosclerosis (hardening of the bone). A prosthesis or artificial stapes may be implanted, 448

Stapes, one of the three ossicles of the middle ear. It is attached to the oval window leading to the inner ear. Also called the *stirrup,* 441*f*, 442, 442*f*

STD, 340

Stent, a stainless steel tube placed within a blood vessel or a duct to widen the lumen, 144, 144*f*

Sterility, inability to father children due to a problem with spermatogenesis, 336

Sterilization, process of rendering a male or female sterile or unable to conceive children, 339

Sternal, pertaining to the sternum or breast bone, 94

Sternocleidomastoid, muscle named for its attachments, the sternum, clavicle, and mastoid process, 107

Sternum, also called the *breast bone.* It is part of the axial skeleton and the anterior attachment for ribs, 84, 85, 86*f*

Steroid sex hormones, a class of hormones secreted by the adrenal cortex. It includes aldosterone, cortisol, androgens, estrogens, and progestins, 358*t*, 360

Stethoscope, instrument for listening to body sounds, such as the chest, heart, or intestines, 144

Stillbirth, viable-aged fetus dies before or at the time of delivery, 327

Stirrup, 441*f*, 442

Stomach, a J-shaped muscular organ that acts as a sac to collect, churn, digest, and store food. It is composed of three parts: the fundus, body, and antrum. Hydrochloric acid is secreted by glands in the mucous membrane lining of the stomach. Food mixes with other gastric juices and the hydrochloric acid to form a semisoft mixture called chyme, which then passes into the duodenum, 27*t*, 33*t*, 243*f*, 244, 248, 248*f*, 250*f*

Stool culture, a laboratory test of feces to determine if there are any pathogenic bacteria present, 261

Stool guaiac, 260

Strabismus, an eye muscle weakness resulting in each eye looking in a different direction at the same time. May be corrected with glasses, eye exercises, and/or surgery. Also called *lazy eye* or *crossed eyes,* 428*f*, 435

Strabotomy, incision into the eye muscles in order to correct strabismus, 437

Strain, trauma to muscle from excessive stretching or pulling, 111

Stratified squamous epithelium, the layers of flat or scalelike cells found in the epidermis. *Stratified* means multiple layers and *squamous* means flat, 50

Strawberry hemangioma, congenital collection of dilated blood vessels causing a red birthmark that fades a few months after birth, 57, 57*f*

Stress fracture, a slight fracture caused by repetitive low-impact forces, like running, rather than a single forceful impact, 97

Stress testing, method for evaluating cardiovascular fitness. The patient is placed on a treadmill or a bicycle and then subjected to steadily increasing levels of work. An EKG and oxygen levels are taken while the patient exercises, 149, 149*f*

Striated muscle, another name for skeletal muscle, referring to its striped appearance under the microscope, 106, 106*f*

Stricture, narrowing of a passageway in the urinary system, 291

Stridor, harsh, high-pitched, noisy breathing sound that is made when there is an obstruction of the bronchus or larynx. Found in conditions such as croup in children, 220

Stroke, 401

STSG, 65

Stye (sty), 434

Subarachnoid space, the space located between the arachnoid layer and pia mater. It contains cerebrospinal fluid, 395, 395*f*

Subcutaneous (SC, sc, sub-q, subcu), (1) Pertaining to under the skin. (2) Injection of medication under the skin, 54, 65, 469*f*, 469*t*, 490, 491

Subclavian artery, 140*f*

Subclavian vein, 142*f*, 183*f*

Subcutaneous layer, this is the deepest layer of the skin where fat is formed. This layer of fatty tissue protects the deeper tissues of the body and acts as an insulation for heat and cold, 51*f*, 52, 53*f*

Subdural hematoma, mass of blood forming beneath the dura mater of the brain, 405, 405*f*

Subdural space, the space located between the dura mater and the arachnoid layer, 395, 395*f*

Sublingual (SL), (1) Pertaining to under the tongue. (2) Administration of medicine by placing it under the tongue, 253, 467, 468, 468*f*

Sublingual duct, 251*f*

Sublingual glands, a pair of salivary glands in the floor of the mouth, 250, 251*f*

Subluxation, an incomplete dislocation, the joint alignment is disrupted, but the ends of the bones remain in contact, 99

Submandibular ducts, 245*f*, 251*f*

Submandibular glands, a pair of salivary glands in the floor of the mouth, 250, 251*f*

subq, 65

Substance-related disorders, overindulgence or dependence on chemical substances including alcohol, illegal drugs, and prescription drugs, 475

Sudden infant death syndrome (SIDS), the sudden, unexplained death of an infant in which a postmortem examination fails to determine the cause of death, 222

Sudoriferous glands, the typical sweat glands of the skin, 53

Suffix, a word part attached to the end of a word. It frequently indicates a condition, disease, or procedure. Almost all medical terms have a suffix, 2, 3, 6–8, 523–24

adjective, 7

procedural, 8

surgical, 7

Suffocation, 218

Systemic lupus erythematosus (SLE), chronic disease of the connective tissue that injures the skin, joints, kidneys, nervous system, and mucous membranes. May produce a characteristic butterfly rash across the cheeks and nose, 62, 65, 99

Systemic veins, 132*f*

Systole, the period of time during which a heart chamber is contracting, 135, 136

Systolic pressure, the maximum pressure within blood vessels during a heart contraction, 141

T

T cells, lymphocytes active in cellular immunity, 184, 364, 366

T lymphocytes, a type of lymphocyte involved with producing cells that physically attack and destroy pathogens, 184

T&A, 494

Tachycardia, abnormally fast heart rate, over 100 bpm, 143

Tachypnea, rapid breathing rate, 218

Tagging, attachment of a radioactive material to a chemical and tracing it as it moves through the body, 479

TAH-BSO, 330

Talipes, congenital deformity of the foot. Also referred to as a *clubfoot,* 99

Target organs, the organs that hormones act on to either increase or decrease the organ's activity level, 358

Tarsal, pertaining to the ankle, 94

Tarsals, the ankle bones in the lower extremity, 88, 89*f,* 90, 91*f,* 91*t*

Taste buds, found on the surface of the tongue; designed to detect bitter, sweet, sour, and salty flavors in our food, 244

TB, 227

Tears, fluid that washes and lubricates the anterior surface of the eyeball, 429

Teeth, structures in mouth that mechanically break up food into smaller pieces during chewing, 244, 245*f,* 246–47

Temporal bone, a cranial bone, 84, 85, 87*f,* 87*t,* 441*f*

Temporal lobe, one of the four cerebral hemisphere lobes. It controls hearing and smell, 392, 393, 393*f*

Tenaculum, a long-handled clamp surgical instrument, 492*t*

Tendinitis, inflammation of tendon, 110

Tendinous, pertaining to a tendon, 110

Tendons, the strong connective tissue cords that attach skeletal muscles to bones, 23, 106

Tendoplasty, surgical repair of a tendon, 110

Tendotomy, incision into a tendon, 110

Tennis elbow, 111

Tenodesis, surgical procedure to stabilize a joint by anchoring down the tendons of the muscles that move the joint, 112

Tenodynia, pain in a tendon, 110

Tenoplasty, surgical repair of a tendon, 110

Tenorrhaphy, suture a tendon, 110

TENS, 489

Testes, the male gonads. The testes are oval glands located in the scrotum that produce sperm and the male hormone, testosterone, 28*t,* 332*f,* 333–34, 333*f,* 339*f,* 358, 359*t,* 364, 365*f*

Testicles, also called *testes* (singular is testis). These oval-shaped organs are responsible for the development of sperm within the seminiferous tubules. The testes must be maintained at the proper temperature for the sperm to survive. This lower temperature level is controlled by the placement of the scrotum outside the body. The hormone testosterone, which is responsible for the growth and development of the male reproductive organs, is also produced by the testes, 333

Testicular, pertaining to the testes, 336

Testicular carcinoma, cancer of one or both testicles, 337

Testicular torsion, a twisting of the spermatic cord, 337

Testis, 357*f,* 364*f*

Testosterone, male hormone produced in the testes. It is responsible for the growth and development of the male reproductive organs, 333, 334, 359*t,* 364, 365*f*

Tetany, a condition that results from a calcium deficiency in the blood. It is characterized by muscle twitches, cramps, and spasms, 370

Tetralogy of Fallot, combination of four congenital anomalies: pulmonary stenosis, an interventricular septal defect, abnormal blood supply to the aorta, and hypertrophy of the right ventricle. Needs immediate surgery to correct, 146

TFT, 373

THA, 102

Thalamic, pertaining to the thalamus, 399

Thalamus, a portion of the diencephalon. It is composed of gray matter and acts as a center for relaying impulses from the eyes, ears, and skin to the cerebrum. Pain perception is also controlled by the thalamus, 362, 363*f,* 392, 392*f,* 393

Thalassemia, a genetic disorder in which the person is unable to make functioning hemoglobin; results in anemia, 175

lates the level of cell metabolism. The greater the level of hormone in the bloodstream, the higher cell metabolism will be, 359*t*, 366

TIA, 408

Tibia, also called the *shin bone.* It is a lower extremity bone, 88, 89*f*, 90, 91*f*, 91*t*

Tibial, pertaining to the tibia or shin bone, 94

Tidal volume (TV), the amount of air that enters the lungs in a single inhalation or leaves the lungs in a single exhalation of quiet breathing, 215*t*

Tinea, fungal skin disease resulting in itching, scaling lesions, 62

Tinea capitis, fungal infection of the scalp; commonly called *ringworm.* 62

Tinea pedis, fungal infection of the foot; commonly called *athlete's foot.* 62

Tinnitus, ringing in the ears, 445

Tissues, tissues are formed when cells of the same type are grouped to perform one activity. For example, nerve cells combine to form nerve fibers. There are four types of tissue: nerve, muscle, epithelial, and connective, 23

　connective, 23

　epithelial, Pertaining to the epithelium, 23

　muscle, 23

　nervous, 23

TKR, 102

TLC, 227

Tolerance, development of a capacity for withstanding a large amount of a substance, such as foods, drugs, or poison, without any adverse effect. A decreased sensitivity to further doses will develop, 470

Tongue, a muscular organ in the floor of the mouth. Works to move food around inside the mouth and is also necessary for speech, 211*f*, 244, 245*f*, 251*f*

Tonic-clonic seizure, type of severe epileptic seizure characterized by a loss of consciousness and convulsions. The seizure alternates between strong continuous muscle spasms (tonic) and rhythmic muscle contraction and relaxation (clonic). It is also called a *grand mal seizure,* 403

Tonometry, measurement of the intraocular pressure of the eye using a tonometer to check for the condition of glaucoma. After a local anesthetic is applied, the physician places the tonometer lightly upon the eyeball and a pressure measurement is taken. Generally part of a normal eye exam for adults, 436

Tonsillar, pertaining to the tonsils, 187

Tonsillectomy, surgical removal of the tonsils, 187

Tonsillitis, inflammation of the tonsils, 187

Tonsils, the collections of lymphatic tissue located in the pharynx to combat microorganisms entering the body through the nose or mouth. The tonsils are the pharyngeal tonsils, the palatine tonsils, and the lingual tonsils, 26*t*, 180*f*, 181, 184, 184*f*

Tooth cavity, 254

Topical, applied directly to the skin or mucous membranes. They are distributed in ointment, cream, or lotion form. Used to treat skin infections and eruptions, 467, 468

Topical anesthesia, topical anesthesia is applied using either a liquid or gel placed directly onto a specific area. The patient remains conscious. This type of anesthetic is used on the skin, the cornea, and mucous membranes in dental work, 490, 491

Torticollis, severe neck spasms pulling the head to one side; commonly called *wryneck* or a *crick in the neck.* 111

Total abdominal hysterectomy - bilateral salpingo-oophorectomy (TAH-BSO), removal of the entire uterus, cervix, both ovaries, and both fallopian tubes, 329

Total calcium, blood test to measure the total amount of calcium to assist in detecting parathyroid and bone disorders, 372

Total hip arthroplasty (THA), surgical reconstruction of a hip by implanting a prosthetic or artificial hip joint; also called *total hip replacement.* 100

Total hip replacement (THR), 100

Total knee arthroplasty (TKA), surgical reconstruction of a knee joint by implanting a prosthetic knee joint; also called *total knee replacement.* 101

Total lung capacity (TLC), the volume of air in the lungs after a maximal inhalation, 215*t*

Total parenteral nutrition (TPN), providing 100% of a patient's nutrition intravenously. Used when a patient is unable to eat, 262

Toxemia, 327

Toxic shock syndrome (TSS), rare and sometimes fatal staphylococcus infection that generally occurs in menstruating women, 325

Toxicity, extent or degree to which a substance is poisonous, 470

Toxins, substances poisonous to the body. Many are filtered out of the blood by the kidney, 184

TPN, 264

Trachea, also called the *windpipe.* It conducts air from the larynx down to the main bronchi in the chest, 27*t*, 33*t*, 209*f*, 210, 211*f*, 212, 212*f*, 214*f*, 245*f*, 362*f*, 365*f*, 366*f*

Tracheostenosis, narrowing and stenosis of the lumen or opening into the trachea, 218

Tracheostomy, surgical procedure used to make an opening in the trachea to create an airway. A tracheostomy tube can be inserted to keep the opening patent, 226, 226*f*

Tracheotomy, surgical incision into the trachea to provide an airway, 218, 226

Trachoma, chronic infectious disease of the conjunctiva and cornea caused by bacteria. Occurs more commonly in people living in hot, dry climates. Untreated, it may lead to blindness when the scarring invades the cornea. Trachoma can be treated with antibiotics, 434

Tract, a bundle of fibers located within the central nervous system, 390, 392

Traction, process of pulling or drawing, usually with a mechanical device. Used in treating orthopedic (bone and joint) problems and injuries, 101, 487

Tractotomy, incision into a spinal cord tract, 407

Trademark, a pharmaceutical company's brand name for a drug, 465

Transcutaneous electrical nerve stimulation (TENS), application of a mild electrical stimulation to skin via electrodes placed over a painful area, causing interference with the transmission of the painful stimuli. Can be used in pain management to interfere with the normal pain mechanism, 487

Transdermal, route of drug administration; medication coats the underside of a patch that is applied to the skin. The medication is then absorbed across the skin, 467, 468

Transfusion reaction, 175

Transient ischemic attack (TIA), temporary interference with blood supply to the brain, causing neurological symptoms such as dizziness, numbness, and hemiparesis. May lead eventually to a full-blown stroke (CVA), 403

Transurethral resection of the prostate (TUR), surgical removal of the prostate gland by inserting a device through the urethra and removing prostate tissue, 339

Transverse colon, the section of colon that crosses the upper abdomen from the right side of the body to the left, 249, 249f, 250f

Transverse fracture, complete fracture that is straight across the bone at right angles to the long axis of the bone, 98, 98f

Transverse plane, a horizontal plane that divides the body into upper (superior) and lower (inferior) sections. Also called the *horizontal plane,* 30, 30f, 31

Transverse section, sectional view of the body produced by a cut along the transverse plane, 30, 31

Treadmill test, 149, 149f

Tremor, involuntary quivering movement of a part of the body, 400

Trendelenburg position, a surgical position in which the patient is lying face up and on an incline with the head lower than the legs, 492f, 492t

Trephine, a surgical saw used to remove a disk-shaped piece of tissue, 491t

Trichomoniasis, genitourinary infection that is usually without symptoms (asymptomatic) in both males and females. In women the disease can produce itching and/or burning and a foul-smelling discharge, and can result in vaginitis, 338

Trichomycosis, abnormal condition of hair fungus, 55

Tricuspid valve, a valve between the right atrium and ventricle of the heart. It prevents blood from flowing backwards into the atrium. A tricuspid valve has three cusps or flaps, 135, 136f, 137f

Trigeminal nerve, 396t

Triiodothyronine (T₃), a hormone produced by the thyroid gland known as T_3 that requires iodine for its production. This hormone regulates the level of cell metabolism. The greater the level of hormone in the blood stream, the higher cell metabolism will be, 359t, 366

Trochanter, the large blunt process that provides the attachment for tendons and muscles, 83, 84, 85f

Trochlear nerve, 396t

Trunk, the torso region of the body, 31, 32f

TSH, 373

Tubal ligation, surgical tying off of the fallopian tubes to prevent conception from taking place. Results in sterilization of the female, 329

Tubal pregnancy, 316

Tubercle, a small, rounded process that provides the attachment for tendons and muscles, 83, 84

Tuberculin skin tests (TB test), applying a chemical agent (Tine or Mantoux tests) under the surface of the skin to determine if the patient has been exposed to tuberculosis, 224

Tuberculosis (TB), infectious disease caused by the tubercle bacillus, *Myocobacterium tuberculosis.* Most commonly affects the respiratory system and causes inflammation and calcification of the system. Tuberculosis is again on the uprise and is seen in many patients who have AIDS, 222

Tuberosity, a large, rounded process that provides the attachment to tendons and muscles, 83, 84

Tumor, abnormal growth of tissue that may be benign or malignant. Also called a *neoplasm,* 496

TV, 227

Two-hour postprandial glucose tolerance test, blood test to assist in evaluating glucose metabolism.

The patient eats a high-carbohydrate diet and fasts overnight before the test. A blood sample is then taken two hours after a meal, 372

Tympanectomy, excision of the eardrum, 445

Tympanic, pertaining to the eardrum, 444

Tympanic membrane, also called the eardrum. As sound moves along the auditory canal, it strikes the tympanic membrane causing it to vibrate. This conducts the sound wave into the middle ear, 441, 442*f*

Tympanitis, eardrum inflammation, 444

Tympanometer, instrument to measure the eardrum, 444

Tympanometry, measurement of the movement of the tympanic membrane. Can indicate the presence of pressure in the middle ear, 447

Tympanoplasty, another term for the surgical reconstruction of the eardrum. Also called *myringoplasty,* 444

Tympanorrhexis, ruptured eardrum, 445

Tympanotomy, incision into the eardrum, 445

Type A blood, one of the ABO blood types. A person with type A markers on his or her RBCs. Type A blood will make anti-B antibodies, 172

Type AB blood, one of the ABO blood types. A person with both type A and type B markers on his or her RBCs. Since it has both markers, it will not make antibodies against either A or B blood, 172

Type B blood, one of the ABO blood types. A person with type B markers on his or her RBCs. Type B blood will make anti-A antibodies, 172

Type O blood, one of the ABO blood types. A person with no markers on his or her RBCs. Type O blood will not react with anti-A or anti-B antibodies. Therefore, it is considered the universal donor, 172

Type and crossmatch, lab test performed before a person receives a blood transfusion; double checks the blood type of both the donor's and recipient's blood, 177

U

U/A, UA, 297

Ulcer, open sore or lesion in skin or mucous membrane, 59, 59*f*

Ulcerative colitis, ulceration of unknown origin of the mucous membranes of the colon. Also known as *inflammatory bowel disease* (IBD), 259

Ulna, one of the forearm bones in the upper extremity, 88, 89*f*, 90, 90*f*

Ulnar, pertaining to the ulna, one of the lower arm bones, 94

Ulnar artery, 140*f*

Ulnar nerve, 397*f*

Ulnar vein, 142*f*

Ultrasound (US), the use of high-frequency sound waves to create heat in soft tissues under the skin. It is particularly useful for treating injuries to muscles, tendons, and ligaments, as well as muscle spasms. In radiology, ultrasound waves can be used to outline shapes of tissues, organs, and the fetus, 481, 481*f*, 487

Ultraviolet (UV), 65

Umbilical, an anatomical division of the abdomen; the middle section of the middle row, 34*t*

Umbilical cord, a cord extending from the baby's umbilicus (navel) to the placenta. It contains blood vessels that carry oxygen and nutrients from the mother to the baby and carbon dioxide and wastes from the baby to the mother, 318, 319*f*, 320

Unconscious, condition or state of being unaware of surroundings with the inability to respond to stimuli, 400

Ungual, 55

Unit dose, drug dosage system that provides prepackaged, prelabeled, individual medications that are ready for immediate use by the patient, 470

Universal donor, type O blood is considered the universal donor. Since it has no markers on the RBC surface, it will not trigger a reaction with anti-A or anti-B antibodies, 172

Universal recipient, a person with type AB blood has no antibodies against the other blood types and therefore, in an emergency, can receive any type of blood, 172

Upper extremity (UE), the arm, 31, 88, 89*f*, 90, 90*f*, 486

Upper gastrointestinal (UGI) series, administering a barium contrast material orally and then taking an X-ray to visualize the esophagus, stomach, and duodenum, 261

Uptake, absorption of radioactive material and medicines into an organ or tissue, 479

Urea, a waste product of protein metabolism. It diffuses through the tissues in lymph and is returned to the circulatory system for transport to the kidneys, 170

Uremia, an excess of urea and other nitrogenous waste in the blood, 282, 289, 291

Ureteral, pertaining to the ureter, 289

Ureterectasis, dilation of the ureter, 289

Ureterolith, a calculus in the ureter, 289

Ureterostenosis, narrowing of the ureter, 289

Ureters, organs in the urinary system that transport urine from the kidney to the bladder, 27*t*, 33*t*, 34*t*, 281*f*, 282, 283, 283*f*, 284*f*

Urethra, the tube that leads from the urinary bladder to the outside of the body. In the male it is

also used by the reproductive system to release semen, 27t, 33t, 281f, 282, 284f, 285,
286f, 314f, 333f

Urethral, pertaining to the urethra, 289

Urethralgia, urethral pain, 289

Urethritis, inflammation of the urethra, 289

Urethrorrhagia, rapid bleeding from the urethra,
289

Urethroscope, instrument to view inside the urethra, 289

Urethrostenosis, narrowing of the urethra, 289

Urgency, Feeling the need to urinate immediately,
291

Urinalysis (U/A, UA), laboratory test that consists of
the physical, chemical, and microscopic examination of urine, 287, 287t, 293

Urinary, pertaining to urine, 289

Urinary bladder, organ in the urinary system that
stores urine, 27t, 33t, 281f, 282, 284, 284f,
286f, 314f, 319f, 333f

Urinary incontinence, involuntary release of urine.
In some patients an indwelling catheter is inserted into the bladder for continuous urine
drainage, 291

Urinary meatus, the external opening of the urethra, 285, 317, 317f, 334

Urinary retention, an inability to fully empty the
bladder, often indicates a blockage in the urethra, 291

Urinary system, system that filters wastes from the
blood and excretes the waste products in the
form of urine. Organs include the kidneys,
ureters, urinary bladder, and urethra, 27t,
279–309, 281f
abbreviations, 297
anatomy and physiology, 282–87
diagnostic procedures, 293–94
homeostasis, kidneys and, 285
kidneys, 282–83
pathology, 291–93
pharmacology, 296
therapeutic procedures, 294–96
ureters, 283
urethra, 285
urinary bladder, 284
urinary production stages, 285–86
urine, 286–87
vocabulary, 290–91
word building, 288–90

Urinary tract infection (UTI), infection, usually from
bacteria such as *E. coli*, of any organ of the urinary system; most often begins with cystitis
and may ascend into the ureters and kidneys;
most common in women because of their
shorter urethra, 293

Urination, the release of urine from the urinary
bladder, 284

Urine, the fluid that remains in the urinary system
following the three stages of urine production: filtration, reabsorption, and secretion,
282, 285–87, 286f
production, 286–87, 286f

Urine culture and sensitivity (C&S), laboratory test
of urine for bacterial infection; attempt to
grow bacteria on a culture medium in order to
identify it and determine which antibiotics it is
sensitive to, 293

Urinometer, instrument to measure urine, 289

Urologist, a physician specialized in treating conditions and diseases of the urinary system and
male reproductive system, 289, 291

Urology, branch of medicine specializing in conditions of the urinary system and male reproductive system, 27t, 28t, 291

Urticaria, hives, a skin eruption of pale reddish
wheals (circular elevations of the skin) with severe itching. Usually associated with food allergy, stress, or drug reactions, 57, 188

US, 483, 489

Uterine, pertaining to the uterus, 323

Uterine tubes, tubes that carry the ovum from the
ovary to the uterus; also called *fallopian tubes*
or *oviducts*, 315

Uterus, also called the *womb.* An internal organ of
the female reproductive system. This hollow,
pear-shaped organ is located in the lower
pelvic cavity between the urinary bladder and
rectum. The uterus receives the fertilized
ovum and it becomes implanted in the uterine
wall, which provides nourishment and protection for the developing fetus. The uterus is divided into three regions: fundus, corpus, and
cervix, 28t, 33t, 286f, 313f, 314, 314f, 316–17,
316f, 319f

UTI, 297

Utricle, found in the inner ear. It plays a role in
equilibrium, 442

UV, 65

Uveitis, inflammation of the uvea of the eye, 432

Uvula, structure that hangs down from the posterior edge of the soft palate, helps in the production of speech, and is the location of the
gag reflex, 244, 245f

V

Vaccination, providing protection against communicable diseases by stimulating the immune system to produce antibodies against that
disease. Children can now be immunized for
the following diseases: hepatitis B, diphtheria,
tetanus, pertussis, *Haemophilus influenzae*
type b, polio, measles, mumps, rubella, and
chickenpox. Also called *immunization*, 184,
185, 192

Pearson Education, Inc.

YOU SHOULD CAREFULLY READ THE TERMS AND CONDITIONS BEFORE USING THE CD-ROM PACKAGE. USING THIS CD-ROM PACKAGE INDICATES YOUR ACCEPTANCE OF THESE TERMS AND CONDITIONS.

Pearson Education, Inc. provides this program and licenses its use. You assume responsibility for the selection of the program to achieve your intended results, and for the installation, use, and results obtained from the program. This license extends only to use of the program in the United States or countries in which the program is marketed by authorized distributors.

LICENSE GRANT

You hereby accept a nonexclusive, nontransferable, permanent license to install and use the program ON A SINGLE COMPUTER at any given time. You may copy the program solely for backup or archival purposes in support of your use of the program on the single computer. You may not modify, translate, disassemble, decompile, or reverse engineer the program, in whole or in part.

TERM

The License is effective until terminated. Pearson Education, Inc. reserves the right to terminate this License automatically if any provision of the License is violated. You may terminate the License at any time. To terminate this License, you must return the program, including documentation, along with a written warranty stating that all copies in your possession have been returned or destroyed.

LIMITED WARRANTY

THE PROGRAM IS PROVIDED "AS IS" WITHOUT WARRANTY OF ANY KIND, EITHER EXPRESSED OR IMPLIED, INCLUDING, BUT NOT LIMITED TO, THE IMPLIED WARRANTIES OR MERCHANTABILITY AND FITNESS FOR A PARTICULAR PURPOSE. THE ENTIRE RISK AS TO THE QUALITY AND PERFORMANCE OF THE PROGRAM IS WITH YOU. SHOULD THE PROGRAM PROVE DEFECTIVE, YOU (AND NOT PRENTICE-HALL, INC. OR ANY AUTHORIZED DEALER) ASSUME THE ENTIRE COST OF ALL NECESSARY SERVICING, REPAIR, OR CORRECTION. NO ORAL OR WRITTEN INFORMATION OR ADVICE GIVEN BY PRENTICE-HALL, INC., ITS DEALERS, DISTRIBUTORS, OR AGENTS SHALL CREATE A WARRANTY OR INCREASE THE SCOPE OF THIS WARRANTY.

SOME STATES DO NOT ALLOW THE EXCLUSION OF IMPLIED WARRANTIES, SO THE ABOVE EXCLUSION MAY NOT APPLY TO YOU. THIS WARRANTY GIVES YOU SPECIFIC LEGAL RIGHTS AND YOU MAY ALSO HAVE OTHER LEGAL RIGHTS THAT VARY FROM STATE TO STATE.

Pearson Education, Inc. does not warrant that the functions contained in the program will meet your requirements or that the operation of the program will be uninterrupted or error-free.

However, Pearson Education, Inc. warrants the diskette(s) or CD-ROM(s) on which the program is furnished to be free from defects in material and workmanship under normal use for a period of ninety (90) days from the date of delivery to you as evidenced by a copy of your receipt.

The program should not be relied on as the sole basis to solve a problem whose incorrect solution could result in injury to person or property. If the program is employed in such a manner, it is at the user's own risk and Pearson Education, Inc. explicitly disclaims all liability for such misuse.

LIMITATION OF REMEDIES

Pearson Education, Inc.'s entire liability and your exclusive remedy shall be:
1. the replacement of any diskette(s) or CD-ROM(s) not meeting Pearson Education, Inc.'s "LIMITED WARRANTY" and that is returned to Pearson Education, or
2. if Pearson Education is unable to deliver a replacement diskette(s) or CD-ROM(s) that is free of defects in materials or workmanship, you may terminate this agreement by returning the program.

IN NO EVENT WILL PRENTICE-HALL, INC. BE LIABLE TO YOU FOR ANY DAMAGES, INCLUDING ANY LOST PROFITS, LOST SAVINGS, OR OTHER INCIDENTAL OR CONSEQUENTIAL DAMAGES ARISING OUT OF THE USE OR INABILITY TO USE SUCH PROGRAM EVEN IF PRENTICE-HALL, INC. OR AN AUTHORIZED DISTRIBUTOR HAS BEEN ADVISED OF THE POSSIBILITY OF SUCH DAMAGES, OR FOR ANY CLAIM BY ANY OTHER PARTY.

SOME STATES DO NOT ALLOW FOR THE LIMITATION OR EXCLUSION OF LIABILITY FOR INCIDENTAL OR CONSEQUENTIAL DAMAGES, SO THE ABOVE LIMITATION OR EXCLUSION MAY NOT APPLY TO YOU.

GENERAL

You may not sublicense, assign, or transfer the license of the program. Any attempt to sublicense, assign or transfer any of the rights, duties, or obligations hereunder is void.

This Agreement will be governed by the laws of the State of New York.

Should you have any questions concerning this Agreement, you may contact Pearson Education, Inc. by writing to:

Director of New Media
Higher Education Division
Pearson Education, Inc.
One Lake Street
Upper Saddle River, NJ 07458

Should you have any questions concerning technical support, you may contact:

Product Support Department: Monday–Friday 8:00 A.M. –8:00 P.M. and Sunday 5:00 P.M.-12:00 A.M. (All times listed are Eastern). 1-800-677-6337

You can also get support by filling out the web form located at http://247.prenhall.com

YOU ACKNOWLEDGE THAT YOU HAVE READ THIS AGREEMENT, UNDERSTAND IT, AND AGREE TO BE BOUND BY ITS TERMS AND CONDITIONS. YOU FURTHER AGREE THAT IT IS THE COMPLETE AND EXCLUSIVE STATEMENT OF THE AGREEMENT BETWEEN US THAT SUPERSEDES ANY PROPOSAL OR PRIOR AGREEMENT, ORAL OR WRITTEN, AND ANY OTHER COMMUNICATIONS BETWEEN US RELATING TO THE SUBJECT MATTER OF THIS AGREEMENT.